Volume I

THE SPINE

SECOND EDITION

Edited by

RICHARD H. ROTHMAN, M.D., Ph.D.

Professor of Orthopaedic Surgery,
The University of Pennsylvania School of Medicine;
Chief of Orthopaedic Surgery,
The Pennsylvania Hospital, Philadelphia

and

FREDERICK A. SIMEONE, M.D.

Professor of Neurosurgery,
The University of Pennsylvania School of Medicine;
Chief of Neurosurgery,
The Pennsylvania Hospital;
Director of Neurosurgery,
Elliott Neurological Center of Pennsylvania Hospital, Philadelphia

1982

W.B. SAUNDERS COMPANY

Philadelphia   London   Toronto
Mexico City   Rio de Janeiro   Sydney   Tokyo

W. B. Saunders Company: West Washington Square
Philadelphia, PA   19105

1 St. Anne's Road
Eastbourne, East Sussex BN21 3UN, England

1 Goldthorne Avenue
Toronto, Ontario M8Z 5T9, Canada

Apartado 26370 – Cedro 512
Mexico 4, D.F., Mexico

Rua Coronel Cabrita, 8
Sao Cristovao Caixa Postal 21176
Rio de Janeiro, Brazil

9 Waltham Street
Artarmon, N.S.W. 2064, Australia

Ichibancho, Central Bldg., 22-1 Ichibancho
Chiyoda-Ku, Tokyo 102, Japan

Library of Congress Cataloging in Publication Data

Main entry under title:

The Spine.

1. Spine – Surgery.   2. Spine – Diseases.   3. Spine –
   Wounds and injuries.   4. Spine – Abnormalities.
   I. Rothman, Richard H.   II. Simeone, Frederick A., 1936–
   [DNLM: 1. Spinal diseases. WE275 S759]

RD533.S68 1981   617'.56   77–25569

ISBN 0–7216–7719–3 (vol. 1)

ISBN 0–7216–7720–7 (vol. 2)

ISBN 0–7216–7718–5 (set)

Listed here is the latest translated edition of this book together
with the language of the translation and the publisher.

Italian (*1st Edition*) – Aulo Gaggi Editore, Bologna, Italy

Volume I   ISBN   0-7216-7719-3
Volume II   ISBN   0-7216-7720-7
The Spine   Complete Set ISBN   0-7216-7718-5

Last digit is the print number: 9   8   7   6   5   4   3   2   1

A new edition of this text has caused us to reflect on the changes in the management of patients with spine-related disorders in these intervening years. Technical advances such as computed tomography, new instrumentation, and perfected pharmacologic agents are obvious. Less perceptible, however, is the progress in hands-on nursing care. This has resulted in a measurable reduction in those complications so devastating to our patients. Bedsores, urinary tract infections, pneumonia, nutritional derangements, and bedside misadventures are no longer accepted as the unavoidable consequences of spinal disease. With greater authority and specialization, the nursing profession is intolerant to these secondary problems that may supervene the primary illness in severity.

This edition, therefore, is dedicated to nursing; to those individuals who bring to ultimate fruition a successful operation or who ease the tragedy of a failure; to the delicate balance between expertise and compassion.

For qualities not unrelated to these, we are indebted also to our wives, Marsha and Kate.

CONTRIBUTORS

ROBERT W. BAILEY, M.D.

Professor of Surgery, University of Michigan Medical School; Active Staff in Orthopedic Surgery, St. Joseph Mercy Hospital, Ann Arbor, Michigan.

Surgical Considerations in Arthritis of the Cervical Spine

M. VALLO BENJAMIN, M.D.

Associate Professor of Clinical Neurosurgery, New York University School of Medicine; Attending Physician, University Hospital; Associate Director, University Hospital; Visiting Attending Physician, Bellevue Hospital; Consultant Physician, Veterans Hospital, New York, New York.

Thoracic Disc Disease

PHILLIP BERNINI, M.D.

Assistant Clinical Professor of Orthopaedic Surgery, Dartmouth Medical School, Hanover, New Hampshire.

Lumbar Disc Disease

DIETRICH BLUMER, M.D.

Chairman, Department of Psychiatry, Henry Ford Hospital; Clinical Professor of Psychiatry, University of Michigan Medical School, Detroit, Michigan.

Psychiatric Aspects of Chronic Pain

HENRY H. BOHLMAN, M.D.

Associate Professor of Orthopaedic Surgery, Case Western Reserve University School of Medicine; Associate in Orthopaedics, University Hospitals, Cleveland, Ohio.

Spine and Spinal Cord Injuries

DAVID S. BRADFORD, M.D.

Professor of Orthopedic Surgery, University of Minnesota; Professor of Orthopedic Surgery, Department of Orthopedic Surgery, University of Minnesota Hospitals; Administrative Director and Director of Fellowship Program, Twin Cities Scoliosis Center; Attending Staff, Fairview Hospital, Minneapolis Children's Hospital, Minneapolis Health Center, Minneapolis, Minnesota.

Scoliosis

THOMAS DUCKER, M.D.

Professor and Head, Division of Neurosurgery, University of Maryland Hospital, Baltimore, Maryland.

Spine and Spinal Cord Injuries

HOWARD DUNCAN, M.B., B.S.

Clinical Professor of Internal Medicine, University of Michigan Medical School; Division of Rheumatology, Bone and Mineral Research Laboratory, Detroit, Michigan.

Metabolic Bone Disease Affecting the Spine

GARY E. FRIEDLAENDER, M.D.

Associate Professor of Surgery (Orthopaedics and Oncology), Yale University School of Medicine; Attending in Orthopaedic Surgery, Yale-New Haven Hospital, New Haven; Consultant in Orthopaedic Surgery, West Haven Veterans Administration Hospital, West Haven; Chief of Orthopaedic Service, Community Health Care Plan, New Haven, Connecticut.

Tumors of the Spine

RICHARD N. HARNER, M.D.

Associate Professor of Neurology, University of Pennsylvania School of Medicine; Chairman, Department of Neurology, Graduate Hospital; Associate Neurologist, Hospital of The University of Pennsylvania; Neurologist, Presbyterian-University of Pennsylvania Medical Center; Consultant in Neurology, Pennsylvania Hospital and Children's Hospital of Pennsylvania, Philadelphia, Pennsylvania.

Differenial Diagnosis of Spinal Disorders

ROBERT N. HENSINGER, M.D.

Associate Professor of Surgery, Department of Surgery, Section of Orthopaedic Surgery, University of Michigan Medical School, Ann Arbor; University of Michigan Hospital, Ann Arbor; Wayne County General Hospital, Westland, Michigan.

Congenital Anomalies of the Spine

JOHN H. HUBBARD, M.D.

Clinical Assistant Professor of Neurological Surgery, Albert Einstein College of Medicine, New York, New York; Attending Neurosurgeon, Montefiore Hospital and Medical Center, New York, New York, Hackensack Hospital, Hackensack, Holy Name Hospital, Teaneck, Pascack Valley Hospital, Westwood, New Jersey.

Chronic Pain of Spinal Origin

ROLLIN M. JOHNSON, M.D.

Associate Clinical Professor of Orthopaedic Surgery, Yale University School of Medicine, New Haven, Connecticut; Attending Orthopaedic Surgeon, Cooley Dickinson Hospital, Northampton, Massachusetts; Consultant Orthopaedic Surgeon, West Haven Veterans Administration Medical Center, West Haven, Connecticut.

Surgical Approaches to the Spine

HENRY LA ROCCA, M.D.

Clinical Professor of Orthopaedic Surgery, Tulane University School of Medicine, New Orleans, Louisiana.

Spinal Sepsis

PABLO M. LAWNER, M.D.

Assistant Professor of Neurosurgery; Assistant Chief, Division of Neurosurgery, Harbor/UCLA Medical Center.

Intraspinal Neoplasms

J. T. LUCAS, M.D.

Chief of Neurosurgery, Louisiana State University School of Medicine, Shreveport, Louisiana.

Spine and Spinal Cord Injuries

G. DEAN MacEWEN, M.D.

Clinical Professor of Orthopaedics, Thomas Jefferson University School of Medicine, Philadelphia, Pennsylvania; Medical Director, Alfred I. DuPont Institute; Consultant in Orthopaedics, Wilmington Medical Center; Consultant in Orthopaedics, St. Francis Hospital, Wilmington, Delaware.

Congenital Anomalies of the Spine

IAN MacNAB, F.R.C.S. (Eng.), F.R.C.S. (Can.)

Associate Professor of Surgery, University of Toronto; Chief of Division of Orthopaedic Surgery, Wellesley Hospital, Toronto, Ontario, Canada.

Acceleration Extension Injuries of the Cervical Spine

PAUL E. McMASTER, M.D.

Associate Professor of Orthopaedic Surgery, University of Southern California; Clinical Professor of Orthopaedic Surgery, University of California at Los Angeles; St. John's Hospital, Santa Monica; Staff, U.C.L.A. Medical Center Hospital, Orthopaedic Hospital, Los Angeles; Staff, Senior Consultant, Department of Orthopaedics, Veterans Administration Facility, West Los Angeles; California.

Osteotomy of the Spine for Fixed Flexion Deformity

JOHN H. MOE, M.D.

Professor and Head, Department of Orthopedics, Professor Emeritus, University of Minnesota; Active Staff, Fairview Hospital; Courtesy Staff, St. Mary's Hospital; Consulting/Honorary Staff, Northwest Hospital; Honorary Staff, Hennepin County Medical Center, Metropoliton Medical Center, Minneapolis, Minnesota; Courtesy Staff, St. Joseph's Hospital, Savannah, Georgia.

Scoliosis

A. M. PARFITT, M.B., B.Chir.

Clinical Professor of Medicine, University of Michigan Medical School; Director, Bone and Mineral Research Laboratory, Henry Ford Hospital, Detroit, Michigan.

Metabolic Bone Disease Affecting the Spine

WESLEY W. PARKE, Ph.D.

Professor and Chairman, Department of Anatomy, University of South Dakota School of Medicine, Vermillion, South Dakota.

Development of the Spine
Applied Anatomy of the Spine

JOSEPH RANSOHOFF, M.D.

Professor and Chairman, Department of Neurosurgery, New York University School of Medicine; Director, Neurological Service, Veterans Administration Hospital; Attending Physician, St. Vincent's Hospital and Medical Center, New York, New York.

Thoracic Disc Disease

RICHARD H. ROTHMAN, M.D., Ph.D.

Professor of Orthopaedic Surgery, The University of Pennsylvania School of Medicine; Chief of Orthopaedic Surgery, Pennsylvania Hospital, Philadelphia, Pennsylvania.

Cervical Disc Disease
Lumbar Disc Disease

FREDERICK A. SIMEONE, M.D.

Professor of Neurosurgery, The University of Pennsylvania School of Medicine; Chief of Neurosurgery, Pennsylvania Hospital; Director of Neurosurgery, Elliott Neurological Center of Pennsylvania Hospital, Philadelphia, Pennsylvania.

Cervical Disc Disease
Lumbar Disc Disease
Intraspinal Neoplasms

NATHAN SMUKLER, M.D.

Professor of Medicine, Thomas Jefferson University School of Medicine; Attending Physician, Thomas Jefferson University Hospital, Philadelphia, Pennsylvania.

Arthritic Disorders of the Spine

WAYNE O. SOUTHWICK, M.D.

Professor of Orthopaedic Surgery, Yale University School of Medicine, New Haven, Connecticut.

Surgical Approaches to the Spine
Tumors of the Spine

E. SHANNON STAUFFER, M.D.

Professor and Chairman, Division of Orthopaedic Surgery and Rehabilitation, Department of Surgery, Southern Illinois University School of Medicine; Active Staff, Memorial Medical Center, St. John's Hospital, Springfield, Illinois.

Rehabilitation of the Spinal Cord–Injured Patient

MICHAEL A. WIENIR, M.D.

Clinical Instructor, University of California at Los Angeles School of Medicine; Neurologist, Medical Center of Tarzana, Tarzana; Encino Hospital, Encino; and Northridge Hospital, Northridge, California.

Differential Diagnosis of Spinal Disorders

ROBERT B. WINTER, M.D.

Professor, Department of Orthopedic Surgery, University of Minnesota, Minneapolis; Chief of Spinal Service, Gillette Children's Hospital, St. Paul; Director of Orthopaedic Education, Fairview Hospital, St. Mary's Hospital, Minneapolis; University of Minnesota Hospitals, Minneapolis Children's Health Center, Minneapolis; St. Paul Children's Hospital, St. Paul-Ramsey Hospital and Medical Center, St. Paul, Minnesota.

Scoliosis

PREFACE

Advancements in medicine generally follow broader scientific and even social trends. The treatment of spine diseases is no exception. Consequently, increments of new information have been added to the general body of knowledge in spotty but predictable areas. These new developments constitute the raison d'être for this second edition. The dramatic progress in radiologic imaging stands out as the most useful innovation. By the time these volumes reach readers' hands, it is likely that computed tomography of the spine will supplement and even replace myelography in the treatment of lumbar spine disease. Logic indicates that the next generation of scanners will delineate all thoracic and cervical disc lesions. Spinal trauma is managed better since the advent of computed tomography. Infections, tumor infiltration, and congenital malformations are being better understood as experience grows. Even older techniques, such as myelography, have been greatly refined with the use of water-soluble contrast agents. Other common, more classical aspects of diagnosis, such as the neurologic examination, remain virtually unchanged.

The therapeutics of spinal disorders have also been led by experience with remedies used for other conditions. Antibiotics that cross the blood-bone barrier, microsurgery for certain spinal disorders, and improved overall postoperative management are but a few.

Some developments, however, do not relate to specific technological improvement, but rather to greater experience with larger numbers of patients who suffer similar problems. Consequently, an extensive analysis of spinal cord injuries is both timely and practical.

Each contributor has demonstrated his commitment to summarizing the most recent information in a manner useful to students and clinicians alike, and for this the editors are proud and appreciative. Mr. Carroll Cann of W. B. Saunders Company is thanked in a special way for his encouragement during the preparation of these volumes.

CONTENTS

CHAPTER 1

Development of the Spine

WESLEY W. PARKE, Ph.D.
University of South Dakota School of Medicine

INTRODUCTION

The role of metamerism in the evolution of vertebrate morphology is remarkably illustrated in the development of the spine. This biologic principle, whereby the organism is formed by the linear repetition of many anatomically similar segments (metameres), was evolved in the higher invertebrates. However, it is only in the chordates that the segments are formed from a series of mesenchymal condensations flanking a longitudinal notochord and dorsal neural tube (Fig. 1–1). The resulting body sections, including their neural and notochordal regions, form the somites.

Primitively, all the post-cranial somites have the same developmental potential, and in the lower aquatic vertebrates they formed a definitive spine that showed minimal regional differentiation. With the evolution of limbs the variety of postures and modes of locomotion required more specific regional differences, and another biologic principle, Stromer's law, was superimposed over the original segmentation. As applied to metamerism, this "law" is actually an observed adaptive trend in which the many similar segments (isomerism) of the primitive animal decrease in number through deletion or fusion, while the remaining segments increase their diverse functional and anatomic specialization (anisomerism).

Despite this evolutionary overlay, the higher vertebrate spine still shows a monot-

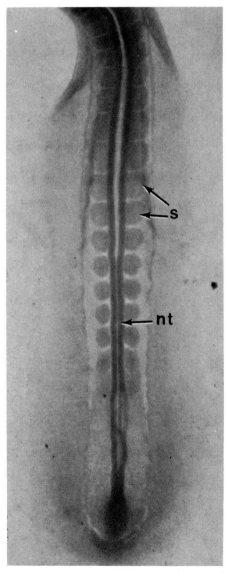

Figure 1–1. Chick embryo at the 20 somite stage. The formation of the cuboidal somites (s) lateral to the neural tube (nt) is apparent. Each somite is separated by the intermyotomic septum.

onous similarity of the somites in its early stages of development, and by following the embryologic acquisition of the regional peculiarities, the common homologies of the various components of the different adult vertebrae are revealed. Therefore, the initial part of this discussion will be devoted to the development of a typical vertebral element, and the regional specialization will be discussed subsequently.

Early Development of the Somites

The development of the human spine starts with the onset of the triploblastic stage of the embryo and ends in the third decade of life. On the seventeenth day of gestation cells at the center of the dorsal layer of the bilaminar embryonic disc invaginate to form the primitive pit. The cells around this opening form the primitive knot and further proliferate cranially between the ectoderm and endoderm as the tubular notochordal process. The cells underlying the hollow axis of this process and their contiguous layer of endoderm both degenerate so that the upper half of the notochordal process comes to lie directly in contact with the contents of the yolk sac and forms the flat notochordal plate. Starting cranially, the lateral edges of this plate then curl under until they meet. This reunites the endoderm and produces the true notochord. The presence of the notochordal cells induces a thickening in the overlying ectoderm (neurectoderm), which forms the neural plate. On the eighteenth day the edges of this plate curl upward, and their union creates the dorsal neural tube.

In the higher vertebrates the notochord determines the longitudinal axis of the early embryo and induces ectodermal and mesodermal differentiation, but in prevertebrate chordates and the cyclostomes it persists as a firm, flexible rod that is the essential part of the axial skeleton.

With the elaboration of the notochord and neural tube, the intraembryonic mesoderm lateral to these structures thickens to form two longitudinal columns, the paraxial mesoderm. Further lateral proliferation of this cell mass results in two other areas so that by the nineteenth day three distinct areas of the mesoderm are evident. These consist of the medial paraxial columns, a bilateral pair of intermediate mesodermal columns, and the most lateral mesodermal plates. The lateral mesoderm forms the layers that encase the coelomic cavities, while the intermediate columns give rise to urogenital structures.

The somites arise from the paraxial mesoderm. On approximately the twentieth day the cells in the anterior parts of these columns condense into pairs of blocklike segments. The first pair appears just caudal to the rostral end of the notochord, and an additional 38 pairs of somites continue to form in a craniocaudal sequence throughout the next 10 days, which is called the somite period. Eventually 42 to 44 somites appear. Externally, they are evident as a series of elevated beads (Fig. 1–5) along the dorsolateral surface of the embryo and, in section, are wedge-shaped with an ephemeral central cavity, the myocoele.

During the somite stage the more cranial, older somites show internal specializations. The cells dorsolateral to the myocoele become the dermomyotome. The lateral group of these cells, the cutis plate, will give rise to the integument, and the more medial group, the muscle plate, establishes the dorsal musculature. The ventromedial cell mass, the sclerotome, exhibits cell migration in three directions in anticipation of forming skeletal structures (Figs. 1–2 to 1–6).

The development and migration of these sclerotome cells indicates the formation of the first of three successive vertebral columns. In the precartilaginous stage the scleratogenous mesenchyme that aligns itself along the notochord and neural tube forms the membranous vertebral column (Fig. 1–6). Chondrification results in the cartilaginous column, and endochondral ossification eventually produces the definitive skeleton column (Figs. 1–6B and 1–7).

The cell population of the early sclerotome is not homogeneous in its distribution; rather, each sclerotome consists of a cranial mass of loosely packed cells and a caudal mass of more densely packed cells (Fig. 1–3). Upon their migration a transverse division, the sclerotomic fissure, appears to separate the two groups of cells, so that the caudal dense cell mass of one sclerotome unites with the cranial loose cell mass of the next caudal somite as they surround the notochord. Thus, the mesenchymal cells destined to form a single centrum actually create an intersegmental structure that receives equivalent contributions from adjacent somites. This is further exemplified by the fact that the segmental branches of the aorta that course lateral to the interval between the somites eventually run

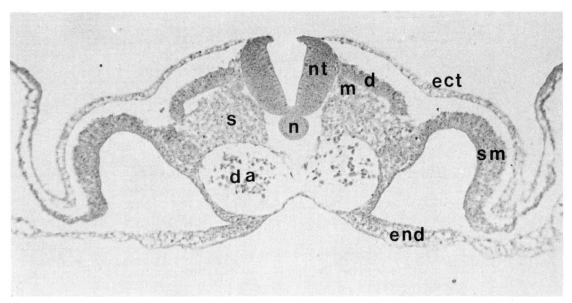

Figure 1–2. Cross section of a thoracic somite in a chick embryo of the 20 somite stage. Notochord (n) underlies neural tube (nt). The somite is divided into dermatome (d), myotome (m) and sclerotome (s). Lateral to this the somatic mesoderm (sm), endoderm (end) and ectoderm (ect) are displayed. Ventral to the sclerotomes lie the paired dorsal aortae (da). Transient myocoele is apparent on right side between the dermatome and myotome.

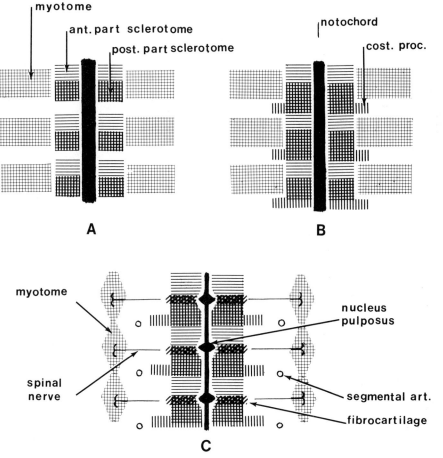

Figure 1–3. Schematic representation of the development of the vertebrae.

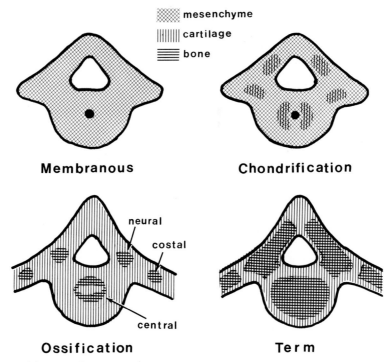

Figure 1–4. Schematic illustration of the sequential development of the typical vertebral element.

around the midsection of each vertebral body, while the spinal nerves and the muscles from their respective myotome become related to two vertebrae and their interposed disc. This provides developmental reinforcement for the structural and functional concept of the motor segment unit as described in Chapter 2.

The second mass of scleratogenous cells migrates dorsally in close approximation to the neural tube and eventually will form the neural or vertebral arch. A third group of cells moves ventrolaterally to establish the costal centers of chondrification and ossification (Fig. 1–6A and B). In this manner the individual vertebrae are all derived from three cell mass extensions of the original sclerotome, and all phyletically and ontogenetically are capable of bearing ribs. In mammals only the thoracic vertebrae normally display true articulated ribs, but elements from the costal centers are nevertheless incorporated in the structure of all other vertebrae except in the coccyx (Fig. 1–16).

Articulated cervical ribs are the rule in most reptiles, and the occasional presence of

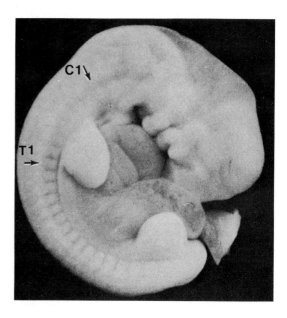

Figure 1–5. Human embryo of 5.5 mm crown-rump length. Note that the somites are externally represented as a series of dorsolateral swellings, and that at least two somites may be discerned rostral to the atlantal (C1) segment.

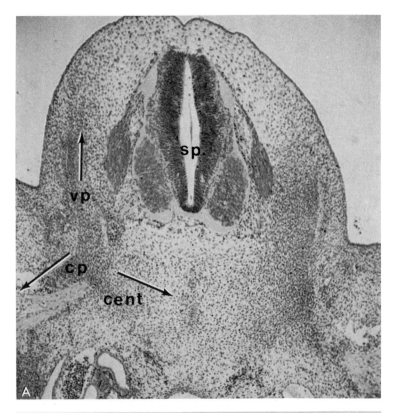

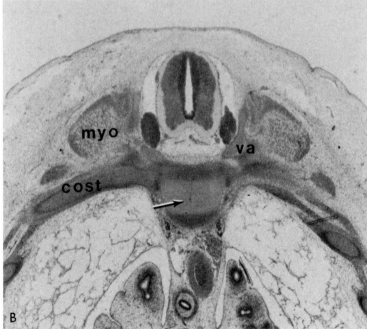

Figure 1–6. *A,* Cross section of a membranous vertebra in a pig embryo of 9 mm. The arrows indicate the directions of somite cell migration to form the vertebral process (vp), the costal process (cp) and the centrum (cent). The neural tube at this stage shows the anterior horn masses and the dorsal root ganglia. *B,* This section shows the chondrification of the pig vertebrae at 18 mm. The cartilaginous vertebral arch (va) and costal process (cost) are evident as is the myotomic precursor to the spinal muscles (myo). The arrow indicates the intracentral vestige of the notochord, called the mucoid streak.

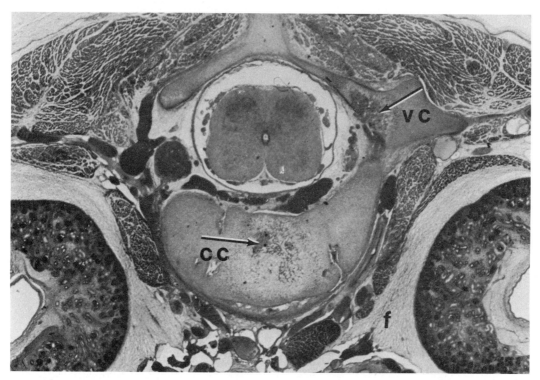

Figure 1–7. A vertebra of a human fetus at 38 mm CRL showing centers of ossification. The section is slightly oblique so that only the right center for the vertebral arch (vc) and the center for the centrum are obvious. Level of section is approximately at T2.

cervical or, less frequently, lumbar ribs in humans should be no surprise.

Fate of the Notochord

Where the notochord becomes surrounded by the precartilaginous cells that will establish the vertebral column, it degenerates. Between the vertebrae, however, notochordal cells develop into a gelatinous mass that becomes the nucleus pulposus of the intervertebral disc. Nevertheless, notochordal "rest" cells may persist in any part of the axial skeleton that once contained the embryonic structure. In the adult, this notochordal "track" commences in the sphenoid bone just posterior to the hypophyseal fossa. It leaves the bone and runs caudally along the ventral surface of the basisphenoid in close relation to the pharynx. Re-entering the bone in the basiocciput, it courses through the centers of the apical odontoid ligament and the odontoid process (Fig. 1–12). From here, it threads its way down the center of each vertebral body to the coccyx. Fortunately, notochordal remnants are usually impossible to demonstrate

outside of the nucleus pulposus in the adult, for where they may still persist the potential occurrence of a malignant chordoma is present. This slow-growing neoplasm occurs most frequently in the base of the skull, where its neurologic consequences are prolonged and disastrous.

Chondrification of a Typical Vertebra

In the sixth week centers of chondrification appear in the mesenchyme of the membranous vertebral column. At the end of the embryonic period two of these centers appear lateral to the notochord and fuse around it to complete the chondrous centrum. Two centers condense lateral to the neural tube, and their dorsal fusion establishes the neural arch and spinous process, while the additional two centers appear at the unions of the arch and centrum and their lateral extensions provide the transverse processes (Fig. 1–4).

During the seventh and eighth weeks the anterior and posterior longitudinal ligaments form from an interstitial matrix that surrounds the cartilaginous vertebrae. Their relationship to the chondrous bodies is identical to the adult condition: Namely, the anterior ligament becomes strongly adherent to the anterior surfaces of the centra, while the posterior ligament becomes attached only at the edges of the discs.

During the process of cartilage formation a thick ring of nonchondrous cells establishes the anulus fibrosus around the beaded segments of the notochord that will become the nucleus. Further chondrification in the centra "squeezes" that part of the notochord so that, prior to ossification, only the prechordal sheath remains as the mucoid streak.

Ossification of a Typical Vertebra

As with other bones of the skeleton, ossification of the vertebrae involves both primary and secondary centers. Each vertebra is derived from three primary centers, one for the centrum and two for the vertebral arch. Around the ninth week the preparation for ossification is heralded by anterior and posterior excavations of the chondrous centrum produced by the invasion of pericostal vessels. These vessels produce ventral and dorsal vascular lacunae, which support the initial ossification (Fig. 1–5). What is regarded as a single ossification center for the centrum shows, for a short time, a dorsal and a ventral component that are briefly separated by an ephemeral plate of cartilage. By the sixteenth week ossification is well under way, but the centers do not appear simultaneously or follow a craniocaudal sequence that one might expect. The centers for the centra usually appear first in the lower thoracic and upper lumbar regions and develop more rapidly to-

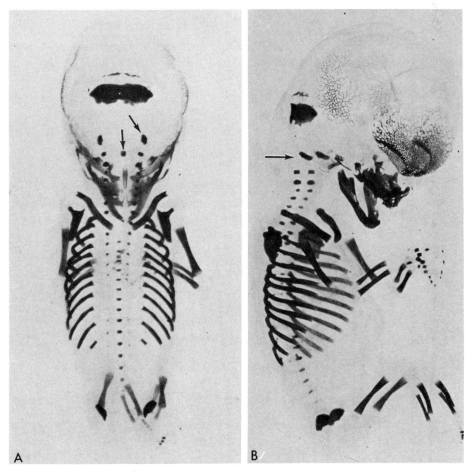

Figure 1–8. *A,* Posterior view of cleared fetus of 54 mm CRL. Specimen has been stained with alizarin to show areas of ossification. The differential appearance of the central ossification in the lower thoracocolumbar region and the vertebral arch centers in the cervical region are well illustrated. *B,* Lateral view of same specimen. Arrows in both *A* and *B* indicate the ossification of an occipital somite.

ward the caudal rather than the cranial vertebrae. This situation is exemplified by the fact
that the two vertebral arch centers show well-
advanced ossification in the cervical vertebrae
much sooner than any detectable ossification
in the centra (Fig. 1–8).

From week 20 to week 24, enlargement of
the ossification center for the centra divides
the body into two chondrous plates that demonstrate endochondral ossification where they
face the intervertebral discs. These plates
receive a number of radiating vessels that
penetrate the cartilage and form a crown of
isolated vascular lacunae. Because of the confusion as to where these epiphyseal-type
plates stop and the early anulus fibrosus
begins, there have been numerous statements

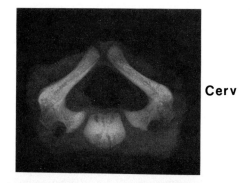

Cerv

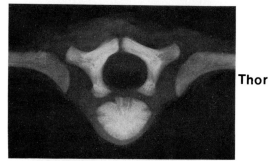

Thor

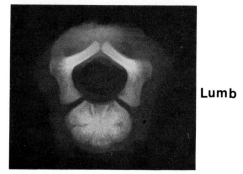

Lumb

Figure 1–10.   Vertical radiograms of individual vertebra of a 34 week fetus. The contributions of the vertebral
arches to the dorsolateral parts of the bodies are apparent. The cartilaginous line between the central ossification and the arches marks the neurocentral synchondroses. The union between the thoracic rib and the vertebral components shows the costovertebral arthroses.

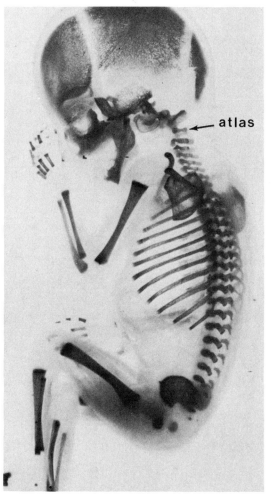

← atlas

Figure 1–9.   An oblique lateral view of a fetus of 125
mm CRL. The separate neural arch and central ossifica-
tions are still obvious. Again note similarity of occipital
and vertebral ossification.

about the presence of vessels in the fetal discs,
but recent analysis has shown that the radiating vascular tufts in the body cartilage stop
short of the developing anulus. Therefore the
disc, both in the fetus and in the adult, is
avascular and derives is nutrition by diffusion
(Fig. 1–18).

Around the ventral and lateral periphery
of the centrum-disc interface, a C-shaped cartilaginous ring develops, to form the ring
apophysis that ossifies during the second postnatal decade. This structure firmly anchors the

anulus to the body and, when ossified, receives the Sharpey's fibers of the anulus laminations.

Ossification becomes evident in the vertebral arches around the eighth week. Two centers, each forming half of the arch, appear first in the cervical region prior to the centers for the bodies. However, the laminae of the arches first unite in the lumbar region, and the subsequent unions progress cranially. During the fifteenth or sixteenth year secondary centers of ossification appear at the tips of the transverse processes and the spinous processes. These eventually fuse in the middle of the third decade (Fig. 1–11).

The transverse processes of the lower cervical vertebrae, particularly the seventh, may show an additional costal center of ossification that produces the troublesome cervical rib; this reinforces the concept that all vertebrae primitively had the potential of forming ribs.

The upper lumbar vertebrae also exhibit a tendency to extra costal centers, but much less frequently than do the cervical. Lack of fusion of these centers then produces a truly articulated lumbar rib, which may confuse the radiologist in the accurate identification of the vertebral levels. In addition, the lumbar vertebrae show accessory centers for the mamillary processes that surmount the articular projections.

Throughout the vertebrae the eventual fusion of the vertebral arches and the centra occurs well anterior to the pedicles at the site of the neurocentral synchondroses. The definitive vertebral body then includes more than just the bone derived from the ossific center of

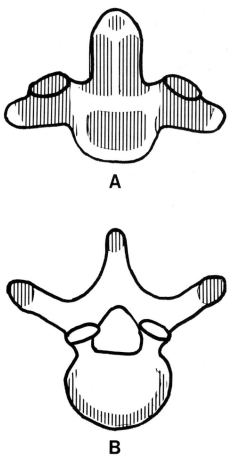

A

B

Figure 1–11. *A,* The centers of ossification of the axis. The lateral and central centers for the body of C2 are like those of subsequent vertebrae, but the odontoid shows two bilateral primary centers and a single secondary apical center. *B,* The secondary centers of ossification of a thoracic vertebra. The centers at the tips of the processes appear at 16 years and fuse approximately at 25 years. The ring apophysis at the edge of the centrum ossifies at approximately 14 years and fuses at 25 years.

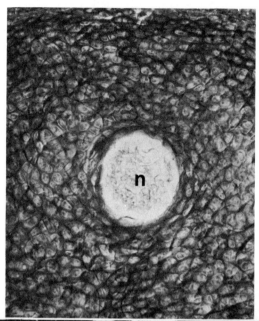

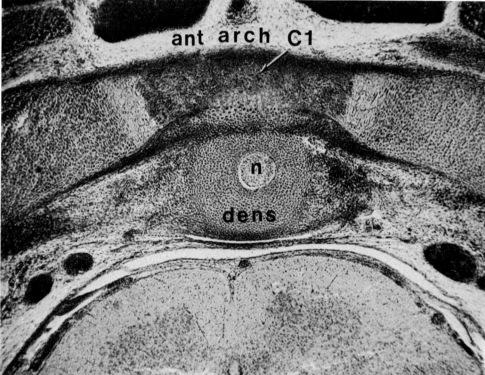

Figure 1–12. Section through the developing odontoid process of the neonatal rat shows the chondrous apex of the process and the ossification of the anterior arch of the atlas. The persistence of the notochord in the odontoid affirms its origin in the homologue of the centrum of C1. Upper illustration shows chondrous cells surrounding loose cellular remnants of notochord.

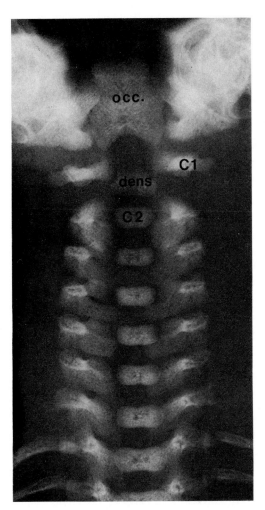

Figure 1–13. A-P radiogram of the cervical spine of a fetus of 30 weeks. The bilobed ossification of the dens and its separation from the body of C2 are quite apparent. Fusion of these two elements occurs in the second decade and completes ossification of the axis.

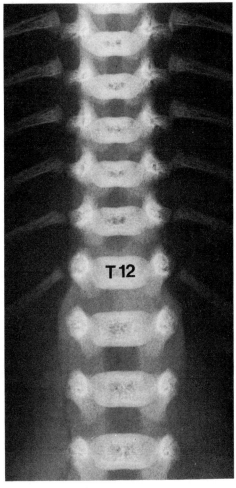

Figure 1–14. A-P radiogram of the mid-thoracolumbar region of a 30 week fetus. The oblate spheroid of the central ossification is particularly well illustrated. The costovertebral articulation is shown to form in relation to adjacent vertebrae and their intervening discs. In the region of the fibrocartilaginous anulus, the central radiolucent area indicates the formation of the nucleus pulposus from the notochord.

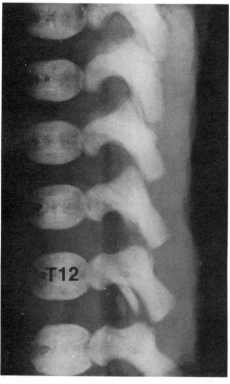

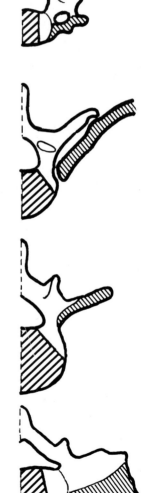

Figure 1–15. Lateral radiogram of a sagittal section of a 34 week spine. The pulley-sheave appearance of the central ossification is due to the ventral and dorsal vascular lakes that almost bisect each centrum. The radiolucent line where the spinal cord was removed marks the position of the spinal canal in relation to the neural arches. Note that the bases of the arches extend ventral to the canal and so contribute to the formation of the vertebral body.

Cervical

Thoracic

☐ neural
▨ costal
▥ central

Lumbar

Figure 1–16. Schematic representation of the relative contributions of the ossific centers to the different regional vertebrae. This emphasizes the ever-present rib-bearing potential of all vertebrae. Note that the neurocentral synchondroses lie well within the vertebral body in all cases, but are most medial in the cervical and sacral regions. Normally the costovertebral synchondroses develop a true diarthroses only in the thoracic region.

Sacral

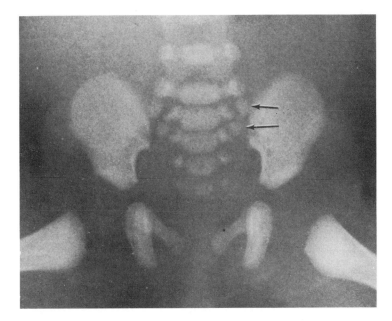

Figure 1–17. A-P radiogram of 34 week fetal pelvis showing two of the eventual three ossific centers for the costal contributions to the alae. These form in the cartilage that anchors the fetal sacrum to the auricular processes of the ilia.

the centrum, so that the terms "body" and "centrum" are not accurately interchangeable as some writings would indicate (Figs. 1–10 and 1–16).

OSSIFICATION OF THE MORE SPECIALIZED VERTEBRAL REGIONS

Atlas and Axis

The formation of these two bones differs markedly from that of other vertebrae. Although the atlas shows three centers of ossification, it bears no recognizable centrum. Two lateral centers establish the lateral masses and are equivalent to the centers for the neural arch in other vertebrae. Since the lateral masses are highly modified forms of the articular pillars found in the succeeding cervical vertebrae, this is a rather obvious homology. The third atlantal center forms the anterior arch and is of less certain homology. It is radiologically visible at birth in 20 per cent of neonates and can usually be demonstrated at the end of the first year in the balance of the specimens.

Five primary and two secondary centers ossify to form the axis. Its body and neural arch develop in the conventional manner, with a single center for the centrum and two for the arch. Following the typical pattern of cervical

ossification, the two centers for the arch appear around the eighth week and that of the centrum some eight to 10 weeks later. The odontoid process (dens) appears as a chondrous rostral projection of the second cervical body. From the twentieth to the twenty-fourth fetal week, two bilateral ossification centers become evident in the base of this process, giving it a bilobed appearance in cross section. The medial union of these centers occurs

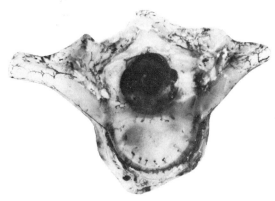

Figure 1–18. Section through the cartilaginous end of the vertebra of 30 weeks. This specimen had been injected to show the coronal vascular pattern in the cartilage. Each tuft consists of a central artery entwined by recurrent veins. It ends in a chondrous lacuna as a terminal A-V anastomotic glomus, from which nutrients diffuse into the surrounding tissue. These vessels do not enter the presumptive disc.

around parturition, but the superior end of the fused centers may still show a separating cleft. A separate apical center of ossification forms postnatally at the end of the second year. Since the odontoid process was phyletically derived from the centrum of the first cervical vertebra, the cartilaginous plate that intervenes between the ossifying odontoid and the body of the second cervical vertebra is homologous to an intervertebral disc. Obliteration of this cartilage usually occurs during the middle of the second decade, along with fusion of the apical center. Ossification of this plate, like that of the discs of the sacrum, commences around its periphery, so that persistence of a central remnant may give a confusing radiologic picture suggesting fracture. Complete failure of ossific fusion results in a congenitally separate os odontoideum. The stability of the atlantoaxial joint then depends on the degree of fibrous union between the dens and the body of C2.

The Sacrum

Ossification of the bodies of the sacral vertebrae is unique in that in addition to the single central ossific zone, two true epiphyseal plates later provide accessory ossification to the superior and inferior surfaces of each segment. The central centers for the superior three sacral vertebrae are evident at week nine, while these centers for the fourth and fifth segments do not appear until after week 24. Each vertebral arch of the sacrum shows the conventional bilateral centers, but in addition six centers produce the sacral alae. Between week 24 and week 32 these centers appear anterolateral to the anterior sacral foramina of the upper three sacral vertebrae. They are expressions of the ever-present potential of the vertebral anlagen to produce costal equivalents (Fig. 1–17).

In the early postnatal years the sacral vertebrae are still separated by intervertebral discs, and the lower two are the first to fuse in late adolescence. Prior to this the ossific centers for the superior and inferior epiphyseal plates of the bodies appear, and between the eighteenth and twentieth year lateral epiphyseal plates form on the auricular surfaces of the sacral alae. By the middle of the third decade the entire sacrum should be fused, although internal remnants of the intervertebral plates remain throughout life. These may be visualized in a sagittal section or in radiograms taken at the appropriate A-P angle.

The coccygeal segments lack neural arch equivalents and form from a single ossific center for their bodies. The first usually appears before the fifth year of life, and the succeeding three then ossify during consecutive five year intervals.

COMPARATIVE COMMENTS

The earliest evidence of vertebral element formation was found in Agnatha. In the extant members of this group, the cyclostomes, small cartilaginous neural arches surmount the notochord in hagfish, and superior and inferior sheets of cartilage reinforce the caudal notochord of lampreys. Aside from the interposition of accessory arches in the shark, in which they form an uninterrupted conduit over the spinal cord, the neural arch has remained functionally and morphologically constant throughout the vertebrate lineage. A second series of elements, the haemal arches, appeared on the ventral aspect of the caudal notochord to provide protection for the dorsal aorta and concurrent vein.

In contradistinction to the straightforward evolution of the arches, the phyletic history of the centrum is a mess, being replete with variations and odd complexities in the preamniotes. It starts out simply enough with four ossicles forming bases for the attachment of the neural and haemal arches to the sides of the notochord. Thus, two *dorsal arch bases* lie superolateral to the notochord, and two *ventral arch bases* lie ventrolateral, as exhibited in the bowfin, *Amia*. These arch bases can be demonstrated developmentally in most forms of fishes, in which the definitive spool-shaped centrum results from additional ossification around and between the bases.

In earlier texts the evolution of the centrum from the fish to the amniote involved the postulation of an original four pairs of "arcualia" — or primitive ossicles that through a complex system of rearrangements could account for all the varieties of centrum types encountered. Unfortunately, this concept was more convenient than accurate.

An iteration of the number of types of centra that have occurred, particularly in the adaptive radiation of the amphibians, is not germane here, but at the risk of oversimplification, a general theme may be traced from the fish to the amniote. Two pairs of ossicles are found lateral to the notochord of the crossopterygian. The ones on each side just below the neural arch are regarded as the equivalent of the *pleurocentrum* of the early amphibian and homologous to the original dorsal arch bases. Inferior to these on the ventral aspect of the notochord a prism-shaped ossicle represents the *intercentrum* and the derivative of the ventral arch bases. The pleuracentra, through comparative evidence, are assumed to be the antecedents of the true amniote centrum. However, the intercentrum predominates as the major vertebral component in most reptiles and reveals its homology by bearing the haemal arches. Thus, we arrive at the amniote condition with a single centrum derived from the pleurocentra and an intercentrum that is found in the caudal vertebrae of most mammals and as small ventral intervertebral ossicles throughout the spine of some Insectivora (*Blarina,* etc.). In the caudal region of most tailed mammals, the intercentrum bears a typical haemal arch called a chevron bone. In most non-caudate mammals, the only discernible remnant of the intercentrum lies in the anterior arch of the atlas.

Without regard to the development or phyletic composition of the vertebrae, a convenient system of descriptive classification is based on the shapes of the articulating surfaces of the centra. For example, the bodies of the human vertebrae generally articulate through mutually flat surfaces and are therefore called *acoelus,* meaning "no cavity" at either end of the centrum. In forms in which much of the notochordal material is still present in spindle-shaped masses between the vertebrae, the centra are biconcave and are designated as *amphicoelus.* In many amniotes either the rostral or the caudal end of the body is concave and articulates with a reciprocal convexity of the next element. These are referred to as *procoelus* and *opisthocoelus* vertebrae, respectively. Most unique are the biaxial articulations seen in the saddle-shaped cervical intervertebral joints of birds, which give these vertebrae the term *heterocoelus.*

REGIONAL COMPARATIVE ANATOMY

Atlantoaxial Complex

It has been previously stated that the human embryo exhibits a total of 42 to 44 somites. Yet only 33 or 34 segments can be accounted for in the adult spine. Deletion of caudal elements explains the loss of most of these, but the incorporation of rostral somites into the formation of the skull and the evolution of the craniocervical articulations are good examples of Stromer's law.

In the generalized fish, the head and trunk move in unison, and the first vertebra simply articulates with a projection on the skull that resembles the posterior aspect of another centrum. Thus, the range of craniocervical movement is approximately equal to that allowed between the individual vertebrae. With the advent of terrestrial life in the amphibia, all but the more primitive forms show a splitting of this single projection into two lateral occipital condyles. The resulting articulation provides a hingelike flexion-extension that may have facilitated the raising and lowering of the head to give greater range to jaw movement, but still restricted lateral mobility (Fig. 1–19).

Most reptiles and birds display a single, rounded occipital condyle, but the cranial two vertebrae have been modified into an atlas and axis. The former is a ringlike structure that formed from the union of the neural arch and intercentrum. The true centrum of C1 tends to remain disassociated from the ring but still does not fuse with C2. Often the proatlas, an extra bone of uncertain origin, though probably derived from neural arch homologues, is intercalated between the skull and the atlas. This articulation gives considerable universal motion but differs from the equivalent joint in mammals in that both the flexion-extension and rotatory actions are achieved between the single condyle and the concave apex of the C1 centrum (odontoid homologue). Other than lending stability to the encircled ball and socket, the manner in which the atlantal ring participates in the joint action seems obscure.

In the mammalian atlantoaxial structure, the atlas also represents the neural arch-intercentrum complex. However, the lateral masses of the atlantal ring articulate directly with the bilateral occipital condyles so that most craniocervical flexion-extension is confined to the atlanto-occipital articulation. The homologue of the centrum of the atlas, the odontoid process, becomes fused to the body of C2 and provides the rotatory pivot, but its apex remains free of any axial thrust.

One must not assume that the evolution of the atlantoaxial complex resulted from progressive changes in vertebrae of equivalent segmental levels, for a simultaneous incorporation of rostral somites into the base of the

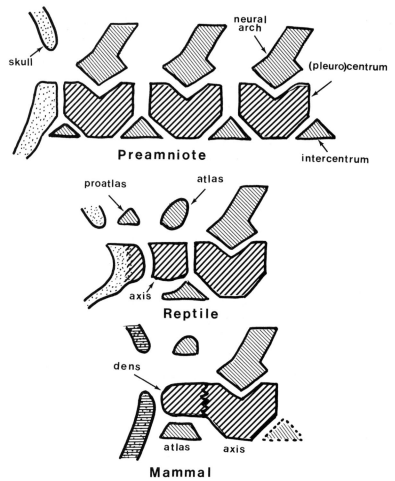

Figure 1–19. Highly schematic depiction of the evolution of the craniocervical articulations. The different fate of the three major contributions (centrum, intercentrum and neural arch) in the formation of atlantoaxial complex is shown without regard to accuracy of relative sizes. The fact that primitive cervical segments were incorporated in the formation of the occipital skull has been indicated by the progressive reduction in number of vertebral elements illustrated.

skull accompanied its phyletic development. The fact that the human embryo shows at least three somites rostral to the definitive level of the craniocervical articulation offers ample evidence of this phenomenon (Fig. 1–5). In the cleared specimen of 14 weeks' gestation (Fig. 1–8), illustrating alizarin-stained areas of ossification, what appears to be the ossific centers of the most cranial cervical vertebrae are actually those of the occipital region of the skull. In addition, the transition from anamniote to mammal involved the inclusion of two additional spinal nerves into the cranial nerve sequence, a certain indication that their corresponding somite levels became involved in the formation of the skull.

It is noteworthy that throughout all spe-cies of mammals the cervical region always shows seven vertebrae: a remarkable consis-tency, considering the numerical variations that may be encountered in other regions. This situation is most emphasized in whales and porpoises (Cetacea), in which the return to the aquatic environment reselected the vertebral adaptations of the fish. This does not imply a reverse evolution but rather an adaptive su-perimposition on the characteristics of higher vertebrates of those that morphologically and functionally meet the requirements of the marine environment. Thus, when the head and trunk again move as a single unit, the cervical vertebrae develop as a stack of seven wafer-thin plates that have the overall dimensions and mobility of a single vertebral element.

Comparative Sacralization

In the evolution of the tetrapod limbs the pectoral girdle of the forelimbs achieves only remote connections with the spine, but the pelvic girdle, from early amphibians on, has established various degrees of direct articulation with vertebrae. The modification of the vertebrae to accommodate this articulation produces the sacrum. In its simplest form, as in the amphibians, only a single vertebral segment became involved, and this usually entailed the modification of a single costal equivalent to form a lateral projection for articulation with the ilium.

In the generalized reptile and all extant legged members of this class, two vertebrae became involved in the spinopelvic articulation. Among the dinosaurs, however, particularly in the ornithischian group, greater numbers of vertebrae became incorporated. The minimum number of vertebral elements forming the mammalian sacrum is three, with additional members being added as adaptive requirements dictated. The Cetacea, in whom the sacrum has been secondarily lost, are an obvious exception.

The results of sacralization reach their epitome in the class Aves (birds), in which not only do those elements regionally associated with the pelvis become fused but also the entire thoracocolumbar spine is united to the pelvis as the inflexible *synsacrum*. It is apparent that this rigid fuselage has considerable significance in the dynamics of flight, yet no similar tendency is observed in the mammalian bats.

References

1. Noback, C. R., and Robertson, G. C.: Sequence of appearance of ossification centers in the human skeleton during the first five prenatal months. Am. J. Anat. *89*:1–28, 1951.
2. Peacock, A.: Observations on the prenatal development of the intervertebral disc in man. J. Anat. *85*:260–275, 1951.
3. Romer, A. S.: The Osteology of the Reptiles. Chicago. University of Chicago Press, 1956.
4. Schufeldt, R. W.: Osteology of birds. Bull. New York State Mus. *130*:5–381, 1909.
5. Sensenig, E. C.: The early development of the human vertebral column. Contr. Embryol. Carneg. Inst. *33*:21–51, 1949.
6. Stromer, E.: Gesicherte Ergebnisse der Paläozoologie. Abh. Bayer. Akad. Wissensch. *54*:1–114, 1944.
7. Williams, E. E.: Gadow's arcualia and the development of tetrapod vertebra. Quart. Rev. Biol. *34*:1–32, 1959.

CHAPTER 2

Applied Anatomy of the Spine

WESLEY W. PARKE, Ph.D.
University of South Dakota School of Medicine

The spine is the segmental column of vertebrae that constitutes the major subcranial part of the axial skeleton. Its individual elements are united by a series of intervertebral articulations to form a firm but flexible shaft that supports the trunk and its appendages while providing a protective covering for the spinal cord. The entire column typically consists of 33 vertebrae. Seven cervical, twelve thoracic, and five lumbar vertebrae compose the movable presacral section of the spine, while five fused elements form the inflexible sacrum that articulates with the pelvic girdle. Caudal to the sacrum four or five irregular ossicles make up the coccyx.

THE VERTEBRAE

Since 97 diarthroses and an even greater number of amphiarthroses are involved in the movements of the spine, the individual vertebra must bear multiple processes and surface markings that indicate the attachments of the numerous ligamentous and tendinous structures. Yet, despite the fact that these characteristics may vary considerably from one region to the next, the homologous segmental origin of the vertebrae provides that a single generalized description can be applied to the basic morphology of all but the most superior and inferior elements.

The typical vertebra consists of two major components: a roughly cylindrical ventral mass of cancellous bone, the body, and the dorsal vertebral arch. The vertebral bodies vary considerably in size and sectional contour, but they exhibit no salient processes or unique external features other than the facets for rib articulation in the thoracic region. Contrarily, the vertebral arch has a more complex structure. It is attached to the dorsolateral aspects of the body by two stout pillars, the pedicles. These are united dorsally by a pair of arched flat laminae that are surmounted in the midline by a dorsal projection, the spinous process. The pedicles, laminae and dorsum of the body thus form the vertebral foramen, a complete osseous ring that encloses the spinal cord.

Near the junction of the pedicles and the laminae are found the lateral transverse processes and the superior and inferior articular processes. The transverse processes extend from the sides of the vertebral arches, and, as all vertebrae are phyletically and ontogenetically associated with some form of costal element, they either articulate with or incorporate a rib component.

The articular processes (zygopophyses) form the paired diarthrodial articulations between the vertebral arches. The superior processes (prezygopophyses) always bear an articulating facet whose surface is directed dorsally to some degree, and complementarily, the inferior articulating processes (postzygopophyses) direct their articulating surfaces ventrally. Variously shaped bony prominences (mammillary processes or parapophyses) may be found lateral to the articular processes and serve in the multiple origins and insertions of the spinal muscles.

The superior-inferior dimensions of the pedicles are roughly half that of their corresponding body, so that in their lateral aspect the pedicles and their articulating processes form the superior and inferior vertebral notches. As the base of the pedicle arises somewhat superiorly from the dorsum of the body, the inferior vertebral notch appears more deeply incised. In the articulated spine, the opposing superior and inferior notches form the intervertebral foramina that pass the neural and vascular structures between the corresponding levels of the spinal cord and their developmentally related body segments.

Regional Characteristics

Although the 24 vertebrae of the presacral spine are divided into three distinct groups, in which the individual members may be recognized by one or two uniquely regional features, there is also a gradual craniocaudal change, so that in a number of ways the vertebrae found above and below the point of regional demarcation will be transitional and bear some of the characteristics of both areas.

The Cervical Vertebrae

Of the seven cervical vertebrae, the first two and the last require special notation, but the third through the sixth are fairly uniform and can be covered by a common description.

As the cervical vertebrae bear the least weight, their bodies are relatively small and thin with respect to the size of the vertebral arch and vertebral foramen. In addition, their diameter is greater transversely than in the anteroposterior direction. The lateral edges of the superior surface of each body are sharply turned upward to form the uncinate processes that are characteristic of the cervical region. However, the most obvious diagnostic feature of the cervical vertebrae is the transverse foramina that perforate the transverse processes and transmit the cervical arteries. The anterior part of the transverse processes represents fused costal elements that arise from the sides of the body. The lateral extremities of the transverse processes bear two projections, the anterior and posterior tubercles. The former serve as origins of anterior cervical muscles, while the latter provides both origins and insertions for posterior cervical

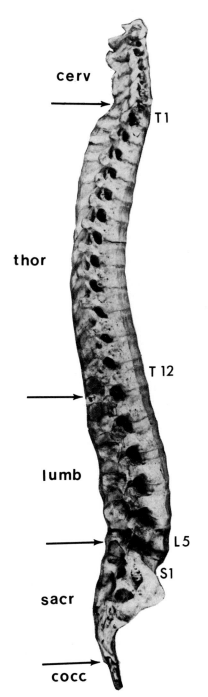

Figure 2–1. Lateral view of dried preparation of the spine with anterior longitudinal and supraspinous ligaments intact.

cerv

T1

thor

T 12

lumb

L5

S1

sacr

cocc

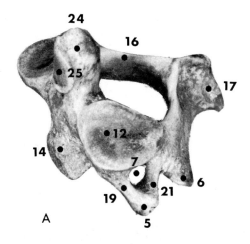

A

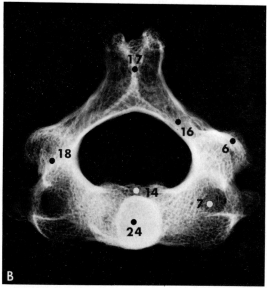

B

Figure 2–2. The atlas, axis, and a typical vertebra of each region is illustrated photographically and radiographically. The following numerical key is applicable to all subdivisions of this figure. *A,* Oblique view of atlas, *B,* Ventral radiographic view of atlas.

 1. lateral mass of atlas
 2. superior articulating process
 3. posterior arch
 4. anterior arch
 5. transverse process
 6. inferior articulating process
 7. transverse foramen
 8. alar tubercle
 9. groove for vertebral artery
10. neural arch element of transverse process
11. costal element of transverse process
12. superior articulating process
13. pedicle

14. body
15. uncinate process
16. lamina
17. spinous process
18. articular pillar
19. anterior tubercle of transverse process
20. neural sulcus
21. posterior tubercle of transverse process
22. superior demifacet for head of rib
23. inferior demifacet for head of rib
24. odontoid process
25. articular facet for anterior arch of atlas

Figure 2–2 continued on opposite page.

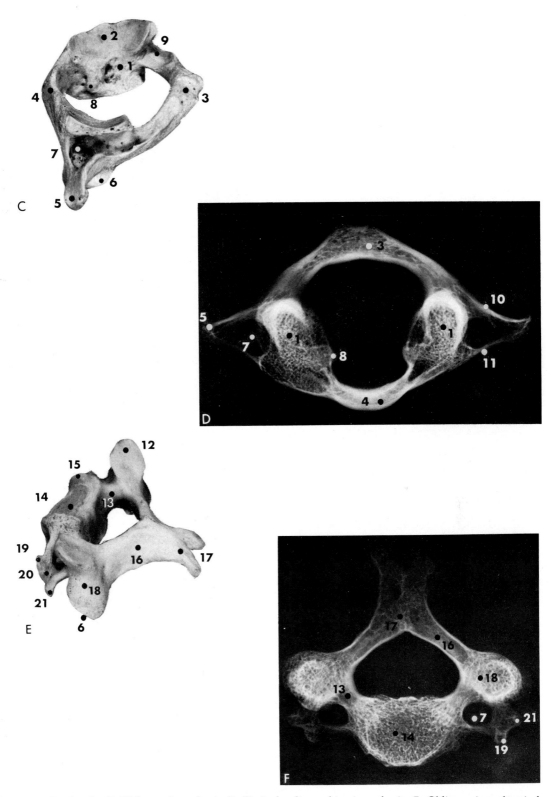

Figure 2–2 *Continued.* C, Oblique view of axis. D, Vertical radiographic view of axis. E, Oblique view of typical (4th) cervical vertebra. F, Vertical radiographic view of typical cervical vertebrae.

Figure 2–2 continued on following page.

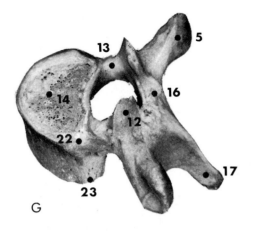

G

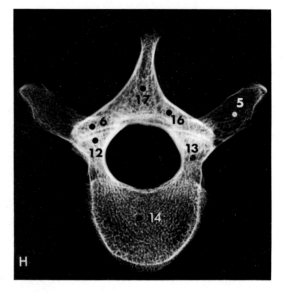

H

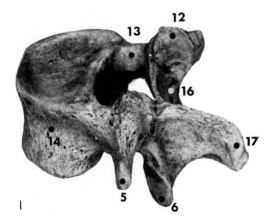

I

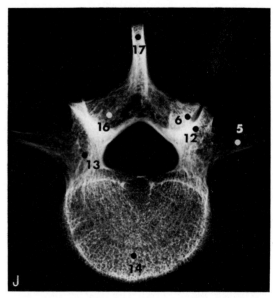

J

Figure 2–2 *Continued.* *G,* Oblique view of typical (5th) thoracic vertebra. *H,* Vertical radiographic view of thoracic vertebra. Note that the plane of the articular facets would readily permit rotation. *I,* Oblique view of typical (3rd) lumbar vertebra. *J,* Vertical radiographic view of lumbar vertebra. Note that the plane of the articular facets is situated to lock the lumbar vertebrae against rotation.

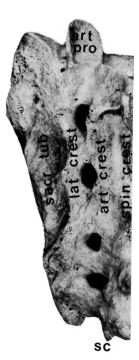
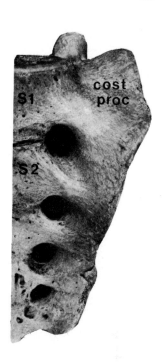

SC

Figure 2–3. Composite anterior-posterior view of the sacrum. The roughened crests on the dorsum (left side of illustration) indicate longitudinal fusions of vertebral arch structures. Note that the articular process is directed backward to buttress the vertebral arch of the 5th lumbar vertebra.

muscles. A deep groove between the upper aspects of the tubercles transmits the cervical spinal nerves.

Both the superior and inferior articular processes appear as obliquely sectioned surfaces of short cylinders of bone which, when united with the adjacent vertebrae, form two osseous shafts posterolateral to that of the stacked vertebral bodies. Thus, the cervical vertebrae present a tripod of flexible columns for the support of the head.

The laminae are narrow and have a thinner superior edge, and at their mid-dorsal junction, they bear a bifid spinous process that receives the insertions of the semispinalis cervicis muscles.

THE ATLANTOAXIAL COMPLEX

The first two cervical vertebrae are structurally and developmentally peculiar. Together they form a complex articular system that permits both the nutational and rotational movements of the head. The first cervical vertebra, or atlas, is a bony ring consisting of an anterior and a posterior arch, which are connected by the two lateral masses. Close inspection, however, reveals that it has all the homologous features of a typical vertebra with the exception of the body. The lateral masses correspond to the combined pedicles and ar-

ticular pillars of the lower cervical vertebrae, but both the superior and inferior articular facets are concave. The superior articular surfaces face upward and internally to receive the occipital condyles of the skull whereas the inferior articulating surfaces face downward and internally to rotate on the sloped "shoulders" of the axis.

The posterior arch consists of modified laminae that are more round than flat in their sectional aspect, and a posterior tubercle that represents an attenuated spinous process and gives origin to suboccipital muscles. Immediately behind the lateral masses on the superior surface of the posterior arch, two smooth grooves serve to pass the vertebral arteries as they penetrate the posterior atlanto-occipital membrane. These arteries take a tortuous course from the transverse processes of the atlas. The anterior arch, which is of uncertain homology, forms a short bridge between the anterior aspects of the lateral masses and bears an anterior tubercle that is the site of insertion of the longus colli muscle. On the posterior surface of the anterior arch, a semicircular depression marks the synovial articulation of the odontoid process; and internal tubercles on the adjacent lateral masses show the attachments of the transverse atlantal ligaments that hold the odontoid against this articular area.

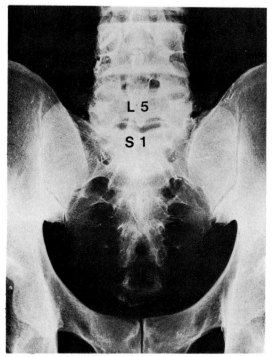

Figure 2–4. Anterior radiographic view of the lumbosacral and sacroiliac articulations. The load transfer from the lumbar spine to the iliac bones via the costal processes of the first and second sacral segments is obvious.

The second cervical vertebra, or axis, provides a bearing surface upon which the atlas may rotate, but its most distinctive characteristic is the vertically projecting odontoid process that serves as a pivotal restraint against horizontal displacements of the atlas. This bony prominence represents the phyletically purloined centrum of the first cervical vertebra. It exhibits a slight constriction at its neck and an anterior facet for its articulation with the anterior arch of the atlas. Posteriorly, a groove in the neck of the odontoid marks the position of the strong transverse atlantal ligament.

The apex of the odontoid process is slightly pointed and is the attachment of the apical ligament. Posterior to the apex, two lateral roughened prominences indicate the attachments of the alar ligaments. These structures and the apical ligament connect the odontoid process to the base of the skull. The superior articulating surfaces of the axis are convex and are directed laterally to receive the direct thrust of the lateral masses of the atlas. The inferior articulating surfaces, however, are typical of those of the cervical verte-

brae and serve as the commencement of the articular columns. The lateral processes of the axis are directed downward, and their posterior or noncostal elements are often quite thin. Anteriorly, the inferior aspect of the body of the axis forms a liplike process that descends over the first intervertebral disc and the body of the third cervical vertebra.

The seventh cervical vertebra is transitional, and the inferior surface of its body is proportionately larger than the superior surface. It bears a long, distinct spinous process that is easily palpable in the living body. The superior and inferior articulating facets are more steeply inclined and presage the form of these structures in the thoracic region. Blunt transverse processes show heavy posterior roots and much lighter anterior roots that

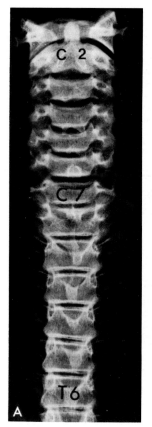
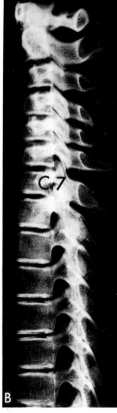

Figure 2–5. *A*, A-P radiograph of dried preparation of cervical and upper thoracic spine. Note the greater relative thickness of the cervical discs and the more lateral disposition of the cervical articular pillars. *B*, Lateral view of preceding specimen. Unfortunately, the normal curvatures did not survive the preparation, but the gradual increase in size of both the bodies and the intervertebral foramina is well illustrated.

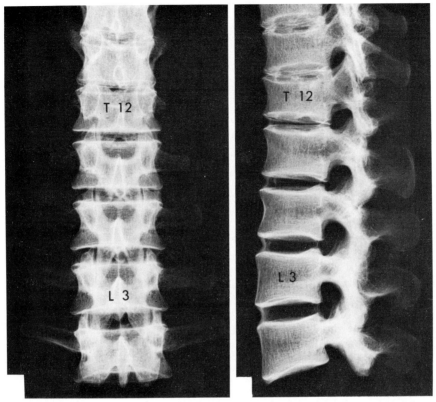

Figure 2–6. A-P and lateral radiographs of lower thoracic–upper lumbar region of articulated dried preparation.

surround transverse foramina that are often bilaterally unequal and seldom pass the vertebral arteries. Not infrequently, one or both of the anterior roots realize their true potential as a costal element and develop into the often troublesome cervical rib.

The Thoracic Vertebrae

All 12 thoracic vertebrae support ribs and thus show facets for the diarthrodial articulations of these structures. The first and last four have specific peculiarities in the manner of costal articulations, but the second through the eighth may be covered by a common description.

The body of a midthoracic vertebra is heart-shaped, and its length and width are roughly halfway between that of the cervical and lumbar centra. Often a flattening of the left side of the body indicates its contact with the descending aorta. In the midthorax, the heads of the ribs form a joint that spans the invertebral disc so that the inferior lip of the

body of one vertebra and the corresponding site of the superior lip of the next inferior element share in the formation of a single articular facet for the costal capitulum. Thus, the typical thoracic vertebra bears two demifacets on each side of its body.

The thoracic vertebral arch encloses a small, round vertebral foramen that will not admit the first joint of the index finger, even when the specimen is derived from a large adult. Because the pedicles arise more superiorly on the dorsum of the body than they do in the cervical region, the inferior vertebral notch forms an even greater contribution to the intervetebral foramen. The superior articular facets form a stout shelflike projection from the junction of the laminae and the pedicles. Their ovoid surfaces are slightly convex and almost vertical in their plane of articulation. They face dorsally and slightly superolaterally, and in bilateral combination present the segment of an arc whose center of radius lies at the anterior edge of the vertebral body. They thus permit a slight rotation around the axis of this radius. The inferior articular facets are borne by the inferior edges of the laminae, and the geometry of their articular surfaces is complementary to that of the superior processes.

On the ventral side of the tip of the strong transverse processes another concave facet receives the tuberculum of the rib whose capitulum articulates with the superior demi-facet of the same vertebra. The spinous processes of the thoracic vertebrae are long and triangular in section. Those of the upper four are more bladelike and are directed backward at an angle of about 40 degrees from the horizontal. The middle four thoracic spines are longer but directed downward at an angle of 60 degrees, so that their spines completely overlap the next lower segment. The four most inferior spines resemble the first four in direction and shape.

The first thoracic vertebra exhibits a complete facet on the side of its body for the capitulum of the first rib and an inferior demi-facet for the capitulum of the second rib. The costal articulations of the ninth to twelfth thoracic vertebrae again tend to confine themselves to the sides of the bodies of their respective segments. On the last two thoracic vertebrae, transitional characteristics are evident in the diminution of the transverse processes and their failure to buttress the last two ribs.

The Lumbar Vertebrae

The lumbar vertebrae are the lowest five of the presacral column. All their features are expressed in more massive proportions, but their essential diagnostic characteristics are negative; that is, they may be easily distinguished from other regional elements by their lack of a transverse foramen or costal articular facets. The body is large, having a width greater than its anteroposterior diameter, and is slightly thicker in front than behind. All structures associated with the vertebral arch are blunt and stout. The thick pedicles are widely placed on the dorsolateral aspects of the centrum, and with their laminae they enclose a triangular vertebral foramen. Although the inferior vertebral notch is deeper than the superior, both make substantial contributions to the intervertebral foramen. The transverse processes are flat and winglike in the upper four lumbar segments, but in the fifth they are presented as thick, rounded stumps. Aside from their relative size, the lumbar vertebrae

may always be recognized by their articular processes. The superior pair arise in the usual manner from the junction of the pedicles and laminae, but their articular facets are concave and directed dorsomedially, so that they almost face each other. The inferior processes are extensions of the laminae that direct the articulating surfaces ventrolaterally and thus lock themselves between the superior facets of the next inferior vertebra in an almost mortise-and-tenon fashion. This arrangement obviously restricts both rotation and flexion in the lumbar region. The lumbar segments also have the most pronounced mammillary processes for the origins and insertions of the thick lower divisions of the epaxial muscles.

The Sacral Vertebrae

The sacrum consists of five fused vertebrae that form a single triangular complex of bone that supports the spine and forms the posterior part of the pelvis. It is markedly curved and tilted backward, so that its first element articulates with the fifth lumbar vertebra at a pronounced angle (the sacrovertebral angle).

Close inspection of both the flat, concave ventral surface and the rough, ridged convex dorsal surface reveals that, despite their fusion, all the homologous elements of typical vertebrae are still evident in the sacrum. The heavy, laterally projecting alae that bear the articular surfaces for articulation with the pelvis are fused anterior costal and posterior transverse processes of the first three sacral vertebrae. These lateral fusions require that separate dorsal and ventral foramina provide egress for the anterior and posterior divisions of the sacral nerves. The ventral four pairs of sacral foramina are larger than their dorsal counterparts as they must pass the thick sacral contributions to the sciatic nerve. Although the ventral surface of the sacrum is relatively smooth, since it must accommodate the birth canal and pelvic viscera, it still displays four transverse ridges that mark the fusions of the vertebral bodies and enclose cryptic remnants of the intervertebral discs. Lateral to the bodies of the second, third, and fourth elements, the ridges of bone that separate the anterior sacral foramina are quite prominent and give origin to the piriformis muscle.

The dorsal aspect of the sacrum is convex, rough, and conspicuously marked by five longitudinal ridges. The central one, the middle sacral crest, is formed by the fusion of the spinous processes of the sacral vertebrae. On either side, a sacral groove separates it from the medial sacral articular crest that represents the fused articular process. The superior ends of these crests, however, form the functional superior articular processes of the first sacral vertebra, which articulate with the inferior processes of the fifth lumbar vertebra. They are very strong, and their facets are directed dorsally to resist the tendency of the fifth lumbar vertebra to be displaced forward at the sacrovertebral angle. Inferiorly, the articular crests terminate as the sacral cornua, two rounded projections that bracket the inferior hiatus where it gives access to the sacral vertebral canal. More laterally, the lateral crests and sacral tuberosities form uneven elevations for the attachments of the dorsal sacroiliac ligaments.

The sacrum and its posterior ligaments lie ventral to the posterior iliac spines and form a deep depression that accommodates and gives origin to the inferior parts of the epaxial muscles that extend the spine. The grooves between the central spinous crest and the articular crests are occupied by the origins of the multifidus muscles, while dorsal and lateral to these are attached the origins of the iliocostal and iliolumbar muscles.

The Coccyx

The coccyx is usually composed of four vertebral rudiments, but situations exhibiting one less or one greater than this number are not uncommon. It is the vestigial representation of the tail or caudal vertebrae of the human.

The first coccygeal segment is larger than the succeeding members and resembles to some extent the inferior sacral element. It has an obvious body that articulates with the homologous component of the inferior sacrum, and it bears two cornua, which may be regarded as vestiges of superior articulating processes. The three inferior coccygeal members are most frequently fused and present a curved profile continuous with that of the sacrum. They incorporate the rudiments of a body and transverse processes but possess no components of the vertebral arch.

The coccyx contributes no supportive function to the spine but serves as an origin for the gluteus maximus posteriorly and muscles of the pelvic diaphragm anteriorly.

ARTHROLOGY OF THE SPINE

The articulations of the spine include the three major types of joints: synarthroses, diarthroses, and amphiarthroses. The synarthroses are found during development and the first decade of life. They are best represented by the neurocentral synchondrosis, a type of nearly immovable joint in which a thin plate of cartilage joins two bones. The neurocentral joints are the two unions between the centers of ossification for the two halves of the vertebral arch and that of the centrum. They are usually obliterated during the second decade. The early unions between the articular processes of the sacral vertebrae also form ephemeral synchondroses.

The diarthroses are the true synovial joints, formed mostly by the articular processes and costovertebral joints, but also include the atlantoaxial and sacroiliac articulations. All of the spinal diarthroses are of the arthrodial or gliding type, with the exception of the trochoidal or pivot joint found in the median atlantoaxial articulation.

The nonsynovial, slightly movable connective tissue joints are of two types: the symphysis, as exemplified by the fibrocartilage of the intervertebral disc, and the syndesmosis, as represented by all the ligamentous connections between both the adjacent bodies and the adjacent arches.

Articulations of the Vertebral Arches

The joints formed by the articular processes of the vertebral arches possess a true joint capsule and are capable of a limited gliding articulation. The capsules are, therefore, thin and lax and are attached to the bases of the engaging superior and inferior articulating processes of opposing vertebrae. Since it is mostly the plane of articulation of these joints that determines the types of motion characteristic of the various regions of the spine, it would be expected that the fibers of the articular capsules would be longest and most loose in the cervical region and become increasingly taut in an inferior progression.

The syndesmoses between the vertebral arches are formed by the paired sets of the ligamenta flava, the intertransverse ligaments, the interspinous ligaments, and the unpaired supraspinous ligament.

The ligamenta flava bridge the spaces between the laminae of adjacent vertebrae from the second cervical to the lumbosacral interval. The lateral extent of each half of a paired set commences around the bases of the articulating processes and can be traced medially where they nearly join at the roots of the spines. This central deficiency serves to transmit small vessels and facilitates the passage of a needle during lumbar punctures. The fibers of the ligamenta flava are almost vertical in their disposition, but they are attached to the ventral surface of the upper lamina and to the superior lip of the next lower one. This shingle-like arrangement conceals the true length of the ligaments because of the overlapping of the superior lamina. Therefore, their morphology is best appreciated from the ventral aspect as in Figure 2–7B. The yellow elastic fibers that give the ligamenta flava their name maintain their elasticity even in embalmed specimens, in which, if a series of three or four laminae and their intervening ligaments are removed intact, they will still stretch and retract to a surprising degree. It has been stated in some texts that the elasticity of the ligamenta flava serves to assist in the maintenance of the erect posture. However, a more probable reason for this property is simply to keep the ligament taut during extension, where any laxity would permit redun-

dancy and infolding toward the ventrally related nervous structures.

The intertransverse ligaments are fibrous connections between the transverse processes. They are difficult to distinguish from extensions of the tendinous insertions of the segmental muscles and, in reality, they may be just that in some regions. Between the cervical transverse processes they appear as a few tough, thin fibers, and in the thoracic area they blend with the intercostal ligaments. Being most distinct between the lumbar transverse processes, they may be isolated here as membranous bands.

The interspinal ligaments (Fig. 2–7A) are membranous sets of fibers that connect adjoining spinous processes. They are situated medial to the thin pairs of interspinal muscles that bridge the apices of the spine. The fibers of the ligaments, however, are arranged obliquely so that they connect the base of the superior spine with the superior ridge and apex of the next next inferior spinous process. When we realize that virtually all somatic segmented structures are bilateral in origin, it is less surprising that these midline ligaments are found in pairs with a distinct dissectible cleft between them.

The supraspinal ligament (Fig. 2–7A) is a

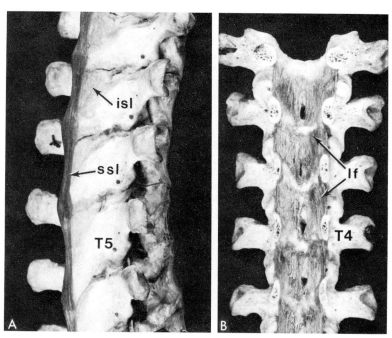

Figure 2–7. *A,* Dried preparation of the thoracic vertebrae showing the supraspinous ligament (SSL) and interspinous ligaments (ISL) *B,* Anterior view of the upper thoracic vertebral arches showing the disposition of the ligamenta flava (LF).

continuous fibrous cord that runs along the apices of the spinous processes from the seventh cervical to the end of the sacral spinous crest. Like the longitudinal ligaments of the vertebra, the more superficial fibers of the ligament extend over several spinal segments, while the deeper, shorter fibers bridge only two or three spines. In the cervical region the supraspinal ligament assumes a distinctive character and a specific name, the ligamentum nuchae. This structure is bowstrung across the cervical lordosis from the external occipital protuberance to the spine of the seventh cervical vertebra. Its anterior border forms a sagittal fibrous sheet that divides the posterior nuchal muscles and attaches to the spinous processes of all cervical vertebrae. The ligamentum nuchae contains an abundance of elastic fibers, and in quadripeds it forms a strong truss that supports the cantilevered position of the head.

SPECIAL ARTICULATIONS

The atlanto-occipital articulation consists of the diarthrosis between the lateral masses of the atlas and the occipital condyles of the skull, and the syndesmoses formed by the atlanto-occipital membranes. The articular capsules around the condyles are thin and loose and permit a gliding motion between the condylar convexity and the concavity of the lateral masses. The capsules blend laterally with ligaments that connect the transverse processes of the atlas with the jugular processes of the skull. Although the lateral ligaments and the capsules are sufficiently lax to permit nodding, they require that the atlas and skull must rotate as a unit.

The anterior atlanto-occipital membrane is a structural extension of the anterior longitudinal ligament that connects the forward rim of the foramen magnum to the anterior arch of the atlas and blends with the joint capsules laterally. It is dense, tough, and virtually cord-like in its central portion.

The posterior atlanto-occipital membrane is homologous to the ligamenta flava and unites the posterior arch of the atlas. It is deficient laterally where it arches over the groove on the superior surface of the arch. Through this aperture, the vertebral artery enters the neural canal to penetrate the dura. Occasionally the free edge of this membrane is ossified to form a true bony foramen around the artery.

The median atlantoaxial articulation is a

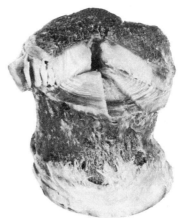

Figure 2–8. Photograph of a dissected third lumbar disc. Note that lamellar bands are still visible when the section is cut deep into bony apophyseal ring. A layer of spongiosa was left attached to the superior surface of the disc to show that only a thin chondral plate intervenes between the vascular trabeculae and the disc. The inward buckling of the lamellae near the cavity of the extirpated nuclear material is well shown (male specimen, 52 years old).

pivot (trochoidal) joint with an intriguing developmental and evolutionary history (Figs. 2–9 and 2–10). The essential features of the articulation are the odontoid process (dens) of the axis and the internal surface of the anterior arch of the atlas. The opposition of the two bones is maintained by the thick straplike

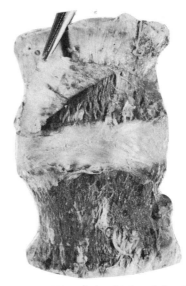

Figure 2–9. Bodies of the third and fourth lumbar vertebrae from a 58 year old male. The spiral course of fibers of the outer lamellae is evident. The periosteal attachment of the reflected anterior longitudinal ligament is well shown, in addition to the delineation of the loosely attached area raised from the surface of the disc.

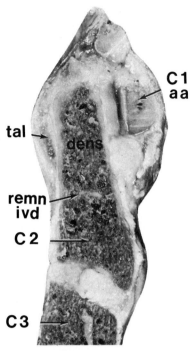

Figure 2–10. Sagittal section through adult odontoid process showing articular relationships with the anterior arch of the atlas (aa) and transverse atlantal ligament (tal). Despite the fact this patient was over 50 years old, a cartilaginous remnant of the homologue of an intervertebral disc may be discerned. Radiologically this might be confused with fracture or a non-union status.

transverse atlantal ligament. Both the ligament and the arch of the atlas have true synovial cavities intervening between them and the odontoid process. Alar expansions of the transverse ligament attach to tubercles on the lateral rims of the foramen magnum, and a single, unpaired cord, the apical odontoid ligament, attaches the apex of the process to the anterior rim of the foramen. The entire joint is covered posteriorly by a cranial extension of the posterior longitudinal ligament that takes the name membrana tectoria in this region. Since the atlas freely glides over the superior articulating facets of C2, the atlanotoaxial pivot is essential for preventing horizontal displacements between C1 and C2. Thus, fracture of the odontoid or, less likely, rupture of the transverse ligament, will produce a very unstable craniospinal articulation.

Articulations of the Vertebral Bodies

The vertebral bodies are connected by the two forms of amphiarthroses. Symphyses are represented by the intervertebral discs, and syndesmoses are formed by the anterior and posterior longitudinal ligaments.

THE INTERVERTEBRAL DISC

The intervertebral disc is the fibrocartilaginous complex that forms the articulation between the bodies of the vertebrae. Although it provides a very strong union ensuring the degree of intervertebral fixation that is necessary for effective action and the protective alignment of the neural canal, the summation of the limited movements allowed by each disc imparts to the spinal column as a whole its characteristic universal motion. The discs of the various spinal regions may differ considerably in size and in some detail, but they are basically identical in their structural organization. Each consists of two components — the internal semifluid mass, the nucleus pulposus, and its laminar fibrous container, the anulus fibrosus.

THE NUCLEUS PULPOSUS. Typically, the nucleus pulposus occupies an eccentric position within the confines of the anulus, usually being closer to the posterior margin of the disc. Its most essential character becomes obvious in either transverse or sagittal preparations of the disc where, as evidence of internal pressure, it bulges beyond the plane of section. Palpation of a dissected nucleus of a young adult shows that it responds as a viscid fluid under applied pressure, but it also exhibits considerable elastic rebound and assumes its original physical state upon release. It is somewhat surprising to find that these properties may still be demonstrated in the spine of a cadaver that has been embalmed for many months.

Histologic analysis provides a partial explanation for the characteristics of the nucleus. As the definitive remnant of the embryonic notochordal tissue, it is similarly composed of loose delicate fibrous strands embedded in a gelatinous matrix. In the center of the mass these fibers show no geometric preference in their arrangement but form a felted mesh of undulating bundles. Only those fibers that are in approximation to the vertebral chondral plates display a definite orientation. These approach the cartilage at an angle, and become embedded in its substance to afford an attachment for the nucleus. A considerable number of cells are suspended in the fibrous network. Many of these are fusiform and resemble typical reticulocytes, but vacuolar and darkly nucleated chondrocytes are also interspersed in matrix. Even in the absence of vascular elements the profusion of cells should accentuate the fact that the nucleus pulposus is composed of vital tissue.

There is no definite structural interface between the nucleus and the anulus. Rather, the composition of the two tissues blends imperceptibly, a fact that frustrates any attempt to cleanly extirpate the entire nucleus in a fresh dissection.

THE ANULUS FIBROSUS. The anulus is a concentric series of fibrous lamellae that encase the nucleus and strongly unite the vertebral bodies. Whereas the essential function of the nucleus is to resist and redistribute compressive forces within the spine, one of the major functions of the anulus is to withstand tension, whether the tensile forces be from the horizontal extensions of the compressed nucleus, from the torsional stress of the column, or from the separation of the vertebral bodies on the convex side of a spinal flexure. Without optical aid, simple dissection and discernment will reveal how well the anulus is constructed for the performance of this service. On horizontal section it is noted that an individual lamella encircling the disc is composed of glistening fibers that run an oblique or spiral course in relation to the axis of the vertebral column. Since the disc presents a kidney- or heart-shaped horizontal section, and the nucleus is displaced posteriorly, these lamellae are thinner and more closely packed between the nucleus and the dorsal aspect of the disc. The bands are stoutest and individually more distinct in the anterior third of the disc, and here when transected they may give the impression that they are of varying composition, because every other ring presents a difference in color and elevation with reference to the plane of section. However, teasing and inspection at an oblique angle will show in the freed lamellae that this difference is due to an abrupt change in the direction of the fibers of adjacent rings. Previous descriptions of the anulus have claimed that the alternating appearance of the banding is the result of the interposition of a chondrous layer between each fibrous ring.[2] Contrarily, our personal observations have shown that the alternations of glistening white lamellae with translucent rings result from differences in the incidence of light with regard to the direction of the fiber bundles. This repeated reversal of fiber arrangement within the anulus has obvious implications in the biomechanics of the disc that will be discussed later.

The disposition of the lamellae on sagittal section is not consistently vertical. In the regions of the anulus approximating the nucleus pulposus, the first distinct bands curve inward, with their convexity facing the nuclear substance. As one follows the successive layers outward, a true vertical profile is assumed, but as the external laminae of the disc are approached, they may again become bowed, with their convexity facing the periphery of the disc.

The attachment of the anulus to its respective vertebral bodies deserves particular mention. This is best understood when a dried preparation of a thoracic or lumbar vertebra is examined first. In the adult the articular surface of the body presents two aspects — a concave central depression that is quite porous and an elevated ring of compact bone that appears to be rolled over the edge of the vertebral body. Often a demarcating fissure falsely suggests that the ring is a true epiphysis of the body, but postnatal studies of ossification have indicated that it is a traction apophysis for the attachment of the anulus and associated longitudinal ligaments.[4]

In life the depth of the central concavity is filled to the level of the marginal ring by the presence of a cribriform cartilaginous plate. Unlike other articular surfaces, there is no closing plate of compact osseous material intervening between this cartilage and the cancellous medullary part of the bone, but the trabeculations of the spongiosa blend into the

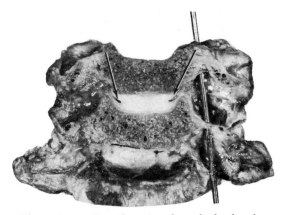

Figure 2–11. Frontal section through the fourth to fifth cervical vertebrae showing a typical cervical disc and its joints of Luschka (arrows). A probe has been passed through the vertebral arterial canal to show its relations to the uncovertebral joints.

internal face of the chondrous plate, while fibers from the nucleus and inner lamellae of the anulus penetrate its outer surface. As intimate as this union between the central disc and vertebra may appear, it is the outer bony ring that affords the disc its firmest attachment, for the stoutest external lamellar bands of fibers actually penetrate the ring as Sharpey's fibers, and scraping the disc right down to the bone will show the concentric arrangements reflecting the different angles at which the fibers insert (Fig. 2–12). The fibers of the outermost ring of the anulus have the most extensive range of attachment, for they extend beyond the confines of the disc and blend with the vertebral periosteum and the longitudinal ligaments.

REGIONAL VARIATIONS OF THE DISC. The discs in aggregate make up approximately one fourth of the length of the spinal column exclusive of the sacrum and coccyx, but their degree of contribution is not uniform in the various regions. According to Aeby,[1] the discs provide more than one fifth of the length of the cervical spine, approximately one fifth

of the length of the thoracic column, and approximately one third of the length of the lumbar region.

The discs are smallest in the cervical spine, and their lateral extent is less than that of the corresponding vertebral body because of the uncinate processes. Here, as in the lumbar region, they are wedge-shaped, the greatest width being anterior. The thoracic discs are somewhat heart-shaped on section, the nucleus pulposus being more centrally located than in the lumbar region. Both the thickness and the horizontal dimensions of the thoracic disc increase caudally with the corresponding increase in size of the vertebral bodies. The normal thoracic kyphosis results from a disparity between the anterior and posterior heights of the vertebral bodies as the discs are of uniform thickness. The lumbar discs are reniform and are both relatively and absolutely the thickest in the spine. The progressive caudal increase in the degree of the lumbar lordosis is due to the equivalent increase in a differential between the anterior and posterior thickness of the disc, a situation that makes the disc of the lumbosacral union the most wedge-shaped.

ANTERIOR LONGITUDINAL LIGAMENT

The anterior longitudinal ligament is a strong band of fibers that extends along the ventral surface of the spine from the skull to the sacrum. It is narrowest and cordlike in the upper cervical region, where it is attached to the atlas and axis and their intervening capsular membranes, but it expands in width as it descends the column to the extent, in the lower lumbar region, of covering most of the anterolateral surfaces of the vertebral bodies and discs before it blends into the presacral fibers. The anterior longitudinal ligament is not uniform in its composition or manner of attachment. Its deepest fibers, which span only one intervertebral articulation, are covered by an intermediate layer that unites two or three vertebrae and a superficial stratum that may connect four or five articular units. Where the ligament is adherent to the anterior surface of the vertebra, it also forms its periosteum, but it is most firmly attached to the articular lip at the end of each body. It is most readily elevated at the point of its passage over the midsection of the discs, where it is loosely attached to the connective tissue band that encircles the anulus (Fig. 2–8).

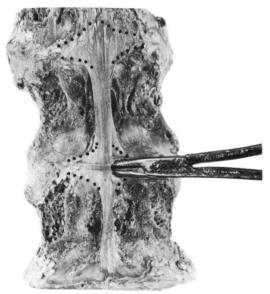

Figure 2–12. Photographic illustration of the posterior longitudinal ligament traversing the bodies of the 3rd and 4th lumbar vertebrae. The central strap of long fibers can be seen passing over the hemostat. The lines of strong attachment of the fibers of the lateral expansions are indicated by the black dots as they outline the rhomboid area, where the fibers are readily dissected from the dorsal surface of the disc. In this case the instrument was inserted into an actual fascial cleft, and the points show the weakest area of the lateral expansion.

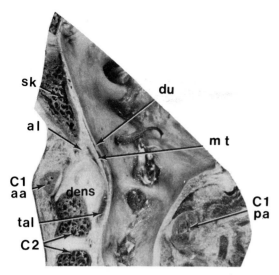

Figure 2–13. Sagittal section through the atlantoaxial articulation of a 4 year old. Note that the major ossific centers of the odontoid process are still separated from the body of C2 by a well differentiated disc. The cartilaginous apex of the process shows a condensation marking the apical ossific center. C1aa and C1pa mark the anterior and posterior atlantal arches. The dura (du) overlies the membrana tectoria (mt), a superior extension of the posterior longitudinal ligament. The transverse atlantal ligament (tal) and apical ligament are also indicated.

THE POSTERIOR LONGITUDINAL LIGAMENT

The posterior longitudinal ligament differs considerably from its anterior counterpart with respect to the clinical significance of its relations to the intervertebral disc. Like the anterior ligament, it extends from the skull to the sacrum, but being within the vertebral canal its central fiber bundles must diminish in breadth as the size of the spinal column increases. The segmental denticulate configuration of the posterior longitudinal ligament is one of its most characteristic features. Between the pedicles, particularly in the lower thoracic and lumbar regions, it forms a thick band of connective tissue that is not adherent to the posterior surface of the vertebral body. Instead, it is bowstrung across the concavity of the dorsum of the body and permits the large vascular elements to enter and leave the medullary sinus located beneath its fibers.

In approximating the dorsum of the disc, the posterior longitudinal ligament displays two strata of fibers. The superficial, longer strands form a distinct strong strap whose filaments bridge several vertebral elements. A second, deeper stratum spans but two vertebral articulations and forms lateral curving extensions of fibers that pass along the dorsum of the disc and out through the intervertebral foramen. It is these deeper intervertebral expansions of the ligament that have the most significant relationship with the disc.

We have found that these fibers are most firmly fixed at the margins of their lateral expansions. This produces a central rhomboidal area of loose attachment or in some cases an actual fascial cleft of equivalent dimensions on the dorsum of the disc. At dissection this characteristic may be readily demonstrated by inserting a blunt probe beneath the intervertebral part of the longitudinal ligament and exploring the area to define the margins of the space where the fibers are strongly inserted (Fig. 2–12). This situation is particularly pertinent to problems involving dorsal or dorsolateral prolapse of the nucleus pulposus. With a dorsocentral protrusion of a semifluid mass, the strong midline strap of posterior longitudinal fibers tends to restrain the herniation. However, if an easily dissectible cleft offers a space for lateral expansion, the mass then extends to either side, dissecting the loose attachment with interruption of numerous nerve fibers. The thinnest part of the lateral expansion of the posterior longitudinal ligament occurs at the convergence of its lines of attachment, and here it is most likely to permit a more dorsal protrusion from internal pressures.

Trabeculations of connective tissue bind the dura to the dorsal surface of the posterior longitudinal ligament, this attachment being the firmest along the lateral edges of the long superficial strap of fibers. Numerous venous cross connections of the epidural sinuses pass between the dura and the ligament, accounting for the fact that venous elements are the most ubiquitous structures among the components related to the vertebral articulations.

Relations of the Roots of the Spinal Nerves

The dorsal and ventral nerve roots pass through the subarachnoid space and converge to form the spinal nerve at approximately the level of its respective intervertebral foramen. Owing to the ascensus spinalis — the apparent developmental rise of the spinal cord resulting from the delayed caudal differential growth of the lower parts of the vertebral column — the course of the nerve roots becomes longer and more obliquely directed as

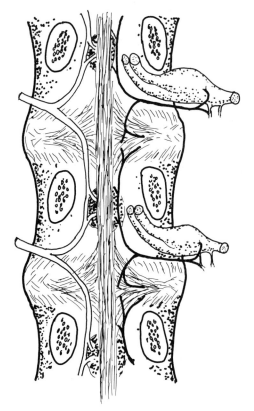

Figure 2–14. Schema of the distribution of the major channels of the branches of the spinal arteries to intravertebral elements (left) and the ramifications of the vertebral branches of the sinuvertebral nerve (right).

one approaches the lower segments. Therefore, in the cervical region the nerve root and the spinal nerve are both posteriorly related to the same corresponding intervertebral disc, but because of the peculiarity of cervical nerve nomenclature, the nerve designation is one number greater than that of the disc. In the lumbar region, however, a different situation prevails. The nerve roots contributing to the cauda equina travel an almost vertical course over the dorsum of one intervertebral disc to exit with the spinal nerve of the foramen one segment lower. Thus, in both the cervical and lumbar regions, dorsal protrusions of disc material affect the nerve root that is numerically designated one number greater than that of the offending disc, but not for a consistent anatomic reason.

Once the meningeal coverings blend with the epineurium, the nerve components become extrathecal. The actual point of this transition is variable, but it usually occurs in relation to the distal aspect of the dorsal root ganglion.

The Intervertebral Foramen

The intervertebral foramen is the aperture that gives exit to the segmental spinal nerves and entrance to the vessels and nerve branches that supply the bone and soft tissues of the vertebral canal. It is superiorly and inferiorly bounded by the respective pedicles of the adjacent vertebrae, but its ventral and dorsal relations involve the two major intervertebral articulations. The dorsum of the intervertebral disc, covered by the lateral expansion of the posterior longitudinal ligament, provides a large part of its ventral boundary, while the joint capsule of the articular facets and the ligamentum flavum contribute the major parts of its dorsal limitation. For obvious reasons the caliber of the foraminal open-

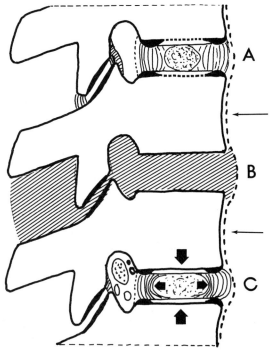

Figure 2–15. Schematic representation showing three aspects of the relational anatomy of the disc. *A* shows the topographic arrangement of the normal disc with the apophyseal ring and perforated chondral plate in relation to the nucleus pulposus and the anulus. *B* indicates, in the cross-hatched area, the inclusions of the motor segment as originally described by Junghanns. The arrows define the limits of the motor segment proposed here as they include the entire developmental somite. *C* indicates the dissipation by the lateral thrust in a compressed disc. The related anatomy of the intervertebral foramen is also indicated. The two structures passing ventral to the spinal nerve are the sinuvertebral nerve and the artery. The other vessels are veins.

ing is larger than the collective size of the structures that pass through it. The remaining space is then obturated by loose areolar tissue and fat to accommodate the slight relative motions of these components (Fig. 2–15).

However ample the overall dimensions of the intervertebral foramen may be, it is its elliptical nature that is responsible for many of its relational problems. In the lumbar region the vertical diameter of the foramen varies from 12 to 19 mm. This undoubtedly accounts for the fact that a complete collapse of the disc may produce little or no evidence of nerve compression. However, the transverse diameter, from the ligamentum flavum to the vertebral body and disc, may be as little as 7 mm. Since the diameter of the fourth lumbar nerve can be just slightly less than 7 mm., the tolerance for pathologic alteration of the bony or connective tissue relations is very restricted.[17]

The existence of any additional ligamentous elements in relation to the intervertebral foramen could be critical. Unfortunately, such structures, known as the transforaminal ligaments, are frequently found in the lumbar region.[13] The transforaminal ligaments are strong, unyielding cords of collagenous tissue that pass anteriorly from various parts of the neural arch to the body of the same or the adjacent vertebra and may be as much as 5 mm. wide.

INNERVATION OF THE SPINE

The sinuvertebral nerve, a recurrent branch of each spinal nerve, is reflected back through the intervertebral foramen to supply fibers to the articular connective tissue, periosteum, meninges, and vascular structures associated with the vertebral canal. The nerve originates just distal to the dorsal root ganglion, where its frequent union with a branch from the ramus communicans reveals its dual spinal and autonomic composition. Occasionally, these two components remain distinct when they enter the foramen, but usually they are reflected as a common bundle that may be 0.5 to 1 mm. thick in the lumbar region (Fig. 2–14).[32]

The sinuvertebral nerve passes through the superior part of the intervertebral foramen, usually between the dorsolateral surface of the vertebral body and its respective spinal nerve roots. Curving upward around the base of the pedicle, it divides into a superior and an inferior branch on approaching the posterior longitudinal ligament. Throughout the course of the nerve and its more conspicuous subdivisions, numerous filaments are distributed to the periosteum, the posterior longitudinal ligament, the dura, and the epidural vessels. Although Roofe[26] maintained that the sinuvertebral nerve coursed only downward along the posterior longitudinal ligament to innervate the disc two vertebrae below the level of origin, a pattern of branching that roughly corresponds with the arterial distribution is more generally reported. The attempt to reconcile the observed extent of the nerve ramifications with clinical and experimental findings has generated speculation concerning the degree of mutual innervation between the areas covered by the segmental nerves. Pedersen and associates[23] traced sinuvertebral fibers in sections of fetal spinal columns and concluded that the branches from each level "anastomose" with those of the adjacent segments. This supports Wiberg's observation that the disc corresponding to an anesthetized spinal nerve may still elicit pain when palpated.[32] Since an overlap in the levels of the sinuvertebral nerve ramifications is certainly consistent with the mutual overlapping of segmental sensory nerve distribution in other areas of the body, it is quite probable that discogenic pain from a single level may involve more than one recurrent branch of the spinal nerves.

Sensory innervation of the more dorsal intervertebral articulations is derived from the posterior ramus of the spinal nerves. This branch supplies filaments to the articular capsules of the facets and to the ligamentum flavum and interspinous ligaments.

For the regional relations of the ultimate terminations of the sinuvertebral nerves, an analysis of the histologic evidence is required. Free nerve endings and complex unencapsulated terminations are demonstrable in the posterior and anterior longitudinal ligaments and in the periosteum of the vertebra.[14] Small encapsulated endings have also been found in the synovial capsules encasing the articular facets. Correlation of the origin of pain with the gross and microscopic distribution of nerve fibers requires some unsubstantiated speculation. The sensory modality mediated by a given type of nerve ending must here be deduced from conclusions about the function of similar endings in other areas of the body. The types of receptors in which myelinated nerves form highly coiled terminations entwined around and within a dense matrix most likely transform a mechanical deformation into a nerve impulse. It is not surprising then that this type of nerve ending is common in the longitudinal ligaments that span the slightly mobile amphiarthrosis of the disc. The function of tension reception would be particularly appropriate to the posterior longitudinal ligament, with its two strata of fibers. The shorter, deeper fibers would be stretched by changes in width or by torsion of the disc, whereas the longer, superficial strap of fibers would be more sensitive to the relative motion of several vertebrae.

It is unlikely that the myelinated fibers associated with these complex nerve endings are involved with any conscious sensations, but in accordance with Hilton's law they are the proprioceptive fibers providing sensory feedback to the given nerve level whose motor fibers move that specific joint. When one considers the precision with which the cerebellum must constantly monitor the position and motion of the spine, particularly with regard to the complex antigravity system required by an erect posture, the significance of these components of the sinuvertebral nerve may be appreciated.

It is in the arborizations of the numerous fine free fibers that the pain of disc disorders most likely originates, and these fibers are amply distributed in the longitudinal ligaments and the periosteum. They are demonstrable in the thin lateral expansions of the posterior longitudinal ligaments that pass through the intervertebral foramen and blend with the thin connective tissue layer that adheres to the periphery of the disc.

The lack of any nervous elements within the nucleus pulposus and the inner laminae of the anulus is almost universally recognized, but the presence of nerve endings within the outer laminae has been alternately demonstrated and denied by various investigators. The distinction here may be immaterial with regard to the origin of discogenic pain, for mechanical and pathologic distortions of the external lamellae would also produce tensions in the overlying connective tissue, and irritation of sinuvertebral nerve fibers could occur whether they do or do not penetrate the external lamella for a short distance. A particularly obvious instance of nerve irritation may be envisioned when a posterior central prolapse of nuclear material elevates the loosely attached central area of the posterior longitudinal ligament. Then, by a lateral extension of

the substance, the highly innervated lateral attachment of the ligament would be progressively dissected from the anulus.

It was probably in recognition of the fact that the vertebral epidural sinuses receive numerous nerve branches that Luschka named their segmental origins the sinuvertebral nerves. Since these thin-walled venous elements show little or no smooth muscle, the numerous fine free nerve endings, so readily demonstrable in methylene blue treated fresh preparations, can reasonably be regarded as sensory terminations. If, as in other parts of the body, these fibers are responsible for the pain elicited when venous structures are compressed or inflamed, the large venous elements directly related to the posterolateral surface of the disc and found between the posterior longitudinal ligament and the dura might well be an additional source of the pain attending disc disorders.

THE MOTOR SEGMENT

With respect to a single vertebral level, the inclusion of all articular tissue, the overlying spinal muscles, and the segmental contents of the vertebral canal and intervertebral foramen into a single functional and anatomic unit was first suggested by Junghanns.[16, 28] This motor segment unit is a useful concept that stresses the developmental and topographic interdependence between the fibrous structures that surround the intervertebral foramen and the functioning of the structures that pass through it. Although the 23 or 24 individual motor segments must be considered in relation to the spinal column as a whole, no congenital or acquired disorder of a single major component of a unit can exist without affecting first the functions of the other components of the same unit and then the functions of other levels of the spine.

Although Junghanns defined the unit primarily in terms of the movable structures comprising the intervertebral articulations, a logical, if not necessary, extension of the motor segment concept should include some aspect of the vertebral elements. DePalma and Rothman[10] included both adjacent vertebrae in their illustration of the unit, but we believe that the unit concept would be improved by incorporating only the opposing superior and inferior halves of each vertebra. Thus, redundancy is eliminated, and the motor segment would represent an embryonic somite as well as a musculoskeletal complex (Fig. 2–15).

In visualizing the motor segment unit as a musculoskeletal complex surrounding a corresponding level of nervous structures, it must be realized that the intervertebral disc is but one form of the articulations involved. The articular facets form the diarthrodial joints of the arthrodial or gliding type. All other intervertebral articulations are generically amphiarthroses. The interosseous fibrous connections that include the interspinous, intertransverse, costovertebral, and longitudinal ligaments as well as the ligamentum flavum are varieties of syndesmoses. Because of the semiliquid nature of the nucleus pulposus and the vacuities that may be demonstrated in the nucleus of aging specimens, Luschka[18] attempted to classify the intervertebral disc as a diarthrosis in which the vertebral chondral plates were the articular cartilages, the anulus provided the articular capsule, and the fluid and ephemeral spaces within the nucleus corresponded to the synovia and the joint cavity. Although the intervertebral disc forms a joint that should be classified in its own exclusive category because its development, structure, and function are generally different from that of any other joint, it most closely conforms to an amphiarthrosis of the symphysis type.

The cervical intervertebral discs have also been a source of controversy because of the so-called "joints of Luschka" or uncovertebral joints. These articular modifications are found on both sides of the cervical discs as oblique cleftlike cavities between the superior surfaces of the uncinate processes and the corresponding lateral lips of the inferior articular surface of the next superior vertebra. Since they initially appear in the latter part of the first decade and are not universally demonstrable in all cervical spines or even in all subaxial discs of the same cervical spine, we here prefer to call them "accommodative joints" that have developed in response to the shearing stresses of the torsions of cervical mobility (Fig. 2–11).

The Nutrition of the Intervertebral Disc

Most descriptive accounts of the intervertebral disc dismiss the subject of its vascular nutrition with a brief mention of the general agreement that the normal adult disc is avascular. Unfortunately, the demonstrable truth of this statement may give the impression that the substance of the disc is rather inert biologically. Actually, experimental evidence has indicated that the normal disc tissue is quite vital and has a surprisingly high rate of metabolic turnover.[7] Unlike the nonvascular cartilage in the diarthroses, the cellular elements of the disc cannot receive the blood-borne nutrients through the mediation of the synovial fluid but must rely on a diffusional system that provides a metabolic exchange with the vessels that lie within the vertebral bodies. Therefore, the exchange of metabolites between the disc and its nearest vasculature must occur through the perforated cartilaginous plate that intervenes between the disc and the spongiosa. This physiologically precarious arrangement suggests that the vitality of the disc is very dependent upon the condition of the vascularity within the adjacent spongiosa, and any change from the optimal state may be reflected in the marked predisposition to degenerative damage that is characteristic of the aging disc.

Unfortunately, a pattern of distribution of the interosseous vascularity in the adult spongiosa is not apparent, and the direct effects that osteoporosis or trauma might have upon the vascular nutrition of the disc may only be surmised.

BLOOD SUPPLY OF THE VERTEBRAL COLUMN

The descriptions and terminology of the nutritional vessels of the vertebrae vary considerably in the current anatomy texts. Generally, like the reports they are based upon, the texts illustrate and discuss the vascularity of a typical thoracic or lumbar vertebra and show a lack of agreement on such basic issues as whether the vertebral body does (Ferguson[11]) or does not (Willis[33]) receive an anterior supply. In addition, discussions of the vascularization of the atypical (craniocervical, cervical, and sacral) vertebral regions are either superficial or entirely lacking. Therefore, much of the information presented here is the result of a *de novo* investigation by the author and associates, and the terminology ascribed to the vessels is derived from a selection of what appears to be the most descriptive names previously used in other reports and our own contributions. It is hoped that the resulting system of terminology to be both comprehensible and comprehensive.

Shortly after the publication of the first edition of this chapter, Crock and Yoshizawa[9] released a photographically illustrated volume showing many injection preparations of the vertebral column and spinal cord. Owing to the similarity of methods used, the high degree of agreement in their depiction of the vascular patterns should not be unexpected, although the independence of the two investigations understandably produced some disparity in the terminology. A major value of this type of work lies in the fact that the reader may visualize the actual specimens rather than interpretive schematizations.

Despite the fact that regional variations may at first appear to thwart the perception of a common pattern of vertebral vascularization, the homologous origin of all vertebral elements nevertheless provides a certain constancy that may be expressed as follows:

From a segmental artery or its regional equivalent, each vertebra receives several sets of nutritional vessels, which consist of anterior central, posterior central, prelaminar, and postlaminar branches. The first and last of these are derived from vessels external to the vertebral column, whereas the posterior central and prelaminar branches are derived from spinal branches that enter the intervertebral foramina and supply the neural, meningeal, and epidural tissues as well. In the midspinal region the internal arteries (i. e., the posterior central and prelaminar branches) provide the greater part of the blood supply to the body and vertebral arch, but reciprocal arrangements may occur, particularly in the cervical region.

This general pattern of the vasculature is best demonstrated in the area between the second thoracic and fifth lumbar vertebrae, where the segments are associated with paired arteries that arise directly from the aorta (Fig. 2–16). Typically, each segmental artery leaves the posterior surface of the aorta and follows a dorsolateral course around the middle of the vertebral body. Near the transverse processes it divides into a lateral (intercostal or lumbar) and a dorsal branch. The dorsal branch runs lateral to the intervertebral foramen and the articular processes as it continues backward between the transverse processes to eventually reach the spinal muscles. Since the segmental artery is closely applied to the anterolateral surface of the body, its first spinal derivatives are two or more anterior central branches that directly penetrate the cortical bone of the body and that may be traced radiologically into the spongiosa (Figs. 2–19 and 2–20). The same region of the segmental artery also sup-

plies longitudinal arteries to the anterior longitudinal ligament (Fig. 2–24).

After the segmental artery divides into its dorsal and lateral branches, the dorsal component passes lateral to the intervertebral foramen, where it gives off the spinal branch that provides the major vascularity to the bone and contents of the vertebral canal. This branch may enter the foramen as a single vessel, or it may arise from the dorsal segmental branch as a number of independent rami. In either case, it ultimately divides into a triad of posterior central, prelaminar, and intermediate neural branches. The posterior central branch passes over the dorsolateral surface of the intervertebral disc and divides into a caudal and a cranial branch, which supply the two adjacent vertebral bodies. Coursing in the same plane as the posterior longitudinal ligament, these branches vascularize the ligament and the related dura before entering the large concavity in the central dorsal surface of the vertebral body. It is apparent, then, that the dorsum of each vertebral body is supplied by four arteries derived from two intervertebral levels. As these vessels tend to converge toward the dorsal central concavity, where they are cross-connected with their bilateral counterparts, their connections with other vertebral levels give the appearance of a series of rhomboidal anastomotic loops (Fig. 2–23) that illustrate the extent of collateral supply to a single vertebra.

The prelaminar branch of the spinal artery follows the inner surface of the vertebral arch, giving fine penetrating nutrient branches to the laminae and ligamenta flava while also supplying the regional epidural and dorsal tissue.

The neural branches that enter the intervertebral foramen with the above described vessels supply the pia-arachnoid complex and the spinal cord itself. In the fetus and the adult the neural or radicular branches are not segmentally uniform in their size or occurrence. Although all spinal nerves receive fine twigs to their ganglia and roots, the major contributions to the cord are found at irregular intervals. Several larger radicular arteries may be discerned in the cervical and upper thoracic regions, but the largest, the arteria radicularis magna, is an asymmetrical contribution from one of the upper lumbar segmental arteries. It travels obliquely upward with a ventral spinal root to join the anterior spinal artery in the region of the conus medullaris. Radicular contributions to the dorsal spinal plexus may

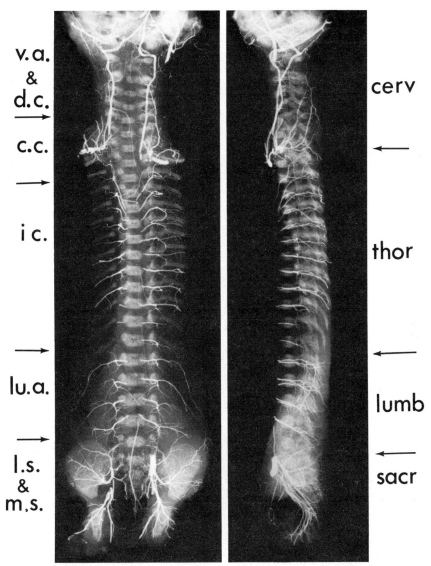

Figure 2–16. A-P and lateral radiography of spine of 8 month fetus injected with finely divided barium sulfate. The traditional regional subdivisions of the spine are indicated on the left, and the regional arteries that provide the segmental branches to the individual vertebrae are indicated on the right. The upper cervical region is supplied by vertebral and deep cervical arteries (v.a. and d.c.). The lower cervical and upper two thoracic segments are supplied by the costocervical trunk (c.c.), while the remaining thoracic vertebrae receive intercostal vessels (i.c.). The lumbar arteries (lu.a.) supply their regional vertebrae, and the sacral segments are provided with branches from lateral sacral (l.s.) and middle sacral (m.s.) arteries.

usually be distinguished by their more tortuous course. Unusual illustrations of the segmental vascularity to the lower spinal cord may be seen in Figures 2–23 and 2–24.

After the dorsal branch of the segmental artery has provided the vessels to the intervertebral foramen, it passes between the transverse processes, where it gives off a fine spray of articular branches to the joint capsule of the articular processes. Immediately distal to this point it divides into dorsal and medial branches; the larger, dorsal branch ramifies in the greater muscle mass of the erector spinae, while the medial branch follows the external contours of the lamina and the spinous process. This postlaminar artery supplies the musculature immediately overlying the lamina and also sends fine nutrient branches into the

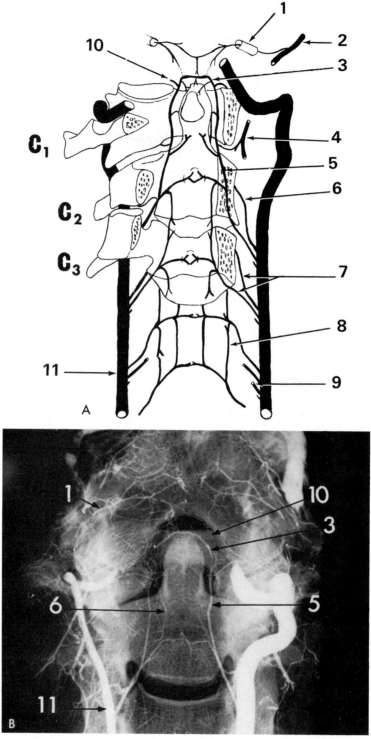

Figure 2–17. *A,* Schema of the arterial supply to the bodies of the upper cervical vertebrae and the odontoid process. Numerical designations apply to the same structures in Figure 2–17*B*. 1, Hypoglossal canal passing meningeal artery. 2, Occipital artery. 3, Apical arcade of odontoid process. 4, Ascending pharyngeal artery giving collateral branch beneath anterior arch of atlas. 5, Posterior ascending artery. 6, Anterior ascending artery. 7, Precentral and postcentral arteries to typical cervical vertebral body. 8, Anterior spinal plexus. 9, Medullary branch of vertebral artery. Radicular, prelaminar, and meningeal branches are also found at each level. 10, Collateral to ascending pharyngeal artery passing rostral to anterior arch of the atlas. 11, Left vertebral artery.

Figure 2–18. Vertical radiograph of section through fourth cervical vertebra of a 6 year old, showing vascularity. The deep cervical artery (dc) provides the posterior laminar branches (plb). The vertebrals show numerous anastomoses with other cervical arteries and send spinal branches (sb) that form posterior central branches (pcb) of the body and anterior lamina branches of the arch. The anterior central branches (acb) may arise independently from the vertebral arteries.

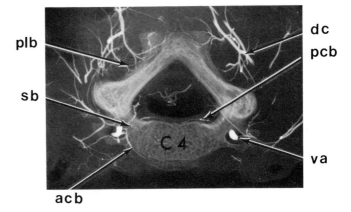

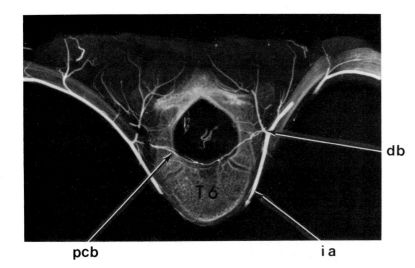

Figure 2–19. Ventral radiograph of a section through T6 of a specimen of a 6 year old injected with barium sulfate. The intercostal arteries (ia) give rise to dorsal branches (db) that provide spinal branches to the vertebral canal and posterior branches to the arch and dorsal musculature. The posterior central branches (pcb) are well shown as they send vessels into the vertebral body. Fine anterior central and anterior laminar and posterior laminar vessels can be seen. Note the neurocentral synchondrosis.

Figure 2–20. Vertical radiograph of section through lumbar vertebra of a 6 year old. The vascuality of the lumbar vertebra may be regarded as the archetypal pattern from which other regions evolved variations. The segmental lumbar artery (la) gives rise to a number of anterior central branches that penetrate the cortical bone of the body. The spinal branch (sb) sends prominent posterior central branches to the dorsum of the body while the dorsal branch (db) supplies both the anterior (alb) and posterior (plb) laminar branches. Neural branches (nb) follow the nerve roots to the cord. In this section the arteria radicularis magna is seen as a neural branch on the right side.

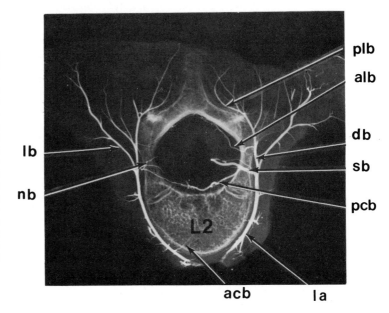

bone. The largest of these branches penetrates the lamina through a nutrient foramen located just dorsomedial to the articular capsule.

Regional Variations in Spinal Vasculature

In an overview of the vascular sources to the spine, it becomes apparent that only those vertebrae related to the aorta have access to direct segmental branches. Thus, the cervical, upper thoracic, and sacral regions have different patterns in their segmental supply that affect to various extents the arrangements of the finer vessels. In the arteriogram of the entire fetal spine (Fig. 2–16) it can be seen that the greater part of the cervical region is supplied by the vertebral arteries and the deep cervical arteries. An intermediate area that usually includes the lower two cervical and upper two thoracic vertebrae is supplied by costocervical branches of the subclavian that are of variable pattern and often bilaterally dissimilar. From T2 to L5 the typical segmental arrangement prevails, but in the sacral area lateral sacral branches of the hypogastric artery and branches of the middle sacral assume the function of supporting the nutritional vasculature to the vertebral elements.

THE CERVICAL REGION

The general pattern of the arterial supply with respect to the typical cervical vertebrae is schematically represented in Fig. 2–17A.[21] Here it can be noted that the vertebral arteries represent a lateral longitudinal fusion of the original segmental vessels and provide a ventrally coursing anterior central artery and a medially directed posterior central artery to each subaxial vertebral element. The anterior spinal plexus is most greatly developed in the cervical region, where it exhibits a rectangular mesh of vessels in which the transverse members (anterior central arteries) run along the upper ventral edges of their respective intervertebral discs. The conspicuousness of this plexus reflects the fact that it also serves the cervical prevertebral musculature. The thyrocervical and costocervical trunks assist in the lower cervical region, and the upper cervical part of the plexus receives contributions from the ascending pharyngeal arteries.

THE ATLANTOAXIAL COMPLEX

With their complex phyletic and developmental history, the components of the atlantoaxial articulation display the most atypical vascular pattern of all the vertebrae. Although the odontoid process represents the definitive

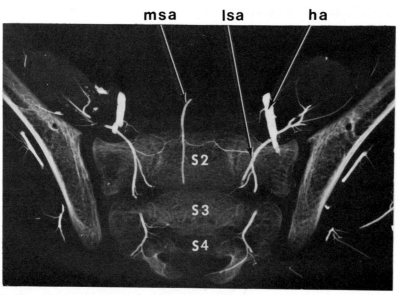

Figure 2–21.   Radiograph of a horizontal section through the sacroiliac joint. The natural curvature of the sacrum provided oblique sections through segments 2, 3, and 4. The hypogastric artery (ha) gives off the lateral sacral artery (lsa) that sends anastomotic branches to join the middle sacral artery (msa); from these the sacral segments receive the penetrating anterior central branches. The dorsal branches pass into the anterior sacral foramina to provide posterior, central, neural and prelaminar branches. The dorsal then leave through the posterior sacral foramina to supply the muscles and posterior laminar branches.

centrum of the first cervical vertebra, it develops and remains as a projecting process of the axis that is almost completely isolated from the rest of the atlas by synovial joint cavities. Its fixed position relative to the rotation of the atlas and the adjacent sections of the vertebral arteries prevents formation of a major vascularization by direct branches at its corresponding segmental level. One might assume that the nutrition of its tissues would easily be accomplished by interosseous vessels derived from the spongiosa within the supporting body of the axis. It is axiomatic, however, that the vascular patterns of bones were developmentally established to supply the original ossification centers within the nonvascular cartilage matrices, and despite the eventual obliteration of the separating cartilage, the original patterns of vascularity generally prevail throughout life. The transient cartilaginous plate, which represents an incipient intervertebral disc between the atlas and axis, does not calcify until the latter half of the first decade

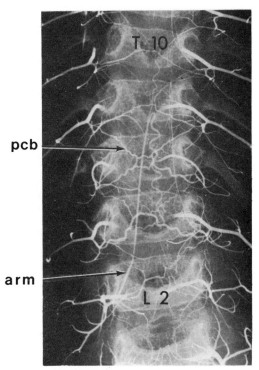

Figure 2–23. A-P arteriogram of the lower thoracic and upper lumbar vertebrae. The interlocking anastomotic pattern formed by the posterior central branches (pcb) and the manner in which four branches converge over the center of the dorsum of the body of each vertebra are well shown. The arteria radicularis magna that forms a major contribution to the anterior spinal artery of the cord can be seen arising at L2. (Six year old child.)

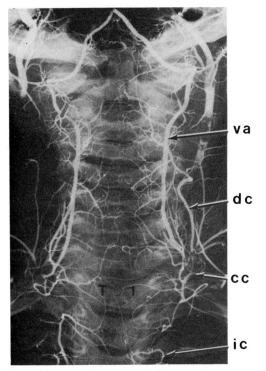

Figure 2–22. Arteriogram of the cervical and upper thoracic regions of the same 6 year old spine seen in Figures 2–18 to 2–20. Note that both the vertebral artery (va) and the deep cervical branch (dc) of the costocervical trunk (cc) supply segmental branches to each vertebra. The costocervical artery also typically supplies T1 and T2, but in this case T2 receives a high intercostal (ic) branch on the left side.

and effectively prevents the development of any significant vascular communication between the axis centrum and the odontoid process. Occasionally noncalcified remnants of this plate may persist in the adult, and although there may be a stable union between the two elements, a radiolucent area may suggest a fracture nonunion or a "false" os odontoideum.

In considering the foregoing facts, it was not unexpected that the investigations of Schiff and Parke[27] revealed that the odontoid process was supplied primarily by pairs of anterior and posterior central branches that coursed upward from the surfaces of the body of the axis and were derived from the vertebral arteries at the level of the foramen of the third cervical nerve. The posterior ascending arteries are the larger members of these two sets of vessels and usually arise independently from the posteromedial sides of their respective vertebral arteries. The individual artery enters the vertebral canal through the foramen

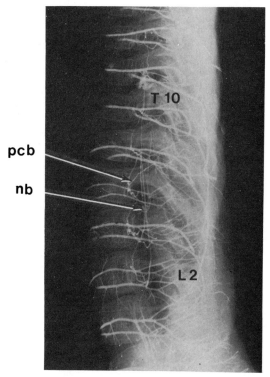

Figure 2–24. Lateral view of preceding illustration. The longitudinal anastomoses of the posterior central branches (pcb) can be appreciated, and the disposition of neural branches (nb) is clarified. The lumbar arteries also supply small longitudinal branches to the anterior longitudinal ligament.

between the second and third vertebrae and trifurcates on the dorsum of the axis body. The typical posterior central perforators are sent medially to pass deep to the posterior longitudinal ligament (called the tectorial membrane in the craniocervical region) to penetrate deep into the spongiosa of the axis, and a small descending branch is sent downward to anastomose with vessels of the next lower segment. The major part of the posterior ascending artery crosses the dorsal surface of the transverse ligament of the atlas about 1.5 mm. lateral to the neck of the odontoid process (Fig. 2–17A and B). Continuing dorsal to the alar ligament, it sends an anterior anastomotic branch over the cranial edge of this ligament to form collateral connections with the anterior ascending artery. The posterior ascending artery then continues on a medial course to meet its opposite counterpart and thus to form the apical arcade that arches over the apex of the odontoid process.

The smaller anterior ascending arteries arise from the anteromedial aspect of the vertebral arteries and pass to the ventral surface of the axis body. Fine medial branches send perforators into the substance of the vertebral body and then meet in a median anastomosis typical of the anterior central branches of the lower cervical region. The rostral continuance of the anterior ascending arteries brings them dorsal to the anterior arch of the atlas. Here each artery sends a number of fine perforators into the anterolateral surfaces of the neck of the odontoid process and terminates in a spray of vessels that supply the synovial capsule of the median atlantoaxial joint.

Fine branches from the anterior and posterior ascending arteries also assist in the nutrition of the syndesmotic relations of the atlantoaxial and craniovertebral articulations, but the main blood supply to the atlanto-occipital joint is provided by a complex of vessels derived from the vertebral and occipital arteries.

In the original observations published by Schiff and Parke,[27] it was noted that collateral vessels passed both over and under the anterior arch of the atlas to anastomose with the apical arcade and ascending arteries, respectively. It was correctly assumed that these were derived from some component of the external carotid system, but since the studies were done with trimmed specimens of the upper cervical spine, they were cautiously referred to as "cleft perforators," implying that they originated anterior to the retropharyngeal cleft. In later observations on injected specimens of the entire neck region of fetuses near term, it was seen that these vessels were actually branches of the ascending pharyngeal artery and that they did not perforate the cleft. Instead, the ascending pharyngeal artery, which has a nearly ubiquitous distribution in the upper pharyngeal region, sends a branch along the inner aspect of the carotid sheath that upon reaching the base of the skull becomes recurrent and descends deep to the prevertebral fascia to supply the upper prevertebral cervical muscles and anastomose with the anterior spinal plexus. These observations also showed that the numerous small bore vessels that descend from the rim of the foramen magnum to anastomose with the apical arcade were not also cleft perforators as originally labeled but were derivatives of a meningeal branch of the occipital artery that enters the skull through the hypoglossal canal (Fig. 2–17A and B). Its descending branches supply not only the periforaminal dura but also the tectorial membrane and alar and apical ligaments and the fine anastomoses to the arcade.

THE SACRUM

As in the cervical region, the segmental vessels to the sacral bone and contents of the vertebral canal (sacral canal) are derived primarily from two longitudinal arteries that course ventrolateral to the vertebral bodies. These lateral sacral arteries may be medial branches of the superior gluteal arteries or, less frequently, they are formed by several more direct branches of the hypogastric arteries (Figs. 2–16, 2–21, and 2–25). As the lateral sacral arteries follow the ventral contour of the sacrum just lateral to the anterior sacral foramina, they send a segmental branch dorsally through each foramen. This foraminal artery corresponds to the dorsal branch of the typical lumbar or intercostal artery, and its first branch runs around the ventral surface of each body segment to supply the penetrating anterior central branches and cross-anastomose with the middle sacral artery and the anterior central branches of the opposite side. The main foraminal branch continues dorsally past the intervetebral foramen, where it provides the typical spinal branches to the sacral canal and then exits through the posterior sacral foramen, to supply the lower back muscles and the equivalent of postlaminar branches to the fused neural arches that cover the sacral canal. Of the spinal branches, the posterior central arteries are the longest and, as in the lumbar and thoracic regions, these anastomose to form an internal set of longitudinal arcades that give penetrating branches to the centrum. The neural branches follow the radicular elements of the cauda equina and, thus, extend up into the lumbar region.

The middle sacral artery contributes to the anterior central branches and to vessels supplying the anterior longitudinal ligaments. This derivative of the aortic bifurcation is the caudal artery of tailed quadrupeds, but it is inconsistant in length and course in the human (compare Figs. 2–16 and 2–25). Of peculiar interest is its association with the glomus coccygeum (Luschka's gland), which lies anterior to the coccyx (Fig. 2–25). Conventionally, the terminations of the middle sacral, lateral sacrals, and other vessels of this region converge on this knot of arteriovenous anastomoses. Particularly in fetal preparations, high pressure injections show that efferent vessels of this glomus form the inferior commencement of the spinal epidural venous plexus.

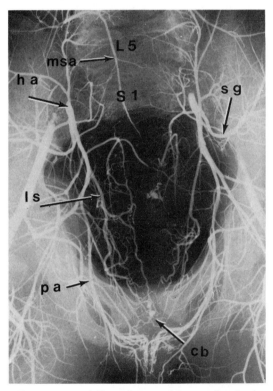

Figure 2–25. A-P arteriogram of the sacral region in a seven year old. The lateral sacral arteries (ls) can be seen coming from the hypogastric vessels (ha). The middle sacral artery (msa) is atypical in this specimen as it stops at S1. Just anterior to the coccyx the coccygeal bodies are indicated as small knots of arteriovenous anastomoses. Pudendal arteries (pa) are well injected.

Venous System of the Vertebral Column

Both an external and an internal plexus of veins are associated with the vertebral column, and the distribution of the two systems roughly coincides with the areas served by the external and internal arterial supplies. Thus, the external venous plexus also consists of an anterior and a posterior set of veins. The small anterior external plexus is coextensive with the anterior central arteries and receives tributaries that perforate the anterior and lateral sides of the vertebral body, while the more extensive posterior external veins drain the regions supplied by posterior (muscular and

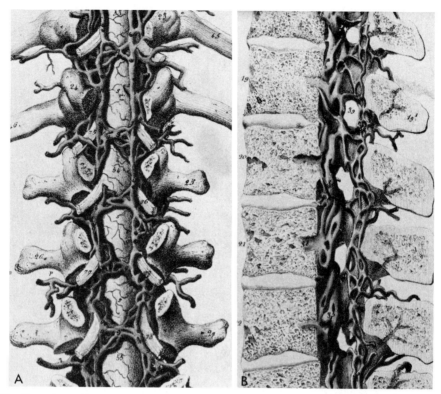

Figure 2–26.   Posterior and lateral illustrations of the spinal epidural venous plexus taken from hand-colored copies of Breschet's original work (*ca.* 1835 — Courtesy Scott Memorial Library, Jefferson Medical College).

postlaminar) branches of the segmental artery. The posterior external veins form what is essentially a paired system, which lies in the two vertebrocostal grooves but which has cross anastomoses between the spinous processes. It is a valveless venous complex that receives the draining segmental tributaries of the internal veins through the intervertebral foramina and communicates ultimately with the lumbar and intercostal tributaries of the caval and azygos system. The posterior external plexus becomes most extensive in the posterior nuchal region, where it receives the intraspinous tributaries via the vertebral veins and drains into the deep cervical and jugular veins.

The internal venous plexus is of more functional and anatomic interest. This plexus is essentially a series of irregular, valveless epidural sinuses that extends from the coccyx to the foramen magnum. Its channels are embedded in the epidural fat and are supported by a network of collagenous fibers, but their walls are so thin that their extent or configuration cannot be discerned by gross dissection. This latter property may account

for the fact that the epidural venous sinuses have been periodically "rediscovered," and it is relatively recently that their functional aspects have been generally appreciated. Although the epidural vertebral veins were known to Vesalius and his contemporaries and were described and beautifully illustrated in the first part of the nineteenth century by Breschet,[6] it has only been within the past several decades that Batson,[3] Clemens,[8] and others have made the functional and pathological significance of these vessels apparent (Figs. 2–26*A* and *B*).

The plexus does not entwine the dura in a completely haphazard fashion but is arranged in a series of cross-connected expansions that produce anterior and posterior ladderlike configurations up the vertebral canal. The main anterior components of the epidural plexus consist of two continuous channels that course along the posterior surface of the vertebral bodies just medial to the pedicles. These channels expand medially to cross-anastomose over the central dorsal area of each vertebral body and are thinnest where they overlie the intervertebral discs. Thus, when injected with a contrast medium, the main channels may appear as a segmental chain of rhomboidal beads. Where the main anterior sinuses cross-connect they receive the large unpaired basivertebral sinus that arises within the dorsal central concavity of the spongiosa and drains the intraosseous labyrinth of sinusoids. Regional visualization of the epidural plexus can be accomplished by introducing a radiopaque medium directly into the spongiosa or the cancellous bone of the spinous process (intraosseous venography). Many drawn cross-sectional illustrations of the vertebral body and its veins show large venous channels passing directly through the spongiosa to connect the basivertebral sinus with veins of the anterior external plexus.

The major external connections of the epidural plexus consist of the veins that pass through the intervertebral foramen and eventually empty into the segmentally available intercostal or lumbar veins. However, since these sinuses are valveless one cannot refer accurately to directions of drainage and flow, for the greatest functional significance of these vessels lies in their ability to pass blood in any direction according to the constantly shifting intra-abdominal and intrathoracic pressures. Breschet[6] surmised that the epidural plexus served as a collateral route for the valveless caval and azygos systems, and this ability has been amply demonstrated by the experimental ligation of either the superior or inferior venae cavae. In addition, the Queckenstedt maneuver, which tests the patency of the spinal subarachnoid space by compressing the jugulars or intra-abdominal veins, causes an increase in the CSF pressure through dural compression from the expansion of the collaterally loaded epideral plexus. The plexus is evidently capable of passing large quantities of blood without developing varices. Clemens claimed this feature to be due to the intricate network of collagenous fibers that supports the thin walls of the sinuses. Also, passive congestion of the spinal cord is prevented by minute valves in the radicular branches draining the spinal cord.[8] This latter fact is anatomically unique since valves exist nowhere else in the venous channels associated with the central nervous system.

An ancillary function of the epidural plexus may be to act in a mechanical capacity as a hydraulic shock absorbing sheath that helps buffer the spinal cord during movements of the vertebral column.

The vertebral sinuses are largest in the suboccipital and upper cervical region. Here they also receive numerous nerve endings from the sinuvertebral nerves, and are associated with glomerular arteriovenous anastomoses, which suggests a possible baroceptive function.[22] The patency of these anastomoses is most easily demonstrated in the fetus, in which arterial injections of a contrast medium may also fill the upper cervical epidural sinuses. Similarly, the coccygeal bodies of the same specimen will pass the arterial injection directly into the epidural veins of the lower sacral region.

The detrimental aspects of the vertebral epidural veins have been well stated by Batson.[3] Retrograde flow from venous connections to the lower pelvic organs provides an obvious route of metastasis for pelvic neoplasms, both to the spine itself and to the regions of the trunk associated with valveless connections to the plexus. Batson claims that direct metastatic transfer can occur between the pelvic organs and the brain via the vertebral epidural route.

BIOMECHANICS OF THE SPINE

The spine is capable of ventroflexion, extension, lateral flexion, and rotation. This remarkable universal mobility may seem at odds with the fact that its most essential function is to provide a firm support for the trunk and appendages. The apparent contradiction may be resolved when one realizes that the total ranges of motion are the result of a summation of limited movements permitted between the individual vertebrae and that the total length of the spine changes very little during its movements. The role of the musculature in the performance of the supportive functions cannot be minimized, as the disastrous scolioses that result from their unilateral loss in a few motor segment units may attest.

Obviously, the degree and combination of the individual types of motion described above vary considerably in the different vertebral regions. Although all subaxial–presacral vertebrae are united in a tripod arrangement consisting of the intervertebral disc and the two zygapophyseal articulations, the relative size and shape of the former and the articular planes of the latter determine the range and types of motion that an individual set of intervetebral articulations will contribute to the total mobility of the spine. In general, flexion is the most pronounced movement of the vertebral column as a whole. It requires an anterior compression of the intervertebral disc and a gliding separation of the articular facets, in which the inferior set of an individual vertebra tends to move upward and forward over the opposing superior set of the adjacent inferior vertebra. The movement is checked mainly by the posterior ligaments and epaxial muscles. Extension tends to be a more limited motion, producing posterior compression of the disc with the inferior articular process gliding posteriorly and downward over the superior set below. It is checked by the anterior longitudinal ligament and all ventral muscles that directly or indirectly flex the spine. Also, the laminae and spinous processes may sharply limit extension. Lateral flexion is accompanied by some degree of rotation. It involves a rocking of the bodies upon their discs, with a sliding separation of the diarthroses on the convex side and an overriding of those related to the concavity. The rotational component brings the anterior surface of the bodies toward the convexity of the flexure and the spinous processes toward its concavity. This phenomenon is well illustrated in a dried preparation of a scoliotic spine.

Lateral flexion is checked by the intertransverse ligaments and the extensions of the ribs or their costal homologues.

Pure rotation is directly proportional to the relative thickness of the intervertebral disc and is mainly limited by the geometry of the planes of the diarthrodial surfaces. The architecture of the disc, while permitting limited rotation between the bodies, also serves to check this movement by its resistance to compression. The consecutive layers of the anulus fibrosus have their fibers arranged in an alternating helical fashion, and rotation in either direction can be accompanied only by increasing the angularity of the opposing fibers to the horizontal, which in turn requires compression of the disc.

The entire vertebral column rotates approximately 90 degrees to either side of the sagittal plane, but most of this traversion is accomplished in the cervical and thoracic sections. It flexes nearly the same amount, using primarily the cervical and thoracic regions. Roughly a total of 90 degrees of extension is permitted by the cervical and lumbar regions, while lateral flexion with rotation is allowed to the extent of 60 degrees to both sides again, primarily by the cervical and lumbar areas.

Specific Regional Considerations

The atlanto-occipital joints mostly permit flexion and extension with a limited lateral action, all being checked by the suboccipital musculature and the atlanto-occipital ligaments. The atlantoaxial articulations allow only rotation, with the pivoted joint being stabilized and checked by the alar ligaments and the ligaments forming the capsules of the atlantoaxial diarthroses.

One half of the rotational mobility of the entire cervical region takes place between the atlas and the axis, and the remainder is distributed among the joints of the subaxial vertebrae. The atlanto-occipital joint also accounts for approximately half of the cervical flexion. However, the remaining 50 per cent is not evenly distributed among the cervical vertebrae but is greater in the upper section.

The subaxial part of the cervical region shows the freest ranges of motion of all the presacral vertebrae. The discs are quite thick in relation to the heights of the vertebral bodies and contribute about one fourth of the height of this part of the column. In addition, a sagittal section shows the middle part of the cervical disc to be lenticular in shape, so that the anteroinferior lips of the bodies are more capable of sliding slightly forward and overriding one another. The range of spinal flexion is greatest in the cervical region, and although the posterior nuchal ligaments and muscles may tend to resist this motion, it is ultimately checked by the chin coming to rest on the chest.

The cervical spine is normally carried in a moderately extended position, and it shows a median variation of 91 degrees between extension and flexion. Extension is checked by the anterior longitudinal ligament and the combined resistances of the anterior cervical musculature, fascia, and visceral structures, all three of which may be traumatized in hyperextension injuries.

Cervical lateral flexion is quite limited by the articular pillars and the intertransverse ligaments, and thus most lateral motion involves considerable rotation. The nearly horizontal position of the planes of the cervical articular facets provides good supportive strength to the articular pillars but increases the lateral rigidity so that hyperextension injuries may be more disastrous if the head is rotated at the time of impact from the rear.

The mobility of the thoracic region is also

not uniform throughout its length. Although the upper segments resemble the cervical vertebrae in respect to the size of the bodies and the discs, the ribs attached to the sternum greatly impair the ranges of motion. The circumferential arc of the plane of the articular facets shows that rotation is the movement least restricted by these structures.

Flexion and extension become freer in the lower thoracic region, where the discs and vertebral bodies progressively increase in size, and the more movable become less restrictive. However, the last few thoracic vertebrae are transitional in respect to the surfaces of the articular facets. These begin to turn more toward the sagittal plane and tend to limit rotation and permit greater extension.

The articulations of the lumbar region permit ventroflexion, lateral flexion, and extension, but the facets of the synovial joints lie in a ventromedial to dorsolateral plane that virtually locks them against rotation. This lumbar non-rotatory rigidity is a feature shared with most mammals and achieves its greatest manifestation in certain quadrupeds in which the inferior articulation fits like a cylindrical tenon into the semicircular mortise of the corresponding superior process of the vertebra below. It thus provides a gliding action that only permits the neural arches to separate or approximate each other during extension and flexion. The morphology of the joints can be well appreciated in an appropriate cut of loin chop or T-bone steak.

The synovial articulations at the lumbosacral junctions are unique. Unlike the more superior lumbar joints, the facets of the inferior articulating processes of the fifth lumbar vertebra face forward and slightly downward, to engage the reciprocally corresponding articular processes of the sacrum. Because of the position of these joint surfaces, a certain amount of rotation should be possible between the fifth lumbar segment and the sacrum, but the presence of the strong iliolumbar ligaments quite likely restricts much motion of this type.

The most essential function of the synovial lumbosacral articulations involves their role as buttresses against the forward and downward displacement of the fifth lumbar vertebra in relation to the sacrum. When one considers that each region of the spine has its own characteristic curvature, the tracing of the vertical line indicating the center of gravity shows that it intersects the column through the bodies of the transitional vertebrae. Therefore, the normal cervical lordosis places most of the cervical vertebrae anterior to the center of gravity, and the compensating thoracic kyphosis places the thoracic vertebrae posterior to the center of gravity. Again, the lumbar lordosis brings the middle lumbar vertebrae anterior to the line. Thus, the transitional vertebrae between each region intersect the center of gravity and appear to be the most unstable regions of the spine. This is emphasized by the fact that disc problems and fractures most frequently occur in the transitional vertebrae.

Because the sacrovertebral angle produces the most abrupt change of direction in the column, and the center of gravity, which passes through the fifth lumbar body, falls anterior to the sacrum, there is a marked tendency for the thick, wedge-shaped fifth lumbar disc to give way to the shearing vector that the lumbosacral angularity produces. The resulting condition, spondylolisthesis, most frequently reveals a deficiency in the laminae (spondylolysis) that fails to anchor the fifth vertebral body to the sacrum and allows its forward displacement. There has been considerable discussion as to whether spondylolysis is congenital or acquired, but the spondylolisthesis seldom occurs without the laminar deficiencies as a preceding condition.

Biomechanics of the Intervertebral Disc

It is axiomatic in mechanical engineering that a well designed machine will automatically reveal its function through the analysis of its structure. There are few instances in biologic circumstances in which this statement is more applicable than in the case of the intervertebral disc. Even when the disc is simply divided with a knife and examined grossly, it is apparent that one is dealing with an organ that is remarkably constructed to simultaneously alleviate shock and yet transmit forces from every conceivable combination of vectors. Moreover, this appreciation of the functional competency of the disc increases as its structure is analyzed at the finer levels of organization.

The internal composition of the disc has evolved to withstand great stresses through the liquid and elastic properties of nucleus and anulus acting in combination. The nucleus is distorted by compression forces, but being liquid in nature it is in itself incompressible. It serves to receive primarily vertical forces from the vertebral bodies and redistribute them radially in a horizontal plane. It is, therefore, the distortion of the anulus by the internal pressure of the nucleus that gives the disc its compressibility, and its resilience makes possible the recovery from pressure.

Were the nucleus pulposus simply a cavity filled with water, it would momentarily act in the same capacity, but the ability to maintain the appropriate quantity of fluid during the continual compression and recovery cycle would be lacking. It is this ability to absorb and retain relatively large amounts of water that is the unique property of the living tissue of the nucleus. It is known that the essential compound involved in this process is a protein-polysaccharide gel, which through a high imbibition pressure will bind nearly nine times its volume of water. It is apparent that the hydrophilia is not a form of biochemical bonding because a quantity of water can be expressed from the nucleus by prolonged mechanical pressure. This accounts for the diurnal decrease in the total length of the spine and its recovery in the supine position at night.

The anulus must receive the ultimate effects of most forces transmitted from one vertebral body to another. Since the major loading of the intervertebral disc is in the form of vertical compression, it may seem paradoxic that the anulus is best constructed to resist tension, but the nucleus transforms the vertical thrust into a radial pressure that is resisted by the tensile properties of the lamellae. Although the basic plan of alternating bands of fibers is one of the obvious sources of the tensile strength of the anulus, this arrangement is not uniform with respect to the directions of the fibers or the degrees of resistance and resilience encountered throughout the anulus. The fibers generally become longer, and the angle of their spiral course becomes more horizontal near the circumference of the disc, for it is here that the shearing stresses of vertebral torsions would be most effective. Experimental analysis has also shown that various parts of the anulus do not respond equally to the same degree of tension, and the discrepancies were related to the plane of section and the location of the sample.[12] The anulus proved to have the greatest resistance and the greatest recovery in horizontal sections of the peripheral lamellae, whereas both vertical and more medial sections were more distensible.

Because the spine acts as a flexible boom to the guy-wire actions of the erector spinae muscles, it is essentially the fulcrum of a lever system of the first class, in which the loading has a considerable mechanical advantage. Pure vector analysis has indicated that a theoretical pressure of approximately three fourths of a ton could be applied to a disc when 100 lb. is lifted by the hands,[5] but this is considerably in excess of the actual pressures achieved. Increased intrathoracic and intra-abdominal pressures alleviate much of the fulcrum compression of the discs by effectively counteracting the load of the anterior lever arm.

The actual pressure variations occurring with postural changes have been recorded by inserting transducers into the third lumbar disc.[20] This procedure indicated that the internal disc pressure increases from approximately 100 kg. in a standing position with the spine erect to 150 kg. when the trunk is bent forward, and to 220 kg. when a 70 kg. man lifts a 50 kg. weight. It was particularly revealing that the pressure showed a considerable increase when the equivalent maneuvers were repeated in a sitting position, and the weight lifting ultimately created a pressure of 300 kg. on the third lumbar disc.

The disc is also "preloaded." The inherent tensions of the intervertebral ligaments and the anulus exert a pressure of about 15 kg., since this weight is required to restore the original thickness of the disc after the ligaments have been divided.[24] From a comparative standpoint this preloading probably offers increased stability to the spine as a functional flexible rod. One is almost induced unconsciously to use teleological thinking in terms of the vertical thrust resistance when regarding the structure of the disc. In perspective, however, the intervertebral disc shows a rather consistent morphology in all mammals, and yet man is the only species that truly stands erect. Although analysis of muscular action would most likely show that all mammalian discs must dissipate and transfer axial thrusts, the preloading would enhance the "beam strength" that is obviously necessary to the vertebral column of quadrupeds.

References

1. Aeby, C.: Die Alterverschiedenheiten der menschlichen Wirbelsaule. Arch. Anat. Physiol. (Anat. Abst.), *10*:77, 1879.

2. Beadle, O. A.: The intervertebral discs. London, Medical Research Council, Special Report No. 160, pp. 6–9, 1931.

3. Batson, O. V.: The function of the vertebral veins and their role in the spread of metastases. Am. Surg. *112*:138–145, 1940.

4. Bick, E. M.: The osteohistology of the normal human vertebra. J. Mt. Sinai Hosp. *19*:490–527, 1952.

5. Bradford, D. L., and Spurling, R. G.: The Intervertebral Disc. Springfield, Illinois, Charles C Thomas, 1945.

6. Breschet, G.: Essai sur les Veines der Rachis. Paris, Mequigon-Morvith, 1819.

7. Brown, M. D.: The pathophysiology of the intervertebral disc: Anatomical, physiological and biomedical considerations. Doctoral thesis, Jefferson Medical College, Philadelphia, 1969.

8. Clemens, H. J.: Die Venesysteme der menschlichen Wirbelsaule, Berlin. Walter de Gruyter, 1961.

9. Crock, H. V., and Yoshizawa, H.: The Blood Supply of the Vertebral Column and Spinal Cord in Man. New York, Springer-Verlag, 1977.

10. DePalma, A. F., and Rothman, R. H.: The Intervertebral Disc. Philadelphia, W. B. Saunders Co., 1970.

11. Ferguson, W. P.: Some observations on the circulation in fetal and infant spines. J. Bone Joint Surg. *32*:640–645, 1950.

12. Galante, J. O.: Tensile properties of the human lumbar annulus fibrosus. Acta. Orthop. Scand. (suppl.), *100*:1–91, 1967.

13. Golub, B. S., and Silverman, B.: Transforaminal ligaments of the lumbar spine. J. Bone Joint Surg., *51A*:947–956, 1969.

14. Hirsch, C.: Studies on mechanism of low back pain. Acta. Orthop. Scand., *22*:184–231, 1953.

15. Jung, A., and Brunschwig, A.: Recherches histologiques sur l'innervation des articulations et des corps vertebreaux. Presse Med. *40*:316–317, 1932.

16. Junghanns, H.: Der Lumboscralwinkel. Deutsch. Z. Chir., *213*:332, 1929.

17. Larmon, A. W.: An anatomic study of the lumbosacral region in relation to low back pain and sciatica. Ann. Surg., *119*:892, 1944.

18. von Luschka, H.: Die Halbgelenke des menschlichen Körpers. Berlin, Karpess, 1858.

19. von Luschka, H.: Die Nerven des menschlichen Wirbelkanales. Tubingen, H. Laupp, 1850.

20. Nachemson, A.: The load on lumbar discs in different positions of the body. Clin. Orthop. *45*:107–122, 1966.

21. Parke, W. W.: The vascular relations of the upper cervical vertebrae. Orthop. Clin. North Am. *9*(4):879–889, 1978.

22. Parke, W. W., and Valsamis, M. P.: The ampulloglomerular organ: An unusual neurovascular complex in the suboccipital region. Anat. Rec. *159*:193–198, 1967.

23. Pedersen, H. E., Blunck, C. F. J., and Gardner, E.: The anatomy of the lumbosacral posterior rami and meningeal branches of spinal nerves (sinu-vertebral nerves). J. Bone Joint Surg. *38A*:377–391, 1956.

24. Petter, C. K.: Methods of measuring the pressure of intervertebral discs. J. Bone Joint Surg. *15*:365, 1933.

25. Puschel, J.: Der Wassergehalt normaler und degenerierter Zwischenwirbelscheiben. Beitr. Path. Anat., *84*:123–130, 1930.

26. Roofe, P. G.: Innervation of anulus fibrosus and posterior longitudinal ligament. Arch. Neuro. Psych. *44*:100–103, 1940.

27. Schiff, D. C. M., and Parke, W. W.: The arterial supply of the odontoid process. Anat. Rec. *172*:399–400, 1972.

28. Schmorl, G., and Junghanns, H.: The Human Spine in Health and Disease. New York, Grune & Stratton, Inc., 1959.

29. Siberstein, C. E.: The evolution of degenerative changes in the cervical spine and an investigation into the "joints of Luschka." Clin. Orthop. *40*:184–204, 1965.

30. Tombol, T.: Über die Ontegenese der vertebralen Blutzirkulation. Verh. Anat. Ges., 7:85–92, 1964.

31. Tsukada, K.: Histologische Studien uber die Zwichenwirbelscheibe des Menschen. Alterveranderungen Akad. Kioto, *25*:1–29, 207–909, 1939.

32. Wiberg, G.: Back pain in relation to nerve supply of intervertebral disc. Acta Orthop. Scand. *19*:211–221, 1949.

33. Willis, T. A.: Nutrient arteries of the vertebral bodies. J. Bone Joint Surg., *31*:538–541, 1949.

The vascular studies presented here were supported by N.I.H. research grant HL-14035.

CHAPTER 3

Differential Diagnosis of Spinal Disorders

RICHARD N. HARNER, M.D.

MICHAEL A. WIENIR, M.D.
University of Pennsylvania

INTRODUCTION

The nervous system and the spine interact in several ways which may produce confusing symptoms or findings when the patient comes for a diagnostic evaluation. These include spinal deformities secondary to neuromuscular disorders, skeletal anomalies associated with anomalies of the central nervous system (usually on a congenital basis), congenital or acquired disorders of the spine which may produce neurological abnormalities, and spinal disorders and primary neurological disorders with similar symptoms.

In the following discussion, there will be no attempt to discuss all spinal disorders or all neurological disorders which may affect the spine. Instead, the orientation will be toward (1) presenting symptoms or symptom complexes, (2) the most frequent types of disorders which may produce such symptoms, and (3) the findings on history, physical examination and special studies, which are important in differential diagnosis. The problems to be considered are listed in Table 3–1.

During the physical examination, one cannot omit the obvious. Most frequently omitted is either an adequate examination of the back or an appropriate examination of the nervous system.

To examine the back, the patient must be undressed completely. The back is inspected in full view, in good light, with the patient in the erect posture, while the examiner is seated. The symmetry of the soft tissues, including the buttocks, is inspected. The spinous processes are located and palpated, and their alignment is determined by making a small mark over each one. The spinal and paraspinal areas are palpated and percussed to determine discrete localization of pain. Mobility of the spine is checked in six directions: flexion, extension, right bending, left bending, left rotation, and right rotation. It is important to note the effect of such movement on any preexisting deformity. Knowledge of the effect of axial traction or axial compression, particularly in the cervical region, can be helpful in determining the presence of radicular components to the pain.

The neurological examination is familiar to most; however, certain points require emphasis, particularly when reflexes, strength, and sensation to pin prick are normal in arms

TABLE 3–1. PRESENTING SYMPTOMS IN
DIFFERENTIAL DIAGNOSIS OF
SPINAL DISORDERS

Spinal deformity
Back pain
Radiating pain or sensory disturbance
Acute paraplegia or quadriplegia
Monoparesis
Impairment of gait
Bladder disturbances

and legs. Check position sense in the toes; check the thoracic and sacral regions for sensory loss; then test bulbocavernosus, anal, and cremasteric reflexes. Straight leg raising and cervical flexion, alone and in combination, are useful in detecting root irritation or meningeal irritation.

As a result of these examinations, accurate localization of the symptoms to bone, paraspinal organs, muscle, nerve roots, spinal cord, or combinations of these structures can usually be made and the search for a specific cause will be facilitated.

SPINAL DEFORMITY

Spinal deformity can result from a variety of causes, congenital and acquired. Those instances in which spinal deformity becomes evident through association with more prominent neurological symptoms are discussed later, in the appropriate section. In the remaining cases, the deformity itself may be a presenting problem, and in these the age of onset can be very helpful in differential diagnosis.

Spinal deformities present in recognizable form *at birth* are almost always manifestations of embryological maldevelopment. Such "dysraphic states" may be secondary to incomplete development of the dorsal aspect, or to the reopening of the previously closed neural tube.[81, 111]

The most frequent clinical presentation at this age is that of *meningomyelocele* with associated hydrocephalus. The characteristic presentation of a bulging, translucent sac in the lumbosacral region, filled with a tangled mass of meninges, nerve roots, and spinal cord, presents little diagnostic difficulty. Enlargement of the head, separation of the cranial sutures, and the characteristic appearance of lückenschädel on the skull roentgenogram are often present. The latter may suggest a poor prognosis.[133]

In the past, recognition of this severe dysraphic syndrome has been associated with an extremely poor prognosis in terms of paraplegia, incontinence, infection, progressive hydrocephalus and death. However, recent experience suggests that closure of the sac within 24 hours to prevent infection, appropriate shunting procedures to relieve hydrocephalus, and an intensive program of rehabilitation can produce functional recovery in some children.[5, 85, 86]

The presence of *hemivertebra* may occasionally be detected at birth or in early infancy when shortening or persistent torsion of the neck or tilting of the head leads to roentgenographic examination of the cervical spine. This anomaly does not produce neurological deficits at birth but can produce acute spinal cord compression in later years.

Throughout the remainder of infancy and up to the age of four years, *idiopathic scoliosis* is by far the most common cause of spinal deformity.[60, 61, 65] At this age, scoliosis is often progressive and is located in the thoracic region and convex to the left. Neurological deficits are rare in these patients, in spite of curvatures that may exceed 70 degrees.

An important cause of scoliosis in early childhood is *intraspinal tumor*. In a series of 115 children, 70 per cent had spinal deformity which included torticollis, scoliosis and kyphosis. In six the initial diagnosis was idiopathic scoliosis. Underlying tumors were often benign and were present at all levels of the spinal cord.[135]

By the time spinal deformity occurs, most intraspinal lesions will also have produced neurological deficit, characterized in the majority by weakness or spasticity of the lower extremities, or both, and variable sensory disturbance which may extend up to the level of the lesion. However, these findings may be mild or they may be difficult to evaluate. In such instances, Pantopaque myelography is essential.[49]

Throughout the remainder of the first and second decades there are four causes of scoliosis that can present diagnostic difficulty: (1) juvenile idiopathic scoliosis; (2) scoliosis associated with spinocerebellar degeneration; (3) scoliosis secondary to an intraspinal lesion; and (4) scoliosis due to peripheral neuromuscular disorders.

JUVENILE IDIOPATHIC SCOLIOSIS. This deformity usually has a right thoracic curvature and occurs more frequently in girls, whereas the infantile variety is more often left thoracic and occurs with equal sex incidence.[100, 101] Neurological examination is normal in almost every case, in spite of severe degrees of curvature. This often provides useful distinction from the remaining categories in which neurological abnormalities can be detected (however, see Gold et al., 1970[49]).

SPINOCEREBELLAR DEGENERATION. Spinocerebellar degeneration, of which the classic example is Friedreich's ataxia, and its related chronic hereditary polyneuropathies are often familial.[35] Mild scoliosis may predate the appearance of impaired coordination and difficulty in walking.[97] The deep tendon reflexes may be normal, increased, decreased or absent. A patient may have an impaired sense of position and vibration in the feet, optic atrophy, pigmentary degeneration of the retina, and myocardial abnormalities (characteristic, inverted T waves). Because the spinal deformity can antedate associated neurological changes, it is best to consider it an associated anomaly rather than one due directly to the neurological involvement itself. In any case, the family history and the details of neurologic examination will distinguish these cases from the larger group of patients with idiopathic scoliosis in almost every instance.

INTRASPINAL LESIONS.   Scoliosis and kyphoscoliosis can also result from intraspinal lesions. For example, in years past, a major cause of kyphoscoliosis in this age group was poliomyelitis, the spinal deformity being produced by asymmetrical weakness of paraspinal musculature caused by involvement of anterior horn cells by the virus.[100] The same mechanism may still be implicated, but now intramedullary lesions of the spinal cord such as syringomyelia, ependymoma, or arteriovenous malformation are relatively much more common.

Perhaps the most common of these lesions is *syringomyelia,* a cystic enlargement of the spinal cord that is often maximal in the cervicothoracic region and sometimes associated with other anomalies such as the Arnold-Chiari malformation.[8, 42, 44] The neurological symptoms in syringomyelia appear most often after the age of 20 but scoliosis may appear a decade earlier and be otherwise asymptomatic.[12, 18, 39, 95] It is important to emphasize that syringomyelia frequently does not possess the "classical" features of a symmetrical mantle of diminished pain and temperature sensation involving the neck, arms and upper thoracic region. Equally common in our experience is the finding of impaired pain and temperature sensation in a segmental distribution, involving multiple cervical and thoracic dermatomes and characterized by a sensory level both above and below the sensory loss. Muscle weakness and atrophy are variably present in a similar distribution.

PERIPHERAL MUSCULAR DISORDERS. Finally, scoliosis can occur at this age as a result of primary myopathy due to a wide variety of causes or as a result of anterior horn cell or peripheral nerve involvement. In the presence of muscular weakness and atrophy, the occurrence of scoliosis favors involvement of nerve or anterior horn cells as opposed to primary myopathic disorders. However, exceptions are well recognized.

From the third decade onward, congenital spinal deformity becomes evident clinically as the result of secondary neurological symptoms due to nerve root or spinal cord compression, such as in spinal stenosis or in achondroplasia with shortening of the anteroposterior dimension of the spinal canal. Spinal deformities occurring in this age as a result of trauma, metabolic bone disease, pelvic asymmetry, arthritis, and other conditions are discussed elsewhere in this volume.

In summary, most cases of scoliosis with spinal deformity secondary to or associated with disease of the neuromuscular system are associated with objective neurological abnormalities. However, this is not always the case and myelography may, at times, be essential for correct diagnosis. Large volume contrast myelography should be considered in evaluating scoliosis when pain is the presenting complaint, when motor or sensory disturbances suggest the possibility of a lesion in the spinal canal, and when the findings in a patient with presumed idiopathic scoliosis have an unusual pattern, for example, an adolescent boy with rapidly progressing left thoracic scoliosis.

BACK PAIN

Local back pain is usually described as a non-radiating, aching, deep, dull soreness of the back muscles, associated with variable degrees of spasm, and influenced by posture. Local pressure or percussion may elicit tenderness.

Most local spinal pain is secondary to involvement of vertebral bodies, intervertebral discs, and ligamentous structures, with secondary spasm of paravertebral muscles. Far too often, the symptoms of neck or back pain are quickly translated into evidence for diagnosis of arthritis or disc disease without adequate examination of the patient or full consideration of the numerous causes of this symptom, ranging from meningeal and spinal cord disorders to disease of internal structures such as aorta, heart, lung, pancreas, kidney, and pelvic organs.

In infancy and childhood, back and neck

pain are not common, but when they occur, differential possibilities are intriguing. *Discitis,* occurring as a local bacterial infection of disc space in the thoracolumbar region with radiographic changes which are characteristic but late to develop, is an important consideration.[69] *Meningismus* or meningitis, particularly in infants and very young children whose sensorium may be difficult to evaluate, can present as neck or back pain due to meningeal inflammation and associated muscle spasm. *Lymphomatous infiltration* or an *abscess* (see below) in the epidural space may become painful well before neurological symptoms are evident.[131, 146] Even a *herniated disc* may become symptomatic.

Throughout the first decade, back pain, often ill-defined and poorly localized, is the most common presenting symptom of *primary intraspinal tumors*.[51, 135] Pain is often accentuated by physical activity, sneezing, coughing, straining, flexing the neck or back, or with straight leg raising. Recurrent back pain with consistent localization in a child is usually important, and deserves complete evaluation.

In the third to sixth decades lumbosacral pain is most often caused by postural or other mechanical disturbances.

Backache, exacerbated by cough, strain and movement is most commonly the symptom of protrusion of a lumbar intervertebral disc and usually antedates sciatic pain by months or years. Kyphosis, scoliosis, lordosis, spondylolysis, spondylolisthesis, spina bifida and vertebral anomalies also may be found on examination, and can become progressively symptomatic.

Next in frequency are inflammatory disease, including rheumatoid arthritis, ankylosing spondylitis, osteomyelitis and discitis.

In this population, Dodge (1951) has emphasized that low back pain (with or without sciatic pain) can be a presenting symptom of *primary intraspinal neoplasm* and may occur without evidence of specific neurologic signs.[34] Over a two-year period, 1242 patients underwent surgery for removal of a herniated intervertebral disc. Twenty-seven patients subsequently were proved to have tumors. Twelve of these patients had no sensory, motor, sphincter or reflex changes. Moersch (1951) reported 37 similar cases.[102]

With advancing age, spondylosis (especially cervical), metabolic bone disease and metastatic involvement of the spine become increasingly frequent causes of back pain.

Metastases to the bone or epidural spaces are unfortunately common causes of back pain, with lymphomas predominating in the third and fourth decades and carcinoma becoming more frequent thereafter.

Torma (1957) reviewed 250 histologically proved tumors and emphasized the presence of local pain for weeks or even months in 95 per cent of cases of spinal metastasis.[138] He noted that complete myelographic block may be found in those patients, in the absence of neurologic findings. Cerebrospinal fluid protein was always above 100 mg per 100 ml, and spine films showed metastatic changes in 30 to 40 per cent of lymphomas and in 60 per cent of solid tumors. Local back pain lasting greater than one week, without neurologic findings, may lead to needless early morbidity and mortality, particularly in cases of lymphoma, Hodgkin's disease, breast and rectal cancer and myeloma.[14, 106] At this time radiotherapy can be particularly effective.[116, 121]

A rare but important cause of axial pain is *spinal epidural abscess*.[3] One to two weeks after the development of a carbuncle or furuncle the patient (who may be of any age) complains of a persistent spinal ache, exacerbated by movement, coughing or straining. After several days or even months, radicular pain may develop (three of eight cases) followed by paraplegia, sensory level in the thoracic region and loss of sphincter control. Spinal tenderness is frequently present, along with fever and stiff neck. Roentgenograms frequently show vertebral osteomyelitis and a soft tissue mass. If spinal puncture is done in the lumbar area, the needle should be aspirated frequently so that epidural pus will not be missed and/or deposited in the subarachnoid space. More properly, a cervical or cisternal tap should be utilized if suppuration in the lumbar area is suspected. Cerebrospinal fluid examination will reveal a variable pleocytosis and elevated protein which depends on the presence of subarachnoid block. Unless the infection has spread through the dura, the CSF glucose is normal and the fluid is sterile.

Spinal *subdural empyema* presents with a symptom complex almost identical to epidural abscess except that (1) percussion tenderness is lacking, (2) there is no radiographic evidence of vertebral osteomyelitis and (3) the myelogram shows defects at several levels in addition to the cerebrospinal fluid block.[43]

Spinal spontaneous *epidural hematoma* is a rare but important surgically remediable cause of localized back pain.[6, 92] The pain occurs acutely and is followed within hours by transverse myelopathy. Bleeding dyscrasias are often responsible.

Although uncommon, *acute transverse myelitis (myelopathy)* can be associated with spinal pain.[82, 112] According to Altrocci (1963), local back pain was the initial complaint in 25 per cent.[3, 4]

Other unusual intraspinal causes of lumbar axial pain include spinal cord *arteriovenous malformation* and primary *intracranial subarachnoid hemorrhage* or *meningitis* with local meningeal irritation from blood or pus which has drained into the lumbar area.[55, 75, 109] Signs of meningeal irritation are present, and cerebrospinal fluid is abnormal.

Recurrent low back pain or neck pain without neurologic findings is also a common complaint in young and middle-aged adults who are bored or depressed. Post-traumatic and compensation neurosis is also frequently encountered. However, these diagnoses are a last resort and a thorough search for spinal pathology is always warranted.

SEGMENTAL PAIN OR SENSORY DISTURBANCES

Radicular pain is more common in the lumbosacral than in the cervical area, and is least common in the thoracic region. While radicular pain is usually typical and lightning-like in nature, at times diagnostic difficulty can arise when the pain occurs most prominently in a hand or foot and mimics local involvement. Furthermore, it is important to separate radicular pain and sensory disturbance from symptoms originating from involvement of the peripheral nerve, brachial plexus, sensory tracts within the cord, or even the brain.

Root pain is rarely recognized before the age of three or four and remains quite rare in the first and second decades. True radicular pain developing during this period is likely to result in an unusual diagnosis such as congenital spinal anomaly, A-V malformation, neurofibroma, or other benign tumor involving the roots directly.

At all ages, the location of the pain is of more diagnostic significance than the age of the patient.

To emphasize the frequency of various disorders presenting with root pain, Eaton (1941) reported 100 consecutive cases at the Mayo Clinic.[36] Fifty-four had verified disc protrusion, eight had probable disc protru-

sion, 12 had spinal cord tumors, seven had various mechanical and bony problems, including pathologic fractures, spondylolisthesis with hypertrophy of the ligamentum flavum and Potts' disease, and 18 were undiagnosed by the techniques utilized at that time. One additional patient had a subarachnoid hemorrhage, with blood pooling in the caudal region.

It is evident that *discogenic disease* is by far the most common cause of radicular pain in the lumbosacral region.

The lumbar disc syndrome[87, 120, 142] may be due to herniation of the nucleus pulposus, as first shown by Mixter and Barr (1934), to an accumulation of degenerative changes in the spine resulting in segmental narrowing of the vertebral canal, or to a generalized narrowing of the spinal canal, which although usually not the sole cause of the syndrome, may be a contributing factor in as many as 30 per cent of cases.[99, 113] Under these circumstances, the nerve roots can become compressed or irritated with subsequent edematous changes.

The main diagnostic challenge then is to remain alert to find the specific symptoms and signs of the more unusual but often remediable and important disorders that can present with root pain. A major alternative is *intraspinal tumor.*[88] The classical history for tumor is the insidious onset of pain which is progressive without intermittency until the patient is incapacitated. However, acute or intermittent symptoms also can occur as a result of vascular compression.

In the middle aged or elderly diabetic patient, *ischemic neuropathy of the lumbosacral plexus* is an additional diagnostic problem.[119] Characteristically, the disorder presents with the acute onset of severe anterior or posterior leg pain or both, often beginning at night. Within a short period of time, weakness and wasting appear, often in the distribution of both femoral and sciatic nerves.

In the cervical area, radicular pain radiating into the arms is most commonly the result of *spondylotic changes* at the C6 or C7 level that develop with advanced age or trauma.[20, 23, 145] The presence of root pain in other than the C6 or C7 distribution should make one consider more carefully the possibility that the cause for root irritation is other than disc or spondylotic disease.

Corbin (1968) noted that, in patients with root irritation, diligent questioning can often elicit the history of initial scapular pain which suggests that the lesion is proximal to the exit of the root from the intervertebral foramina.[28] The absence of scapular pain favors a more distal location of the lesion, such as in the brachial plexus.

Cervical root pain is more commonly seen in men than in women, and usually has its onset from the fourth decade onward. Radicular pain in this area may infrequently be caused by *primary spinal tumors*,[29, 84] *A-V malformation*,[107] or *metastatic tumors*.[14, 130, 138, 149]

Syringomyelia may on occasion present with a "boring" type of upper limb pain, which can be mistaken for true nerve root irritation.[18, 39] More commonly, there is a combination of pain and paresthesia in a dermatomal distribution involving one arm.

The *thoracic outlet syndrome* usually occurs in women in their third to fifth decade (80 per cent) and often affects those with an asthenic build.[140] Pain and paresthesias develop insidiously, and in 95 per cent are in the distribution of the ulnar nerve. Loss or diminution of the radial pulse is often found with Adson's maneuver, in addition to the radicular or ulnar sensory, motor and reflex changes. Bruits can sometimes be heard over the subclavian artery. One should also be alert for Horner's syndrome in these patients, for it may be secondary to a superior sulcus pulmonary tumor or some other disturbance of the spinal sympathetic outflow.[28]

Brachial plexus neuropathy or neuralgic amyotrophy is an uncommon disorder of unknown etiology that presents with a typical pattern of symptoms and signs.[139] The disorder can occur at any age, although the majority of patients are in the third through seventh decades. Males are affected more than females, with a ratio of 2.4 to 1. About 25 per cent of the patients give a history of antecedent flu-like illness, and a history of recent vaccination or immunization is often obtained. The first symptom is almost invariably intense pain which comes on suddenly and is described as sharp, stabbing, throbbing or aching, and less commonly as deep aching, gnawing or burning. The pain is usually constant and is exacerbated by any arm movement but, unlike root pain, not by coughing or straining. In occasional familial cases, recurrent attacks are common and the presence of residual focal neurological abnormalities may indicate the occurrence of a previous attack, even in the absence of appropriate antecedent symptoms.[46, 47, 129]

Finally, *median nerve compression* at the wrist and focal involvement in the opposite *parietal lobe* may mimic root pain.[59, 105] In the first case, evidence of increasing pain with flexion or extension of the wrist will suggest local involvement and in the second case predominant loss of discriminative sensation and hyperreflexia will be most helpful.

In the thoracic region, radicular pain is more likely to be due to extramedullary tumors than to disc protrusion.[83, 89, 127] *Meningiomas* typically occur in the fifth to seventh decades, with women involved three to four times more often than men. *Neurofibromas* occur in younger adults and produce radiological findings in 40 per cent.[24, 84]

Lymphomas and *metastatic carcinoma* form another large group of patients, as discussed in the section on local back pain.

Spinal cord arteriovenous malformations occur at any age, and are most common in the thoracic region. Radicular pain is often the first symptom.[107] Myelography may demonstrate the abnormal collection of vessels on the dorsal surface of the cord, but an alternative screening procedure is the noninvasive radioisotope scan of the cord.[31, 32] In some cases DiChiro (1973) suggests passing directly to spinal cord angiography after isotopic scan.[33] Recent successful surgical management of these lesions has made their early recognition more imperative.[73, 75, 90, 109]

Tabes dorsalis commonly presents with multiple, recurrent, knifelike pains in the anterior chest and abdomen in the distribution of multiple roots. In the series reported by Merritt (1968), these lancinating pains eventually occurred in 75 per cent of the patients.[97] Examination may reveal isolated patches of hypalgesia in the distribution of the pain (Hitzig spots), impaired pain and position sense in the feet, and absent Achilles reflexes.

Herpes zoster segmental radiculitis is a common disorder that can cause difficulty in diagnosis for three or four days until the erythema and typical clusters of vesicles make their appearance in the distribution of the involved roots. This is rarely followed by segmental zoster paresis, or myelitis.[57, 136]

Occasionally intramedullary lesions produce segmental sensory disturbances which may or may not be interpreted as painful. Multiple sclerosis,[26] syringomyelia,[39] subacute combined degeneration,[141] arteriovenous malformation, radiation myelopathy,[68] and intramedullary tumors,[71, 148] as well as myelopathy associated with spinal cord compression,[37] fall into this category. In some instances paresthesias extending into the extremities and down the spine can be produced by neck flexion (Lhermitte's sign). Demyelination with axonal preservation in the cervical region may be the common factor.[68]

ACUTE PARAPLEGIA OR QUADRIPLEGIA

Sudden onset of severe weakness involving arms, legs, or both occurs most frequently as a result of *trauma* to the spine and spinal cord and is primarily a therapeutic problem, beyond the scope of this discussion. When the history of trauma is unclear, or when the course and constellation of symptoms are unusual, important diagnostic considerations are necessary.

At the outset one must distinguish supraspinal disorders and disorders of the peripheral neuromuscular system from those directly involving the spinal cord.

Quadriplegia in the first year of life is most commonly the result of congenital degeneration of anterior horn cells, *Werdnig-Hoffmann disease.* A paucity of spontaneous movements is noted shortly after birth. Preservation of sensation in the legs is important in distinguishing this disease from direct spinal cord injury at birth, which is rare but which can occur as a sequela of breech delivery.

The acute onset of muscular weakness, usually involving both legs and arms, can be due to peripheral neuromuscular disorders as well. The *Guillain-Barré syndrome* is a good example of the manner in which rapidly ascending muscular weakness can mimic cord compression.[11, 54, 93, 144] The preservation of nearly normal sensation in these patients and most others with acute weakness due to a peripheral neuromuscular disorder can be diagnostically useful.

Beyond the age of 50, acute *infarction in the pontomedullary* region may produce quadriplegia in a patient who is seemingly alert, although usually unable to talk or swallow properly.[41, 108] On examination, such patients usually have defective eye movements and impaired pharyngeal reflexes as indications of brainstem involvement.

Sudden paraplegia or quadriplegia due to *spinal cord compression* usually presents a characteristic clinical picture. Bilateral weakness, urinary retention, and impaired sensation below the level of spinal involvement may de-velop instantly or over the course of a few hours or days. Reflexes may be increased or decreased, and the Babinski response is variable. When progression is slower, an ascending pattern of sensorimotor involvement often occurs, owing to the fact that the sacral and lumbar segments are located more peripherally in the sensory and motor columns of the spinal cord than are the thoracic and cervical segments, which are more central. Lesions of the central cord are also common and can present with symptoms primarily in the cervical segments, as in the cases due to trauma described by Schneider and colleagues (1958, 1961).[124, 125]

At this point, we emphasize the need to consider the possibility of spinal cord injury in every person who has sustained severe trauma and is unconscious. These patients are unable to complain of pain in the injured spine, and severe quadriplegia of spinal origin may go unrecognized. It is essential that all such patients be protected from unnecessary spinal movement until lateral roentgenograms of the cervical spine are obtained in the supine position.

If trauma is excluded, extradural spinal cord compression due to encroachment by tumor or bone is the most common cause of what has come to be called the "transverse myelopathy syndrome."

Up to the age of 40 years, *extradural lymphoma* or *leukemic deposits* must be suspected first. With a prior diagnosis of a hematopoietic or lymphatic disorder, the presence of spinal pain followed by rapidly developing weakness and sensory loss below that level must indicate immediate myelography, followed by local radiotherapy or surgery in association with steroids or chemotherapeutic agents.[131, 146]

In these early decades, extradural bony compression can occur as a result of congenital anomalies. *Hemivertebra* in the cervical region is a good example of a disorder in which symptoms are not present at birth but are delayed for one or more decades, sometimes being precipitated by minor trauma. A similar situation occurs in *achondroplastic dwarfism.*[2, 132] The anteroposterior diameter of the spinal canal is narrowed by shortening of the vertebral pedicles in such patients, who may develop acute paraplegia owing to spinal compression in the thoracic region following relatively minor trauma. (Similar sequelae occur in an animal model of this disorder, the dachshund.)

Above the age of 50, cord compression due to *extradural metastases* become increasingly common and may be the first manifestation of a primary parenchymal tumor.[14] In most instances, spinal pain is present for a prolonged period prior to acute spinal cord compression. *Cervical spondylosis* can also cause acute quadriplegia following seemingly minor trauma.[20, 23, 145]

The syndrome of *acute idiopathic transverse myelitis* can occur at any age but peaks in frequency during the first and second decades.[4, 82] The onset is abrupt, and the symptoms of leg weakness, sensory loss, back pain, root pain, and sphincter disturbances are indistinguishable from those associated with spinal cord compression. The thoracic location is most common but 22 per cent of cases occur in the cervical region.

Myelography is essential to rule out extradural compression. Occasionally, localized cord swelling caused by the inflammatory process can be seen. Cerebrospinal fluid cell count and protein are elevated in the majority of patients.

The etiology of this disorder is obscure, but the history of viral infection in approximately one third of cases suggests an infectious element. A relationship to multiple sclerosis has not been established.

Next most common as a cause of the transverse myelopathy syndrome, particularly in older patients, is *spinal cord infarction.* This may be preceded by symptoms of spinal cord ischemia or may occur suddenly without prodromata.[58, 67] Arteriosclerotic involvement of a major radicular artery along its course from the aorta to the vertebral foramen is the rule,[58] but aortic surgery,[1,128] dissecting aneurysm of the aorta,[137] embolization,[147] thrombophlebitis, compression by tumor in the vertebral foramen, or luetic arteritis may also occur.[45, 56]

Sometimes acute paraplegia will occur in the course of radiotherapy for a neoplasm, when the portal includes the spinal column. This is probably due to vascular occlusion, as well.[114]

Sudden transverse myelopathy will occasionally be the first manifestation of an arteriovenous malformation of the spinal cord caused by sudden subarachnoid hemorrhage, hematomyelia, or watershed infarction caused by a change in hemodynamics. The syndrome of subacute, necrotizing myelitis of Foix and Alajounine, consisting of sudden spastic then flaccid paraplegia with an ascending spinal level, has been shown to be secondary to arteriovenous malformation.[21, 33, 107]

Finally, infection of the epidural space should be considered. In the case of *abscess* pain, local tenderness, stiff neck, fever, lymphocytosis and elevated cells of protein in the spinal fluid are characteristic.[4] Roentgenograms of the spine show evidence of vertebral osteomyelitis and a preceding staphylococcal infection is often present. With *spinal epidural empyema,* tenderness may be absent and vertebral osteomyelitis may not be evident radiographically.[43]

Spinal *epidural hematoma* is an unusual but treatable disorder in which symptoms and findings of cord transection develop progressively in a very short time, usually after trauma and severe back pain.[6, 123] These lesions can occur spontaneously as well as in association with extradural arteriovenous malformation and following anticoagulant therapy.

An important complication of mesenteric angiography or aortography is *injury to the spinal cord caused by contrast material.* Particularly when peripheral hypotension and constriction of the splanchnic bed are present, shunting of contrast material into spinal radicular arteries results in sudden paraplegia with marked disinhibition of reflex activity below the level of involvement. The slightest touch will produce uncontrollable spasms of both legs. In such cases, large amounts of organic iodide can be found in the spinal fluid and must be removed to prevent ascending sensory and motor involvement of the spinal cord owing to diffusion through the cerebrospinal fluid. The patient must be maintained in the sitting position and at least 100 ml. of spinal fluid exchanged with an equal amount of saline over the course of 30 minutes.

An unusual cause of extradural bony compression occurs as a result of incompetence of either the *odontoid process* or the transverse atlantal ligament secondary to congenital, traumatic, neoplastic, or inflammatory disorders, especially rheumatoid arthritis.[52]

MONOPARESIS

Weakness of an arm or leg without pain is not commonly due to involvement of the spinal cord. More frequent at all ages are disorders of the plexuses or peripheral nerves. Ulnar, median, peroneal, and radial nerves may be affected and produce weakness and atrophy in the distribution of the specific nerve, often with surprisingly little sensory loss. Acute compression or chronic, recurrent trauma should be suspected whenever sensory and motor findings are limited to the distribution of a single nerve.[105] Less commonly, diabetes, collagen vascular disease, toxins, or local injections may be responsible. The most useful diagnostic test is peripheral nerve conduction velocity, which will be markedly slowed across the point of compression or injury.

Next most common are lesions of the spinal cord. In the first two decades, *spinal cord tumor*[135] or *extradural lymphoma*[131, 146] are most common and are discussed elsewhere in this chapter.

In the second through fourth decades multiple sclerosis, syringomyelia, and progressive muscular atrophy must be considered as well. Monoparesis is actually rare in *multiple sclerosis* but the disease is common and 20 per cent of patients in the series of Carter and others (1950) complained of weakness or were found to have objective signs in one arm or hand.[26] In contradistinction, *syringomyelia* is a rare disease in which painless monoparesis is characteristic, occurring in one third of patients.[18, 39] *Progressive muscular atrophy* caused by primary anterior horn cell degeneration is common at this age and often begins in one arm.[9, 17, 25, 74, 96]

Rarely, intramedullary or extramedullary *cervical tumors* can present with painless weakness of an extremity.[71, 148]

In older patients, *amyotrophic lateral sclerosis* becomes a common spinal cord cause of monoparesis, and occurs in 26 to 41 per cent of patients with that disorder.[80, 104] Characteristically, weakness and atrophy are asymmetric in the beginning and may remain so for many months. When combined upper and lower motor neuron findings are associated with involvement of the tongue and other bulbar musculature, the diagnosis is clear. Otherwise, complete myelography is essential to rule out *cervical spondylosis* and other disorders that may mimic motor neuron disease.

Infrequently, a *focal lesion of the cerebral hemisphere* may produce the symptom of monoparesis at any age. Children are more likely to disregard minor associated disability in a less affected extremity on the same side. The presence of hyperreflexia in the affected arm or leg and subtle findings of hemiparesis are usually present on examination and point to the correct localization.

IMPAIRMENT OF GAIT

There hardly exists an orthopedic or neurological disorder which cannot produce abnormalities of gait at some time in its course. If we exclude those cases in which orthopedic abnormalities are obvious on inspection or in which pain or severe muscular weakness is evident, a group of patients remain in whom the causes of gait impairment are predominantly neurological in origin. These include, in descending order of frequency, disorders of the corticospinal pathways (spasticity), basal ganglia (Parkinsonism), cerebellum and connections (ataxia), cerebral cortex (gait apraxia), neuromuscular system (weakness) and sensation (ataxia).

At birth, spontaneous movements of the legs are normally present and constitute the first of a series of milestones in the development of neuromuscular skills necessary for walking. Most often, delayed walking is preceded by a corresponding delay in other neuromuscular accomplishments such as head control, rolling over, and sitting. Cerebral causes are most common, ranging from anoxia at birth to severe developmental abnormalities. Direct indices of cerebral function are nearly absent at this age. This may be emphasized by noting the occasional case of hydranencephaly (with essentially no cortex) whose neuromuscular, "emotional," and even electroencephalographic development may be nearly normal during the first months of life.

When spontaneous movements are impaired early in life, or when muscular weakness is found on examination (for example, the child who slips through your fingers when supported in the axillae), *anterior horn cell degeneration* or *congenital myopathy* must be suspected.[66, 117]

As development proceeds, loss of previously acquired neuromuscular skills, including walking, is an important sign of a progressive intracranial process such as one of the inherited metabolic disorders or increased intracranial pressure caused by ventricular obstruction, subdural hematoma, arteriovenous malformation or tumor. Of the former, *metachromatic leukodystrophy* is of particular interest since associated involvement of peripheral nerves may produce leg weakness as a predominant symptom. It is clear that the physical examination plays an important role in distinguishing the spasticity and hyperreflexia, which occur as a result of common supraspinal defects in gait, from the rare peripheral neuromuscular disorders which produce weakness and hyporeflexia.

Throughout the remainder of the first decade, a different spectrum of disorders is seen with approximately equal frequency. *Acute cerebellar ataxia,* most commonly occurring in childhood, is seen after exanthematous diseases, particularly chickenpox, and can occur in the absence of proved viral infection.[16, 22, 72] The onset is acute, a history of prior infection may be present, and the findings on examination are limited to ataxia of gait, dysmetria of the arms and nystagmus. Similar symptoms may occur in posterior fossa tumor, particularly *medulloblastoma,* but the onset is usually more insidious and is often associated with nausea, vomiting and headache, as signs of increased intracranial pressure.

Several heredofamilial disorders can present with clumsy gait or frank ataxia at this age. Most common are the variants of spinocerebellar degeneration, especially Friedreich's ataxia.[35, 97] *Ataxia telangiectasia* is a rare, related disorder which produces very slowly progressive ataxia, telangiectases over the sclera and face and behind the ears, and which is associated with chronic upper respiratory infections and deficiency in gamma globulin (IgA).[94]

Disorders of the basal ganglia can produce gait disturbances at this age. *Dystonia musculorum deformans* begins primarily with intorsion of one leg.[38] *Sydenham's chorea,* now uncommon, causes gait disturbance in association with involuntary movements of the arms, face, and tongue.[10]

Congenital midline spinal defects often become symptomatic at this age, when a child is referred for peculiar gait or poor posture associated with shortening of one leg.[62] Deformities of the foot develop later. Neurological findings are dependent on the level of the defect and the duration of symptoms. Early neurological findings are slight and sometimes limited to hypalgesia in the saddle region. Later, loss of deep tendon reflexes, sensory disturbances, and atrophy may develop in the legs. If a lesion is located higher, in the lumbar or thoracic cord, hyperreflexia may also be present. The overlying skin may show a dimple sinus, angioma, nevus, or subcutaneous lipoma. Pathologically, mesodermal elements are found at the thoracolumbar or sacral levels which compress, separate, or are located primarily within the spinal cord. A bony protrusion splitting the cord (diastematomyelia,[63, 64])

may be seen on plain radiographs, particularly with tomography, and produces symptoms progressively as a result of growth-related traction on the spinal cord.

Spinal cord tumors cause gait disturbance at this age but are usually preceded by pain.[135]

During the second through fourth decades, *multiple sclerosis* is a frequent cause of gait disturbance in the general population.[26] A history of remissions, visual disturbances, high CSF gamma globulin or IgA, and abnormal central evoked potentials point strongly to this diagnosis. Impaired gait results from involvement of cerebellar pathways, loss of position sense or spasticity, alone or in combination. However, when all findings can be explained by a lesion in the spinal cord, when the history is more progressive than recurrent, or when pain develops in a spinal or radicular distribution, an *intraspinal tumor,* such as a neurofibroma, meningioma, neurenteric cyst, or A-V malformation must be considered.

With increasing age, chronic spinal cord compression related to *cervical spondylosis* becomes a frequent cause of gait impairment.[20, 23, 30, 145] When pain in the neck is a prominent symptom and examination reveals decreased range of motion of the neck, weakness and wasting in the hands, and spasticity, hyperreflexia and loss of position sense in the legs, the diagnosis is easy. When the syndrome is incomplete, or when it is complicated by the appearance of leg pain or fasciculation of the legs, difficulties arise.[77]

Second in frequency to cervical spondylosis is *amyotrophic lateral sclerosis* which also presents a variable mixture of wasting and atrophy, more in the arms, and spasticity and hyperreflexia, more in the legs.[80, 91, 104] A careful check for fasciculations in the tongue may be helpful. On the other hand, the presence of moderate loss of position sense in the feet excludes this disorder effectively. Uncommonly, a tumor[15, 29, 134, 143] involving the spinal cord as high as the foramen magnum, or a vitamin B_{12} deficiency[141] may be present, with spasticity, loss of position sense, and paresthesias in the legs.

Experienced clinicians seek laboratory confirmation in every case, utilizing electromyography of legs and arms, and complete myelography.

From the fifth decade onward, cerebral causes of impaired gait again predominate, and *Parkinsonism* with characteristic short steps is the most frequent. *Diffuse encepha-*

lopathy may also produce a gait characterized by very short steps, with the feet appearing to be stuck to the floor — gait "apraxia."[98]

In the past, *tabes dorsalis* was a frequent cause of disturbance of sensation, and resulted in a broad based, ataxic gait, made worse in the dark or when visual cues were otherwise absent. Such cases develop 10 to 20 years after initial syphilitic infection and may become frequent again.[97]

Astasia abasia, described by Blocq in 1888, is a bizarre disturbance of gait in which standing and walking are seemingly impaired but falling is avoided by remarkable feats of balance. When considered, the hysterical basis of this remarkable symptomatology is easily recognized.[110]

BLADDER DISTURBANCES

Incontinence and other disturbances of urinary bladder function are occasionally the first manifestations of disease of the spinal cord as well as the rest of the nervous system. In this section we will stress the importance of associated neurologic findings in delineating these lesions.

The physiology of micturition is complex but has been well reviewed.[76, 115] The terms "atonic bladder" or "spastic bladder" are no longer useful in describing different levels of neurological involvement and are related mainly to local factors in the bladder wall. Rather, localization of impaired micturition depends on (1) loss of bladder sensation; (2) perineal sensory loss; (3) patulous anal sphincter; (4) absence of the bulbocavernosus and anocutaneous reflexes; and (5) sensory, motor, and/or reflex changes in the lower extremities. An associated history of impotence or rectal incontinence should clearly suggest the presence of a common neurogenic cause for urinary incontinence, and the additional presence of sacral pain should suggest tumor in the sacral region.

Sensory loss restricted to the bladder and the skin of the anogenital region (S2, S3, S4) suggests involvement of sacral dorsal roots. Ventral root involvement is suspected when anogenital reflexes are impaired but sensation is preserved. Combined sensory and motor impairment restricted to the S2, S3, S4 segments may occur with lesions of the conus medullaris or with more peripheral involvement of dorsal and ventral sacral roots. Associated sensory or motor impairment in the legs or trunk occurs when the responsible lesions affect the spinal cord above the conus. With cerebral lesions, impaired inhibition of the micturition reflex produces incontinence when diffuse encephalopathy is present or, rarely, when there is localized involvement of the parasagittal or frontal regions.[7] Specific sacral sensory or motor impairment is not present in such cases.

In the first years of life, failure to achieve toilet training in children without cerebral impairment is most likely to be because of congenital *obstructive uropathy,* which may be complicated by infection or distention. In these cases, careful urologic examination and intravenous pyelography will usually disclose the lesion.

Primary *intramedullary tumors* such as ependymoma or midline teratomas must also be considered in this age group.[53, 71, 148] Secondary medulloblastoma, implanting from a primary tumor in the posterior fossa, is a well-recognized complication.

In the first and second decades, congenital obstructive uropathy with overflow dribbling is the most common cause of incontinence, and is unassociated with neurologic signs and symptoms. *Occult dysraphic states* that become symptomatic during this time are not usually first manifested by bladder disturbances,[62, 64] although bladder disturbances may develop later on (but see Cooper, 1968[27]).

Benign tumors such as epidermoids, dermoids, and lipomas may also first manifest themselves with bladder disturbances in this age group. *Lipomas* involving the sacral segments and the cauda equina characteristically present with slowly progressive sphincter disturbances, in association with mild unilateral talipes equinovarus. In addition, examination will often reveal enlargement (lipoma) of one buttock, decreased Achilles reflex, mild leg weakness, reduced sacral sensation, and impaired anocutaneous and bulbocavernosus reflexes. Plain spine radiographs reveal abnormalities in 80 to 90 per cent, including spina bifida occulta, widened spinal canal, massive defects in the sacrum, and scoliosis.[48]

In the third and fourth decades, neurologic disease presenting as urgency and reflex incontinence is most likely to be *multiple sclerosis.* The most prominent defect of detrusor function is loss of the ability to inhibit reflex contraction once it has been evoked by distention.[103] In some cases, potentiation of reflex contraction of external sphincter leads to urinary retention, but in most instances this does not prevent reflex voiding.[19] In the series of Carter and coworkers, 11 per cent of the cases presented with the urinary sphincter disturbances while 78 per cent eventually developed some disorder of micturition.[26]

Throughout the rest of adult life urinary incontinence is most commonly due to non-neurologic disorders. In males, acquired obstruction is usually apparent from a careful urologic examination. In women, intermittent stress incontinence, occasionally with retention and poor sensation, is seen after pelvic stretching during repeated pregnancies. The cystometrogram shows a poor contractile response with elevated or unobtainable micturition reflex thresholds. Neurologic examination is normal, and relief may be provided by a variety of procedures for pelvic suspension or lengthening of the internal sphincter.

In later life, the most common specific neurologic cause of incontinence is *sacral neuropathy,* resulting from diabetes mellitus, polyneuritis, midline disc protrusion, tumors invading the sacral roots, tabes dorsalis, subacute combined degeneration of the cord, amyloid neuropathy and herpes zoster. Examination will reveal a combination of sensory and reflex changes in the legs, sacral sensory loss, impaired sacral reflexes, and patulous sphincter. Cerebrospinal fluid examination may reveal an increase in protein, and tumors may show erosion on plain roentgenograms.

A *pure conus medullaris lesion,* with an autonomous dilated bladder, reduced sphincter tone, impotence, and sacral hypalgesia, with or without symmetric sensory motor changes in the legs is usually secondary to a small intramedullary glioma (most commonly an ependymoma), metastatic lesion, or cyst.[71, 148]

Sensory and motor disturbances of the bladder and, in some cases, pure motor paralytic bladder can also result from *lesions of the cauda equina,* the most common being a myxopapillary ependymoma originating in the filum terminale.[40, 70] Retention and urinary incontinence may be the first and only manifestation of these lesions for a long time. In most cases, however, pain, weakness and numbness are apparent in the gluteal region and legs. Recently, cauda equina lesions have been demonstrated in ankylosing spondylitis and rheumatoid arthritis.[50, 122]

Retention and overflow incontinence can also be the presenting complaint of degenerative lesions of the nervous system caused by general inattention, or associated with specific autonomic failure. In cases of *idopathic orthostatic hypotension,* Shy and Drager (1960) found cell loss in multiple sites including the intermediolateral (sympathetic) cell column of the spinal cord.[126] In some cases the findings are limited to the pigmented neurons of the brain and are identical to the findings in idiopathic Parkinsonism.[13] The presenting complaint is often that of overflow incontinence or difficulty in voiding as the micturition reflex is interrupted. Orthostatic hypertension, fixed heart rate, anhydrosis, and sexual impotence are characteristic in association, with variable degrees of pyramidal, cerebellar and extrapyramidal disturbances. The latter, in the form of Parkinsonism, is often incapacitating but may not develop until some time after the autonomic impairment.

Occasionally, chronic spinal cord compression or intramedullary tumors in the cervical or thoracic area may produce early bladder disturbances, but usually a history of paresthesia or pain can also be obtained, and neurologic examination will reveal leg weakness and sensory disturbances.

CONCLUSION

Effective diagnosis and treatment of a spinal disorder are aided by early consideration of the most frequent causes of a specific symptom at a given age, and by the recognition of common patterns of disease in the midst of conflicting symptoms and signs. If the age of onset, symptoms, findings or clinical course are unusual, a detailed search for an uncommon disorder (or an atypical manifestation of a common disorder) must be undertaken.

References

1. Adams, H. D., and van Geertruyden, H. H.: Neurologic complications of aortic surgery. Ann. Surg. *144*:574–610, 1956.
2. Aegerter, E. E., and Kirkpatrick, J. A., Jr.: Orthopedic Diseases: Physiology, Pathology, Radiology, 4th ed. Philadelphia, W. B. Saunders Co., 1975.
3. Altrocchi, P. H.: Acute spinal epidural abscess vs. acute transverse myelopathy. Arch. Neurol. 9:17–25, 1963.
4. Altrocchi, P. H.: Acute transverse myelopathy. Arch. Neurol. 9:111–119, 1963.
5. Ames, M. D., and Schut, L.: Results of treatment of 171 consecutive myelomeningoceles, 1963–1968. Pediatrics 50:466–470, 1972.
6. Amyes, E. W., Vogel, P. J., and Raney, R. B.: Spinal cord compression due to spontaneous epidural hemorrhage. Bull. L. A. Neurol. Soc. *20*:1–8, 1955.
7. Andrew, J., and Nathan, P. W.: Lesions of the anterior frontal lobes and disturbances of micturition and defaecation. Brain 87:233–262, 1964.

8. Appleby, A., Foster, J. B. Hankinson, J., et al.: The diagnosis and management of Chiari anomalies in adult life. Brain 91:131–140, 1968.

9. Armstrong, R. M., Fogelson, H. H., and Silberberg, D. H.: Familial proximal spinal muscular atrophy. Arch. Neurol. 14:208–212, 1966.

10. Aron, A. M., Freeman, J. M., and Carter, S.: The natural history of Sydenham's chorea. Am. J. Med., 38:83–95, 1965.

11. Asbury, A. K., Arnason, B. G., and Adams, R. D.: The inflammatory lesion in idiopathic polyneuritis. Medicine 48:173–215, 1969.

12. Ballantine, H. T., Ojemann, R. G., and Drew, J. H.: Syringohydromyelia. Progr. Neurol. Surg. 4:227–245, 1971.

13. Bannister, R., and Oppenheimer, D. R.: Degenerative diseases of the nervous system associated with autonomic failure. Brain 95:457–474, 1972.

14. Barron, K. D., Hirano, A., Araki, S., et al.: Experiences with metastatic neoplasms involving the spinal cord. Neurol. 9:91–106, 1959.

15. Bennett, A. E., and Fortes, A.: Meningioma obstructing the foramen magnum. Arch. Neurol. Psych., 53:131–134, 1945.

16. Blaw, M. E., and Sheehan, J. C.: Acute cerebellar syndrome of childhood. Neurol. 8:538–542, 1958.

17. Bobowick, A. R., and Brody, J.: Epidemiology of motor-neuron diseases. N. Engl. J. Med. 288:1047–1055, 1973.

18. Boman, K., and Iivanainen, M.: Prognosis of syringomyelia. Acta Neurol. Scand. 43:61–68, 1967.

19. Bradley, W. E., Logothetis, J. L., and Timm, G. W.: Cystometric and sphincter abnormalities in multiple sclerosis. Neurol. 23:1131, 1973.

20. Brain, W. R., Northfield, D., and Wilkinson, M.: The neurological manifestations of cervical spondylosis. Brain 75:187–225, 1952.

21. Brion, S., Netsky, M. G., and Zimmerman, H. M.: Vascular malformations of the spinal cord. AMA Arch. Neurol. Psychiat. 68:339–361, 1952.

22. Brumlik, J., and Means, E. D.: Tremorine-tremor, shivering, and acute cerebellar ataxia in the adult and child — a comparative study. Brain 92:157–190, 1969.

23. Bucy, P. C.: Syndromes produced by disorders of the cervical intervertebral disks. Med. Clin. N. Amer. 42:515–521, 1958.

24. Bull, J. W. D.: Spinal meningiomas and neurofibromas. Acta. Radiol. 40:283–300, 1953.

25. Byers, R. K., and Banker, B. Q.: Infantile muscular atrophy. Arch. Neurol. 5:140–164, 1961.

26. Carter, S., Sciarra, D., and Merritt, H. H.: The course of multiple sclerosis as determined by autopsy proven cases. Res. Publ. Ass. Res. Nerv. Ment. Dis. 28:471–511, 1949.

27. Cooper, D. G. W.: Detrusor action in children with myelomeningocele. Arch. Dis. Child. 43:427–432, 1968.

28. Corbin, K. B.: Common neurologic brachial pain problems. Med. Clin. N. Amer. 52:773–779, 1968.

29. Craig, W. M., and Shelden, C. H.: Tumors of the cervical portion of the spinal cord. Arch. Neurol. Psychiat. 44:1–161, 1940.

30. Crandall, P. H., and Batzdorf, U.: Cervical spondylitic myelopathy. J. Neurosurg. 25:57–66, 1966.

31. Di Chiro, G.: Recent successes and failures in radiographic and radio-isotopic angiography of the spinal cord. Brit. J. Radiol. 45:553–560, 1972.

32. Di Chiro, G., Jones, A. E., Johnston, G. S., et al.: Radioisotope angiography of the spinal cord. J. Nucl. Med. 13:567–569, 1972.

33. Di Chiro, G., and Werner, L.: Angiography of the spinal cord. J. Neurosurg. 39:1–29, 1973.

34. Dodge, H. W., Svien, H. J., Camp, J. D., et al.: Tumors of spinal cord without neurologic manifestations, producing low back and sciatic pain. Proc. Mayo Clin. 26:88–95, 1951.

35. Dyck, P. J., and Lambert, E. H.: Lower motor and primary sensory neuron diseases with peroneal muscular atrophy. Arch. Neurol. 18:603–618, 1968.

36. Eaton, L. McK.: Pain caused by disease involving the sensory nerve roots. J.A.M.A. 117:1435–1439, 1941.

37. Edelson, R. N., Deck, M. D., and Posner, J. B.: Intramedullary spinal cord metastases. Neurology 22:1222–1231, 1972.

38. Eldridge, R.: The torsion dystonias: Literature review and genetic and clinical studies. Neurology 20(11):1–78, Part 2, 1970.

39. Ellertsson, A. B.: Syringomyelia and other cystic spinal cord lesions. Acta Neurol. Scand. 45:403, 1969.

40. Elsberg, C. A., and Constable, K.: Tumors of the cauda equina. Arch. Neurol. Psychiat. 23:79–105, 1930.

41. Feldman, M. H.: Physiological observations in a chronic case of locked-in syndrome. Neurology 21:459–478, 1971.

42. Foster, J. B., Hudgson, P., and Pearce, G. W.: The association of syringomyelia and congenital cervico-medullary anomalies: Pathological evidence. Brain 92:25–34, 1969.

43. Fraser, R. A. R., Ratzan, K., Wolpert, S. M., et al.: Spinal subdural empyema. Arch. Neurol. 28:235–238, 1973.

44. Gardner, W. J.: Hydrodynamic mechanism of syringomyelia: Its relationship to myelocele. J. Neurol. Neurosurg. Psychiat. 28:247–259, 1965.

45. Garland, H., Greenberg, J., and Harriman, D. G.: Infarction of the spinal cord. Brain 89:645–662, 1966.

46. Geiger, L.: Personal communication.

47. Geiger, L., Mancall, E., Penn, A., and Tucker, S.: Familial neuralgic amyotrophy. Brain 97:121–136, 1974.

48. Giuffré, R.: Intradural spinal lipomas. Acta Neurochir. (Wien) 14:69–95, 1966.

49. Gold, L. H. A., Leach, C. G., Kieffer, S., et al.: Large-volume myelography. Radiology 97:531–536, 1970.

50. Gordon, A. L., and Yudell, A.: Cauda equina lesion associated with rheumatoid spondylitis. Ann. Int. Med. 78:555–557, 1973.

51. Grant, F. C., and Austin, G. M.: The diagnosis, treatment and prognosis of tumors affecting the spinal cord in children. J. Neursurg. 13:535–545, 1956.

52. Greenberg, A. D.: Atlanto-axial dislocations. Brain 91:655–683, 1968.

53. Haymaker, W.: Bing's Local Diagnosis in Neurological Diseases, 15th ed. St. Louis, C. V. Mosby Co., 1969.

54. Haymaker, W., and Kernohan, J. W.: The Landry-Guillain-Barré syndrome. Medicine 28:59–141, 1949.

55. Henson, R. A., and Croft, P. B.: Spontaneous spinal subarachnoid hemorrhage. Quart. J. Med. 25:53–66, 1956.

56. Henson, R. A., and Parsons, M.: Ischemic lesions of

the spinal cord: An illustrated review. Quart. J. Med., *36*:205–222, 1967.

57. Hogan, E. L., and Krigman, M. R.: Herpes zoster myelitis. Arch. Neurol. *29*:309–311, 1973.

58. Hughes, J. T.: The pathology of vascular disorders of the spinal cord. Int. J. Paraplegia *2*:207–213, 1965.

59. Hunt, G. M., Abbott, K. H., and Roberts, W. H.: The median nerve and carpal tunnel syndrome. Bull. L. A. Neurol. Soc. *25*:211–222, 1960.

60. James, J. I. P.: Idiopathic scoliosis. J. Bone Joint Surg. *36B*:36–49, 1954.

61. James, J. I. P.: Two curve patterns in idiopathic structural scoliosis. J. Bone Joint Surg. *33B*:399–406, 1951.

62. James, C. C. M., and Lassman, L. P.: Spinal dysraphism. Arch. Dis. Child. *35*:315–327, 1960.

63. James, C. C. M., and Lassman, L. P.: Diastematomyelia. Arch. Dis. Child. *33*:536–539, 1958.

64. James, C. C. M., and Lassman, L. P.: Diastematomyelia. Arch. Dis. Child. *39*:125–130, 1964.

65. James, J. I. P., Lloyd-Roberts, G. C., and Pilcher, M. F.: Infantile structural scoliosis. J. Bone Joint Surg. *41B*:719–735, 1959.

66. Jepsen, R. H., Johnson, E. W., Knobloch, H., et al.: Differential diagnosis of infantile hypotonia. Am. J. Dis. Child. *101*:8–17, 1961.

67. Jellinger, K.: Spinal cord arteriosclerosis and progressive vascular myelopathy. J. Neurol. Neurosurg. Psychiat. *30*:195–206, 1967.

68. Jones, A.: Transient radiation myelopathy. Br. J. Radiol. *37*:727–744, 1964.

69. Keiser, R. P., and Grimes, H. A.: Intervertebral disk space infections in children. Clin. Orthop. *30*:163–166, 1963.

70. Kernohan, J. W., Woltman, H. W., and Adson, A. W.: Gliomas arising from the region of the cauda equina. Arch. Neurol. Psychiat. *29*:287–307, 1933.

71. Kernohan, J. W., Woltman, H. W., and Adson, A. W.: Intramedullary tumors of the spinal cord. Arch. Neurol. Psychiat. *25*:679–701, 1931.

72. King, G., Schwarz, G. A., and Slade, H. W.: Acute cerebellar ataxia of childhood. Report of nine cases. Pediatrics *21*:731–745, 1958.

73. Krayenbühl, H., Yasargil, M. G., and McClintock, H. G.: Treatment of spinal cord vascular malformations by surgical excision. J. Neurosurg. *30*:427–435, 1969.

74. Kugelberg, E., and Welander, L.: Heredofamilial juvenile muscular atrophy simulating muscular dystrophy. AMA Arch. Neurol. Psychiat. *75*:500–509, 1956.

75. Kunc, Z., and Bret, J.: Diagnosis and treatment of vascular malformations of the spinal cord. J. Neurosurg., *30*:436–445, 1969.

76. Kuru, M.: Nervous control of micturition. Physiol. Rev. *45*:425–494, 1965.

77. Langfitt, T. W.: Cervical spondylosis: The neurological mimic. West Va. Med. J. *65*:97–100, 1969.

78. Laurence, K. M.: The survival of untreated spina bifida cystica. Devel. Med. Child. Neurol. *8*(Suppl. 11):10–19, 1966.

79. Laurence, K. M., and Tew, B. J.: Follow-up of 65 survivors from the 425 cases of spina bifida born in south Wales between 1956 and 1962. Devel. Med. Child. Neurol. *9*(Suppl. 13):1–3, 1967.

80. Lawyer, T., and Netsky, M. G.: Amyotrophic lateral sclerosis, clinico-anatomic study of 53 cases. Arch. Neurol. Psychiat. *69*:171–192, 1953.

81. Lichtenstein, B. W.: "Spinal dysraphism." Spina bifida and myelodysplasia. Arch. Neurol. Psychiat. *44*:792–810, 1940.

82. Lipton, H. L., and Teasdall, R. D.: Acute transverse myelopathy in adults. Arch. Neurol. *28*:252–257, 1973.

83. Logue, V.: Thoracic intervertebral disc prolapse with spinal cord compression. J. Neurol. Neurosurg. Psychiat. *15*:227–241, 1952.

84. Lombardi, G., and Passerini, A.: Spinal cord tumors. Radiology *76*:381–392, 1961.

85. Lorber, J.: Results of treatment of myelomeningocele. Devel. Med. Child. Neurol. *13*:279–303, 1971.

86. Lorber, J.: Spina bifida cystica. Arch. Dis. Child. *47*:854–873, 1972.

87. Love, J. G.: Protruded intervertebral disks. Surg. Gynec. Obst. *77*:497–509, 1943.

88. Love, J. G.: The differential diagnosis of intraspinal tumors and protruded intervertebral disks and their surgical treatment. J. Neurosurg. *1*:275–290, 1944.

89. Love, J. G., and Schorn, V. G.: Thoracic-disk protrusions. J.A.M.A. *191*:627–631, 1965.

90. Luessenhop, A. J., and Dela Cruz, T.: The surgical excision of spinal intradural vascular malformations. J. Neurosurg. *30*:552–559, 1969.

91. Mackay, R. P.: Course and prognosis in amyotrophic lateral sclerosis. Arch. Neurol. *8*:117–127, 1963.

92. Markham, J. W., Lynge, H. N., and Stahlman, G.: The syndrome of spontaneous spinal epidural hematoma. J. Neurosurg, *26*:334–342, 1967.

93. Masucci, E. F., and Kurtzke, J. F.: Diagnostic criteria for the Guillain-Barré syndrome. J. Neurol. Sci. *13*:483–501, 1971.

94. McFarlin, D. E., Strober, W., and Waldmann, T. A.: Ataxia-telangiectasia. Medicine *51*:281–314, 1972.

95. McIlroy, W. J., and Richardson, J. C.: Syringomyelia. Canad. Med. Assn. J. *93*:731–734, 1965.

96. Meadows, J. C., Marsden, C. D., and Harriman, D. G. F.: Chronic spinal muscular atrophy in adults. Part 1: The Kugelberg-Welander syndrome; pages 527–550. Part II: Other forms; pages 551–566. J. Neurol. Sci., Volume 9, 1969.

97. Merritt, H. H.: A Textbook of Neurology, 4th ed. Philadelphia, Lea & Febiger, 1968.

98. Meyer, J. S., and Barron, D. W.: Apraxia of gait: A clinico-physiological study. Brain *83*:261–284, 1960.

99. Mixter, W. J., and Barr, J. S.: Rupture of the intervertebral disc with involvement of the spinal canal. New Eng. J. Med. *211*:210–215, 1934.

100. Moe, J. H.: Fundamentals of the scoliosis problem for the general practitioner. Postgrad. Med. *23*:518–532, 1958.

101. Moe, J. H.: In American Academy of Orthopaedic Surgeons (Instructional Course Lectures), pp. 196–240 (Vol. 18), Symposium on the Spine. Cleveland, Ohio, 1967. St. Louis, C. V. Mosby Company, 1969.

102. Moersch, F. P., Craig, W. McK., and Christoferson, L. A.: Spinal cord tumors with minimal neurologic findings. Neurol. *1*:39–47, 1951.

103. Muellner, S. R., Lornan, J., and Alexander, L.: The urinary bladder in multiple sclerosis. J. Urol. *68*:230–236, 1952.

104. Mulder, D. W.: The clinical syndrome of amyotrophic lateral sclerosis. Proc. Staff Mtgs. Mayo Clin. *32*:427–436, 1957.

105. Mulder, D. W., Calverley, J. R., and Miller, R. H.:

Autogenous mononeuropathy: Diagnosis, treatment, and clinical significance. Med. Clin. N. Amer. *44*:989–999, 1960.

106. Mullins, G. M., Flynn, J. P. G., El-Mahdi, A. M., et al.: Malignant lymphoma of the spinal epidural space. Ann. Int. Med. *74*:416–423, 1971.

107. Newman, M. J. D.: Racemose angioma of the spinal cord. Quart. J. Med. *28*:97–108, 1959.

108. Nordgren, R. E., Markesbery, W. R., Fukuda, K., et al.: Seven cases of cerebromedullospinal disconnection: The "locked-in" syndrome. Neurology *21*:1140–1148, 1971.

109. Ommaya, A. K., DiChiro, G., and Doppman, J.: Ligation of arterial supply in the treatment of spinal cord arteriovenous malformations. J. Neurosurg. *30*:679–692, 1969.

110. Osler, W. E.: Diseases of the nervous system. *In* Modern Medicine. Philadelphia. Lea & Febiger, 1910, p. 840.

111. Padget, D.: Development of so-called dysraphism; with embryologic evidence of clinical Arnold-Chiari and Dandy-Walker malformations. Johns Hopkins Med. J. *130*:127–165, 1972.

112. Paine, R. S., and Byers, R. K.: Transverse myelopathy in childhood. Am. J. Dis. Child. *85*:151–163, 1953.

113. Paine, K. W. E., and Haung, P. W. H.: Lumbar disc syndrome. J. Neurosurg. *37*:75–82, 1972.

114. Palmer, J. J.: Radiation myelopathy. Brain *95*:109–122, 1972.

115. Plum, F.: Bladder dysfunction. Mod. Trends Neurosurg. *III*,151–172, 1962.

116. Posner, J. B.: Neurological complications of systemic cancer. Med. Clin. N. Amer. *55*:625–646, 1971.

117. Rabe, E. F.: The hypotonic infant. J. Pediat. *64*:422–440, 1964.

118. Raff, M. C., and Asbury, A. K.: Ischemic mononeuropathy and mononeuropathy multiplex in diabetes mellitus. New Eng. J. Med. *279*:17–22, 1968.

119. Raff, M. C., Sangalang, V., and Asbury, A. K.: Ischemic mononeuropathy multiplex associated with diabetes mellitus. Arch. Neurol. *18*:487–499, 1968.

120. Rothman, R. H.: The clinical syndrome of lumbar disc disease. Ortho. Clin. N. Amer. *2*:463–475, 1971.

121. Rubin, P.: Extradural spinal cord compression by tumor. Radiology *93*:1243–1260, 1969.

122. Russell, M. L., Gordon, D. A., Ogryzlo, M. A., et al.: The cauda equina syndrome of ankylosing spondylitis. Ann. Intern. Med. *78*:551–554, 1973.

123. Russman, B. S., and Kazi, K. H.: Spinal epidural hematoma and the Brown-Séquard syndrome. Neurology *21*:1066–1068, 1971.

124. Schneider, R. C., and Schemm, G. W.: Vertebral artery insufficiency in acute and chronic spinal trauma. J. Neurosurg. *18*:348–360, 1961.

125. Schneider, R. C., Thompson, J. M., and Bebin, J.: The syndrome of acute central cervical spinal cord injury. J. Neurol. Neurosurg. Psychiat. *21*:216–227, 1958.

126. Shy, G. M., and Drager, G. A.: A neurological syndrome associated with orthostatic hypotension. Arch. Neurol. *2*:511–527, 1960.

127. Simeone, F. A.: The modern treatment of thoracic disc disease. Ortho. Clin. N. Amer. *2*:453–462, 1971.

128. Skillman, J. J., Zervas, N. J., Weintraub, R. M., et al.: Paraplegia after resection of aneurysms of the abdominal aorta. New Eng. J. Med. *281*:422–425, 1969.

129. Smith, B. H., Ramakrishna, T., and Schlagenhauff, R. B.: Familial brachial neuropathy. Neurology *21*:941–945, 1971.

130. Smith, R.: An evaluation of surgical treatment for spinal cord compression due to metastatic carcinoma. J. Neurol. Neurosurg. Psychiat. *28*:152–158, 1965.

131. Sparling, H. J., Jr., Adams, R. D., and Parker, F.: Involvement of the nervous system by malignant lymphoma. Medicine *26*:285–332, 1947.

132. Spillane, J. D.: Three cases of achondroplasia with neurological complications J. Neurol. Neurosurg. Psychiat. *15*:246–252, 1952.

133. Stein, S., Schut, L., and Borns, P.: Lacunar skull deformity (Lükenschädel) and intelligence in myelomeningocele. J. Neurosurg. *41*:10–13. 1974.

134. Symonds, C. P., and Meadows, S. P: Compression of the spinal cord in the neighborhood of the foramen magnum. Brain *60*:52–84, 1937.

135. Tachdjian, M. O., and Matson, D. D.: Orthopaedic aspects of intraspinal tumors in infants and children. J. Bone Joint Surg. *47A*:233–248, 1965.

136. Thomas, J. E., and Howard, F. M.: Segmental zoster paresis — a disease profile. Neurology *22*:459–466, 1972.

137. Thompson, G. B.: Dissecting aortic aneurysm with infarction of the spinal cord. Brain *79*:111–118, 1956.

138. Torma, T.: Malignant tumors of the spine and the spinal extradural space. Acta Chir. Scand. Suppl. 225:1957.

139. Tsairis, P., Dych, P. J., and Mulder, D. W.: Natural history of brachial plexus neuropathy. Arch. Neurol. *27*:109–117, 1972.

140. Urschel, H. C., and Razzuk, M. A.: Management of the thoracic-outlet syndrome. New Engl. J. Med. *286*:1140–1143, 1972.

141. Victor, M., and Lear, A.: Subacute combined degeneration of the spinal cord. Am. J. Med. *20*:896–911, 1956.

142. Walsh, M. N., and Love, J. G.: The syndrome of protruded intervertebral disk. Proc. Staff Meet. Mayo Clin. *14*:230–234, 1939.

143. Webb, J. H., Craig, W. McK., and Kernohan, J. W.: Intraspinal neoplasms in the cervical region. J. Neurosurg. *10*:360–366, 1953.

144. Wiederholt, W. C., Mulder, D. W., and Lambert, E. H.: The Landry-Guillain-Barré-Strohl syndrome of polyradiculoneuropathy: historical review report on 97 patients and present concepts. Mayo Clin. Proc. *39*:427–451, 1964.

145. Wilkinson, M.: Cervical Spondylosis: Its Early Diagnosis and Treatment. Philadelphia, W. B. Saunders Co., 1971.

146. Williams, H. M., Diamond, H. D., Craver, L. F., et al.: Neurological Complications of Lymphomas and Leukemias. Springfield, Ill., Charles C Thomas, 1959.

147. Wolman, L., and Bradshaw, P.: Spinal cord embolism. J. Neurol. Neurosurg. Psychiat. *30*:446–454, 1967.

148. Woltman, H. W., Kernohan, J. W., Adson, A. W., et al.: Intramedullary tumors of the spinal cord and gliomas of intradural portion of filum terminale. Arch. Neurol. Psychiat. *65*:378–395, 1951.

149. Wright, R. L.: Malignant tumors in the spinal extradural space: results of surgical treatment. Ann. Surg. *157*:227–231, 1963.

CHAPTER 4

Surgical Approaches to the Spine

ROLLIN M. JOHNSON, M.D.

WAYNE O. SOUTHWICK, M.D.
Yale University School of Medicine

FUNCTION AND SURGICAL ANATOMY OF THE NECK

FUNCTION OF THE NECK

The neck is an extraordinarily versatile link between the head and body that is uniquely suited to three vital functions. It houses the spinal cord and protects it from injury; like a universal joint it offers great flexibility in three planes; and it acts as a shock absorber to protect the brain from the rougher movements of the rest of the body. The normal neck moves as much as 130 degrees in flexion and extension (Hohl, 1964; Johnson et al., 1980, Lysell, 1969), 75 degrees in lateral bending, and 160 degrees in rotation (Johnson et al., 1980). Under normal conditions, the ligaments and bony elements of the vertebrae protect the spinal cord and nerve roots even in these extremes of motion. As the head accounts for only seven per cent of body weight (Ruff, 1950; Verbiest, 1969), the neck is not required to support large forces; rather, it serves as a flexible link, providing the movement needed to use the senses of sight, smell, and hearing.

In the developing embryo, the spinal axis forms a large "C" curve, as shown in Figure 4–1. However, as the spine matures, it becomes a double "S" curve, as viewed in the sagittal plane, with two segments of the curve convex to the front and two convex posteriorly. This double "S" shape appears to act as a springlike shock absorber, an effect that is enhanced by the cushioning of the intervertebral articulations. The posterior convex curves, at the thorax and sacrum, are the most rigid areas of the spine, whereas the lordotic curves of the cervical and lumbar levels are more flexible, accounting for a greater proportion of the spine's motion. This difference in flexibility appears to predispose the more mobile segments to the effects of injury and degeneration. The most common sites of disc degeneration occur in the lower cervical and lower lumbar segments, just above the more rigid thoracic and sacral levels. In the lower cervical spine, the C5-6 articulation has the greatest range of sagittal plane motion (Johnson et al., 1980), and this is the cervical level that is subject to the highest incidence of spinal injury and disc degeneration (Bosch, 1972; Simeone and Rothman, 1975).

The cervical spine has six degrees of freedom of motion. The traditionally appreciated motions are flexion and extension (sagittal plane), lateral bending (frontal plane), and rotation. In addition, the spine may distract or compress along the longitudinal axis,

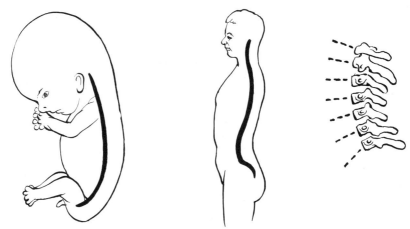

Figure 4–1. The spine begins as a "C" curve in the embryo and develops a double "S" curve by adulthood. The cervical and lumbar curves are convex anteriorly and are more mobile, accounting for the principal movements of the vertebrae. The lower cervical intervertebral discs are angled obliquely forward. (From Robinson, R. A., and Southwick, W. O.: Surgical Approaches to the Cervical Spine. *In* the American Academy of Orthopaedic Surgeons: Instructional Course Lectures, Vol. XVII. St. Louis, The C. V. Mosby Co., 1960.)

translate anteriorly or posteriorly along the sagittal plane, or move laterally along the frontal plane. As demonstrated by Fielding (1964) and White (1969), these latter motions are fine movements that occur in conjunction with normal flexion and extension. However, in clinical practice, roentgenograms are required to appreciate these small degrees of "coupled" motion (Fig. 4–2). For example, in normal flexion the facets of the upper vertebra glide forward and superiorly, producing rotation of the upper vertebra in the sagittal plane, longitudinal distraction of the posterior elements, compression of the disc space anteriorly, and anterior displacement of the upper vertebra. Thus, flexion is the result of "coupled" motion in three planes. The phenomenon of "coupling" one motion with another has been extensively studied in the thoracic, cadaver, bone–ligament construct by Panjabi and coworkers (1976) and White (1969).

Sagittal plane motion at the individual intervertebral articulations has been studied in the normal young adult (Table 4–1; Johnson et al., 1980). The greatest flexion and extension is found at the occipitoatlantal joint (25 degrees, mean) and in the lower cervical segments between the fifth and sixth cervical vertebrae (21 degrees). The least flexion and extension is found between the second and third cervical vertebrae and at the transition between the lowest cervical and first thoracic segment. Overall, the range of flexion from the neutral position almost equals extension. However, at the occipitoatlantal joint, the range of extension is significantly greater than

flexion, whereas in the lower cervical segments, relatively more flexion is observed.

Accurate measurements of lateral bending and rotation at the individual segmental levels have been hampered by inadequate methods of measuring these motions clinically. Hohl (1964) found on cineroentgenographic studies that no rotation or lateral bending occurred at the occipitoatlantal joint and that approximately half of the normal cervical rotation occurs at the atlantoaxial joint. Lysell (1969) studied motion in human cadaver spines and found that a total of 90 degrees of rotation was permitted in the lower cervical spine, coupled with 48 degrees of lateral bending. He also found that a total of 98 degrees of lateral bending was permitted in the lower cervical spine, coupled with 56 degrees of rotation. The obligate coupling of lateral

TABLE 4–1. SAGITTAL PLANE FLEXION-EXTENSION OF THE NORMAL ADULT CERVICAL SPINE 20 TO 40 YEARS OF AGE AT EACH SEGMENTAL LEVEL

Cervical Level	Mean	± 2S. D.*	Low	High
Occiput-C1	25.5	± 11.2	15	41
C1-2	15.6	± 8.8	4	25
C2-3	12.0	± 5.1	6	19
C3-4	17.5	± 6.7	10	25
C4-5	19.5	± 6.4	10	26
C5-6	20.8	± 7.3	13	29
C6-7	20.5	± 6.9	13	29
C7-T1	11.9	± 6.1	4	19

*± 2 standard deviations of the mean.

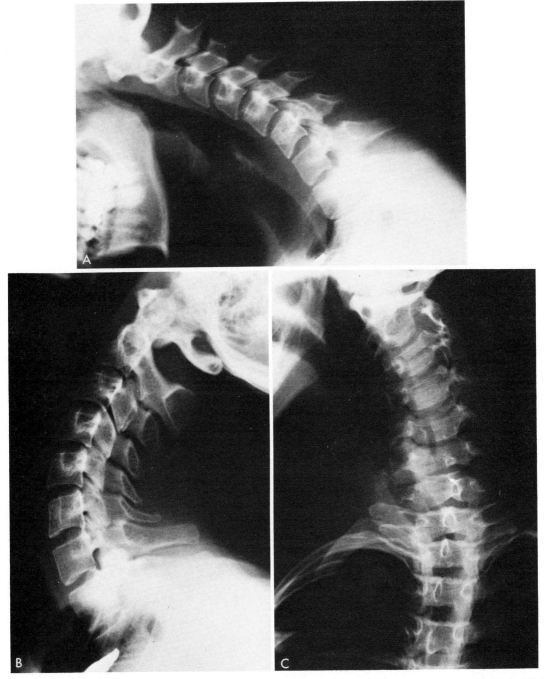

Figure 4–2. Radiographs of the cervical spine in maximal flexion *(A)*, extension *(B)*, and rotation to the right *(C)*. In flexion *(A)*, the facets glide anteriorly and superiorly on the facets below, resulting in rotation of the vertebra in the sagittal plane. Concomitantly, the posterior elements separate, the intervertebral disc is compressed anteriorly, and one vertebra moves forward horizontally on the vertebra below. In extension *(B)*, the reverse occurs with distraction at the intervertebral disc anteriorly. In rotation *(C)*, there is obligate coupling of lateral bending with rotation, as the facet on one side moves forward and superiorly while the opposite facet moves posteriorly and inferiorly.

bending with rotation is due to the 45 degree oblique relationship of the facet joints in the sagittal plane. In rotation, one superior facet glides forward and superiorly, and the other glides posteriorly and inferiorly (Fig. 4–2C). Thus, as one vertebral body rotates on the other, it also tilts in the frontal plane to produce lateral bending.

In summary, all the cervical vertebral articulations contribute to flexion and extension. One-half of the total rotation occurs at the atlantoaxial joint, and the other half occurs in the lower five articulations. Lateral bending occurs primarily in the lower cervical segments, from the second to the seventh vertebrae.

SURGICAL ANATOMY OF THE NECK

Triangles and Surface Anatomy of the Neck

For convenience of description, the neck is divided into two large triangles by the prominent sternomastoid muscle (Fig. 4–3). These are subdivided by the digastric and omohyoid muscles into several smaller triangles, which take their names from local anatomic features, such as the digastric, carotid, or subclavian triangles.

Certain surface landmarks are useful surgically in localizing the levels of the vertebrae. The third cervical vertebra is at the level of the hyoid bone, the fourth is opposite the upper border of the thyroid cartilage, and the sixth lies opposite the cricoid cartilage, a prominent ring palpable just below the thyroid cartilage. Posteriorly, the first prominence below the occiput is the second cervical spinous process. This is a large, bifid structure, which is ordinarily buried between the paracervical muscles but may be felt with firm pressure over the midline. Below this the sixth cervical spinous process is often palpable, and the seventh is most prominent.

Laterally, the transverse processes may be palpated through the sternomastoid muscle in the upper neck. The transverse process of the atlas is the most prominent transverse process and is found just below and somewhat anterior to the mastoid process. To clearly separate this from the skull, it may be necessary to rotate the neck. With rotation, the atlas will appear to move independently from the

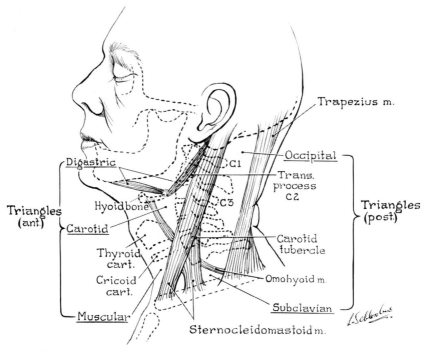

Figure 4–3. Triangles and surface anatomy of the neck. The transverse process of the first cervical vertebra is palpable below the mastoid process deep to the sternomastoid muscle. The hyoid bone is at the level of the third cervical vertebra, the thyroid cartilage opposite the fourth vertebra, and the cricoid cartilage opposite the sixth cervical vertebra. (From Robinson, R. A., and Southwick, S. O.: Surgical Approaches to the Cervical Spine. *In* the American Academy of Orthopaedic Surgeons: Instructional Course Lectures, Vol. XVII. St. Louis, The C. V. Mosby Co., 1960.)

skull. By following a gentle curve anteriorly and down, one can palpate all the transverse processes of the neck. Ordinarily, these are so similar and their margins so obscure that one cannot accurately identify the vertebral level below the atlas from the lateral side of the neck.

Skin, Platysma, Superficial Nerves, and Veins

Anteriorly, the skin of the neck is mobile, soft, and thin and has an excellent blood supply. The anterior skin creases are transverse in the lower neck but tend to run obliquely upward near the mandible. Incisions in the anterior neck should follow these skin creases as these will heal more easily with a less noticeable scar than incisions that traverse these planes. The skin, subcutaneous fascia, and platysma muscle are mobile, allowing significant distortion with retraction. The skin of the back of the neck is much thicker and less mobile than the front, and longitudinal incisions here tend to heal with prominent

scars that may spread because of tension from the trapezius muscle.

Just beneath the skin is a thin layer of superficial fascia that contains the platysma muscles anteriorly. The platysma muscles are rhomboid in shape and extend from the mandible to the superficial fascia over the chest and from the midline to the lateral border of the sternomastoid muscle. Their motor nerve supply is derived from the cervical branch of the facial nerve, and the anterior cutaneous nerves of the neck pierce them to innervate the skin. In anterior surgical exposures the platysma layer should be identified and its muscle fibers cut transversely or split longitudinally. These should be closed as a separate layer to avoid separation with healing and an ugly scar.

Beneath the platysma and embedded within the superficial layers of the deep cervical fascia are four superficial nerves of the neck, which emerge behind the posterior border of the sternomastoid muscle at its midpoint (Fig. 4–4). These nerves fan out radially and carry sensory fibers to the posterior occi-

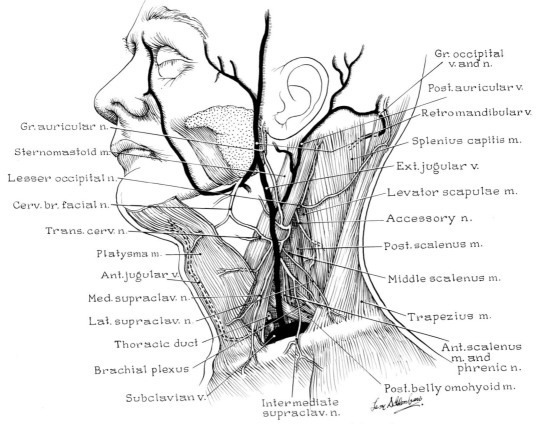

Figure 4–4. Superficial veins and nerves of the neck.

put, the front and sides of the neck, and the cape over the clavicle and upper chest. The lesser occipital nerve is derived from the second cervical root and supplies the skin over the lateral occipital region. The great auricular nerve arises from the second and third cervical roots and appears slightly lower, behind the sternomastoid muscle. It then arches over this muscle, running parallel with the external jugular vein and supplies the area over the parotid gland and the skin about the ear. The anterior cervical cutaneous nerve, arising from the second and third cervical roots, runs anteriorly across the sternomastoid muscle, supplying the region around the hyoid bone. The supraclavicular nerve arises from the third and fourth cervical roots and has three main branches, supplying the skin over the clavicle and anterior trapezius.

Short transverse incisions in the anterior cervical triangle rarely transect these major cutaneous nerve trunks or cause permanent numbness, but longitudinal incisions in the anterior triangle or transverse incisions posterior to the sternomastoid muscle may divide these nerves. The greater and lesser occipital nerves and the great auricular nerve arise from the second cervical nerve root. This root passes between the ring of the atlas and lamina of the axis as it emerges from the spinal canal. With fractures of the posterior arch of the atlas, odontoid process, or neural arch of the axis, this second root may be irritated, causing pain over the back of the head, behind the ear, or over the parotid gland. This may be a valuable diagnostic symptom that should arouse suspicion in patients having a history of injury and pain in these locations.

Beneath the platysma and in the same plane as the superficial nerves lies the external jugular vein (Fig. 4–4). It is formed by the posterior and auricular vein and a branch of the posterior facial vein, which unite below the ear lobe to run vertically caudad. The external jugular vein crosses the sternomastoid muscle at its midpoint, passing into the posterior triangle of the neck, where it pierces the superficial layer of the deep cervical fascia posterior and lateral to the clavicular head of the sternomastoid muscle. The anterior jugular vein is formed by several small veins in the region of the protuberance of the mandible and descends just lateral to the midline to enter the suprasternal space. Just above the sternum it crosses laterally and deep to the sternomastoid muscle to terminate either in the external jugular or in the subclavian vein.

Communicating veins, between the anterior and external jugular veins, pass through the suprasternal space by means of a separate reflection of the superficial layer of the deep fascia.

Fasciae of the Neck

The fascial layers of the neck surround many major anatomic structures and separate these into discrete compartments. These fascial planes may be used as landmarks or paths to guide the surgeon on a safe and simple course through the front of the neck to the vertebral bodies beneath. The fascial layers enclose certain vital structures, such as those of the carotid sheath, and protect the contents from injury during surgical dissection. In addition, the natural cleavage planes between these fascial layers provide pathways for safe dissection between these complex structures. For example, in the anterior approach to the cervical vertebral bodies, the recurrent laryngeal nerve lies in potential jeopardy. This nerve lies deep to the visceral layer of the deep cervical fascia, however. By dissecting within the natural cleavage plane between the alar and visceral fascia and not within the visceral fascial envelope, this nerve may be safely bypassed and there is no need to identify it. Similar protection is provided by the alar fascia surrounding the carotid structures and the prevertebral fascia protecting the phrenic nerve. However, it is important to know the relationship of these fascial layers, using the natural cleavage planes and not violate the integrity of certain fascial sheaths. Grodinsky and Holyoke (1938) described these fascial layers in their classic article.

The cervical fascia is divided into one superficial and four deep layers (Figs. 4–5 and 4–6). The superficial fascia is a continuous plane that surrounds the neck in the subcutaneous tissue and envelops the platysma in its deep portion. The superficial layer of the deep cervical fascia surrounds the neck and encloses the sternomastoid and trapezius muscles. The middle layers of the deep cervical fascia enclose the strap muscles and omohyoid in the anterior cervical region and extend as far laterally as the scapula. The deepest component of this middle layer is the visceral fascia, which surrounds the larynx, trachea, esophagus, and thyroid. The alar fascia spreads like two wings behind the esophagus and surrounds the carotid sheath structures laterally. The deepest layer is the

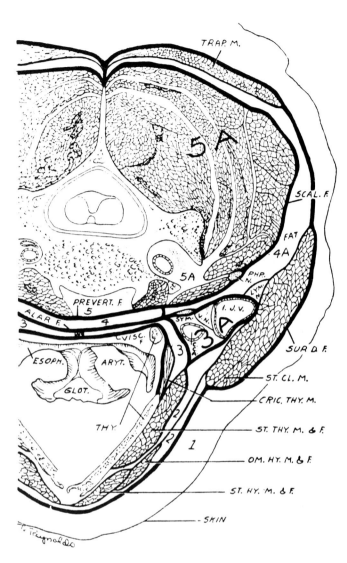

Figure 4–5. Cross-section of the fascial compartments of the neck at the level of the thyroid cartilage. Alar F., alar fascia; prevert. F., prevertebral fascia; Scal. F., scalenus fascia; Sup. D. F., superficial layer of deep fascia; Visc. F., visceral fascia. (From Grodinsky, M., and Holyoke, E. A.: Fasciae and fascial spaces of head, neck and adjacent regions. Am. J. Anat., 63:367, 1938. Reproduced with permission.)

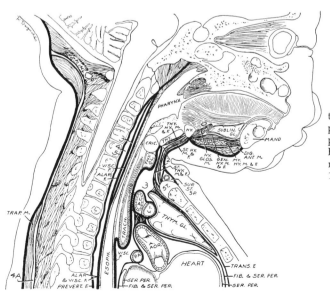

Figure 4–6. Fascial compartments of the neck in the sagittal plane. Note that space "4" between the prevertebral and alar fascia is continuous with the posterior mediastinum. (From Grodinsky, M., and Holyoke, E. A.: Fasciae and fascial spaces of head, neck, and adjacent regions. Am. J. Anat., 63:367, 1938. Reproduced with permission.)

prevertebral fascia, which surrounds the vertebrae and paraspinal muscles, enclosing structures such as the phrenic nerve and scalene muscles.

The superficial fascia is a continuous subcutaneous sheet that surrounds the neck and extends from the head into the thorax. This fascial plane is relatively loose in the front of the neck and contains the platysma in its deeper portion. The next fascial layer is the thicker superficial layer of the deep fascia, which surrounds the neck, fusing with the intermuscular septum posteriorly and the spinous processes of the vertebrae. It splits to surround the sternomastoid and trapezius muscles. Just above the sternum it divides to form the suprasternal or Burn's space, inserting on the anterior and posterior margins of the sternum, and laterally it fuses with the clavicle, acromion, and scapular spine. The superficial nerves and the anterior and external jugular veins are partially contained within the superficial fibers of this plane. Superiorly, at the hyoid, the superficial layer of the deep fascia fuses with the middle layers of fascia.

These extend beyond the hyoid as one common layer of fascia to cover the muscles of the submental triangle and then split to form the capsules of the maxillary and parotid glands.

The suprasternal or Burn's space is a useful landmark for transecting the insertions of the sternomastoid muscle above the sternum and clavicle. Henry (1957) and Nanson (1957) described an approach to the lower cervical and upper thoracic spine through the clavicular head of the sternomastoid muscle (see Part II, Anterior Cervical Approaches). The subclavian and internal jugular veins lie immediately behind this structure and may be injured unless carefully protected. The potential space between the two layers of fascia may be developed by blunt dissection, and the muscle may be transected with a finger, protecting these structures beneath (Fig. 4–7).

The middle layer of the deep cervical fascia is divided into three parts. The first of these is called the omohyoid-sternohyoid layer and forms a sheath around these muscles. Superiorly it attaches to the hyoid, inferiorly to the posterior border of the sternum

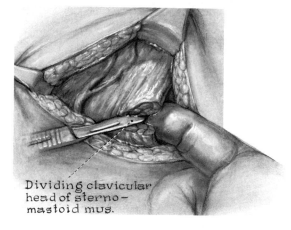

Dividing clavicular head of sterno-mastoid mus.

Figure 4–7. Blunt dissection within Burn's space to protect the structures within the carotid sheath and subclavian vein. The subclavian and internal jugular veins and the carotid artery lie beneath the sternomastoid muscle and can be injured during division of the sternomastoid in approaches through this structure. The potential space between two layers of the deep cervical fascia is developed by blunt dissection, and the muscle is transected with the finger protecting these structures beneath.

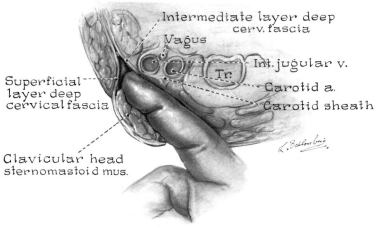

Intermediate layer deep cerv. fascia

Vagus

Int. jugular v.

Tr

Carotid a.

Superficial layer deep cervical fascia

Carotid sheath

Clavicular head sternomastoid mus.

and clavicle, and laterally it fuses with the deep surface of the sternomastoid sheath, a portion of the superficial layer of the deep fascia. Over the midportion of the omohyoid muscle, this fascia becomes thicker, forming a pulley for the omohyoid, which allows this muscle to change dissections as it proceeds laterally to the scapula, holding the central section of this muscle down. The second part of the middle cervical fascia is the relatively thin sternothyroid-thyrohyoid layer, which surrounds these muscles. It too inserts superiorly on the hyoid, inferiorly on the sternum and clavicle, and laterally fuses with the deep surface of the sternomastoid sheath. The third portion of the middle layer of the cervical fascia is the visceral fascia, which surrounds the trachea, esophagus, and thyroid. Posterior to the pharynx, it ascends to the base of the skull, and anteriorly it attaches to the thyroid cartilage and hyoid. Posteriorly and in the upper thorax, it fuses with the alar fascia, surrounds the intrathoracic portion of the trachea and esophagus, and is continuous with the fibrous pericardium. The visceral layer is important as it protects the recurrent laryngeal nerves and esophagus from injury during anterior exposures of the cervical spine.

The alar fascia lies behind the esophagus and spreads laterally as a sheet to surround the carotid structures like two wings. The alar fascia fuses with the prevertebral fascia beneath, over the transverse processes of the vertebrae. This tends to limit the lateral spread of a midline infection within this potential space. Between the alar and prevertebral fascial planes lies a loose potential space that extends from the atlas to the posterior mediastinum deep within the thorax. This space "four" of Grodinsky and Holyoke (1938) is often referred to as the "danger space," as retropharyngeal or prevertebral infections may extend through it into the posterior mediastinum.

The prevertebral fascia surrounds the vertebral bodies, the scalene and paravertebral muscles, and the phrenic nerves. Posteriorly this fascia fuses with the intermuscular septum and inserts on the vertebral spinous processes. Inferiorly it is continuous with the lumbodorsal fascia.

In approaching the middle and lower cervical vertebrae from the front (Part II), one divides the superficial fascia and the platysma muscle. The next layer is the well-developed superficial layer of the deep cervical fascia, which is divided longitudinally by sharp dis-

section at the anterior margin of the sternomastoid muscle. Beneath, the two thin muscular layers of the middle cervical fascia may be divided by finger dissection, medial to the carotid sheath. The plane of dissection then follows the natural cleavage plane between the visceral and alar fascia to the midline, behind the esophagus and over the vertebral bodies. This dissection is made easier if these sheaths are left intact protecting the esophagus and recurrent laryngeal nerves within the visceral fascia from injury. Finally, the alar and prevertebral layers must be divided by sharp, longitudinal dissection to expose the vertebral bodies beneath.

An understanding of the fascial planes of the neck also helps in localizing the source of cervical infections. The prevertebral and alar fascial sheaths are fused laterally over the transverse processes and not in the midline. Therefore, an infection of vertebral origin usually occurs in the midline, spreading laterally to either side. If this infection then breaks through the prevertebral fascia, it may spread inferiorly into the posterior mediastinum through the space between the alar and prevertebral layers. On the other hand, the visceral fascia is usually fused to the alar fascia in the midline so that abscesses of pharyngeal origin tend to occur on one side lateral to the midline. Therefore, retropharyngeal abscesses that occupy a central position are often of vertebral origin, whereas those that are eccentric to one side more commonly arise from the pharynx, limited by these fascial connections.

Anterior Neck Muscles

The superficial muscles of the anterior triangle of the neck are divided by the hyoid bone (Fig. 4–8). Those above the hyoid in the digastric triangle are the stylohyoid, the anterior and posterior belly of the digastric, which is attached to the hyoid bone by a sling at its midportion, and the mylohyoid arising from the mandible. These are innervated by the hypoglossal nerve, which swings downward along the carotid sheath and dives deep to the stylohyoid and posterior belly of the digastric in company with the lingual artery. These structures are not normally encountered except in anterior exposures to the upper cervical vertebrae.

Below the hyoid are the strap muscles, which are attached to the hyoid, thyroid car-

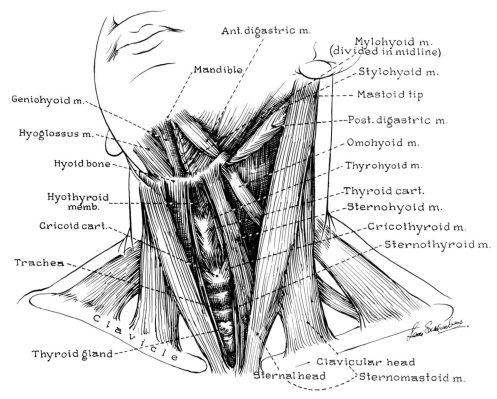

Figure 4–8. Superficial muscles of the anterior neck. The sternomastoid divides the neck into the anterior and posterior triangles, and the hyoid presents a natural division between the muscles of the digastric triangle and the infrahyoid or strap muscles.

tilage, and sternum. The strap muscles are found in two layers: The superficial layer includes the sternohyoid and omohyoid, and the deep layer includes the thyrohyoid and sternothyroid muscles. These infrahyoid muscles are innervated by the ansa hypoglossi as it proceeds along the carotid sheath. Branches from the ansa arch forward to the muscles in the upper neck and can be retracted forward with care in exposures of the middle and lower neck. However, these branches will be stretched or divided in exposures to the upper cervical vertebrae medial to the carotid sheath.

The sternomastoid muscle is the most prominent muscle of the neck and divides the neck into its anterior and posterior triangles. It arises by two heads, the medial one from the manubrium of the sternum and the lateral one from the clavicle. The muscle inserts on the mastoid process in the lateral half of the superior nuchal line of the occipital bone. It is innervated by the spinal accessory nerve, which reaches the upper third of this muscle

along its deep surface. The accessory nerve then emerges from behind the midportion of the sternomastoid and descends beneath the superficial layer of deep fascia to innervate the trapezius. This nerve should be identified and protected in approaches through the posterior triangle of the neck. Immediately subjacent to the sternomastoid muscle is the carotid sheath, surrounded by its alar fascia. Henry (1957) and Whitesides (1966) describe an approach in which the sternomastoid muscle is everted to expose structures of surgical importance in the lateral cervical spine, including the brachial plexus and vertebral artery. The accessory nerve must be identified and protected during this eversion, as described in Part II.

The deepest muscles lie along the anterior surface of the vertebrae, covering the lateral aspect of the vertebral bodies and filling the hollow between the bodies and adjacent transverse processes (Fig. 4–9). The longus colli is the most central of these muscles, extending from the atlas to the third thoracic vertebra. It does not cover the centers of the vertebral bodies except at the atlas. The longus capitis lies just lateral to the longus colli and is primarily a flexor of the head.

The sympathetic trunk lies directly over the longus colli and capitis in a loose reflection of alar fascia at the carotid sheath. Ordinarily, the sympathetic trunk is easily dissected from the carotid sheath and remains with the longus colli and capitis muscles when the carotid

structures are displaced anteriorly. The sympathetic trunk and the superior cervical sympathetic ganglion should be protected in dissections of this area to prevent the development of Horner's syndrome.

Deep to the longus capitis and connecting the transverse processes at each level are the intertransverse muscles (Fig. 4–10). The anterior intertransverse muscles connect the anterior aspects of each gutterlike transverse

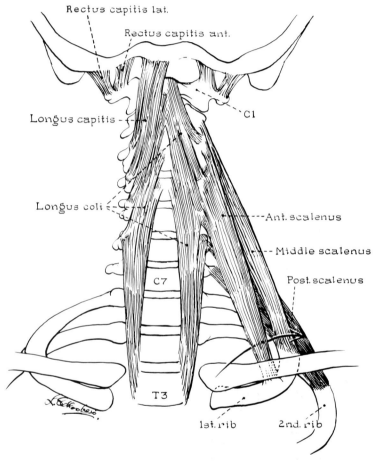

Figure 4–9. The deep muscles of the anterior neck. The deepest muscles are the longus colli and capitis, which lie along the lateral aspect of the vertebrae, filling the hollow between the bodies and adjacent transverse processes. The longus colli is a flexor of the neck and has three components: an inferior oblique part, which arises from the first three thoracic bodies and inserts on the anterior tubercles of the fifth and sixth cervical transverse processes; the superior oblique component, which arises from the third through fifth transverse processes and inserts through a tendon on the anterior tubercle of the atlas in the midline; and the vertical component, which arises from the lower cervical and upper thoracic bodies and inserts on the upper cervical bodies from the second to the fourth vertebrae. The longus capitis lies lateral to the longus colli and is a flexor of the head. It arises from the anterior tubercles of the third through sixth cervical transverse processes and inserts on the basilar portion of the occiput. The scalene muscles arise from the tubercles of the cervical transverse processes and insert on the first and second ribs. The scalenus anterior is separated from the scalenus medius and scalenus posterior by the brachial plexus and subclavian artery. The scalenus anterior arises from the anterior tubercles of the third through the sixth vertebrae and inserts on the first rib between the subclavian artery and vein and beneath the sternomastoid and prevertebral fascia. The scalenus medius arises from the posterior tubercles of the second through sixth cervical vertebrae and inserts on the first rib. The scalenus posterior is often a subdivision of the medius, which inserts on the second rib.

process, one to the next, and the posterior component connects the transverse processes posteriorly, behind the nerve roots. Over the upper spine two specialized muscles perform a similar function, lateral bending of the head and neck (Fig. 4–9). The rectus capitis anterior covers the atlanto-occipital joint, extending from the lateral mass of the atlas to the occipital bone. The rectus capitis lateralis extends from the transverse process of the atlas to the jugular process of the occipital bone. The scaleni and levators, which also arise from the transverse processes, will be described later.

All the capital cervical muscles are innervated by the ventral rami of the segmental cervical nerves close to their level of origin. Perry and Nickel (1959) note that all these muscles contribute to stability of the cervical spine. When these are paralyzed, the major deficits are an inability to move the head, to maintain normal posture, and to support pharyngeal or respiratory function without external support; however, the intrinsic bond between vertebrae is not lost.

The Cervical Vertebrae

The upper two cervical vertebrae and articulations are very different from those of the middle or lower cervical spine. The first cervical vertebra, or atlas, is shaped like a ring with long transverse processes extending laterally from the anterior half of this ring and a short, truncated tubercle extending from the midline posteriorly (Fig. 4–11). Unlike any of the other cervical vertebrae, the atlas has no true spinous process or body, and the bone around the ring is small and delicate in cross section. The transverse processes of the atlas extend farther laterally than any of the other cervical vertebrae, a fact that may be used to identify this vertebra in palpating the lateral sides of the neck. The occipitoatlantal joint is a shallow ball and socket joint that is elongated front to back. The occipital condyles protrude downward to form two truncated balls, which fit into the shallow and elliptical cups of the atlas (Fig. 4–11). The lateral wall of this cup is higher than the medial wall, which effectively limits lateral displacements. The ball and socket shape provides great overall stability but does permit the largest range of flexion and extension of any cervical articulation (25 degrees).

The vertebral artery leaves the transverse foramen of the atlas and curves abruptly back adjacent to the articular condyles of the atlas (Figs. 4–11 and 4–12). It then takes another sharp turn medially over the top of the first cervical ring behind the condyles. It follows a shallow groove on the surface of this ring to a

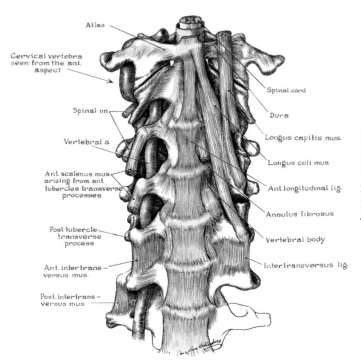

Figure 4–10. Cervical spine, ligaments, and intrinsic muscles seen from the front. Note that the vertebral artery ascends within the costotransverse foramina anterior to the nerve roots. (From Johnson, R. M., et al.: Some new observations on the functional anatomy of the lower cervical spine. Clin. Orthop., 3:192–200, 1975.)

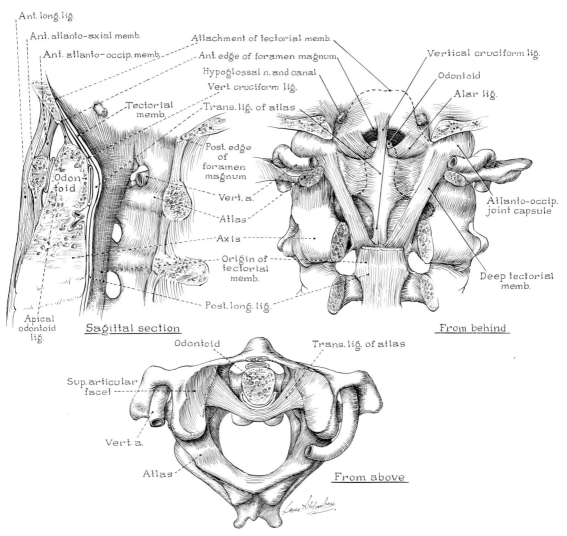

Figure 4–11. The cruciform and tectorial ligaments seen from within the spinal canal looking anteriorly, in sagittal section and from above. The cruciform ligament holds the odontoid in a sling to the anterior ring of the atlas. It is composed of a superior arm, which inserts on the basiocciput, an inferior arm, which reinforces the base of the dens, and two lateral arms, the transverse ligament. The transverse ligament inserts on the ring of the atlas and is one of the primary stabilizers of the atlantoaxial joint. This is reinforced by the tectorial and deep tectorial membranes or ligaments. The odontoid is fixed to the base of the skull through the apical odontoid and alar ligaments.

point about 2 cm. from the midline and dives into a hole in the posterior atlanto-occipital ligament, disappearing from view. In posterior fusions involving the atlas, it should be remembered that this artery and its accompanying venous plexus are less than 2 cm. from the midline.

The second cervical vertebra, or axis, serves as a transition between the upper and lower cervical segments. The lower articulations are similar to those of the middle and lower cervical spine, but the superior articula-

tions are unique. The odontoid extends upward from the second vertebral body, articulates with the anterior ring of the first vertebra, and through its ligamentous connections provides a major bond between the atlas, the first cervical ring, and the occiput. The odontoid serves as a pivot between the first and second vertebrae, permitting almost 45 degrees of rotation to each side. Because this joint is hinged at the odontoid, in front of the spinal canal, rotations in excess of this will narrow the canal and sever the cord.

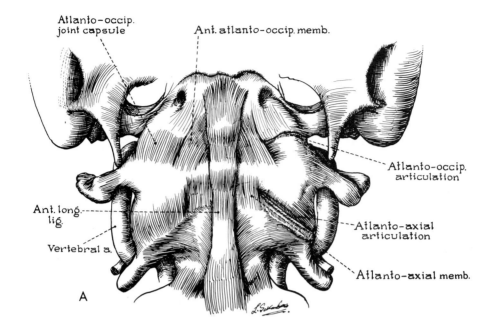

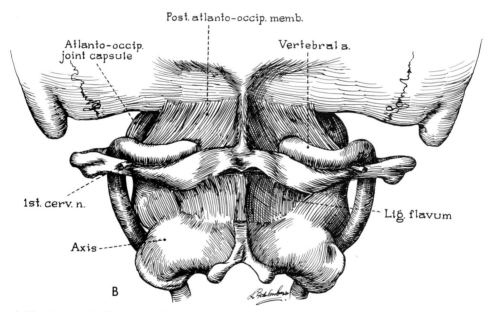

Figure 4–12.   *A,* Anterior ligaments of the upper two cervical vertebrae from the basiocciput to the axis. *B,* Posterior ligaments of the upper cervical vertebrae from the occiput to the axis.

The atlantoaxial articulations sit like sloping shoulders on the lateral masses. Each opposing surface is relatively convex, which reduces the frictional resistance at this joint, increases the range of rotation in the longitudinal axis, and permits over 15 degrees of flexion and extension and small amounts of lateral bending.

The upper two cervical nerve roots are surrounded by bone on three sides as they leave the spinal canal. The first cervical nerve root divides into a large dorsal and smaller ventral ramus before it leaves the spinal canal. These emerge from a hole in the atlanto-occipital ligament just posterior to the articular condyles between the occiput and ring of the first vertebra. The dorsal ramus proceeds beneath the vertebral artery and laterally to enter and supply the muscles of the suboccipital triangle. The smaller ventral ramus proceeds anteriorly, medial to the vertebral artery and over the transverse process. The second cervical nerve root emerges behind the atlantoaxial facet. It supplies the posterior capitocervical muscles and terminates in three major branches, the greater and lesser occipital nerves and the great auricular nerve. Irritation or trauma to this root or nerve trunks will produce pain, headache, or hyperesthesia in their dermal distribution over the occiput and about the ear.

The lower five cervical vertebrae and articulations are similar to one another. The upper pole of the vertebral body is shaped like a cup and appears to cradle the vertebral body above (Fig. 4–13). This effect is created by the joints of Luschka, which articulate with the posterolateral aspect of the vertebral body above. The transverse processes extend laterally from the posterior half of the vertebral body. These are shaped like a gutter and support the nerve roots as they leave the neural foramina. Each of the transverse processes from the first through the sixth vertebrae contains a foramen through which the vertebral arteries ascend into the head (Fig. 4–10). The transverse processes terminate in an anterior and posterior tubercle from which many of the capitocervical muscles arise. The most prominent tubercle is usually found at the sixth vertebra and is known as the carotid or Chassaignac's tubercle. Although this may be a useful landmark to determine the segmental level at surgery, there is enough anatomic variation that roentgenographic confirmation is recommended in the operating room.

The pedicles project posteriorly and laterally to the prominent pillars of the facets behind. The facet joints are angled obliquely at a 45 degree plane, front to back, and in the lower cervical spine the angle of obliquity increases to a more vertical plane. The facet joints permit a gliding motion between their articular surfaces of 4 to 6 mm. with the superior facet gliding forward and up, or backward and down with respect to the lower face. With rotation or lateral bending, the facet on one side moves forward and up and the contralateral facet moves in the opposite direction, accounting for the ''coupling'' of rotation with lateral bending.

The laminae close the spinal canal posteriorly, ending in the spinous processes behind. All of these from the second to the sixth vertebrae are normally bifid. The seventh spinous process is the most prominent projection and is usually single and not bifid.

The intervertebral neural foramina between the second and seventh cervical vertebrae are posterior and lateral to the vertebral body and anterior to the facet pillars. The superior and inferior walls of the foramen are formed by the pedicles of the two adjacent vertebrae. The posterior wall is primarily formed by the superior facet pillar. The anterior wall is formed by the vertebral body, the joint of Luschka, and the vertebral artery and vein and their investing fascia. The transverse processes extend laterally and slightly anterior from the foramina and are shaped like a trough, holding the nerve roots, ganglia, and accompanying vessels. The cervical intervertebral foramina may be visualized roentgenographically with oblique views. The right neuroforamina are outlined with a left posterior oblique roentgenogram, and the left are outlined with a right posterior oblique view.

The lower six cervical nerve roots are surrounded by bone and the intervertebral articulations as they leave the spinal canal. With degeneration of the intervertebral disc, the facet joint, or joints of Luschka, osteophytes may develop, which decrease the size

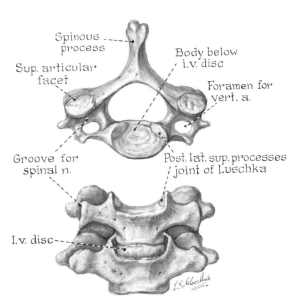

Figure 4–13. Lower cervical vertebrae, showing the relationships of the discs, facets, vertebral foramina, and joints of Luschka. (From Robinson, R. A., and Southwick, W. O.: Surgical Approaches to the Cervical Spine. *In* the American Academy of Orthopaedic Surgeons: Instructional Course Lectures, Vol. XVII. St. Louis, The C. V. Mosby Co., 1960.)

of the foramina. Osteophytes or extravasated disc material may impinge directly on the nerve roots, as demonstrated by Hadley (1957), or they may irritate adjacent soft tissues, which react with edema and secondarily compress or irritate the nerve roots.

Ligaments of the Upper Cervical Spine

The vertebrae and articulations of the upper two cervical vertebrae are morphologically and functionally very different from those of the lower cervical elements. The anterior longitudinal ligament is the superior extension of this same ligament in the lower spine. It narrows appreciably over the body of the second cervical vertebra, is attached to the anterior tubercle of the first cervical ring, and inserts on the basiocciput (Fig. 4–12A). Beneath this is the anterior atlanto-occipital membrane or ligament, which joins the superior ring of the first vertebra to the basiocciput. At the next lower level, the anterior atlantoaxial ligament joins the inferior ring of the atlas to the upper body of the axis. Both of these are broad, dense bands of fibrous tissue that extend laterally to the capsular ligaments.

The capsular ligaments are short but thick ligaments that essentially surround the occipitoatlantal and atlantoaxial articulations. The individual ligament fibers lie perpendicular to the plane of the facet, permitting maximal laxity of the ligament when the facets are in a neutral or fully opposed position. The capsular ligaments of the atlantoaxial joint are remarkably lax and normally permit almost 45 degrees of rotation from the neutral position in either direction.

Within the spinal canal and posterior to the dens, there are a number of ligaments that firmly bond the odontoid to the anterior ring of the atlas and occiput (Fig. 4–11). These are primarily responsible for stability between the occiput and the first and second vertebrae. The cruciform ligament has an upper vertical arm, which inserts on the posterior aspect of the basiocciput. Two transverse arms, the transverse ligament, extend from the dens to the ring of the atlas and hold the dens firmly in a sling to the anterior arch of the atlas. The cross is completed by a vertical inferior arm, which extends down the posterior aspect of the dens to the body of the second vertebra, reinforcing the base of the dens and limiting anterior displacement following fracture at the base of the dens in many cases. The lateral

alar odontoid ligaments are fibrous bands that join the superolateral aspect of the dens to the medial aspect of the occipital condyles. Finally, the apical odontoid ligament joins the tip of the dens to the posterior tip of the basiocciput beneath the vertical cruciform ligament.

The tectorial membrane is an extension of the posterior longitudinal ligament and covers the cruciform ligament as a broad band. The tectorial membrane inserts on the basilar groove of the basiocciput. It has an accessory or deep portion laterally, which joins the anterolateral ring of the atlas to the posterior body of the axis.

Posteriorly, the occiput is joined to the posterior ring of the atlas by a broad but thin and elastic posterior atlanto-occipital ligament (Fig. 4–12B). The posterior ring of the atlas is joined to the lamina of the axis by the analogous ligamentum flavum.

The dens forms a pivotal position between the atlantoaxial joint. The majority of the atlantoaxial ligaments are lax, permitting almost 90 degrees of rotation to both sides and 15 degrees of flexion and extension. The dens and its integral ligaments, particularly the transverse ligament, are primarily responsible for stability at this joint. The intact dens limits posterior displacement of the ring of the atlas, and the ligaments limit anterior and lateral displacements as well as rotation. In our clinical experience, the dens ordinarily fractures before its ligaments give way. Rheumatoid degeneration or pure shearing injuries, such as a violent blow to the back of the head, can produce pure ligament injuries at this joint without fractures (Fielding, 1974).

Fractures of the ring of the atlas (Jefferson, 1920), may be reasonably stable as long as the transverse ligament remains intact. When the transverse ligament has ruptured, the ring may spread laterally, and atlantoaxial stability may be impaired. This can be identified on open-mouth, anteroposterior roentgenograms of the odontoid. Spence (1970) notes that when the transverse measurement of the atlas is 7 mm. wider than the axis, rupture of the transverse ligament should be suspected.

Ligaments of the Lower Cervical Spine

The lower five cervical articulations between the second and seventh cervical vertebrae are similar anatomically. The authors studied the ligaments of the lower cervical spine in 15 fresh cadaver spines, 19 to 73 years of age (1975). Eight intervertebral ligaments were found, four anterior to the spinal canal and four posterior to it.

The anterior longitudinal ligament is a thin, translucent structure, closely adherent to the midportion of the vertebral bodies (Fig. 4–10). The ligament is thickest and widest in the frontal plane over the disc spaces and blends intimately with the underlying anulus fibrosus.

The anulus fibrosus is a dense, fibrous structure firmly bonded to the cartilaginous endplates. It blends completely with the anterior and posterior longitudinal ligaments. In none of the specimens dissected was a discrete nucleus pulposus found. The whole of the intervertebral disc was occupied by dense ligament, the largest ligament of the cervical spine.

The posterior longitudinal ligament is a thick band of dense, fibrous tissue running over the posterior vertebral bodies (Figs. 4–14B and C and 4–15) that is considerably thicker than its anterior counterpart. It is firmly attached to the posterior lips of the vertebral bodies and blends intimately with the fibers of the anulus. In most cases, it is not attached to the concave midportion of the vertebral bodies, leaving a space between the bone and ligament. The nutrient vessels enter this space from the side and disappear into the small nutrient foramina at the midportion of the vertebral bodies. The ligament appears as an undulating band, widest at the disc spaces and narrowest at the midportion of the vertebral body. The ligament is widest in the frontal plane in the upper cervical spine and becomes progressively narrower but thicker in the lower cervical and upper thoracic spine (Fig. 4–15).

Running longitudinally between adjacent costotransverse processes is a thin, fibrous septum that joins the anterior lips of one transverse process to the next (Fig. 4–10).

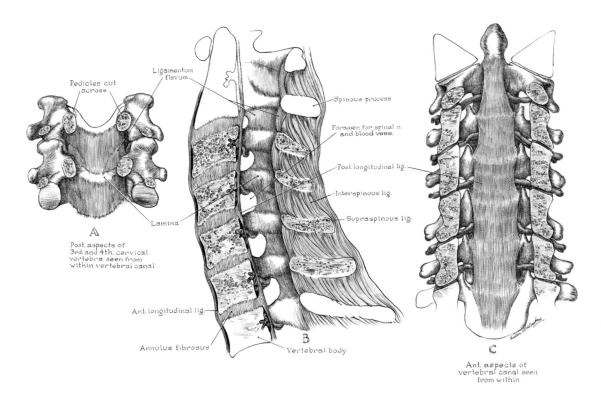

Figure 4–14. *A*, Posterior elements and ligamentum flavum of the third and fourth cervical vertebrae viewed from within the spinal canal looking posteriorly. *B*, Longitudinal cross-section of the cervical spine. *C*, Posterior longitudinal ligament viewed from within the spinal canal looking anteriorly. Note the nutrient vessels entering the space beneath the ligament from the sides. (From Johnson, R. M., et al.: Some new observations on the functional anatomy of the lower cervical spine. Clin. Orthop., 3:192–200, 1975.)

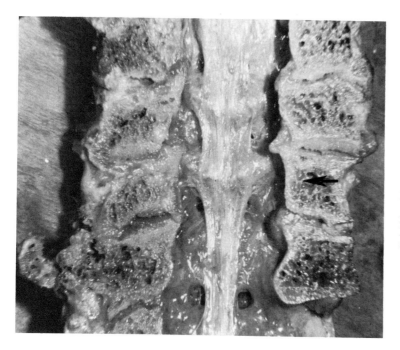

Figure 4–15. Posterior longitudinal ligament viewed from within the spinal canal looking anteriorly. The spine has been divided longitudinally through the pillars of the facets in the lower cervical and upper thoracic spine. The arrow is at the level of the seventh cervical vertebra. Note that the posterior longitudinal ligament narrows significantly in the lower cervical and upper thoracic spine.

This thin, translucent septum lies beneath the overlying intertransverse muscles and is just anterior to the vertebral artery.

The ligamentum nuchae is a fibrous midline intermuscular septum, attached to the spinous processes and paracervical muscles. In humans it has relatively few elastic fibers and appears to provide little intrinsic struc-

tural support, although in bovines it is most prominent and contains many elastic fibers (Fielding, 1976).

The supraspinous and interspinous ligaments connect the spinous processes of the cervical vertebrae (Figs. 4–16 and 4–17). As Halliday (1964) found, these structures are often poorly defined or incomplete in the

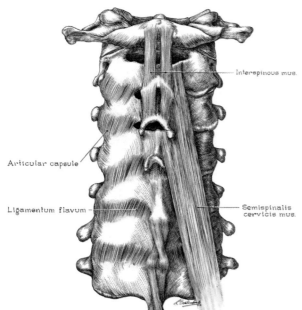

Interspinous mus.

Articular capsule

Ligamentum flavum

Semispinalis
cervicis mus.

Figure 4–16. Cervical spine and ligaments viewed from behind. The supraspinous ligaments are attached to the bifid spinous processes and cross one another at the midline. (From Johnson, R. M., et al.: Some new observations on the functional anatomy of the lower cervical spine. Clin. Orthop., 3:192–200, 1975.)

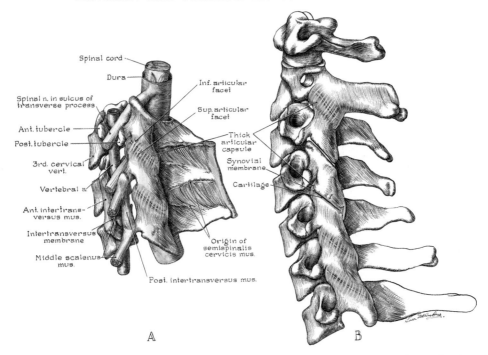

Spinal cord

Dura

Inf. articular facet

Spinal n. in sulcus of transverse process

Sup. articular facet

Ant. tubercle

Thick articular capsule

Post. tubercle

Synovial membrane

3rd. cervical vert.

Cartilage

Vertebral a.

Ant. intertrans-versus mus.

Intertransversus membrane

Origin of semispinalis cervicis mus.

Middle scalenus mus.

Post. intertransversus mus.

A

B

Figure 4–17. Cervical spine, facets, and capsular ligaments viewed from the side. (From Johnson, R. M., et al.: Some new observations on the functional anatomy of the lower cervical spine. Clin. Orthop., 3:192–200, 1975.)

upper cervical spine. In the lower levels they become better and more consistently developed. The supraspinous ligaments are a continuation of the ligamentum nuchae. They overlap and cross at midline, are attached to the bifid spinous processes, and blend with the interspinous ligaments anteriorly. The interspinous ligaments join the inferior aspect of one vertebral spine to the superior aspect of the subjacent spine. The fibers tend to run obliquely from the upper vertebrae, posteriorly to the next lower spine.

The ligamentum flavum joins the lamina of one vertebra to the next (Figure 4–14A). It is a thick, orange-yellow ligament that is grossly elastic. It connects the anterior and inferior aspects of the upper lamina with the superior aspect of the subjacent lamina. Most of this ligament is contained within the spinal canal.

The facet joints are covered with a thin layer of cartilage. Between the facets and beneath the capsular ligament is a thin band of synovial tissue that appears to surround the joint and is loosely attached to the capsule. The capsular ligaments bind the facets together, beginning anterolaterally at the transverse

process and extending posteromedially, in a 180 degree arc, to the lamina (Fig. 4–17). The capsular ligaments are short but thick fibrous structures. The fibers of the ligament are arranged at a 90 degree angle to the plane of the facet joint and are firmly bound to the bony prominence above and below the facet, extending a total length of only 5 to 7 mm.

The anterior longitudinal ligament, although thin and translucent, appears on the basis of our biomechanical studies to effectively limit extension of the spine (Johnson, 1973; Panjabi, 1975; White, 1975). The anulus fibrosus is a thick, dense structure that is more firmly attached to the outer perimeter of the vertebral body than the central cartilaginous plate. Its fibers are arranged in circumferential lamellae, with one layer running 60 degrees obliquely to the next. This arrangement, plus its size, effectively limits shear movements between the vertebrae, for shear displacement in any direction increases the tension along at least a portion of its fibers. With age and degeneration, hemorrhages, tears, and fissures appear in the ligament, which reduces its functional strength. Ultimately, the disc space narrows, and bony osteophytes may bridge the gap between vertebral bodies, increasing strength at the expense of mobility.

The posterior longitudinal ligament appears to limit flexion as well as intervertebral distraction (Johnson, 1973). It is thick and wide and appears to protect the spinal cord at the cervical level from posterior protrusion of disc material. Laterally, the nerve roots are not similarly protected, and disc material may protrude into the neuroforamina and irritate the roots. As long as the posterior longitudinal ligament remains intact, the spinal cord may be protected during anterior surgical dissections of the disc or body, but the nerve roots laterally are not similarly protected.

Halliday (1964) reports that the supraspinous and interspinous ligaments are often poorly defined or incomplete in the upper cervical spine, whereas in the lower cervical levels they become better and more consistently developed. Our gross anatomic observations wee similar; however, biomechanical trials indicated that the ligaments did consistently limit flexion and anterior horizontal displacement (Johnson, 1973; Panjabi, 1975; White, 1975). We must conclude that although the supraspinous and interspinous ligaments are not well defined anatomically, they are active functionally and should be spared, if possible, in posterior surgical approaches.

The capsular ligaments have been described as "thin and lax," contributing little to the strength of the spine. In our study they consistently appeared thick and dense but did permit considerable motion within well-defined limits. This controlled motion would appear to be related to the orientation of the ligament fibers perpendicular to the plane of the facet. When the facet is in a neutral or fully opposed position, the capsular ligament is most lax. As the facet glides forward or back from midposition, the capsular fibers progressively tighten, effectively limiting motion of more than 2 to 3 mm. from the neutral position (Fig. 4–18A). The 45 degree plane of the facets appears to contribute to flexion of the cervical vertebrae and stabilizes the vertebrae by limiting anterior displacements. When the facets were removed, flexion was consistently de-

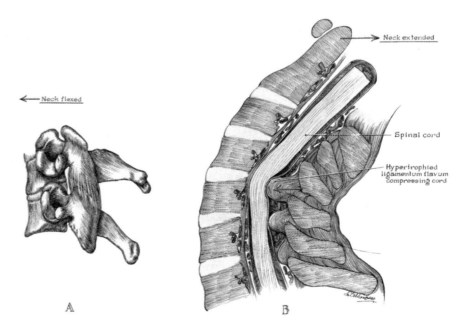

A   B

Figure 4–18.   *A,* Two cervical vertebrae viewed from the side in flexion. Note that in flexion the spinous processes separate, the superior facet glides forward and anteriorly on its subjacent facet, and the disc space separates posteriorly and approximates anteriorly. The fibers of the capsular ligaments are no longer aligned perpendicular to the plane of the facets. They are oriented obliquely and are taut, limiting further gliding anteriorly. *B,* Longitudinal cross-section of the cervical spine in extension illustrating an hypertrophied and relatively inelastic ligamentum flavum protruding into the spinal cord. (From Johnson, R. M., et al.: Some new observations on the functional anatomy of the lower cervical spine. Clin. Orthop., 3:192–200, 1975.)

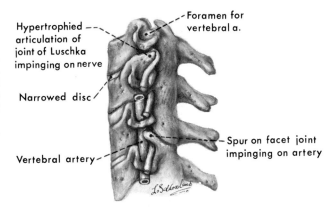

Figure 4–19. Encroachment of the neural foramen and vertebral artery by hypertrophic osteoarthritic spurs. (From Robinson, R. A., and Southwick, W. O.: Surgical Approaches to the Cervical Spine. *In* the American Academy of Orthopaedic Surgeons: Instructional Course Lectures, Vol. XVII. St. Louis, The C. V. Mosby Co., 1960.)

creased, but anterior horizontal displacement increased (Johnson, 1973). Because of this stabilizing effect, the facets and capsular ligaments should be spared, if possible, in posterior surgical approaches to the spine.

A large volume of the ligamentum flavum is found within the posterior spinal canal. Because of its inherent elasticity, the ligament will normally contract on itself when the neck is extended. With age or degeneration, however, this elasticity may be lost, and the ligament may bulge with neck extension and may protrude into the spinal canal and cord (Fig. 4–18*B*).

Deep Anterior Vessels and Nerves

The vertebral artery is the first branch of the subclavian artery. It passes directly to the costotransverse foramen of the sixth cervical vertebra, ascending through successive vertebral foramina (Fig. 4–10) to the first vertebra. At the atlas it leaves the costotransverse foramen and curves posteriorly and medially over the posterior ring of the first vertebra, penetrates the posterior atlanto-occipital ligament, and ascends through the foramen magnum. Here it joins the artery from the opposite side to form the basilar artery, which leads to the circle of Willis at the base of the brain. The vertebral vein draining the suboccipital region enters the transverse process at the first vertebra and descends through the costotransverse foramina in company with the artery. A portion of the sympathetic chain also accompanies the artery and vein through these foramina. Care is required prior to blind ligation of the vertebral artery because the nerve root passes directly behind the artery and could be traumatized during this maneuver. Unilateral ligation of the vertebral artery is ordinarily safe in younger individuals. In older individuals, such ligation may result in basilar artery insufficiency and receptive blindness due to ischemia of the calcarine fissure. The left vertebral artery is ordinarily dominant, but there is enough anatomic variation that preoperative angiography is recommended prior to surgery. If there is a discrepancy in size, the larger vertebral artery should be considered dominant and spared if possible. Hadley (1957) pointed out that spurs arising from the facets or joints of Luschka may impinge on the vertebral arteries (Fig. 4–19). The vertebral artery may be exposed through the anterolateral approach described by Henry (1957), discussed in Part II, Anterior Cervical Approaches. The longus capitis and colli muscles are reflected anteriorly, and the anterior portion of the transverse process over the foramen is removed using rongeurs to expose the artery beneath.

The cervical sympathetic chain is a deep structure, closely associated with the longus capitis and colli muscles. It lies in a loose reflection of the carotid sheath along the anterior surface of the lateral masses and prevertebral muscles. It extends from the second cervical vertebra downward and has three ganglionic enlargements: the superior ganglion, beside the second and third cervical vertebrae; the middle ganglion (sometimes lacking), beside the sixth, and the inferior ganglion. The inferior ganglion is frequently fused with the first thoracic vertebra just below the seventh cervical vertebra to form the stellate ganglion. A simple and effective method of blocking the stellate ganglion is to retract the carotid sheath with a finger at the level of the sixth cervical vertebra and infiltrate a local anesthetic into the space between the prevertebral and alar fasciae (Fig. 4–5), with the patient sitting up. A block is usually effective in a few minutes, when the anesthetic solution rolls down between these fascial layers, and may be recognized by pupillary constriction on the affected side.

The hypoglossal nerve (Fig. 4–20) courses anteriorly over the carotid artery just above the greater horn of the hyoid bone. It rests on the hypoglossus muscle and bends upward under the posterior belly of the digastric. It is usually slightly superior and superficial to the lingual artery, a branch of the external carotid, and is usually not exposed unless one is approaching the upper two cervical vertebrae anteriorly. In this approach it should be identified and protected.

The ansa hypoglossi is a nerve loop derived from the first, second, and third cervical nerve roots and travels as two separate limbs into the neck, the upper root anteriorly and the lower root located more posteriorly on the carotid sheath. The upper root, or descendens hypoglossi, travels with the hypoglossal nerve. It separates from the hypoglossal nerve

at the angle of the mandible and descends over the carotid sheath, giving off branches to the omohyoid, sternothyroid, and sternohyoid muscles. The branches to these muscles are given off in the midcervical region and are not usually disturbed in anterior approaches to the middle and lower neck, as the plane of dissection is between these and the carotid sheath. However, in exposures to the upper vertebrae, anterior and medial to the carotid, these may be stretched or injured. Another smaller branch of the descendens hypoglossi travels with the hypoglossal nerve anteriorly and supplies the geniohyoid and thyrohyoid muscles high in the neck. The upper root of the ansa cervicalis loops posteriorly in the lower neck and joins the lower root of the ansa, which emerges from behind the jugular vein and crosses the carotid artery.

The internal jugular vein and common carotid arteries are buried beneath the sternomastoid muscle within the carotid sheath. The sheath and its contents may be identified by

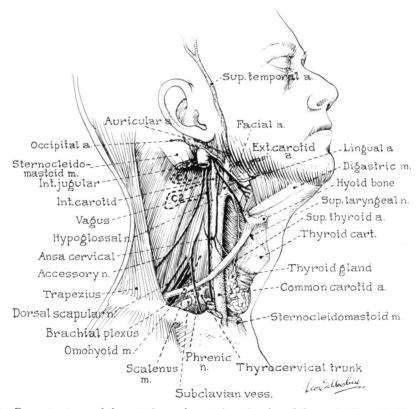

Figure 4–20. Deep structures of the anterior and posterior triangles of the neck. (From Robinson, R. A., and Southwick, W. O.: Surgical Approaches to the Cervical Spine. *In* the American Academy of Orthopaedic Surgeons: Instructional Course Lectures, Vol. XVII. St. Louis, The C. V. Mosby Co., 1960.)

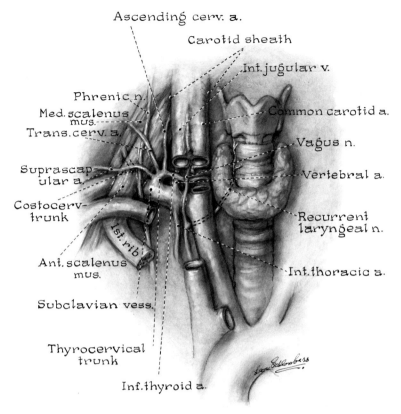

Ascending cerv. a.

Carotid sheath

Int. jugular v.

Phrenic n.

Med. scalenus mus.

Trans. cerv. a.

Common carotid a.

Vagus n.

Suprascapular a.

Vertebral a.

Costocerv-trunk

1st rib

Recurrent laryngeal n.

Ant. scalenus mus.

Int. thoracic a.

Subclavian vess.

Thyrocervical trunk

Inf. thyroid a.

Figure 4–21. Arteries and nerves at the base of the neck on the right side. The right recurrent laryngeal nerve arises from the vagus at the level of the subclavian artery, loops beneath the subclavian artery, and ascends between the trachea and esophagus. The right recurrent laryngeal nerve can recur above the level of the subclavian artery and could be injured in an approach to the middle cervical spine to the right of the midline.

the pulsations of the carotid artery. The carotid divides at the upper border of the thyroid cartilage into the internal and external carotid arteries. The internal carotid remains within the carotid sheath and yields no branches within the neck. The external carotid gives off one branch below the hyoid bone, the superior thyroid artery, which loops conveniently upward before descending to give off its hyoid and superior laryngeal branches. Inferior to this loop, the carotid sheath may be separated from the visceral fascia (containing the trachea and esophagus) to expose the cervical vertebral bodies without ligating a single artery.

The pharyngeal and superior laryngeal branches of the vagus nerve lie deep to the carotid and superior thyroid arteries and supply the trachea, the muscles of the posterior pharynx, and the cricothyroid and provide sensory innervation to the larynx. Since they run in a longitudinal, oblique course, they are not damaged by retraction except in exposures of the upper spine anterior to the carotid

sheath. The recurrent laryngeal nerve on the right (Fig. 4–21) arises from the vagus at the level of the subclavian artery, loops beneath the subclavian artery, and ascends between the trachea and esophagus, protected by the visceral fascia. The left recurrent nerve arises at the level of the aortic arch within the thorax and loops beneath the arch to ascend between the trachea and esophagus. Excessive retraction has caused temporary paralysis of the recurrent nerve following the anterior cervical approaches. Because the right recurrent laryngeal nerve can recur above the level of the subclavian artery, it may be injured in a right anterolateral approach. For this reason, we prefer to approach the neck to the left of the midline.

Structures of the Posterior Triangle

Deep to the superficial layer of the deep fascia, the spinal accessory and third and fourth cervical nerves emerge from the posterior border of the sternomastoid to innervate the trapezius muscle. The posterior belly of the omohyoid is one or two finger breadths above the clavicle and is covered by a thin, additional layer of fascia, the omohyoid-sternohyoid fascia, which forms its sling. The external jugular vein crosses the sternomastoid at the midpoint of the posterior triangle.

The floor of the posterior triangle (Figs. 4–4 and 4–20) is formed by several muscles, the most central being the levator scapulae deep to the spinal accessory nerve. It inserts on the vertebral border of the scapula and originates from the transverse processes of the first four cervical vertebrae. Superior to the levator scapulae is the splenius capitis, and inferior to the levator are the scaleni (Fig. 4–9). The scalene muscles arise from the tubercles of the cervical transverse processes and insert on the first and second ribs. The scalenus anterior is separated from the scalenus medius and posterior by the brachial plexus and subclavian artery. The brachial plexus lies deep to the prevertebral or scalenus fascia. Its cords are covered by a sheath of prevertebral fascia as they descend into the axilla. The plexus is formed from the anterior rami of the fifth cervical to the first thoracic nerves.

The scalenus anterior is occasionally thought to encroach upon the subclavian artery and brachial plexus, particularly in the presence of a cervical rib, and may be sectioned surgically for the relief of pain. This exposure is described later with the Nanson anterolateral approach to the lower cervical vertebrae. The phrenic nerve crosses the midportion of the scalenus anterior, beneath the prevertebral fascia, and should be identified prior to scalenus section. It arises from the anterior ramus of the fourth cervical root, receives twigs from the third and fifth root, crosses the first part of the subclavian artery and enters the thorax to innervate the diaphragm. The thoracic duct is found at the base of the neck on the left, between the phrenic nerve and carotid sheath. It loops over the subclavian artery at the level of the first thoracic vertebra anterior to the scalenus anterior and phrenic nerve and enters the subclavian vein.

The Back of the Neck

The structures of this area are described in the order in which they are encountered surgically, from superficial to deep. Stretching in the midline from the external occipital protuberance to the spinous process of the seventh cervical vertebra is a fibrous intermuscular septum known as the ligamentum nuchae. Lateral to this and deep to the superficial fascia is the trapezius muscle. This is attached to the ligamentum nuchae, the dorsal vertebrae, and the medial border of the superior nuchal line and inserts into the scapula and clavicle. Just lateral to its superior border lies the great occipital nerve and the occipital artery. In the lower part of the neck, the rhomboid minor and serratus posterior superior muscles attach to the ligamentum nuchae and the seventh cervical spinous process to run obliquely downward toward the scapula and ribs. The next deeper muscle

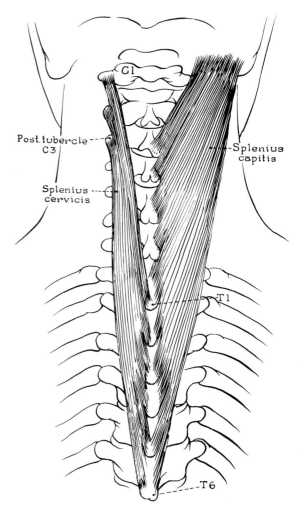

Figure 4–22. Deep muscles of the back of the neck, the splenius capitis and cervicis. These act as extensors of the head and neck respectively.

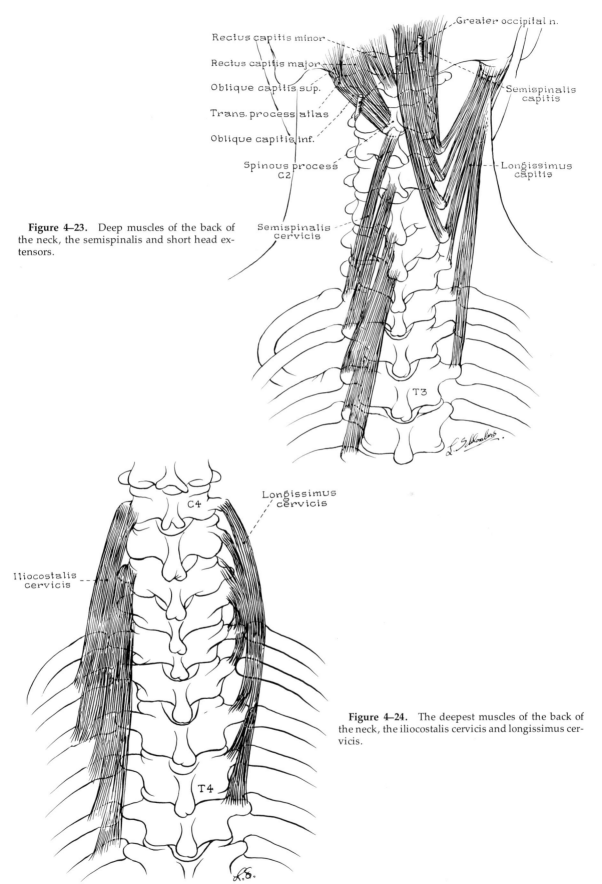

Figure 4–23. Deep muscles of the back of the neck, the semispinalis and short head extensors.

Rectus capitis minor

Rectus capitis major

Oblique capitis sup.

Trans. process atlas

Oblique capitis inf.

Spinous process C2

Semispinalis cervicis

Greater occipital n.

Semispinalis capitis

Longissimus capitis

T3

Figure 4–24. The deepest muscles of the back of the neck, the iliocostalis cervicis and longissimus cervicis.

Longissimus cervicis

C4

Iliocostalis cervicis

T4

encountered is the splenius capitis (Fig. 4–22), arising from the lower half of the ligamentum nuchae and the upper six thoracic vertebrae to attach deep to the sternomastoid on the occiput. The splenius cervicis arises from the upper six thoracic vertebrae, passes deep to the levator scapulae, and inserts on the posterior tubercles of the first, second, and third cervical vertebrae. Deep to the splenius is the semispinalis capitis and cervicis (Fig. 4–23), a long muscle group that originates through a series of tendinous slips from the articular processes of the fourth, fifth, and sixth cervical vertebrae and from the transverse processes of the upper five or six thoracic vertebrae. It has a thick insertion on the occipital bone and is pierced by the greater occipital nerve. The deeper muscles of this group, the iliocostalis and longissimus cervicis, are rarely separated in the usual surgical approaches to the back of the neck (Fig. 4–24).

There are a group of small head extensors, including the rectus capitis posterior major and minor and the superior and inferior capitis obliques, all attaching to the spinous or transverse processes of the axis (Fig. 4–23). These muscles must be mobilized in posterior approaches to the atlas and axis. The inferior oblique muscle has been implicated as a cause of entrapment of the greater occipital nerve as this nerve emerges from beneath this muscle belly.

References

Bosch, A., Stauffer, E. S., and Nickel, V. L.: Incomplete traumatic quadriplegia: A ten year review. Final report, Regional Spinal Cord Injury Rehabilitation Center, Rancho Los Amigos Hospital, Giii–Gv, 1972.

Fielding, J. W.: Normal and abnormal motion of the cervical spine from C2 to C7, cineroentgenography. J. Bone Joint Surg., 46-A:1779–1782, 1964.

Fielding, J. W., Cochran, G. V. B., Lawsing, J. F., and Hohl, M.: Tears of the transverse ligament of the atlas. J. Bone Joint Surg., 56-A:1683–1691, 1974.

Fielding, J. W., Burstein, A. H., and Frankel, V. H.: The nuchal ligament. Spine, 1:3–14, 1976.

Grodinsky, M., and Holyoke, E. A.: The fasciae and facial spaces of the head, neck, and adjacent regions. Am. J. Anat., 63:367–408, 1938.

Hadley, L. A.: Covertebral articulations and cervical foramen encroachment. J. Bone Joint Surg., 39-A:910–920, 1957.

Halliday, D. R., Sullivan, C. R., Hollinshead, W. H., and Bahn, R. C.: Torn cervical ligaments: Necropsy examination of normal cervical region. J. Trauma, 4:219–232, 1964.

Henry, A. K.: Extensile Exposure, 2nd ed. Essex, Longman Group Ltd., Edinburgh, E. 1970, pp. 53–80.

Hohl, M.: Normal motions in the upper portion of the cervical spine. J. Bone Joint Surg., 46-A:1777–1779, 1964.

Jefferson, G.: Fracture of the atlas vertebra. Report of four cases, and a review of those previously recorded. Br. J. Surg., 7:407–422, 1920.

Johnson, R. M.: Biomechanical stability of the lower cervical spine. Thesis: Yale University School of Medicine, Section of Orthopaedic Surgery, pp. 1–58, 1973.

Johnson, R. M., Owen, J. R., and Lerner, E.: Normal motion of the cervical spine in subjects 20 to 40 years of age and spinal instability. 1980, (being prepared for publication).

Johnson, R. M., Crelin, E. S., White, A. A., Panjabi, M. M., and Southwick, W. O.: Some new observations on the functional anatomy of the lower cervical spine. Clin. Orthop., III:192–200, 1975.

Lysell, E.: Motion in the cervical spine. Acta Orthop. Scand., Suppl., 123:1–61, 1969.

Nanson, E. M.: The anterior approach to upper dorsal sympathectomy. Surg. Gynecol. Obstet., 104:118–120, 1957.

Panjabi, M. M., White, A. A., and Johnson, R. M.: Cervical spine mechanics as a function of transection of components. J. Biomech. 8:327–336, 1975.

Panjabi, M. M., Brand, R. A., and White, A. A.: Mechanical properties of the human thoracic spine. J. Bone Joint Surg., 58-A:642–652, 1976.

Perry, J., and Nickel, V. L.: Total cervical spine fusion for neck paralysis. J. Bone Joint Surg., 41-A:37–60, 1959.

Ruff, S.: Brief acceleration: Less than one second. German Aviation Medicine, World War II, Vol. 1, p. 584, 1950. The Surgeon General.

Spence, K. F., Decker, S., and Sell, K. W.: Bursting atlantal fracture associated with rupture of the transverse ligament. J. Bone Joint Surg., 52A:543–549, 1970.

Simeone, F. A., and Rothman, R. H.: Cervical disc disease. In Rothman, R. H., and Simeone, F. A.: The Spine. Philadelphia, W. B. Saunders Co., 1975.

Verbiest, H.: Anterolateral operation for fractures and dislocations in the middle and lower parts of the cervical spine. J. Bone Joint Surg., 51-A:1489–1530, 1969.

White, A. A.: Analysis of the mechanics of the thoracic spine in man. An experimental study in autopsy specimens. Thesis. Acta Orthop. Scand. (Suppl.), 127:1–105, 1969.

White, A. A., Johnson, R. M., Panjabi, M. M., and Southwick, W. O.: Biomechanical analysis of clinical stability in the cervical spine. Clin. Orthop., 109:85–96, 1975.

Whitesides, T. E., Jr., and Kelly, R. P.: Lateral approach to the upper cervical spine for anterior fusion. South. Med. J., 59:879–883, 1966.

SURGICAL APPROACHES
TO THE CERVICAL SPINE

APPROACHES TO THE
CERVICAL SPINE

Anterior Versus Posterior

Under most circumstances, the choice of approach to the cervical spine should be dictated by the site of the primary pathologic condition. For example, to biopsy a tumor of the vertebral body, the most direct approach is anterior. There are, however, certain indications for and limitations to each approach.

ANTERIOR

The anterior approach provides the most direct access to the vertebral body, vertebral artery, and transverse processes. The anterior approach is the most direct means of removing an osteophyte on the posterior wall of the vertebral body that is protruding into the spinal canal or nerve roots. It is also the most appropriate route to decompress the spinal cord when a vertebral body is fractured and displaced posteriorly into the canal (Fig. 4–25). In this situation, the spinal cord may be tethered to or tented over these fragments and may not be adequately relieved by laminectomy alone, and attempts to remove these bony fragments around the cord may only cause further neurologic damage.

The major limitation to anterior expo-

sures is that most fusion techniques from the front do not add to spinal stability immediately after surgery, and in some cases stability is removed. This is particularly true when the primary injury occurs over the posterior elements and the last threads of remaining stability are in the front (Stauffer, 1977). In these conditions, anterior fusion will remove these last elements of continuity and will create a most precarious situation. Figure 4–26A is the preoperative lateral roentgenogram illustrating a fracture through the body of C5. This was wired and fused anteriorly in an attempt to improve stability, but despite this, progressive anterior displacement occurred (Fig. 4–26B). Stabilization was ultimately provided with interspinous wiring and fusion. Figure 4–27A and B are the roentgenograms taken at the time of and immediately after surgery of an unstable spine fused anteriorly between the fourth and fifth cervical vertebral bodies. Because of this posterior instability, the fourth vertebra continued to migrate anteriorly on the fifth (Fig. 4–27C). Posterior interspinous wiring and fusion was required to stop this progressive anterior displacement. Figure 4–28A is an example of what may happen following anterior fusion when the graft is not properly fixed or ''keyed'' into the adjacent vertebrae and there is associated posterior instability. This 20 year old male was struck by a car and sustained a fracture-dislocation of

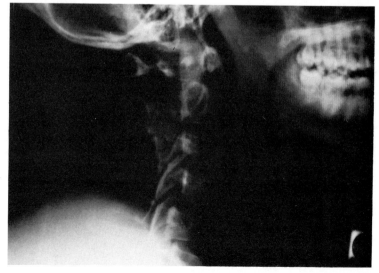

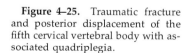

Figure 4–25. Traumatic fracture and posterior displacement of the fifth cervical vertebral body with associated quadriplegia.

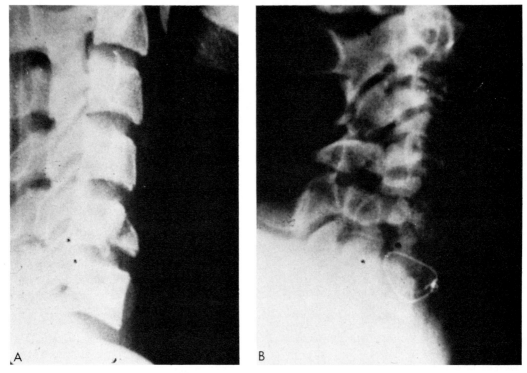

Figure 4–26. *A,* Traumatic fracture of the fifth cervical vertebra. *B,* Despite anterior fusion and wire stabilization, the fifth vertebral body continued to migrate anteriorly on the sixth beneath. Note the position of the marks on the posterior aspect of the fifth and sixth vertebral bodies *(A)* and the subsequent position in *(B)* after anterior subluxation.

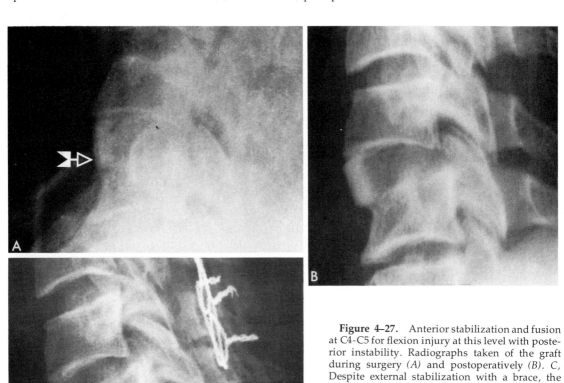

Figure 4–27. Anterior stabilization and fusion at C4-C5 for flexion injury at this level with posterior instability. Radiographs taken of the graft during surgery *(A)* and postoperatively *(B)*. *C,* Despite external stabilization with a brace, the graft and fourth vertebra continued to migrate anteriorly, requiring posterior interspinous wiring and fusion.

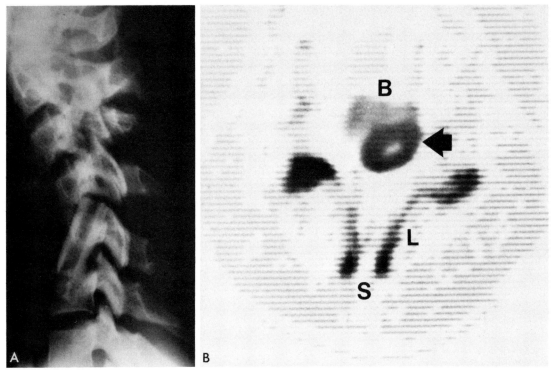

Figure 4–28. Posterior displacement of a vertebral body graft into the spinal canal with associated neural injury. This 20-year-old man was struck by a car and sustained a fracture-dislocation of the fifth cervical vertebra with posterior displacement of the vertebral body into the spinal canal and incomplete spinal cord injury. The vertebral body was excised to decompress the spinal canal, and the body was replaced with a fibular strut graft wedged between adjacent vertebrae. Shortly after surgery, the upper pole of the graft moved posteriorly and to the right into the spinal canal, and all function of the fifth and sixth cervical nerve roots on the right was lost. *A,* Lateral roentgenogram revealing the upper pole of the fibular vertebral body graft displaced posteriorly into the spinal canal and the posterior separation of the spinous processes suggesting associated posterior instability. *B,* Computerized axial tomogram at the upper level of the fifth cervical vertebra and fibular graft. B, vertebral body; L, lamina; and S, spinous process of the fifth cervical vertebra. The arrow points to the fibular graft, which is displaced posteriorly and to the right into the spinal canal. Note the central lucency over the intramedullary canal of the fibular graft. (From Light, T. R., et al.: Correction of spinal instability and recovery of neurologic loss following cervical vertebral body replacement. Spine, in press. Reproduced with permission of the author.)

the fifth cervical vertebra with posterior displacement of the vertebral body into the spinal canal and incomplete spinal cord injury. The vertebral body was excised to decompress the spinal canal, and the body was replaced with a fibular strut graft wedged between the adjacent vertebrae. Shortly after surgery the graft moved posteriorly and to the right into the spinal canal, and all function of the fifth and sixth cervical nerve roots on the right was lost (Fig. 4–28*B*). Nine weeks later the fibular graft was removed and replaced with an iliac graft using keys (Fig. 4–54*A*) to secure the graft to the upper and lower vertebral body. Because of the extensive injury to the posterior ligaments, posterior wiring and fusion were performed to increase the immediate stability and to speed rehabilitation without the use of a halo cast (Fig. 4–54*B* and *C*). Twenty-four

months after this procedure, the patient has regained a significant return of motor and sensory function and is walking with crutches and a short leg brace on the left leg.

POSTERIOR

The posterior approach provides the most direct access to the spinous processes, laminae, and facets. In addition, the spinal canal may be explored and decompressed over a large area with less loss of stability than equivalent anterior decompression would afford. Laminectomy does remove some intrinsic stability, but the immediate integrity of the spine is not usually jeopardized. On the other hand, resection of one or more vertebral bodies creates an obvious problem, and these bodies must be replaced, and the spine must be rigidly supported until fusion is established.

Certain posterior fusion techniques using wire through the spinous processes or facets offer increased strength immediately after surgery through internal stabilization. The anterior elements do not offer similar vantage points for internal fixation, and the surrounding structures, such as the esophagus, may be injured by wires, plates, or screws. Therefore, in very unstable situations where improved strength through internal fixation may be needed, posterior wiring and bone graft will offer the advantage of increased immediate strength, whereas most anterior fusion techniques will not. Once osseous union is complete, however, there does not appear to be any advantage of posterior over anterior methods of fusion.

Selection of Approach and Level of Involvement

The posterior approach through a midline longitudinal incision provides access to the posterior elements at all levels of the cervical spine. The standard anterior approach through a transverse incision provides adequate access from the third through seventh cervical vertebrae. However, the upper and lower anterior cervical elements have to be approached more selectively because of certain anatomic restrictions.

ANTERIOR

The basiocciput may be reached anteriorly through the pharynx by dividing the soft palate and part of the hard palate (Alonso et al., 1971; Southwick and Robinson, 1957). This introduces the element of contamination by pharyngeal organisms and restricted working area but provides direct local access, suitable for biopsy, drainage, or limited resection. DeAndrade and MacNab (1969) described an effective extraoral approach to this region through an oblique incision (Fig. 4–29A) parallel to the anterior border of the sternomastoid and medial to the carotid sheath. This requires retraction or division of certain laryngeal nerves that cross the neck anteriorly and may result in minor but persistent hoarseness.

The first and second cervical vertebrae may be reached directly anteriorly via the pharynx or anterolaterally through the approach described by Henry (1957) and Whitesides (1966), posterior to the carotid sheath. The transcutaneous anterolateral approach is made via an oblique incision at the anterior margin of the sternomastoid (Fig. 4–29B). The sternomastoid muscle is everted at its origin on the mastoid process, and the anterior elements of the spine are approached posterior to the carotid sheath. Because the internal carotid artery, jugular vein, and vagus and hypoglossal nerves are tethered to their foramina at the base of the skull and may not be retracted anteriorly with safety, the upper limit of dissection is restricted to the anterior ring of the first vertebra, and the basiocciput cannot be reached.

The anterior bodies of the third through seventh cervical vertebrae are easily exposed via the anterior approach described by Robinson and Southwick (1957, 1960, 1961), with dissection anterior and medial to the carotid sheath (Fig. 4–29C). The lower cervical and upper thoracic spine, as well as structures of the thoracic inlet, may be reached through the transverse supraclavicular approach (Fig. 4–29D) described by Nanson (1957). This approach provides limited exposure through the thoracic inlet, in many cases as far as the body of the third thoracic vertebra.

POSTERIOR

Satisfactory access to all levels of the posterior cervical spine is afforded by the midline longitudinal incision made over the spinous processes. The incision is extended superiorly over the occiput for occipitocervical fusions and fusions of the atlas and axis.

Occipitocervical fusion is reserved for atlanto-occipital instability or if the ring of C1 is fractured and stability between the odontoid and anterior ring of the first vertebra is lost. It may also be required after extensive resection of the posterior ring of C1 or the anterior elements of the atlas and axis. Fractures of the base of the odontoid and ruptures of the transverse ligament with atlantoaxial dislocation are usually treated by authors with the Brooks' circumlaminar wiring and bone graft at C1-2 (p. 132).

Fusion techniques below the level of the first cervical vertebra are selected dependent upon the amount of bone remaining in the posterior elements. If the spinous processes are intact, a simple interspinous wiring and fusion is performed. If the spinous processes and laminae have been sacrificed for the sake of decompression, the facets are wired and fused. If the laminae and facets are missing, a strut of cortical bone is bridged across the posterior defect and wired to the first intact

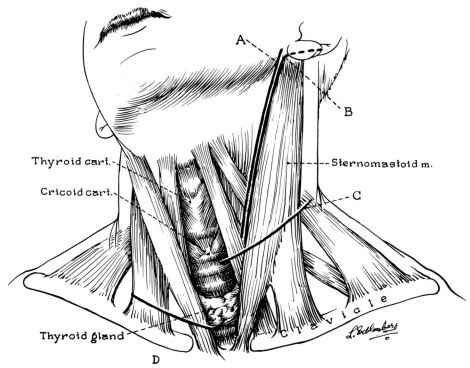

Thyroid cart.

Cricoid cart.

Thyroid gland

Sternomastoid m.

A

B

C

Clavicle

D

Figure 4–29. Anterior approaches to the cervical spine; incisions. *A,* Occiput and upper cervical spine medial to the carotid sheath. *B,* Anterior approach to the first and second vertebrae lateral to the carotid sheath. *C,* Anterior approach to the middle and lower cervical vertebrae medial to the carotid sheath. *D,* Anterior approach to the lower cervical and upper thoracic vertebrae.

spinous processes or facets, but additional anterior interbody fusions may be required to provide long-term stabilization in these cases.

Posterior laminectomy is ordinarily sufficient to expose and decompress the cervical cord posteriorly. Occasionally, part or all of a facet must also be removed to decompress a nerve root. If only one nerve root need be decompressed through the posterior approach, the laminotomy-foraminotomy exposure described by Scoville (1958, 1961) should be considered (p. 132). This exposure is primarily indicated to excise a soft disc protruding into the neural foramen or causing unilateral single nerve root irritation.

PREOPERATIVE PREPARATIONS

Intraoperative Stabilization

Most surgical procedures of the cervical spine require some form of traction stabiliza-tion intraoperatively. The type of stabilization should be selected on the basis of the spinal instability present before surgery and the amount anticipated in the early postoperative period. The obviously unstable spine with associated paraplegia is controlled well with skull tongs of the Crutchfield or Vinke type. These may be used before, during, or after surgery, but a turning frame or bed is required until healing is complete and internal stabiliza-tion is established. If rigid external support is required, which frees the patient from a turn-ing frame and allows him to get out of bed, a halo-cast should be considered. Traction may be applied to the halo before or during sur-gery, and the halo may be fixed to a body jacket or pelvic pins following surgery to mobilize the patient out of bed. Most surgical approaches to the neck may be performed with the halo and body jacket in place, caus-ing only limited inconvenience to the surgeon.

In some circumstances, traction is only required intraoperatively. Posterior cervical wiring and fusion techniques often add enough immediate stability that simple braces are sufficient to protect the spine postoperatively. For most posterior approaches, we prefer a three-point pin headrest with countertraction applied to the shoulders to maintain position and alignment during surgery. With uncomplicated anterior interbody fusion, minimal external support as well as a short period of longitudinal distraction is needed. We use a simple head halter with 5 to 10 pounds of weight and increase the distraction briefly during graft insertion.

CRUTCHFIELD TONGS.　A large area over the top of the head is shaved and surgically prepared. Using sterile marking solution, a line is drawn across the top of the head along the plane of the external auditory meatus. A cross mark is made at the vertex of the skull. The Crutchfield tongs themselves are used as a guide for making the drill holes. The points of the tongs approach the skull at right angles to the plane of the skull. The tongs should be opened three fourths of their maximal width, with 10 to 11 cm. separating the tips of the tongs (Fig. 4–30). If the tongs are not opened wide enough, the points will not satisfactorily penetrate the outer table and may pull out. If they are spread too far, the points of the tongs will approach the skull at an angle almost parallel with the direction of traction and also may pull out.

Using a sterile marking pen, cross marks are made at the points of insertion into the skull. Local anesthetic solution is infiltrated into the skin, subcutaneous tissues, and periosteum. A longitudinal incision is made to the bone with a small scalpel over the points of

insertion. A special drill with safety flanges is used to drill the skull, permitting penetration through the outer table only. The drill depth is 3 mm. in children and 4 mm. in adults. The opened tongs are held by an assistant adjacent to the skin wounds and are used as a guide to proper placement and angle of the drill holes. The points of the tongs are inserted into the drill holes, and the tongs are tightened snugly and locked in place. Traction is applied to the ring at the center of the tongs. The wounds are dressed with small, cut gauze flaps and sealed with collodion.

The tongs should be checked daily and tightened only if loose. If the tongs are tightened too aggressively, they tend to penetrate the inner table. To flex or extend the neck, the traction pulley is placed anterior or posterior to the midsagittal plane. The tongs may be inserted anterior or posterior to the external auditory meatus to encourage flexion or extension, but this procedure limits later adjustments and changes in alignment.

Crutchfield (1954) recommends traction weights according to the level of cervical involvement as outlined in Table 4–2. Traction should be applied within these limits, depending on the size and muscular development of the patient, the amount of paraspinal muscle spasm, and the type of injury. Traction weights exceeding these limits may be required temporarily to reduce a fracture-dislocation or locked facet. However, serial roentgenograms and frequent neurologic examinations should be performed when these limits are exceeded, and the patient should be constantly attended. Initially, roentgenograms

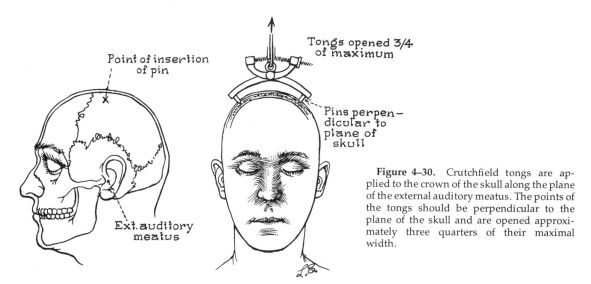

Point of insertion of pin

Ext. auditory meatus

Tongs opened 3/4 of maximum

Pins perpendicular to plane of skull

Figure 4–30. Crutchfield tongs are applied to the crown of the skull along the plane of the external auditory meatus. The points of the tongs should be perpendicular to the plane of the skull and are opened approximately three quarters of their maximal width.

TABLE 4–2. CERVICAL TRACTION WEIGHTS

Level of Injury	Minimum Weight in Pounds	Maximum Weight in Pounds
C1	5	10
C2	6	12
C3	8	15
C4	10	20
C5	12	25
C6	15	30
C7	18	35

should be made every day to check that no level of the cervical spine becomes excessively distracted as the paraspinal muscle spasm subsides. Excessive distraction may impair satisfactory healing or may irritate the spinal cord or nerve roots.

VINKE TONGS. The Vinke tongs are somewhat easier to apply correctly than Crutchfield tongs, and there is less risk of them pulling out or penetrating the inner table of the skull. Because the pins of these tongs are larger and more elaborate, there is, in our experience, a higher incidence of local irritation or pin tract infection than with Crutchfield tongs. The Vinke tongs fit over the horizontal aspect of the skull about the temporal ridge rather than at the apex (Fig. 4–31). Thus,

the traction forces are applied at right angles to the longitudinal axis of the skull and body. The points of the tongs are equipped with a flat, eccentric metal table, which is locked into the space between the outer and inner tables of the skull. This prevents penetration through the inner table and reduces the risk of the tongs pulling out. Included with the tongs is a drill that limits the depth of penetration into the bone. In addition, a tool is provided to undercut the bone between the outer and inner tables.

The tongs are inserted in the plane of the external auditory meatus about the temporal ridge. The skin is shaved locally and prepared surgically over the intended drill holes. Marks are made using sterile marking solution, and local anesthetic is infiltrated into the skin, subcutaneous tissue, and periosteum. A short longitudinal incision is made to the bone over the skin marks, using a small scalpel. The periosteum is elevated slightly, anteriorly and posteriorly, to allow the guide bushing to fit directly against the bone of the skull. The traction frame is closed against the skull and held by an assistant. The special drill is inserted through the guide bushing, and drilling is continued until the drill stop reaches the outer surface of the guide frame to insure that a hole of sufficient depth is made. It is important to remove all bone chips from the drilled hole,

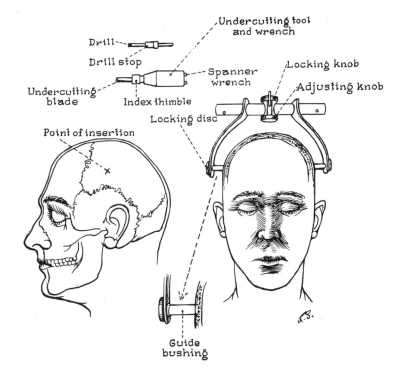

Figure 4–31. Vinke tongs are applied to the widest portion of the skull above the ears. Special tools are provided, such as a drill with a stop to prevent penetration of the inner table of the skull and an undercutting tool to cut the bone between the outer and inner tables of the skull. The points of the tongs are equipped with a flat eccentric metal table, which expands within the space cut between the outer and inner tables and locks the tongs to the skull.

and repeated clearing of the drill or saline irrigations are recommended. The undercutting blade is inserted through the guide bushing into the drill hole with the blade retracted into position 1. The index thimble is progressively advanced to position 5, and the blade is rotated clockwise at least one full revolution to complete the undercut. The undercutting tool is returned to position 1 and removed. The locking pins are inserted through the guide bushing into the skull, with the locks retracted. The locks are extended between the tables of the skull by turning the locking discs 180 degrees in either direction and are then snapped in place. At this point, the tongs are locked securely to the skull. The side frames are adjusted so the patient feels no pressure laterally. The side frames are locked into position with the locking knob, and the knob is tightened using the spanner wrench on the handle of the undercutting tool. The wounds are dressed, and traction is applied to the traction bail or ring on the center bar.

HALO TRACTION. The halo provides four-point skeletal fixation through a circumferential steel ring (Fig. 4–32). This rigidly controls the head and, when attached to a body jacket with steel uprights (Fig. 4–33), permits mobilization of the patient without sacrificing control of the head and neck (DeWald, 1975; Kopits, 1970; Perry, 1959, and 1972). The halo may be used with dynamic traction intraoperatively, or surgery may be performed between the steel uprights of the halo-body assembly. There is a cosmetic objection to the frontal pin placement in the forehead. However, these pin wounds ordinarily heal with a visible but small scar that is not cosmetically objectionable.

The skull pins have a thin, sharp point

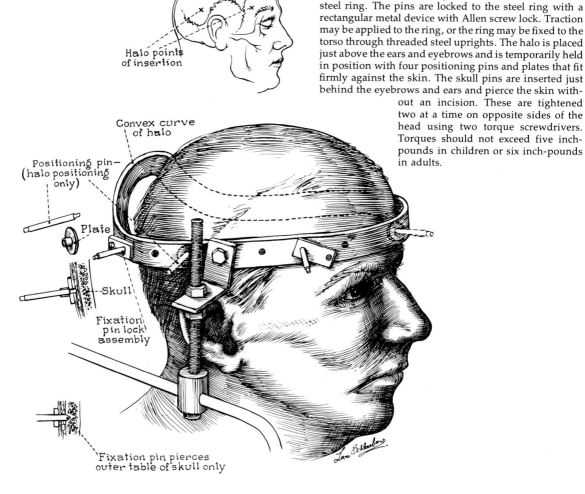

Halo points of insertion

Convex curve of halo

Positioning pin (halo positioning only)

Plate

Skull

Fixation pin lock assembly

Fixation pin pierces outer table of skull only

Figure 4–32. The halo provides four-point skeletal fixation using pins that pierce the outer table of the skull. These pins are attached by threads to a circumferential steel ring. The pins are locked to the steel ring with a rectangular metal device with Allen screw lock. Traction may be applied to the ring, or the ring may be fixed to the torso through threaded steel uprights. The halo is placed just above the ears and eyebrows and is temporarily held in position with four positioning pins and plates that fit firmly against the skin. The skull pins are inserted just behind the eyebrows and ears and pierce the skin without an incision. These are tightened two at a time on opposite sides of the head using two torque screwdrivers. Torques should not exceed five inch-pounds in children or six inch-pounds in adults.

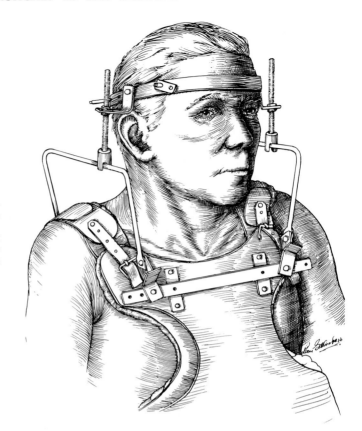

Figure 4–33. The halo ring may be attached to a plastic vest, plaster of Paris body cast, or pins through the pelvis through rigid steel uprights. This rigidly controls the head and neck and allows the patient with an unstable spine to transfer or ambulate, speeding the course of rehabilitation and avoiding the morbidity associated with prolonged bedrest and traction.

that pierces the outer table of the calvarium. These points are fragile and are easily blunted with repeated use. To improve fixation to the skull and to avoid the complication of these pins pulling out, new pins should be used with each application. Physiologic traction to 35 pounds may be applied without difficulty; however, larger loads, as may be required to reduce locked facets, are not recommended, as the pins are not designed for large forces and may pull out of the skull.

A halo ring is selected that is almost 4 cm. larger than the head circumference. This permits a gap between the ring and skull of almost 1.5 cm. The raised portion of the ring is located over the occiput, with the convex curve directed superiorly (Fig. 4–32). The lower rim of the ring should be placed at the level of the eyebrows just above the ear. The skull pins pierce the skin without an incision and should enter the skull perpendicular to its surface. The anterior skull pins are directed at the frontal bone 1 cm. above the eyebrows and 1 cm. anterior to the temporal ridge. The posterior pins enter the skull above and 1 cm. behind the ear. These positions usually corre-

spond to the middle hole in each of the three-hole sets about the ring.

The patient's head is prepared with surgical scrub about the pin sites. The halo is positioned around the skull using the positioning pins and plates (Fig. 4–32). The skin is marked with sterile surgical dye over the sites of intended pin fixation, and local anesthetic is infiltrated into the skin and periosteum over these marks. The skull pins are advanced two at a time, using torque screw drivers, with the surgeon and assistant working simultaneously on diametrically opposed pins to prevent displacement of the ring. The same torques should be registered by the surgeon and assistant. Torques should not exceed 5 inch-pounds in children or 6 inch-pounds in adults. The pins enter the outer table. The most reliable indication of satisfactory pin placement is a gradually increasing bony resistance (Kopits, 1970). A sudden decrease in this resistance is a warning that the pin is entering the space between the tables of the skull. When the halo is secure, the pins are locked in place with a pin-lock assembly.

Traction may be applied to the ring, or the

ring may be attached to the torso with a plastic vest (Fig. 4–31), plaster of Paris body cast, or pins through the pelvis. For the first few days after the halo is applied, the pins should be checked and tightened with a torque screw driver. Ordinarily, irritation about a pin tract is caused by loosening, and this may be easily corrected by tightening the pin to 5 or 6 inch-pounds. If a pin must be removed for any reason, a new pin is inserted in a hole adjacent to the unsatisfactory pin, and the old pin is removed.

THREE-POINT PIN HEADREST. The three-point pin headrest is fixed to the operating table and provides rigid immobilization and distraction of the cervical spine during surgery. We generally employ the pin headrest for posterior cervical fusions in which we anticipate adding enough immediate strength that simple braces are sufficient to protect the spine postoperatively. The pin headrest is composed of a U-shaped frame that is adjustable in width (Fig. 4–34). Two pins are fixed to a hinged yoke on one side of the frame, and the third pin is fixed to the opposite side. The

frame is attached to the operating table through a universal joint that permits a wide variety of positions. The pin headrest is generally applied with the patient supine, and the patient is then turned to the prone position. To avoid confusion when using this assembly for the first time, we recommend a mock placement on a cooperative volunteer.

The patient is anesthetized on a stretcher in the supine position using a noncollapsible endotracheal tube. The hair is thinned, but not shaved, and scrubbed with Betadine. The pins and headrest are sterilized, and the pins are inserted into the frame. The frame is centered over the patient's head, and the surgeon holds the cross bar of the frame in one hand with the back of his fingers resting on the patient's forehead (Fig. 4–35). This insures that the frame does not rest on the patient's skin. The single pin is centered just above the ear, and the double pins are placed at the same level on the opposite side. The frame is closed firmly using the turning knob until fixation is satisfactory.

The surgeon holds and applies traction to

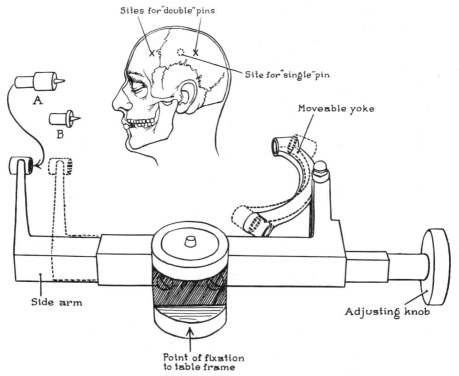

Figure 4–34. The three-point-pin headrest is a U-shaped frame that is adjustable in width. Two pins are fixed to a hinged yoke on one side of the frame and a third pin is fixed to the opposite side. These are placed just above the ear of the patient at the widest point of the skull. Pediatric pins (A) are available that have a longer shank and should be used in children or adults with a narrow head. These decrease the distance between the pins and provide satisfactory fixation even when the skull is narrow.

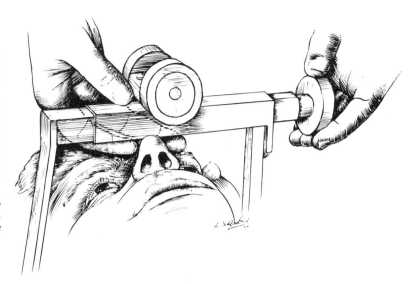

Figure 4–35. To place the pin headrest on the patient, the surgeon holds the center of the frame in one hand with his fingers resting on the patient's forehead. This insures that the frame does not press against the patient's skin. The pins are placed just above the ear at the widest portion of the skull, and the frame is closed firmly using the turning knob until the pins are well seated in the outer table of the skull. The frame should be moved to check that all of the pins are well fixed to bone and do not move within the soft tissues.

the frame with one hand and supports the neck with the second hand. The patient is then rolled like a log onto the operating table, with the surgeon controlling the head and neck and directing the other members of the team. An assistant then secures the frame to the operating table while the surgeon maintains traction until the neck is satisfactorily positioned and stabilized (Fig. 4–36). Countertraction is applied by taping the shoulders to the distal end

of the operating table. A lateral roentgenogram is then obtained to check vertebral alignment. In children or adults with a narrow head, pediatric pins should be used (Fig. 4–34A). These have a longer shank, which decreases the distance between pins and allows secure fixation even when the skull is narrow.

HEAD-HALTER TRACTION. Head-halter traction is used to provide minimal external

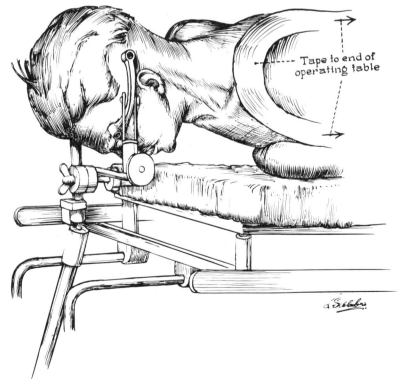

Figure 4–36. The patient is turned onto the operating table with the surgeon controlling the head and neck by holding the pin headrest. The surgeon places the head and neck in the desired position, and an assistant secures the frame to the operating table. Countertraction is then applied to the neck by taping the shoulders to the distal end of the operating table, and a lateral roentgenogram is made to verify that the vertebrae are properly aligned. (From Griswold, D. M., et al.: Atlantoaxial fusion for instability. J. Bone Joint Surg., 60A:285–292, 1978. Reproduced with permission.)

support and short periods of increased longitudinal distraction. We generally use head-halter traction for simple anterior cervical interbody fusions in which the spine is intrinsically stable. The head-halter is placed about the mandible and occiput and is joined with a metal yoke above the head. The traction rope is attached to the yoke and extended over an anesthesia frame at the head of the table, and 5 to 10 pounds of weight are suspended from it. Countertraction is applied by taping the shoulders to the distal end of the table. At the time of bone graft insertion, the anesthesiologist provides additional longitudinal distraction through the head-halter for a short period of time until the graft is in place.

ANTERIOR CERVICAL APPROACHES

Transoral Pharyngeal Approach to the Upper Cervical Spine

The bodies of the upper three cervical vertebrae are separated from the posterior pharynx by four thin layers of tissue (Fig. 4–37) and are readily palpable through this posterior pharyngeal wall. Despite this apparent accessibility, the pharyngeal approach to these vertebrae has not been very popular because of the risk of infection by pharyngeal flora and the confined working area.

Since antiquity, posterior pharyngeal abscesses have been drained through the mouth by local stab incisions. Thompson and Negus (1947) reported the use of the transoral approach to evacuate retropharyngeal abscesses. Crowe and Johnson (Southwick and Robinson, 1957) resected a large osteoma of the second and third cervical vertebrae through this approach in 1944; and Alonso (1971) reported on the resection of a chordoma of the clivus (basiocciput) through a transoral-transpalatal approach.

Fang and Ong (1962) described six cases in which a fairly extensive vertebral body resection and bone grafting were attempted through the mouth. These authors recommend this approach to reduce and fuse chronic atlantoaxial fracture-dislocations that cannot be reduced with skeletal traction. In this series, four of the six patients developed wound infections, and one of these four died of septic encephalomeningitis. Two of the six developed significant intraoperative hemorrhage from tears of the vertebral artery. These were immediately controlled with Gelfoam packing. In another two cases, the surgeons had difficulty closing the wound, which they felt was due to inadequate reduction of the vertebrae and the extra volume of the bone graft.

Our experience with this approach has been less morbid, but we have restricted our procedures to biopsy, incision and drainage, or limited resection and have not attempted more extensive open reductions and bone grafting. Because of the risk of infection and the relatively confined working area through the mouth, we recommend this route primarily for limited or direct procedures, such as drain-

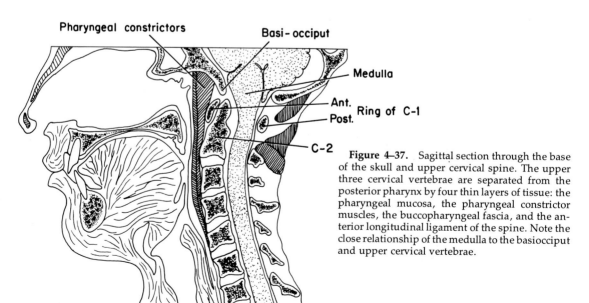

Figure 4–37. Sagittal section through the base of the skull and upper cervical spine. The upper three cervical vertebrae are separated from the posterior pharynx by four thin layers of tissue: the pharyngeal mucosa, the pharyngeal constrictor muscles, the buccopharyngeal fascia, and the anterior longitudinal ligament of the spine. Note the close relationship of the medulla to the basiocciput and upper cervical vertebrae.

age, biopsy, excision, or even resection of the odontoid.

The approach is suitable to expose the basiocciput and the vertebral bodies to the third cervical level. The ring of the first cervical vertebra lies above the soft palate, and considerable retraction or division of the soft palate may be necessary to gain suitable direct vision at this level or above. The third cervical body is at the level of the epiglottis, and the tongue must be firmly depressed to gain proper access to this level or below. The approach is ideally suited to lesions of the body of the second vertebra, which is directly visible through the mouth.

TECHNIQUE

Parenteral prophylactic antibiotics are given, based upon preoperative nasopharyngeal culture and sensitivity studies. Anesthesia is administered by endotracheal intubation using a noncollapsible tube and cuff. If extensive dissection is anticipated, tracheostomy is advisable. Despite the use of a cuffed endotracheal tube, the patient should be placed in the Trendelenburg position to prevent aspiration of blood and debris. A mouth gag of the Davis-Crowe type is placed in the mouth to maintain retraction (Fig. 4–38). The operating surgeon wears a head lamp to light the operative field. The hypopharynx is packed, and often the soft palate is folded back on itself and temporarily sutured to the junction of the hard and soft palates to expose the upper cervical vertebrae. The soft palate may be divided in the midline, and the posterior hard palate may be resected to expose the clivus or basiocciput (Alonso, 1971). The vertebral bodies should be identified by palpation. The ring of the first vertebra has a midline anterior tubercle, and the disc between the second and third vertebra is prominent and provides another localizing landmark. The eustachian tube orifices are at the level of the basiocciput.

A longitudinal incision is made in the midline of the posterior pharynx over the desired level (Fig. 4–38). The incision is carried down through the mucous membrane and soft tissues to bone. The incision should be long enough to provide adequate exposure. Although the midpharynx is relatively avascular, small bleeders will be encountered, which should be clamped and cauterized. Soft tissues may be stripped laterally by subperiosteal dissection as far as the lateral masses of the axis. The soft tissue flaps may be retracted using long stay sutures. Following the procedure, the wound and hypopharynx should be

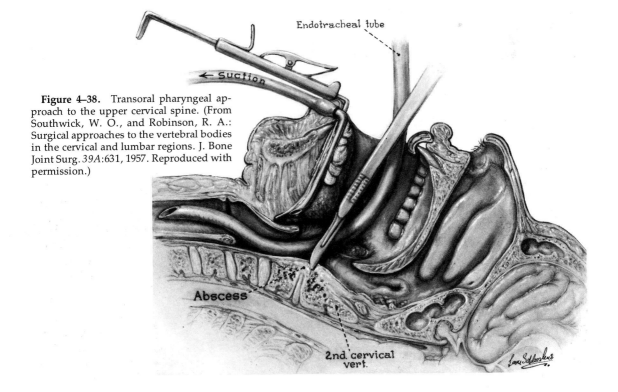

Figure 4–38. Transoral pharyngeal approach to the upper cervical spine. (From Southwick, W. O., and Robinson, R. A.: Surgical approaches to the vertebral bodies in the cervical and lumbar regions. J. Bone Joint Surg. 39A:631, 1957. Reproduced with permission.)

carefully irrigated, and all debris and fluid should be removed. The wound is closed loosely with interrupted absorbable sutures. Drainage may be provided through a small rubber drain attached to heavy silk, which is then passed through the nose and taped to the cheek. Packs are removed, and the pharynx and hypopharynx are inspected to insure that all loose material is removed. Parenteral antibiotics are given prophylactically for a total of at least three days.

This exposure may be augmented by creating an inferiorly based horseshoe-shaped flap of nasopharyngeal and oropharyngeal mucosa and muscle. This is best suited to exposures of the basiocciput and ring of the first cervical vertebra because the posterior nasopharyngeal soft tissues are thicker and more redundant at this level than below.

COMPLICATIONS

Many problems may be encountered. Children with lymphoid proliferation tend to bleed actively. If an atlantoaxial fracture-dislocation is reduced by manipulation, the vertebral arteries may be injured, with life-threatening hemorrhage or basilar artery ischemia, particularly in the elderly. Infection is always a potential problem. The risk of infection increases with the extent of resection and the application of a bone graft. Opening or exposing the dura is hazardous because of the risk of direct contamination and septic encephalomeningitis. For this reason, prophylactic broad-spectrum antibiotics are given parenterally for at least 72 hours postoperatively and are selected on the basis of preoperative nasopharyngeal culture and sensitivity studies.

Wound closure may be a problem, particularly if the incision is extended low on the third cervical body, where the overlying soft tissues are thin, adherent to the underlying bone, and less redundant. Flaps may be created laterally to provide the tissue length necessary for closure, and bone grafts should be recessed within the vertebral body so they do not protrude beyond the anterior margin.

The airway is of prime concern, and for this reason the patient should be placed in the Trendelenburg position even when the trachea is presumably sealed with an endotracheal tube and cuff. Prior to extubation, the pharynx should be carefully irrigated and inspected. Following surgery, the airway remains at risk because of edema, hemorrhage, or continued drainage. For this reason, tracheostomy should be seriously considered if the surgical dissection is extensive or if significant postoperative drainage is anticipated.

Anterior Approach to the Occiput and Upper Cervical Spine, Medial to the Carotid Sheath

DeAndrade and MacNab (1969) described an approach to the basiocciput and upper cervical spine that is an extension of the approach described by Southwick and Robinson (1957) and Bailey and Badgley (1960), entering anterior to the sternomastoid and carotid sheath. The working area is somewhat limited by the mandible and subglottic structures, particularly in patients with short and muscular necks, and one has to accept the risk of injuring the superior laryngeal nerves.

In the standard anterior approach to the middle and lower cervical spine described by Robinson and Smith (1955), Smith and Robinson (1958), and Southwick and Robinson (1957), anterior and medial to the carotid sheath, the dissection proceeds beneath the vascular leash of the superior thyroid artery and vein and the external branch of the superior laryngeal nerve. These structures cross the neck anterior and medial to the carotid artery at the level of the third cervical vertebra and are not distributed in approaches to the middle and lower cervical elements. In exposures of the upper spine and particularly of the basiocciput, however, the superior thyroid artery and vein must be ligated, and the external branch of the superior laryngeal nerve must be divided or severely distorted by retraction. When this nerve is injured or cut, persistent postoperative hoarseness and laryngeal fatigue will occur. In addition, certain other structures may be sacrificed, such as the ansa cervicalis, which provides motor innervation to the strap muscles, the internal branch of the superior laryngeal nerve, the hypoglossal nerve, and the lingual or facial arteries. Because of this and because of the limited working area, this approach should be restricted to the few special circumstances in which access or fusion at this level is required.

It is possible to biopsy a tumor of the basiocciput or fuse the occiput to the atlas through this route without fear of the bacterial contamination that the transpharyngeal approach may cause. Anterior fusion at the atlanto-occipital joint is rarely required, but it is indicated following extensive posterior laminectomy at the upper cervical elements or when a flexion deformity is present at this level. A kyphos or flexion deformity at the atlanto-occipital level subjects a posterior graft to tensile rather than compressive forces, and on this account the graft may attenuate with time. On the other hand, an anterior graft across a kyphos would be relatively compressed and should provide continuing support.

This approach medial to the carotid sheath may also be used to excise lesions of the odontoid or fuse the upper spine, but the route to be discussed next (Henry 1957; Whitesides 1966), lateral and posterior to the carotid sheath, offers safe access without disturbing the superior laryngeal nerves.

TECHNIQUE

Because of the potential of extensive postoperative edema and airway obstruction, tracheostomy should be considered preoperatively. In the presence of instability or if extensive dissection is anticipated, skull traction with tongs or a halo is recommended. Exposure may be made from either side, although we prefer the left to avoid injury to an aberrant recurrent laryngeal nerve on the right. The incision is made along the anterior border of the sternomastoid from the level of the mastoid prominence to the cricoid cartilage (Fig. 4–39A, insert). The platysma and superficial layer of the deep cervical fascia are divided in line with the skin incision. A large communicating branch of the external jugular system is often found imbedded within the superficial layer of the deep cervical fascia along the anterior margin of the sternomastoid muscle and should be ligated and divided. High in the wound, the external jugular vein and great auricular nerve (Fig. 4–4) will be found close together within the superficial layer of the deep cervical fascia, crossing anterior to the sternomastoid muscle and ascending over the parotid gland in front of the ear. These can be retracted posteriorly but may be divided if necessary.

Beneath the superficial layer of the deep cervical fascia, the carotid triangle emerges, with the anterior border of the sternomastoid muscle and subjacent carotid sheath forming the posterior limit (Fig. 4–39A). The posterior belly of the digastric and stylohyoid muscles, the hypoglossal nerve, and the hyoid bone form the superior oblique margin. The inferior margin, running anteriorly and obliquely, is formed by the anterior belly of the omohyoid muscle and the strap muscles beneath. Several major arterial tributaries, veins, and nerves cross this triangle from posterior to anterior. Some of these must be divided to provide proper access to the basiocciput and vertebrae beneath. The superior thyroid, lingual, and facial arteries, all branches of the external carotid artery, cross the triangle in ascending sequence. The ansa hypoglossi, the external and internal branches of the superior laryngeal nerve (a division of the vagus nerve), and the hypoglossal nerve and its muscular branches descend across the triangle obliquely. Damage to the laryngeal nerves will produce minor but persistent laryngeal dysfunction, whereas injury to the hypoglossal nerve will result in unilateral paralysis of the tongue, and persistent difficulty with swallowing and speech may occur.

After opening the superficial layers of the deep cervical fascia, the sternomastoid and strap muscles are developed by sharp and blunt dissection. The spinal accessory nerve is identified and protected as it enters the anterior border of the sternomastoid muscle at its upper third. It is separated from the internal jugular vein and retracted laterally with the sternomastoid. The omohyoid muscle may be divided at its central tendinous portion, and the strap muscles may be retracted medially. The carotid artery is identified by its pulsations, and the carotid sheath is carefully exposed. The superior thyroid and lingual arteries and veins and occasionally the facial artery must be ligated. The external and internal branches of the superior laryngeal nerve should be isolated and retracted superiorly and anteriorly, if possible, but for adequate exposure division may be required. The hypoglossal nerve should be carefully protected.

The retropharyngeal space is entered at the level of the thyroid cartilage and is developed by blunt dissection (Fig. 4–39B and C). Dissection proceeds superiorly along the anterior bodies of the cervical vertebrae posterior to the pharyngeal musculature and fascia. The first cervical vertebra is easily identified by its most prominent transverse processes and central anterior tubercle. Above this is a hollow where the basiocciput ends (Fig. 4–37). The basiocciput is angled anteriorly to create the roof of the pharynx at the basisphenoid. Dissection onto the basisphenoid, the roof of the pharynx, is hindered by the insertion of the pharyngeal muscles on the pharyngeal tubercle. The anterior margin of the foramen magnum may be palpated between the basiocciput and the ring of the first cervical vertebra.

The pharynx is retracted anteriorly and laterally with a broad right-angle retractor, and the underlying anterior vertebrae and basiocciput are exposed (Fig. 4–39C). Four cranial nerves, (the hypoglossal, glossopharyngeal, vagus, and accessory nerves), as well as the internal carotid artery and jugular vein, are tethered to the occiput as they leave their foramina and may be injured by vigorous retraction or dissection. The hypoglossal nerve leaves the occiput from the anterior condyloid foramen just lateral to the midportion of the occipital condyle, and the jugular vein and carotid artery enter the skull just

lateral to this. This leaves only 2 cm. of working area from the midline to these structures laterally at the base of the skull. The pharyngeal and laryngeal branches of the vagus nerve arise shortly below this level and are stretched by anterior retraction of the pharynx. The longus colli and longus capitis muscles lie over the transverse processes and bodies of the first and second cervical vertebrae. The longus colli meets in midline at the anterior tubercle of C1. Beneath is the anterior longitudinal ligament and its extension to the skull. To minimize bleeding from the profuse plexus of veins within the longus colli and capitis muscles, a longitudinal incision is made to the bone in the midline over the first and second vertebrae and basiocciput. The ligament and muscle are dissected subperiosteally

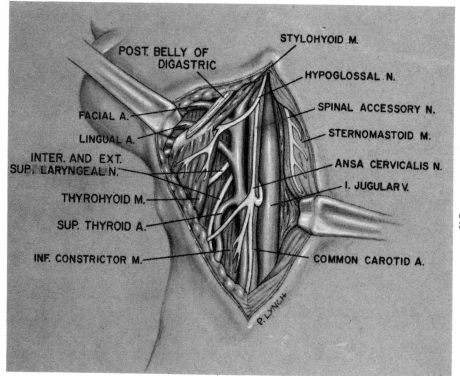
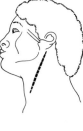

A

Figure 4–39. *A Insert,* Skin incision along the anterior border of the sternomastoid muscle from the mastoid prominence to the level of the cricoid cartilage. The sternomastoid muscle is retracted, and the deep structures of the carotid triangle are exposed. *B,* Cross-section of the neck at the level of the thyroid cartilage showing the plane of dissection anterior to the sternomastoid muscle and carotid sheath. *C,* Vertebrae and associated structures of the retropharyngeal space. Although they will not ordinarily be exposed at this level of the dissection, the internal carotid artery, jugular vein, and vagus and hypoglossal nerves are tethered to the base of the skull and may be injured by harsh dissection.

Illustration continues on opposite page.

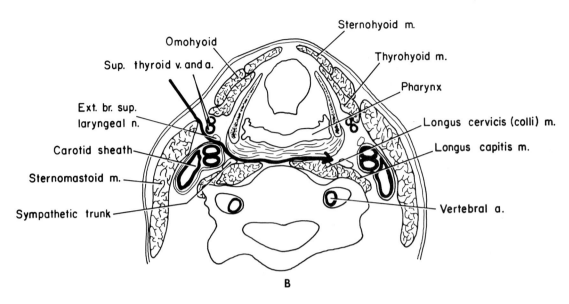

B

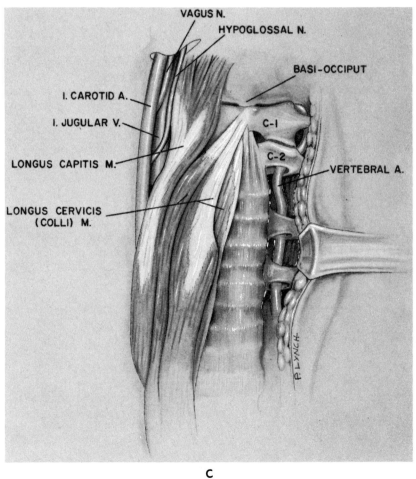

C

Figure 4–39. *Continued.*

and laterally to expose the bone. Through this approach, biopsy, curettage, or fusion is possible.

To fuse the vertebrae at this level, a broad but shallow trough is made in the bone. It should be recalled that the ring of the first vertebra and the basiocciput are thin structures, so the trough should be shallow to avoid injury to the underlying medulla. A thin segment of corticocancellous bone is taken from the iliac crest and laid into the trough. The bone graft should not protrude more than a few millimeters anterior to the vertebra and basiocciput to avoid an excessive bulge into the posterior pharynx. A suction drain may be placed in the inferior retropharyngeal space to reduce postoperative retropharyngeal hematoma and should be removed on the second or third postoperative day. The omohyoid may be reapproximated with interrupted sutures. The platysma and skin are sutured in separate layers to effect a cosmetic closure.

Postoperatively, the patient is placed in a high humidity tent for 48 hours to reduce tracheal and laryngeal swelling. Tracheostomy is recommended to avoid airway obstruction, particularly if considerable dissection, retraction, or bone graft has been applied. Skeletal traction is maintained until the patient's physical condition permits application of a Minerva body jacket or halo cast. External stabilization is maintained until fusion is established roentgenographically in four to six months.

COMPLICATIONS

Airway obstruction caused by edema of the pharynx and larynx or bulging of bone graft into the posterior pharynx is the most immediate threat. We recommend considering tracheostomy either preoperatively or postoperatively to reduce this risk.

Laryngeal and pharyngeal dysfunction may be anticipated in the immediate postoperative period, secondary to retraction of the laryngeal nerves, even if none have been transected. Patients should be advised to expect difficulty with phonation and swallowing, especially in the early postoperative course. Persistent but minor problems will arise if the external branch of the superior laryngeal nerve has been transected. DeAndrade and MacNab (1969) reported persistent postoperative hoarseness, laryngeal fatigue, and an inability to produce high tones in three of five cases in their study.

Other potential complications include injury to the medulla or upper cervical spinal cord. Hemorrhage from the carotid artery, the jugular vein, or their tributaries may be difficult to control without cerebral ischemia or possible air embolism. Because of these many dangers, this approach should be reserved for situations that permit no alternative route.

Anterolateral Approach to the Upper Cervical Spine, Lateral to the Carotid Sheath

Whitesides and Kelly (1966) reported on their experience with the anterolateral approach to the atlantoaxial vertebral bodies originally described by Henry (1957) for exposing the vertebral artery. This approach is anterior to the sternomastoid but lateral and posterior to the carotid sheath. The major branches of the external carotid artery and laryngeal nerves are thus not disturbed. The upper end of the exposure is limited to the ring of the first cervical vertebra. The basiocciput cannot be reached safely through this route lateral and posterior to the carotid sheath without the risk of injuring the internal carotid artery, jugular vein, and vagus, accessory, and hypoglossal nerves. These structures are effectively tethered to the skull posterior to the basiocciput and would be injured if retracted sufficiently to fully expose the basiocciput.

This approach is ideally suited to reach the anterior aspect of the first and second cervical vertebrae without risk of bacterial contamination by nasopharyngeal flora. It also permits direct distal extension to the first thoracic vertebra without permanently affecting laryngeal function.

Because of the many potential hazards, this approach should be restricted to those circumstances that require anterior exploration at this level, such as biopsy and curettage of tumor or infection or resecting the odontoid. Anterior fusion of the first three cervical vertebrae is possible through this exposure but should be considered only in situations in which posterior fusions are impractical, such as following extensive posterior laminectomy or in the presence of a fixed flexion deformity.

In summary, if an extra pharyngeal exposure as high as the basiocciput is needed, the approach should be medial to the carotid sheath, accepting the risk of injuring the superior laryngeal nerves and causing postoperative hoarseness. If access only as high as the first cervical ring is necessary, the route lateral and posterior to the carotid sheath is available, and the superior laryngeal nerves can be spared. However, it is important to remember that the carotid sheath should be retracted forward gently because of the threat of avulsing these vessels as well as certain cranial nerves from the base of the skull.

TECHNIQUE

Because of potential postoperative edema and airway obstruction, either preoperative or postoperative tracheostomy should be considered. If the spine is unstable or if extensive surgical dissection is planned, skull traction with tongs or halo may be needed. A longitudinal incision is made along the anterior margin of the sternomastoid muscle (Fig. 4–40). At the superior end, the incision is carried transversely and back over the mastoid prominence. Deep to the platysma is the broad sheath of the superficial layer of the deep cervical fascia. Embedded within this at the superior pole of the incision is the external jugular vein (Fig. 4-4), which crosses the anterior margin of the sternomastoid muscle. This must be ligated and divided. Posterior to

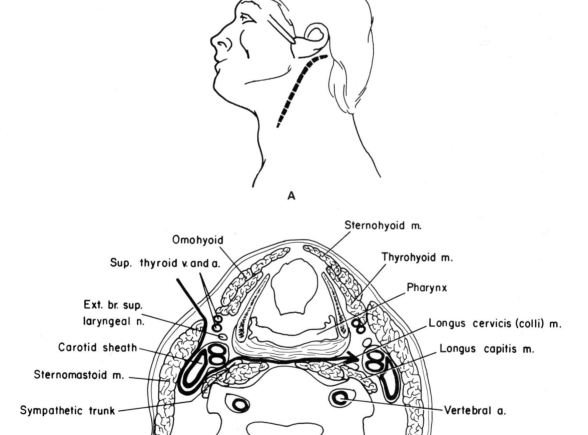

Figure 4–40. *A,* Longitudinal incision along the anterior border of the sternomastoid muscle passing posteriorly over the mastoid prominence. *B,* Cross-section of the neck at the level of the thyroid cartilage showing the plane of dissection posterior to the carotid sheath and anterior to the sympathetic trunk. The sternomastoid muscle is everted, permitting direct access to the posterior aspect of the carotid sheath.

the external jugular vein and running parallel with it in the same tissue plane is the great auricular nerve, which usually divides into its terminal branches at the anterior border of the sternomastoid, providing sensation over the parotid gland and around the ear. Some of these anterior branches may need to be divided. The sternomastoid muscle is divided at its mastoid origin, and the splenius capitis muscle beneath may be partially sectioned if necessary. The superficial layer of the deep cervical fascia is opened anterior to the sternomastoid, and this muscle is mobilized by sharp and blunt dissection. The spinal accessory nerve courses downward, anterior and deep to the sternomastoid muscle, and enters this muscle at its upper third. The accessory nerve should be identified and separated from the jugular vein to provide greater mobility and should be protected throughout the procedure. The sternomastoid branch of the occipital artery is inferior to the accessory nerve but travels in the same plane and should be ligated.

Dissection then proceeds lateral and posterior to the carotid sheath, separating the carotid sheath from the sternomastoid (Figure 4–40B). The sternomastoid muscle and accessory nerve are retracted posteriorly, and the carotid sheath is retracted anteriorly. The transverse processes of all the cervical vertebrae are palpable within this space. Using sharp and finger dissection, the plane between the alar and prevertebral fascia is developed along the anterior aspect of the transverse processes to the vertebral bodies. The dissection plane is anterior to the longus colli and capitis muscles as well as the overlying sympathetic trunk and superior cervical ganglion. The sympathetic trunk tends to remain with the longus capitis muscle during this dissection and is not usually disturbed. The ring of the first cervical vertebra and its anterior tubercle may be identified by palpation. Below this, the next major prominence is at the disc space between the second and third vertebrae (Fig. 4–37). When the vertebral level is accurately identified, a longitudinal incision is made to the bone over the middle of the vertebra through the anterior longitudinal ligament. The ligament and overlying muscles are dissected subperiosteally and laterally.

The upper cervical vertebrae may be visualized through this approach, and by extending the incision distally, the vertebral bodies of the middle and lower spine may be reached in continuity. The basiocciput, clivus, and sphenoid may be palpated but are poorly seen.

Biopsy, curettage, or anterior fusion using corticocancellous strips in a longitudinal trough is possible. The retropharyngeal space should be drained to prevent excessive retropharyngeal hematoma, and the wound should be closed. If stability is in doubt, external stabilization in a brace is recommended until fusion is established roentgenographically.

An alternative approach within the retropharyngeal space is to separate the longus colli and capitis muscles from their bony insertions on the transverse processes and retract these muscles anteriorly. This provides direct exposure of the nerve roots, transverse processes, and vertebral artery but will distrub the sympathetic rami communicantes and may cause a Horner's syndrome.

COMPLICATIONS

Airway obstruction and difficulty with swallowing due to retropharyngeal edema or hematoma are the most immediate threats. We recommend considering tracheostomy either preoperatively or postoperatively to reduce the risk of airway obstruction and suggest nursing the patient in a high humidity tent or with a mask for a few days after surgery to reduce pharyngeal edema. Intravenous feeding may be required for five to seven days because of dysphagia.

The long, oblique skin incision tends to leave an area of hypesthesia around it and the ear. This is more pronounced than one sees around short, transverse incisions in the lower neck but is rarely a problem. The spinal accessory nerve should be carefully identified and protected throughout the procedure to prevent weakness of the sternomastoid and trapezius muscles. The sympathetic trunk and superior cervical ganglion lying over the longus capitis muscle and opposite the second and third cervical vertebrae should be preserved to prevent Horner's syndrome. Prolonged or excessive retraction of the carotid sheath medially can interfere with function of the vagus and recurrent laryngeal nerves on that side.

Hemorrhage can occur from a variety of sources. The vertebral artery is reasonably well protected in its course through the costotransverse foramina, but it may be injured in the interval between transverse processes. Ordinarily, the right vertebral artery is not dominant, but injury to the left or dominant vertebral artery can cause receptive blindness with infarction of the calcarine fissure.

Anterior Approach to the Middle and Lower Cervical Vertebrae, Below C2, Medial to the Carotid Sheath

This approach has been clearly described by Southwick and Robinson (1957, 1960, and 1961) and Bailey and Badgley (1960). Although its origin is unknown, Lahey and Warren (1954) described a similar approach to excise diverticula of the esophagus. Robinson and Smith (1955) successfully used the exposure in a series of anterior interbody arthrodeses of the cervical vertebrae, and it has subsequently gained wide popular acceptance as an approach to the spine. Because of the abundance of vital structures in the neck, a thorough knowledge of the anatomic landmarks is a basic requirement for the safety of the patient. The plane of dissection is beneath the vascular leash of the superior thyroid vessels, the external branch of the superior laryngeal nerve, and through certain natural cleavage planes. The landmarks are well defined, and a relatively safe and straightforward route to the vertebral bodies unfolds without dividing any major structure or vessel.

This approach provides direct access to the bodies of the vertebrae from the third through the first thoracic levels. It may be used to biopsy or excise a lesion of the anterior vertebral body or to drain an abscess. Vertebral bodies may be excised and replaced with bone graft; the disc space may be curetted, and posterior osteophytes compressing the nerve roots or spinal cord may be removed, and the resultant defect may be filled with bone graft.

TECHNIQUE

Although local anesthesia could be used, general endotracheal anesthesia is routinely employed in our center to maintain an unobstructed airway. Head-halter traction (10 to 15 pounds) is generally required, especially for interbody fusion. Countertraction is applied by securing the shoulders with tape to the distal end of the operating table. A small, folded sheet is placed between the scapulae to depress the shoulders; the head is slightly extended and rotated to the right, and a folded towel is placed behind the middle of the neck to support it during dissection and graft insertion.

The area from the mandible to the upper thorax is prepared, and the neck is draped free. If a bone graft is to be used, the anterior iliac crest is also prepared. A short, transverse incision is made within a skin crease two to four finger breadths above the clavicle (Fig. 4–41), depending upon the level of exposure required. Although the incision may be made on either side, an incision to the left of the midline is less likely to injure an aberrant recurrent laryngeal nerve on the right.

The incision is begun at the midline and is extended over the belly of the sternomastoid muscle laterally. The platysma is divided in the same line as the skin incision. Skin flaps are developed superiorly and inferiorly beneath the platysma but superficial to the subjacent deep fascia. The superficial layer of the deep fascia overlying the strap and sternomastoid muscles is incised longitudinally. The margin between the strap muscles medially and the sternomastoid muscle laterally is identified and developed. A plane is then created medial to the carotid sheath and lateral to the thyroid through the thin intermediate layers of the deep cervical fascia (Fig. 4–42) using a combination of sharp and blunt dissection. The carotid artery is easily identified by its pulsations, and the carotid sheath is retracted laterally with a finger to protect it from injury. The dissection then proceeds within the natural cleavage plane between the alar and visceral fascia behind the esophagus to the anterior aspect of the vertebral bodies. This is best performed with blunt finger dissection, preserving the integrity of these fascial sheaths. The alar fascia surrounds the carotid sheath structures, the visceral fascia, the esophagus, and recurrent laryngeal nerves. If these sheaths are left intact, there is less likelihood of entering or injuring these structures. The plane between the alar and visceral fascia should be extended inferiorly and superiorly along the vertebral bodies to allow adequate exposure. The trachea and esophagus are retracted medially, and the carotid sheath is retracted laterally, using smooth deep blade retractors. Care is required to properly identify the smooth-walled esophagus and to protect it during retraction. The vertebral bodies are palpable through the alar and prevertebral fascia. The disc spaces may be identified as they protrude above the level of the vertebral bodies; the vertebral bodies themselves are slightly concave. A longitudinal incision is made with scissors in the prevertebral fascia over the midline of the vertebral bodies, and the fascia is separated laterally by blunt dissection. The thin translucent anterior longitudinal ligament covers the anterior aspect of

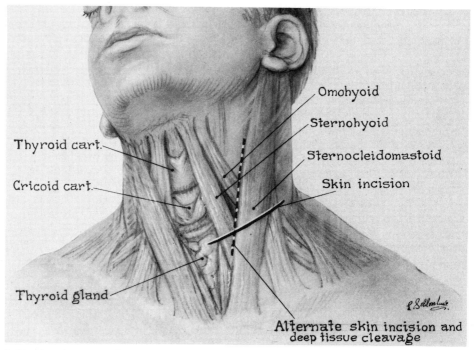

Figure 4–41. Anterior approach to the mid and lower cervical vertebrae. (From Southwick, W. O., and Robinson, R. A.: Surgical approaches to the vertebral bodies in the cervical and lumbar regions. J. Bone Joint Surg., *39A*:634, 1957. Reproduced with permission.)

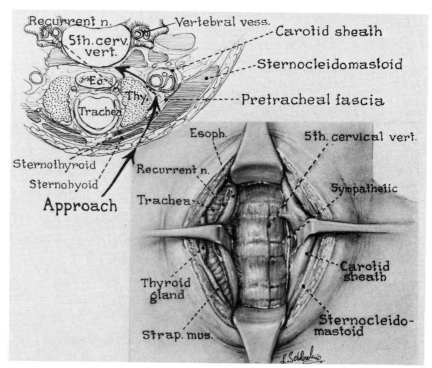

Figure 4–42. Anterior approach to the mid and lower cervical vertebrae, deep dissection. (From Southwick, W. O., and Robinson, R. A.: Surgical approaches to the vertebral bodies in the cervical and lumbar regions. J. Bone Joint Surg., *39A*:634, 1957. Reproduced with permission.)

the vertebrae. Laterally, the longus colli fibers crowd the vertebral bodies and cover the transverse processes. The sympathetic nerves lie over the longus capitis muscles laterally and should not be disturbed.

In order to identify the proper vertebral level, it is recommended that a lateral roentgenogram be obtained in the operating room with a radiopaque marker placed in the disc at the level desired. Other aids to localization are the cricoid cartilage, which is opposite the body of the sixth cervical vertebra, and the carotid (Chassaignac's tubercle), which is the prominent, anterior, transverse process of the sixth cervical vertebra. When osteoarthritic spurs are present along the anterior bodies of the vertebrae, they are usually palpable and may be an aid to localization.

For exposures of the lower cervical vertebrae below C5, the skin incision should be located about two finger breadths above the clavicle, and dissection should proceed beneath the omohyoid muscle. For higher levels of exposure, the skin incision should be located above this, and dissection may proceed above the omohyoid muscle. A common mistake is to locate the skin incision too inferiorly. For example, to approach the C4-5 interspace, an incision above the cricoid cartilage and at least three finger breadths above the clavicle is required.

COMPLICATIONS

There are a number of potential complications associated with this procedure. Perforation of the esophagus may occur directly if the visceral fascia is opened or if the esophagus is not properly identified. The esophagus is a soft, smooth-walled structure, and if its location is in doubt, a soft rubber nasogastric tube may be inserted by the anesthetist and the lumen can be identified. The nasogastric tube should be removed before the esophagus is retracted and the vertebrae are exposed. The esophagus may be injured by vigorous retraction or by the use of retractors with sharp blades, teeth, or self-retaining features. Hand-held retractors with smooth blades are, therefore, recommended. If the esophagus is perforated, it should be repaired immediately with sutures, and bone grafting should be delayed until healing has occurred. Perforations that are overlooked usually result in retroesophageal abscesses with attendant fever, swelling, and dysphagia. The diagnosis may be established by fluoroscopy using a water-soluble, radiopaque dye swallow. Retroesophageal abscesses require prompt drainage and debridement with repair of the defect, if possible, and prolonged nasogastric intubation until continuity and healing are established.

The recurrent laryngeal nerve is ordinarily protected by the visceral fascia, but it may be injured in this approach by harsh dissection or retraction. On the left side, the recurrent laryngeal nerve descends into the thorax within the carotid sheath. It leaves the vagus nerve and carotid sheath within the thorax, loops under the aortic arch, beneath the ligamentum arteriosum, and ascends into the neck beside the trachea and esophagus. On the right side, the course of the recurrent laryngeal nerve is not so constant. Usually, it descends within the carotid sheath and loops beneath the subclavian artery, ascending into the neck between the trachea and esophagus (Fig. 4–21). The recurrent nerve on the right may leave the carotid sheath at a higher level, however, crossing anteriorly behind the thyroid. For this reason, we select the left rather than the right anterior approach to avoid direct injury to an aberrant recurrent nerve.

Horner's syndrome will occur if the sympathetic nerve fibers are irritated or damaged in their course from the stellate ganglion over the longus capitis muscles and the transverse processes. This may be avoided if these muscles are not disturbed or if they are retracted only slightly and subperiosteally from the midline.

The vertebral artery may be injured as it ascends within the costotransverse foramina from one vertebra to the next. Usually, bleeding may be controlled with Gelfoam pack, and no adverse cerebral effects should result if the injury is unilateral.

The superior thyroid artery is the second branch of the external carotid artery and crosses anterior and inferior to the superior pole of the thyroid at the level of the third cervical vertebra. This artery should be protected in dissections of the upper cervical vertebrae. The external laryngeal nerve courses across the neck adjacent and superior to the superior thyroid artery. This nerve innervates the cricothyroid muscle and, when injured, produces hoarseness and laryngeal fatigue. For this reason, it should be identified and protected in dissections of the upper cervical vertebrae.

The inferior thyroid artery, a small branch of the subclavian artery, also crosses the neck and enters the inferior pole of the thyroid gland and should be identified and ligated in dissections of the lower cervical vertebrae.

The thoracic duct ascends from the thorax just lateral to the esophagus, lying on the prevertebral fascia. It loops over the subclavian artery at the level of the first thoracic vertebral body, anterior to the scalenus anterior and phrenic nerve, and enters the subclavian vein (Fig. 4–4). In anterior approaches to the lower cervical and upper thoracic spine, the duct should be protected, or a surgical approach to the right of the midline should be employed.

Postoperative hoarseness or laryngeal edema is occasionally a problem caused by irritation of the trachea or larynx by retraction or endotracheal intubation. This may be minimized by placing the patient in a high humidity tent for 24 to 36 hours after surgery.

Anterior Approach to the Lower Cervical and Upper Thoracic Vertebrae

Nanson (1957) described an approach to the lower cervical and upper thoracic vertebrae through the thoracic inlet. This approach was designed to provide access to the upper thoracic sympathetic ganglia, but the approach may also be used for scalene node dissection, section of the scalenus anterior muscle, and exploration of the soft tissues at the base of the neck. In addition, it provides excellent exposure of the lower cervical vertebral bodies and more limited exposure of the upper thoracic vertebral bodies.

Access within the thorax is dependent upon several variables: the diameter of the thoracic inlet, the height of the clavicles and manubrium anteriorly, and the extent of cervicothoracic kyphos. Preoperatively, the upper margin of the clavicles and manubrium should be compared with the vertebral body level on a standard lateral roentgenogram of the upper thoracic spine. In some patients, the manubrium and thoracic inlet will ride high to the level of the first or second thoracic vertebra, and exposures within the thorax below this level will be limited and impractical. In others, a lower-riding manubrium may permit access as far as the third or fourth thoracic levels. In patients with a narrow anteroposterior chest diameter or significant cervicothoracic kyphos, the intrathoracic exposure will be restricted.

The approach may be made to either side of the midline, although we prefer the right side to avoid the thoracic duct on the left. The recurrent laryngeal nerve on the right should be identified and protected as it loops beneath the subclavian artery (Fig. 4–21). Proximal extension via this exposure along the cervical spine is hampered by the subclavian vessels and recurrent nerve. The subclavian vessels effectively tether the carotid artery and internal jugular vein so that proximal extension lateral to the carotid sheath is impractical. Dissection medial to the carotid sheath jeopardizes the recurrent laryngeal nerve. However, the recurrent nerve may be identified and mobilized sufficiently to permit retraction of the esophagus, trachea, and thyroid and to reach the spine as high as the fifth cervical level without extending the skin incision.

TECHNIQUE

A towel is placed beneath the scapulae to extend the neck, the head is rotated away from the proposed incision, and the arm on the side of the incision is pulled down to open the supraclavicular space. A transverse incision at least 8 cm. in length is made parallel to and 1 cm. above the right clavicle (Fig. 4–43A, insert). The incision extends from the midline to the lateral margin of the sternomastoid muscle. The platysma muscle is divided transversely in line with the incision. The external jugular vein and medial supraclavicular nerve, a cutaneous nerve to the anterior chest, are located within the superficial fascia just lateral to the platysma and sternomastoid and should be spared if possible (Fig. 4–43A). The clavicular head of the sternomastoid is separated from its manubrial head by blunt dissection in line with the muscle fibers.

The internal jugular and subclavian veins lie behind the sternomastoid muscle and are separated from it by the deep cervical fascia and a potential space (known as "Burns' space") between two layers of fascia. To protect these major vessels from injury, the operator should bluntly dissect with a finger behind the clavicular head of the sternomastoid within this potential space (Fig. 4–43B). The clavicular head of the sternomastoid is then divided transversely, close to its clavicular insertion, with a finger behind the muscle, protecting these vessels.

Beneath the sternomastoid is the intermediate layer of deep fascia. The omohyoid muscle is invested in this fascia and crosses the field descending obliquely from medial to lateral. At its midportion it is tendinous and is invested in a well-developed fascial expansion of the intermediate layers of fascia. This fascial expansion serves as a pulley, which permits the muscle to change directions from its oblique descent within the neck to a more lateral course extending to the shoulder. This middle layer of deep fascia is divided transversely, and the omohyoid is released from its pulley and retracted superiorly and laterally. Beneath is a fairly dense fat pad with small lymph nodes overlying the scalenus anterior muscle. This fat pad effectively hides the thyrocervical arterial trunk, phrenic nerve, and scalene muscle and should be cleared to visualize the structures beneath (Fig. 4–43C). By blunt finger dissection, the internal jugular vein and contents of the carotid sheath can be separated from the prevertebral fascia and retracted medially away from the scalenus anterior muscle. Two large arteries cross the field: the suprascapular artery, which crosses low and transversely, and the transverse cervical artery, which crosses obliquely high in the field (Fig. 4–43C). These arteries or the thyrocervical trunk from which they arise should be doubly ligated and divided. The phrenic nerve crosses the scalenus anterior muscle from lateral to medial. It should be carefully mobilized along its entire length within the wound and should be retracted medially.

Both margins of the scalenus anterior muscle are defined, and a right-angle clamp is passed behind this muscle. The muscle is divided sharply by cutting onto this right-angle clamp 1 cm proximal to the muscle's insertion. Often a small branch of the subclavian artery is found entering this muscle, and this should be ligated. Beneath the scalenus anterior muscle is a thin, often translucent layer of fascia (Fig. 4–43D) that covers the dome of the lung known as Sibson's fascia. This is a continuation of the prevertebral fascia lining the intrathoracic surfaces of the ribs. It passes over the dome of the lung and down the anterior side of the pleura and fuses with the lateral wall of the alar fascia at the carotid sheath. Sibson's fascia is opened transversely using scissors, and the visceral pleura and lung beneath are dissected free using a finger. The visceral pleura may be bluntly dissected to the neck of the third rib, and the pleura and lung may be retracted inferiorly and laterally using a moist pad (Fig. 4–43E). Care is required to avoid injuring the pleura, causing a pneumothorax. The stellate ganglion

is visible over the neck of the first rib, and the vertebrae are medial to this. The first thoracic nerve root is seen climbing out of the thorax over the first rib and should be protected. The vertebral level may be identified in reference to the first rib. The first rib articulates with the seventh cervical and first thoracic vertebral bodies and intervening discs. However, lateral roentgenograms should be obtained in the operating room with a radiopaque marker fixed to the vertebra in question to verify the level.

Through this approach, exposures of the seventh cervical and first thoracic vertebrae are usually adequate, but exposures distal to this may be limited by the size and position of the anterior thorax. The distal extent of the exposure may be predicted with preoperative lateral roentgenograms of the upper thoracic spine as discussed earlier. Proximal extension along the cervical spine is hampered by the recurrent laryngeal nerve on the right, but this nerve usually may be mobilized and retracted sufficiently to provide access to the fifth cervical vertebral body. Biopsy, curettage, disc excision, or bone grafting is possible through this approach.

The wound should be flooded with saline before closure, and the lungs should be inflated to check for possible air leak. The scalenus anterior muscle and clavicular head of the sternomastoid muscle may be repaired, and the platysma and skin should be approximated. We recommend inserting a drain through the wound to the dome of the lung to prevent the accumulation of fluid and blood, which might otherwise compromise chest expansion. Prior to extubation, a chest roentgenogram should be obtained in the operating room to check for pneumothorax, and a chest tube should be inserted if one is present.

COMPLICATIONS

All the complications discussed in the section on anterior approaches to the middle and lower cervical vertebrae are possible. In addition, the pleura should be inspected carefully for tears, and these should be repaired if present. The inferior thyroid artery should be identified and ligated if necessary. If the approach is to the left of the midline, the thoracic duct should be identified and ligated if injured. A troublesome chylous effusion may occur if perforations are not identified. The thoracic duct may be divided without incident, as collateral pathways will develop with time, but it should be doubly ligated both proximally and

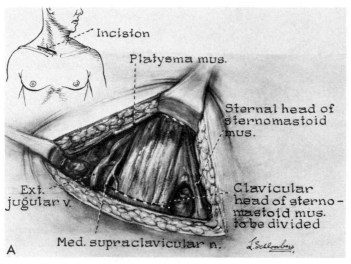

Incision

Platysma mus.

Sternal head of sternomastoid mus.

Ext. jugular v.

Clavicular head of sterno- mastoid mus. to be divided

Med. supraclavicular n.

A

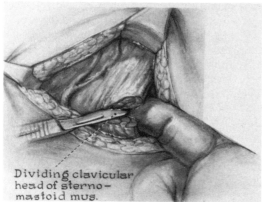

Dividing clavicular head of sterno- mastoid mus.

Figure 4–43. Anterior approach to the lower cervical and upper thoracic vertebrae. *A*, Incision. *Insert*, line of incision across the clavicular head of the sternomastoid muscle. *B*, Dissection within Burns' space behind the sternomastoid muscle. A finger is placed within this space to protect the internal jugular and subclavian veins as well as the carotid artery from injury during the division of the clavicular head of the sternomastoid.

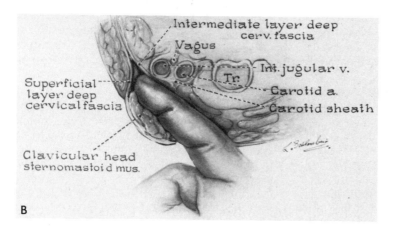

Intermediate layer deep cerv. fascia

Vagus

Int. jugular v.

Tr

Superficial layer deep cervical fascia

Carotid a.

Carotid sheath

Clavicular head sternomastoid mus.

B

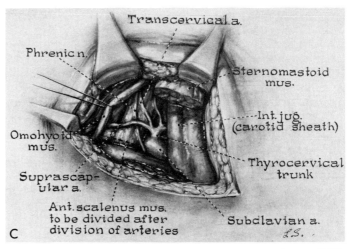

C

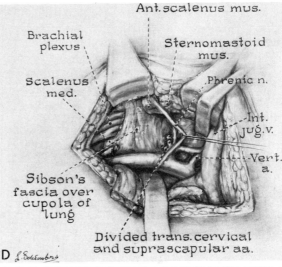

Figure 4–43. *Continued. C,* Arteries and phrenic nerve crossing the scalenus anterior muscle. The omohyoid muscle is retracted upward and laterally. The subclavian vein lies anterior to the scalenus anterior muscle at the bottom of the wound. *D,* The scalenus anterior muscle is divided, exposing Sibson's fascia and the subclavian artery. The dome of the lung lies beneath this thin layer of Sibson's fascia. *E,* The visceral pleura and lung have been retracted laterally and downward and are protected with a moist pad. The posterior thorax, stellate ganglion, and upper thoracic vertebral bodies are now visible looking from above downward through the thoracic inlet.

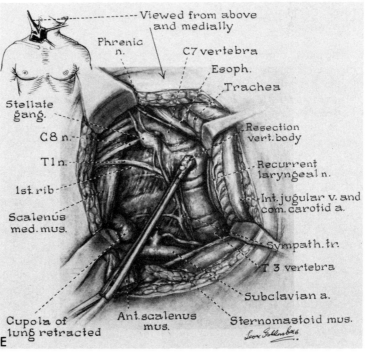

E

119

distally (Lindskog, 1962). It should be noted that although the thoracic duct usually arises in the thoracic inlet to the left of the midline, it may bifurcate or ramify within the thorax and present to the right or on both sides of the midline.

The phrenic and recurrent laryngeal nerves may be injured during retraction, and temporary paralysis of the involved diaphragm or vocal cord can occur. Because of this, special care is required to protect these structures during their mobilization and retraction, and some assistance with ventilation may be required following surgery. The right recurrent laryngeal nerve normally arises below the subclavian artery and crosses the neck anterior to the thyroid gland and trachea (Fig. 4–21). The right recurrent nerve can arise higher in the neck and cross the larynx at almost any level. Therefore, it is important to identify this nerve, particularly when proximal extension along the cervical spine is planned.

Fluid may accumulate postoperatively above the dome of the lung and may depress the lung and thus limit the tidal volume of ventilation. For this reason, it is wise to drain this space and check that collapse of the upper lobe does not occur on follow-up chest roentgenograms.

Biopsy, Curettage, and Drainage Through the Anterior Approach to the Cervical Spine

The most direct and effective means of diagnosing a lesion of the anterior cervical spine is via the transoral, pharyngeal approach or through one of the anterolateral exposures. The operative approach will be dictated by the cervical level and the extent of the proposed dissection. On reaching the vertebral body, a needle should be inserted into the suspected area, and roentgenograms should be made on the operating table to verify the level and position of the lesion. Often the lesion is grossly evident, and a direct biopsy specimen can be obtained using a drill and curettes. Large sterile defects should be grafted primarily.

Osteomyelitis of the vertebral body or disc space infections can be effectively curetted and drained through these anterior exposures. The curettage should be thorough to remove as much diseased bone and divitalized tissue as possible. If the spine is made unstable, the patient should be protected with

traction or a halo cast, and posterior interspinous wiring and fusion should be performed at a later date. If a large anterior defect persists, anterior grafting may ultimately be required to fill this defect. A tuberculous abscess may be drained anteriorly and at the time of drainage and curettage should be grafted primarily with antibiotic coverage. Direct surgical exposure of a suspect lesion offers the best chance to identify the pathologic condition and treat the disease process primarily.

Excision of Intervertebral Discs, Osteophytes, and Interbody Fusion Anteriorly

Herniated intervertebral discs compressing the spinal cord or nerve roots may be treated expeditiously through the anterior approach. In addition, osteophytes of the posterior lip of the vertebral body impinging on the cord or nerve roots may also be removed through this approach.

The radicular pain associated with cervical spondylosis is often caused by compression of the nerve root by herniated disc material or osteophytes. Disc excision, osteophyte excision, or both and interbody fusion will effectively improve persistent symptoms if the involvement is restricted to one or two levels and if there is objective neurologic and myelographic evidence of nerve root impingement. The incidence of successful fusion and satisfactory clinical results tends to decrease with each additional level fused (White, 1973; Williams, 1968).

Despite these optimistic statements about surgery, the authors still feel that the *primary* treatment of most cervical spondylotic or discogenic problems is conservative, using anti-inflammatory drugs, orthoses, or traction for an extended period of time. In most cases symptoms will be significantly improved. Only if these conservative measures fail should surgery be considered.

The rationale for surgery is to remove the disc and posterior osteophyte to relieve the pressure on the spinal cord or nerve root. The disc space is then filled with a bone graft, which distracts the disc space and effectively enlarges the neural foramina. We suspect that small but pathologic motion between vertebrae is responsible for the development of posterior osteophytes. Fusion is performed to maintain the height of the disc space and to eliminate this motion and recurrent osteophyte formation. Fusion alone without osteophyte excision is often sufficient to relieve radicular symptoms, for after osseous union is complete, the osteophytes will usually resorb in nine to twelve months' time and symptoms will subside. However, in order to provide immediate relief of symptoms, offending osteophytes may be removed at the time of anterior interbody fusion.

Anterior fusion should be restricted to those levels that are producing clinical symptoms and objective signs. Often, multiple levels will appear to be involved radiographically, and the myelogram may demonstrate obliteration of the nerve root sleeves at levels that do not appear to be involved clinically. In these situations, we recommend fusing only those levels that are involved clinically. When there is a discrepancy between the myelographic and clinical findings, we advocate fusing only those levels that are involved clinically.

Fusion may also be used effectively to relieve discogenic symptoms in which the pain is localized to the neck and in which there is no radicular component. The problem here is to accurately localize the source of symptoms at a single or perhaps two intervertebral segments, because any of the eight cervical articulations can produce symptoms. Local neck pain may be caused by degeneration of the disc with posterior protrusion of disc material into the posterior longitudinal ligament. This distorts the posterior longitudinal ligament and may irritate local nerve fibers within the ligament. Pain may also be produced by arthritic degeneration of the facet joints. It is hard to differentiate between these causes, although plane roentgenograms may reveal degeneration of the disc and loss of disc space height or narrowing of the articular space between the facets and local spurs or osteophytes. Unfortunately, these are only presumptive pieces of evidence and do not prove that these are the levels of involvement or source of symptoms. Injection of the disc space or involved facet joints with saline, lidocaine (Xylocaine), or steroids may improve the localization, but these techniques are potentially dangerous and are only sometimes helpful. Motion of the neck may aggravate these symptoms, with flexion or rotation of the neck irritating the facets and extension placing increased stress on the posterior disc and ligament. Because of the difficulties in accurately localizing the source of local symptoms, we advocate a very cautious approach to the treatment of discogenic pain. Conservative measures, such as anti-inflammatory

drugs, traction, collars, and braces should be tried for an extended period of time and often will yield satisfactory results. Only if these measures fail and if satisfactory localization is possible should surgical fusion be considered.

Many patients may present with pain radiating up the back of the neck to the occiput above and behind the ear. This pain may be caused by irritation of the greater occipital nerve at the atlantoaxial level. Anterior fusions at a lower cervical level cannot improve this symptom.

TECHNIQUE

The vertebral bodies and interspaces are reached through one of the anterolateral approaches, depending on the level of the spine involved. A needle is placed in the involved disc space, and a control lateral roentgenogram is obtained to verify the level. A rectangular window may be cut in the anterior longitudinal ligament over the interspace. An alternative approach is to develop a flap in the anterior longitudinal ligament over the midvertebral body, which may be replaced after surgery. The bulk of the anulus fibrosus is removed from the disc space using curettes and pituitary rongeurs (Fig. 4–44A). The cartilaginous end plate is removed with angled curettes, but the subchondral cortical end plate is left intact. It is important to remember that the cervical disc space is angled superiorly and that dissection should proceed along this plane, to prevent inadvertent injury of the cortical end plate. The anterior cortical lip of the vertebra is also spared, unless a significant osteophyte is present, and this anterior lip is later used to lock the bone graft in place. The whole of the anulus is removed to the posterior longitudinal ligament. In the cervical spine the posterior longitudinal ligament is a broad, dense ligament which effectively protects the cord during this phase of the dissection. However, the posterior longitudinal ligament does not extend laterally over the neural foramina so the nerve roots are not similarly protected.

To remove a posterior osteophyte, a drill with a small round burr may be used to create a transverse trough in the cortical end plate adjacent to the posterior edge of the vertebra. This weakens the bone around the osteophyte. A small, angled curette is then used to reach behind the osteophyte, break it off, and deliver it into the wound (Figure 4–44B). This maneuver is repeated until the osteophyte is completely removed and the cord and nerve

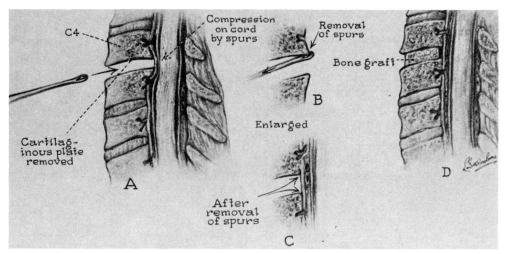

Figure 4–44. Anterior cervical interbody fusion and posterior osteophyte excision. *A,* The anulus fibrosus and cartilage end plates are removed with curets and pituitary rongeurs. The subchondral cortical end plate is left intact. *B* and *C,* The posterior osteophyte is removed. *D,* A horseshoe-shaped plug of iliac bone is tamped into the intervertebral defect. (From White, A. A., Southwick, W. O., DePonte, R. J., et al.: Relief of pain by anterior cervical spine fusion for spondylosis. J. Bone Joint Surg., 55A:525, 1973. Reproduced with permission.)

root are free of impingement (Fig. 4–44C). The osteophyte may also be removed directly using a very fine 60 degree angled rongeur with a cup diameter of only 2 mm. The rongeur is introduced into the disc space using two hands, and the terminal end of the rongeur blade is carefully placed posterior to the osteophyte. The rongeur is pulled firmly against the osteophyte, and the blades are closed to prevent the rongeur from moving posteriorly into the cord or nerve roots. This maneuver is repeated until the osteophyte or transverse bar is completely removed.

The defect in the intervertebral disc space is then measured using a flexible probe. This defect usually measures 15 by 15 by 8 mm., and a graft that is 10 to 12 mm. in depth, 15 mm. wide, and 8 mm. in height will usually fill this defect adequately. To obtain the bone graft, a short incision is made over the anterior iliac crest. Two parallel cuts are made in the ilium through both cortical tables using osteotomes or an oscillating saw with two parallel blades set 8 to 10 mm. apart. A horseshoe-shaped plug of bone with cortex on three margins is removed. The bone graft is then shaped to fit the defect in the disc space. The height of the graft should be somewhat greater than the height of the disc space so that it will fit snugly under compression. The anteroposterior dimension of the graft should be at least 5 mm. less than the depth of the vertebra so that when the graft is recessed behind the lips

of the vertebra, it will not compress the cord posteriorly.

A small transverse trough is cut at the front of the end plate of the upper vertebra to lock the graft in place anteriorly. The neck is carefully extended by the anesthetist, and about 20 lbs. of head-halter traction are applied. The graft is gently tamped into position with a metal punch and mallet. The anterior aspect of the graft should be recessed behind the anterior cortical lip of the vertebra and locked into the transverse trough previously created. This is done to hold the graft and to prevent it from sliding forward into the esophagus (Fig. 4–27). On release of traction, the graft should fit snugly and should be compressed by the remaining cervical ligaments and muscles. A lateral roentgenogram should be obtained to check position and alignment and to verify that the graft is not protruding into the spinal canal posteriorly.

The wound is irrigated, the superficial layer of the deep fascia is repaired loosely, and the platysma is closed with interrupted inverting sutures to prevent a wide scar. The skin is closed, and a narrow, cosmetically pleasing transverse scar that is concealed by adjacent skin folds should result in 10 to 12 weeks. The neck should be protected with external support to prevent hyperextension until bony fusion is established in three to six months.

Although all of the hyaline cartilage plate

is removed, the bony cortical end plates of the vertebral bodies are spared throughout the dissection. The graft is inserted so that the horseshoe of cortical bone abuts with the end plate, effectively distracting the vertebrae. The end plates are spared to provide as much support for the graft as possible and to minimize postoperative compression of the disc space. This distraction creates significant enlargement of the nerve root foramina and reduces nerve root impingement. Although some settling of the graft will occur with time, a satisfactory and permanent enlargement of the foramina can be obtained.

CASE REPORT

P. D., a 45 year old female, was involved in a motor vehicle accident eight years previously and sustained a fracture of the odontoid. She was successfully treated with an atlantoaxial posterior fusion using the Brooks technique (see Posterior Cervical Approaches). Six years later she developed pain in the right shoulder radiating to her right arm. Conservative treatment with intermittent traction, a cervical collar, and aspirin did not provide lasting relief. After two years of such treatment, she was admitted to the hospital for myelography. At this time, a slight sensory deficit in the right C5 and C6 nerve root distribution was noted.

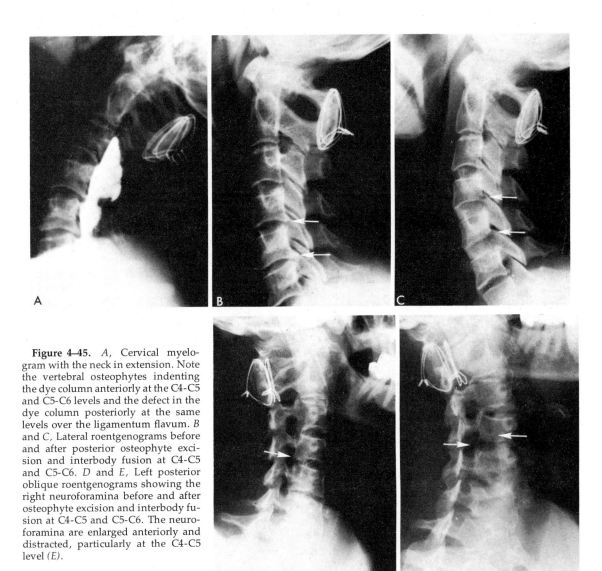

Figure 4–45. *A,* Cervical myelogram with the neck in extension. Note the vertebral osteophytes indenting the dye column anteriorly at the C4-C5 and C5-C6 levels and the defect in the dye column posteriorly at the same levels over the ligamentum flavum. *B* and *C,* Lateral roentgenograms before and after posterior osteophyte excision and interbody fusion at C4-C5 and C5-C6. *D* and *E,* Left posterior oblique roentgenograms showing the right neuroforamina before and after osteophyte excision and interbody fusion at C4-C5 and C5-C6. The neuroforamina are enlarged anteriorly and distracted, particularly at the C4-C5 level *(E).*

There was objective weakness of the right biceps and brachioradialis muscles and an asymmetric deficit in these reflexes.

A myelogram revealed blunting of the C5 and C6 nerve root sleeves, and on lateral views, vertebral body osteophytes indenting the dye column were seen. With extension of the neck, a posterior defect in the dye column over the ligamentum flavum was also noted (Fig. 4–45A). We concluded that this defect in the posterior dye column was due to hypertrophy or loss of the normal elasticity of the ligamentum flavum. With neck extension, the redundant ligamentum flavum protruded anteriorly, effectively reducing the anteroposterior dimension of the canal, forcing the spinal cord against the vertebral bodies and osteophytes.

The therapeutic options were to perform a wide posterior decompressive laminectomy at multiple levels and to fuse the spine. We felt that a simpler and functionally less debilitating approach was to enter the spine anteriorly, remove the osteophytes, relieve the nerve root compression, and fuse the spine to prevent further osteophyte formation. If this was not completely effective, a posterior approach could be performed at a later date.

Decompression and fusion at two levels anteriorly, C4-C5 and C5-C6, were accomplished. Postoperative roentgenograms revealed that the posterior osteophytes were satisfactorily excised (Fig. 4–45B and C) and the foramina were considerably enlarged, particularly at the C4-C5 level (Fig. 4–45D and E). The patient enjoyed complete improvement of her preoperative symptoms and neurologic deficit and established a stable fusion in four months. The nerve root foramina remain open, as demonstrated radiographically, seven years following fusion, and there is no evidence of collapse of the grafts.

Excision of Vertebral Body and Replacement with Bone Graft through the Anterior Approach

Complete excision of one or more vertebral bodies may be required when the body is extensively involved with infection or tumor or when the body is fractured and displaced posteriorly into the spinal canal. In many of these cases the body should be replaced with bone graft to maintain vertebral height and alignment and to provide stability when osseous union is complete. Bone graft replacement should be considered even when the spinal cord is completely and irreversibly damaged, to prevent progressive ascending neurologic damage.

Fractures of the cervical vertebral bodies with posterior displacement and spinal cord injury are most often associated with hyperflexion-compression injuries, such as diving accidents (Braakman and Penning, 1971). In these injuries, the body is often severely comminuted with some fragments displaced posteriorly into the spinal canal, or the fracture occurs at the pedicles, with the vertebral body as a whole displaced posteriorly. The spinal cord may be compressed and draped over these fragments. Posterior laminectomy may effectively decompress the canal; however, the cord may still be draped over the fragments and may continue to be irritated or damaged. Furthermore, it is almost impossible to remove a cervical vertebral body through the posterior approach without injuring the cord more extensively. Finally, posterior laminectomy will remove the last threads of spinal stability remaining and will compound the structural problems present. For these reasons we prefer to treat vertebral body fractures that are displaced posteriorly and in which there is incomplete or progressive neurologic deficit with anterior decompression and fusion.

Anterior fusion techniques rarely add any stability in the immediate postoperative period, and vertebral body resection may seriously contribute to any preexisting instability, even when the body is replaced by a bone graft. A number of authors have advocated notching the graft (Whitecloud, 1976), recessing the graft behind the anterior cortical margin of the vertebra (Bailey and Badgley, 1960; Bailey, 1974; Robinson and Riley, 1975; and Verbiest, 1969), or using sutures, screws, or plates to improve fixation. We advocate carving keys on either end of the graft and fitting these into troughs burred into the end plates of the upper and lower vertebrae. These prevent anteroposterior displacement of the graft into the spinal cord or esophagus. Without these keys, catastrophic displacements can occur (Fig. 4–28; Light, 1980). Despite this, the spine may remain unstable, particularly in flexion or against shear forces between vertebrae. Stauffer and Kelly (1977) have demonstrated that instability is most prevalent following anterior fusion when there is coexistent damage of the posterior elements. For this reason, traction, a halo cast, or subsequent posterior interspinous wiring and fusion may be required to maintain vertebral alignment until anterior osseous union is complete.

TECHNIQUE

Endotracheal anesthesia and skeletal traction are ordinarily required for this procedure. The involved vertebral body is exposed through one of the anterior approaches as dictated by the level of involvement (Fig. 4–29). The involved vertebra is carefully resected using rongeurs and curettes (Fig. 4–46). As the dissection proceeds posteriorly, care is required to prevent further injury to the spinal cord. Most often the posterior longitudinal ligament is torn or frayed and does not present a natural barrier between the vertebral body and the canal. The body is extremely vascular, and considerable hemorrhage is usually encountered. For this reason, it is recommended that as the dissection approaches the canal, the lateral side of the body that is least involved should be resected first. The joint of Luschka is removed laterally, and the nerve root is identified. Using this landmark, the dissection should proceed medially, following the nerve root to the dura. In this manner, the neural elements may be spared.

The intervening anulus fibrosus and cartilaginous end plates on either side of the involved body should be resected, but the subchondral, cortical end plates of the adjacent vertebrae should be spared (Fig. 4–47A and B). These will provide support for the bone graft and will prevent collapse of the graft into the softer cancellous portion of the body. The dura and nerve roots should be carefully inspected to insure that the decompression is adequate.

The bone graft is usually obtained from the anterior ilium. A long plug that has three cortical surfaces and that includes the inner and outer tables of the ilium is removed. The defect is measured, and the graft is fashioned so that it will fit the defect tightly. Keys are shaped at either end of the graft, as illustrated in Figure 4–47C and D. The keys will be fitted into transverse troughs in the end plates of the adjacent vertebrae to prevent anterior or posterior migration of the graft.

Transverse troughs are cut into the end plates of the adjacent vertebrae, as illustrated in Figure 4–47C and D and Figure 4–48. These are fashioned so that the graft may slide into the trough from one lateral side. The cervical spine is slightly extended, and longitudinal traction is increased. The graft is tamped into

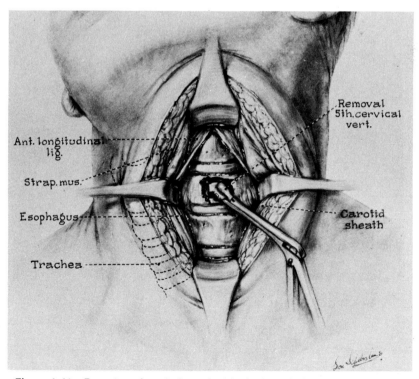

Figure 4–46.   Resection of cervical vertebral body through the anterior approach.

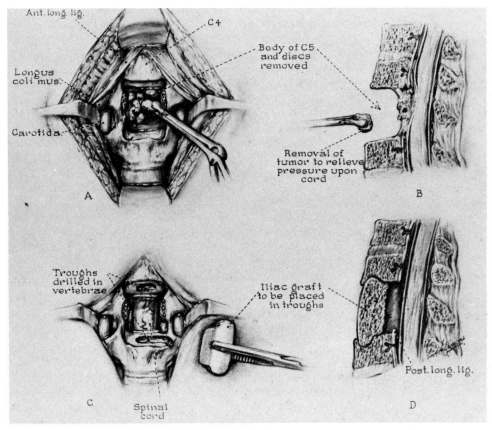

Figure 4–47. *A,* The involved vertebra is resected using rongeurs and curets. *B,* The anulus fibrosus and cartilaginous end plates are resected on either side of the involved vertebra, and the cord is decompressed. The subchondral cortical end plates of the uninvolved vertebrae are left intact to support the graft. *C,* Troughs are drilled in the adjacent vertebrae, and an iliac graft is fashioned with keys at either end. *D,* Sagittal section with iliac graft in place.

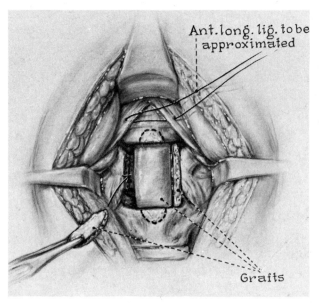

Figure 4–48. Anterior view of iliac graft with additional graft material being placed on either side.

place, and control lateral roentgenograms are obtained to insure that placement is satisfactory and that there is no protrusion of the graft into the canal. A corticocancellous spike of bone may be inserted into the trough and driven into the soft, cancellous vertebral body to lock the graft in place and prevent it from slipping laterally. The wound is carefully irrigated, and the deeper layers are closed loosely to permit drainage. A subcutaneous drain may be used to prevent compressive hematoma and subsequent airway obstruction.

The troughs in the vertebrae and keys in the graft are fashioned to prevent graft migration posteriorly into the spinal canal or anteriorly into the esophagus. These do not prevent distraction, anteroposterior shear displacements, or flexion if the posterior elements are damaged. Therefore, some form of external stabilization, such as longitudinal skeletal traction, a Minerva body jacket, or a halo cast, is required following this procedure until fusion is established. Anterior bone grafting provides little or no immediate postoperative stabilization; however, when osseous union is established, the stability is excellent.

POSTERIOR APPROACHES TO THE CERVICAL SPINE

Posterior-Occipitocervical Fusion

Although occipitocervical fusions are rarely required, there are certain situations in which fusion of the occiput to the upper cervical spine is necessary. Bursting fractures of the ring of the first cervical vertebra (Jefferson, 1920) with associated rupture of the transverse ligament (Spence, 1970) may make the cervical spine extremely unstable. Not only is the posterior ring of the first vertebra separated from the front, but the stability provided by the transverse ligament between the odontoid and anterior ring of the atlas is lost as well. Fusion may be required to bridge the occiput to the second or third vertebrae. Extensive resection of the anterior atlantoaxial elements also creates instability, which may be controlled by occipitocervical fusion. Fractures of the odontoid or ruptures of the transverse ligament at the atlas with atlantoaxial subluxation do not ordinarily require occipitocervical fusion unless the posterior arch of the first or second vertebrae is compromised. Generally, these may be adequately stabilized with a posterior atlantoaxial fusion of the Brooks' type, to be described in the next section (p. 132).

The fusion technique described using corticocancellous struts of bone wired to the involved vertebrae adds immediately to the stability of the atlanto-occipital articulation and upper cervical vertebrae. Ordinarily, sufficient strength is provided so that the patient may be mobilized in a cervicothoracic brace, and traction or a halo brace are not required in the postoperative regimen. Nevertheless, if a significant kyphos or flexion deformity is present at this level, a posteriorly placed graft will be situated under tension and might attenuate with time. In this condition, a posterior fusion may be used to provide immediate postoperative stability, and a second stage anterior fusion may be added to provide long-term support.

TECHNIQUE

Endotracheal anesthesia is required to maintain the airway. The three-point pin headrest (Fig. 4–34 and 4–35) is applied to the skull under aseptic conditions, and the patient is turned to the prone position while maintaining cervical traction through the pin headrest. The pin headrest is attached to the operating table with the spine distracted to maintain stability intraoperatively (Fig. 4–36). Counter traction is recommended by taping the shoulders to the distal end of the operating table. A lateral roentgenogram of the cervical spine is taken to verify that the vertebrae are properly aligned.

A longitudinal midline incision is made, extending from the occipital protuberance to the lower cervical spine (Fig. 4–49A). The incision is extended deeply within the relatively avascular midline structures, the intermuscular septum. Deviation from the midline may result in troublesome hemorrhage. The spinous processes, posterior tubercle of the atlas, and median nuchal line of the occiput are palpated. The incision is carried down to these midline bony prominences using a scalpel. The laminae of the second and third cervical vertebrae are dissected subperiosteally and laterally to the facets, but the capsular ligaments of the facets should be preserved to maintain stability. The posterior ring of the first vertebra is cleared of soft tissues by subperiosteal dissection. Care is required to

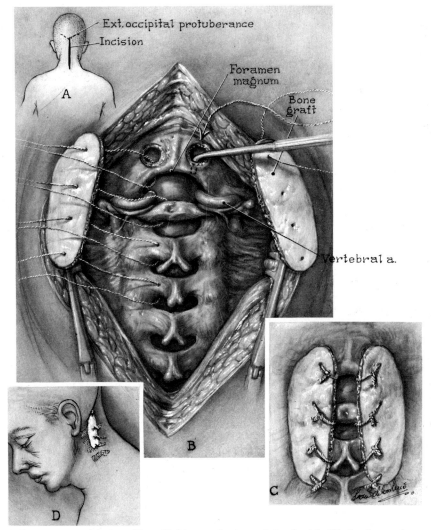

Figure 4–49. Occipitocervical fusion. (From Robinson, R. A., and Southwick, W. O.: Surgical approaches to the cervical spine. *In* the American Academy of Orthopaedic Surgeons: Instructional Course Lectures, Vol. XVII. St. Louis, The C. V. Mosby Co., 1960.)

avoid injuring the vertebral arteries and vertebral venous plexus, which lie on the superior aspect of the first cervical ring less than 2 cm. from midline. The posterior occiput is dissected laterally by sharp subperiosteal dissection to the level of the external occipital protuberance. The posterior lip of the foramen magnum is visible, and the vertebral arteries may be palpated as they enter the atlanto-occipital ligament on their course to the foramen magnum. Two burr holes are made in the posterior occiput about 7 mm. from the foramen magnum and 10 mm. lateral to midline (Fig. 4–49B). The dura is exposed and depressed from

the inner table by gentle, blunt dissection with a right-angled dissector. The posterior atlanto-occipital ligament is separated from the posterior lip of the foramen magnum using fine curets and an elevator. The epidural space between the burr holes and foramen magnum is connected. A twisted wire is passed from the burr holes through the epidural space and out the foramen magnum, using a right angled Mixter clamp and nerve protector.

The ring of the first vertebra is cleared of ligament using straight and angled fine curets. The dura is depressed using a right-angled dissector, and twisted wire is passed around the posterior ring about 1 cm. lateral to midline. The grafts may also be secured to the spinous processes of the second and third cervical vertebrae. Holes are drilled in the outer table of the spinous processes, on either side, adjacent to the laminae (Fig. 4–51A). These holes are connected with a "sweetheart" or towel clip, and two strands of twisted wire are passed through these (Fig. 4–51B and C).

A long, ovoid graft of corticocancellous bone is taken from the iliac crest. Holes are made in the graft at appropriate intervals to accept the twisted wires. Wires are passed through these holes so that the cancellous surface of the graft will lie against the spinous processes, laminae, and occiput. The graft is settled snugly against the laminae, and the wires are tightened and twisted to hold the graft firmly in place. This procedure is duplicated on the opposite side, and the grafts are manipulated to insure that satisfactory stabilization is achieved (Fig. 4–49B and D). Long, thin strips of cancellous iliac bone are laid about the cortical grafts to stimulate osseous fusion.

The grafts and wires should be inspected to insure that they do not impinge on the dura or vertebral arteries. The wound is copiously irrigated with saline and is closed in multiple layers using interrupted absorbable sutures, approximating the intermuscular septum and ligamentum nuchae. The skin is closed cosmetically, the wound is dressed, and the head and neck are splinted to protect the neck during turning, extubation, and transfer to bed. Some form of external support is strongly recommended until fusion is established to prevent motion in all planes. The type of immobilization needed will depend upon the degree of primary instability, but ordinarily a cervicothoracic brace will suffice.

COMPLICATIONS

Care is required in passing the wires to prevent injury to the brain stem or spinal cord. Posterior fusion without decompressive laminectomy tends to constrict the spinal canal. Following trauma to the spine, a certain amount of edema and hemorrhage of the cord and adjacent structures is anticipated. Three weeks following trauma, the swelling begins to subside. Because of this, we recommend a delay following trauma of three to six weeks before fusion without associated laminectomy is attempted. This will help to minimize any compromise of cord or nerve root function that surgery might add immediately following trauma.

The vertebral artery and associated venous plexus should be identified and spared throughout the dissection. The venous plexus, which is closely related to the vertebral artery, can cause particularly troublesome hemorrhage if it is disturbed.

Brooks' Posterior Atlantoaxial Fusion

Fractures of the base of the odontoid (Type II, Anderson and D'Alonzo, 1974) or disruptions of the transverse ligament with atlantoaxial dislocation generally heal poorly. When fractures at the base of the odontoid are treated conservatively, nonunion rates of 5 to 64 per cent are reported (Anderson, 1974; Aymes, 1956; Roberts, 1972; Schatzker, 1971). Because of the high incidence of nonunion, recurrent dislocation, and the ever-present threat of sudden death with insignificant trauma, the treatment of choice in most clinics is early reduction and fusion.

A recent review of our experience with this lesion by Griswold (1978) revealed a 63 per cent nonunion rate after "satisfactory" conservative treatment. Over half of these were symptomatic and required surgical fusion at a later date. Patients with fractures that united satisfactorily were all under 21 years of age. Because of the high incidence of nonunion, conservative treatment is probably indicated only in patients under 21 years of age or in those too old or debilitated to withstand the rigors of a major surgical procedure.

In 1910, Mixter and Osgood reported on posterior stabilization of the first two cervical vertebrae using a fascial loop. Gallie (1937) and others revised this technique, using a wire loop for immediate stabilization and bone graft to induce fusion. The atlantoaxial joint permits more physiologic motion than any other vertebral articulation. Fusion at this level should prevent flexion, extension, and rotation as well as horizontal displacements. The simple posterior wiring technique described by Gallie prevents flexion and anterior horizontal displacement but does not restrict extension, rotation, and posterior or lateral horizontal displacements. For this reason, we have adapted a method described to us by Dr. Arthur Brooks of Vanderbilt University and recently published (Brooks, 1978). Two prism-shaped pieces of corticocancellous iliac graft are secured to the posterior laminae on either side of the midline. The apex of the cancellous portion of the graft fits between the laminae. Each graft is held firmly in position with two loops of twisted wire surrounding the laminae and graft. The wedged-shaped graft functions like a brake shoe, effectively preventing flexion, rotation, and translation. This fusion technique provides enough immediate stability that in most cases a simple cervicothoracic brace is sufficient to protect the spine until osseous union is established. In our experience, the ultimate rate of stable fusion has improved from 67 per cent using other fusion techniques to 97 per cent using Brooks' approach.

Fielding (1976) has described a modification of the Gallie fusion technique using a single butterfly or U-shaped corticocancellous graft secured to the posterior elements of the atlas and axis with a wire loop. He has obtained a very high rate of fusion using this technique, but does protect his patients with traction or a Minerva jacket for the first six weeks following surgery. Leider and Ferlic (1977) have recently reported on the use of the halo-cast to treat fractures of the base of the odontoid and report a union rate of 90 per cent using this technique in 20 patients. The halo-cast appears to offer a significant improvement in the incidence of union compared with other conservative measures; however, additional experience is required to verify this.

TECHNIQUE

The patient is anesthetized on a stretcher next to the operating table using endotracheal intubation and a noncollapsible tube. Care is required during intubation to prevent flexion or extension of the head and neck. The three-point pin headrest is applied to the parietal portion of the skull to provide rigid control of the neck intraoperatively (Figs. 4–34 and 4–35). The patient is rolled like a log onto the operating table. During this maneuver, the surgeon controls the head and neck by holding the pin headrest with one hand, applying firm, longitudinal traction. The surgeon uses his second hand to support the neck and directs the other members of the team in turning the patient. The pin headrest is attached to the table with the neck in a neutral position and the head slightly flexed. The head is flexed by rotating the skull and mandible anteriorly in a military posture, separating the occiput from the posterior ring of the atlas and providing

more room for dissection about the atlas. The neck is distracted gently with the pin headrest, and countertraction is applied by taping the shoulders to the distal end of the operating table (Fig. 4–36). A lateral roentgenogram of the cervical spine is obtained to insure that the vertebrae are properly reduced.

After the skin is prepared, a wide operative field is draped from the occiput to the lower cervical spine. Bleeding may be reduced by infiltrating the midline structures with 10 ml. of a 1:200,000 solution of epinephrine. A midline incision is made from the lower occipital region to the level of the fourth cervical spinous process. The incision is extended deeply within the relatively avascular midline structures, the intermuscular septum or ligamentum nuchae. The spinous processes and posterior tubercle of the atlas are palpated, and the incision is carried down to these midline bony prominences using a scalpel. The ligaments and muscles are dissected from the spinous processes and laminae of the first and second cervical vertebrae by subperiosteal dissection. The small muscular attachments to the bifid spinous process of C2 (Fig. 4–23) can be removed with a curet while holding the vertebra with a Kocher clamp to prevent gross motion. Care is required in dissecting laterally over the atlas to prevent injury to the vertebral arteries and vertebral venous plexus. These lie on the superior aspect of the ring, less than 2 cm. lateral to the midline. We have found this dissection is facilitated by making a transverse incision through the periosteum along the posterior ring of the atlas. The periosteum is raised using a Joseph elevator, and the vertebral vessels are mobilized in continuity with the periosteum. This maneuver protects the vertebral vessels from injury as they are separated from the plane of dissection by an intact layer of tissue. The occiput should not be exposed to avoid inadvertent fusion to the base of the skull. Using right-angled curets and elevators, the first and second cervical laminae are exposed circumferentially. Two strands of #24 gauge stainless steel wire are twisted on themselves in a drill. This increases the strength of the wire while not adding greatly to its stiffness. Two separate wires are passed on each side of the midline beneath the laminae of the first and second vertebrae, using a small right-angled Mixter clamp or aneurysm needle (Fig. 4–50A–E). Great care is required during this maneuver to prevent injury to the dura or cord.

The bone graft is taken from the posterior iliac crest superficial to the sacroiliac joint where the ilium is thick. Ordinarily, there is a longitudinal prominence in this area that parallels the posterior margin of the ilium. A rectangle about 2 by 4 cm. in size is marked in the ilium, centered over this ridge, and a prism-shaped piece of corticocancellous bone is removed from the outer table, as shown in Figure 4–50F. This is divided into two segments, 1.5 by 2.0 cm. in length. The wedge-shaped cancellous apex of the graft is tailored to fit between the laminae of the upper two vertebrae without impinging on the spinal canal or vertebral artery. Notches are fashioned in the upper and lower cortical surfaces to hold the circumferential wires and prevent them from slipping. The grafts are placed snugly against the denuded laminae, and the two wires are tightened and twisted on each side (Fig. 4–50G and H). The wires should be separated so that they encompass the lateral and medial sides of the graft and do not cluster toward the midline. The ring of the atlas is carefully manipulated to insure that stabilization is satisfactory. The wires and grafts are inspected to verify that they do not impinge on the dura or the vertebral arteries.

The wound is copiously irrigated with saline and closed in multiple layers with interrupted absorbable sutures approximating the intermuscular septum. The skin is closed cosmetically and the wound is dressed. The head and neck are splinted during turning, extubation, and transfer of the patient to bed. External support is recommended until fusion is established in three to six months (five months average in our series). Skeletal tongs or a halo brace may be used initially, but a simple cervicothoracic brace provides enough support in most cases.

COMPLICATIONS

In the series reviewed by Griswold (1978), there were several complications. Two patients developed recurrent anterior atlantoaxial subluxation in the early postoperative period. Two developed spontaneous extension of the fusion, one to the third and one to the fourth cervical vertebra. One resulted in an inadequate fusion to the posterior ring of the atlas. This patient had two previous failures of fusion by other techniques and a marginal vascular supply to the posterior ring of the atlas. The early recurrent subluxation could have been prevented by more adequate external bracing in the early postoperative period. We would recommend the Somi brace to prevent this problem based upon our functional studies of cervical orthoses (Johnson, 1977). Spontaneous extension of fusion is a minor problem that may be minimized by careful dissection confined to the areas of intended fusion. All patients ultimately developed stability, and none acquired any neurologic embarrassment.

We are aware of several instances in which the spinal cord has been injured during this procedure, resulting in some permanent neurologic deficit. This presumably occurred while passing the wires about the lamina, and for this reason, care is required during this maneuver. Posterior fusion without decompressive laminectomy tends to constrict the spinal cord. Because of this, we recommend a delay following trauma of three to six weeks before fusion is attempted. This permits the hemorrhage and edema of trauma to subside before constrictive fusion is attempted.

The vertebral artery and associated venous plexus should be identified and spared throughout the dissection. The vertebral venous plexus ordinarily lies superficial to the vertebral artery and can cause particularly troublesome hemorrhage if disturbed.

In our experience, fusion of the atlantoaxial joint results in a loss of almost half of normal cervical rotation, and patients should be advised of this prior to surgery. Many of our patients have noticed this restriction when driving a motor vehicle but have been able to accommodate for this easily. It is possible that the successful treatment of odontoid fractures using a halo-cast may not affect rotation of the atlantoaxial joint as significantly as does fusion, and this factor should be examined in future clinical studies.

Posterior Interspinous Wiring and Fusion of the Lower Cervical Spine, from C2 to the Thorax

Two areas are available for wiring and fusion posteriorly: the spinous processes and facets. The authors have found that in most cases wiring and fusion of the spinous processes is a less complex technique and provides almost as much immediate stabilization as facet posterolateral fusion. For these reasons, we recommend interspinous wiring and fusion and reserve the more complex fusion techniques for those situations in which the spi-

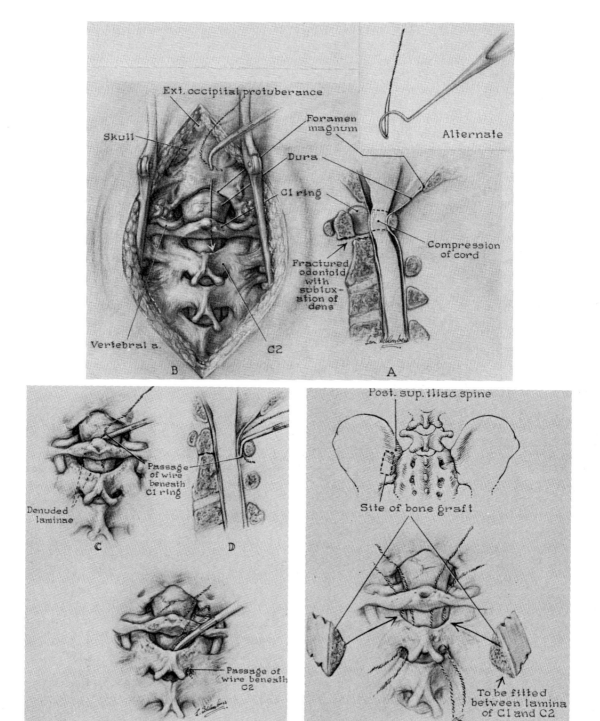

Figure 4–50. *See legend on opposite page.*

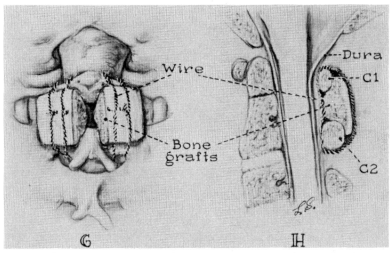

Figure 4–50. *A* and *B*, Brooks' atlantoaxial fusion. *A*, The odontoid should be reduced and its position should be checked with a lateral roentgenogram made in the operating room prior to preparing or draping the patient. This must be done before dissecting around the posterior elements or passing wires to prevent injury to the spinal cord or medulla. *B*, The posterior ring of the atlas and lamina of the axis are cleared of soft tissue by gentle subperiosteal dissection. The base of the occiput is not dissected free as shown to avoid inadvertent fusion to the skull. Twisted 24-gauge stainless steel wires are passed beneath the ring of the atlas and lamina of the axis using a right-angled clamp. An alternative method is to pass an aneurysm needle around the lamina of the axis from above. A heavy silk suture is threaded into the eye of the aneurysm needle, the needle is withdrawn upward, and the suture is retrieved. The silk suture is passed in a similar manner beneath the posterior ring of the atlas. The wires then may be attached to the silk suture and passed atraumatically beneath both posterior rings. *C, D,* and *E,* Two 24-gauge twisted wires are passed beneath the posterior atlantoaxial rings, two on each side of the midline to hold the grafts in place. *F,* A rectangle of bone graft 2 × 4 cm. in size is taken from the posterior ilium superficial to the sacroiliac joint and includes only the outer cortex. This rectangle is centered over the longitudinal ridge, normally present over the posterior ilium. The graft is divided into two prism-shaped pieces, 1.5 × 2.0 cm. in length and 1 cm. deep. The deep surface should be carved to create a triangle, the apex of which will fit snugly between the posterior vertebral rings. The grafts are notched at their upper and lower ends to hold the wires and to keep them from slipping. *G* and *H,* The two wires on either side are separated as far as possible without injuring the vertebral vessels. The wires are then tightened and twisted to wedge the grafts in place between the vertebral rings. This creates a secure bone block, which effectively limits motion in all planes. (From Griswold, D. M., et al.: Atlantoaxial fusion for instability. J. Bone Joint Surg., *60A*:285–292, 1978.)

nous processes, laminae, or facets are deficient or have been removed.

We have found that in many circumstances interspinous wiring and fusion provides effective immediate stabilization and that in most cases a precariously unstable spine may be converted to one in which only a simple cervicothoracic brace is required for protection until osseous fusion is established. In biomechanical studies performed on human cadaver spines, we have found that a mean of 284 newtons may be added to the strength of the spine by this wiring technique alone (Johnson et al., 1980). If the facet joints have not been disturbed, this wiring will effectively restrict flexion and anterior horizontal translation but will not control extension. Therefore, interspinous wiring and fusion should provide the most effective stabilization of flexion injuries of the neck with primary involvement of the posterior ligaments. However, interspinous wiring provides little control over extension injuries in which the anterior stabilizing ligaments have been destroyed. In these situations, additional internal fixation or external support using a halo-cast may be required. When the facet joints have been fractured or removed, interspinous wiring will provide little control over anterior horizontal shear displacements, and interfacet wiring (pp. 138 to 141) may be required to provide satisfactory immediate stabilization.

TECHNIQUE

The authors prefer an interspinous fusion technique similar to the method described by Rogers (1942, 1957). The patient is anesthetized on a stretcher next to the operating table, using endotracheal intubation and a noncollapsing tube. The three-point pin headrest is applied to the skull (Fig. 4–34, 4–35, and 4–36). The patient is turned onto the operating table, and the headrest is fixed to the operating table in moderate distraction. Countertraction is applied by taping the shoulders to the distal end of the operating table, and a control lateral roentgenogram is obtained to verify that the vertebrae are in proper alignment.

The skin over the back of the head and neck is shaved, surgically prepared, and draped from the occiput to the upper thoracic spine. Bleeding may be reduced by infiltrating the midline structures with 10 to 15 ml. of a 1:200,000 solution of epinephrine. A generous midline incision is made over the area of intended fusion and is extended deeply to the spinous processes, through the relatively avascular midline structures. Deviation to either side into the paraspinal muscles will produce troublesome hemorrhage. Throughout this dissection, the spinous processes are palpated to verify their position and level. Scalpel dissection should only be used over these bony prominences and not within the interspinous ligaments or over a suspected spina bifida. The bifid spinous processes are grasped with a Kocher clamp to prevent gross motion or injury during this dissection and are cleared of muscle and tendon insertions using a sharp periosteal elevator. Dissection is extended laterally to the lamina but not to the capsular ligaments and facets. The capsular ligaments surrounding the facets contribute significantly to stability of the spine and should be spared if possible.

Holes are made in the outer cortex of the spinous processes adjacent to the lamina using a 4 mm. drill (Fig. 4–51A). These holes should be centered over the midportion of the spinous processes to prevent the stabilizing wires from cutting out above or below. Drill holes are made on either side of the spinous processes through the outer cortical surface and are connected, using a towel clip or "sweetheart" clamp in a rotary motion, as illustrated in Figure 4–51B. The drill holes or towel clip should not enter the spinal canal or injure the dura. Two strands of #24 gauge stainless steel wire are twisted on themselves in a drill. The twisted wires are passed through these holes in adjacent vertebrae (Fig. 4–51C) and are secured by twisting either end of the wire on itself in a clockwise direction. In this manner, adjacent spinous processes are secured in pairs to each other. One additional wire is used to surround all the vertebrae within the area of intended fusion (Fig. 4–51D). Ordinarily, if instability is confined to one level, three vertebrae are wired together, two surrounding the lesion and one below. If a larger area is involved, the general rule is to fuse one vertebra above and two below the area of involvement. The wiring of one additional segment below the area of involvement provides supplementary strength, which may be useful in certain unstable situations. We have found that when this fusion fails, either clinically or experimentally, the wire usually pulls out of the lower spinous process. By adding this extra level, one can improve the protection of the unstable segment.

The vertebrae are manipulated to insure that the wires are contributing to stability. The wiring should be examined, and a control lateral roentgenogram should be obtained to

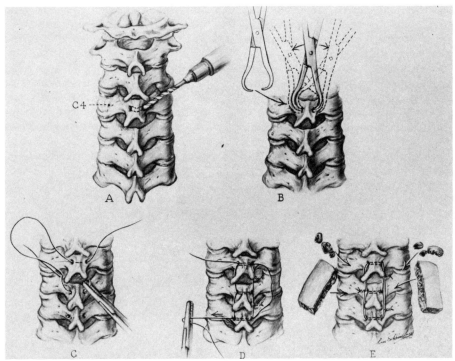

Figure 4–51. Posterior interspinous fusion. *A*, Holes are drilled in the outer cortex of the spinous process adjacent to the lamina. *B*, The drill holes are connected with a towel clip. *C*, Wires are passed through the holes in adjacent vertebrae and are twisted in place. *D*, One additional wire is passed to surround all the vertebrae involved in the area of intended fusion. *E*, Corticocancellous strips of bone graft are laid down about the posterior elements in the area of intended fusion.

verify that the wires are not too tight and that the vertebrae are not held in hyperextension. Hyperextension may compromise the spinal canal or neural foramina; the wires should be loosened if this is present.

Corticocancellous strips of bone are taken from the posterior iliac crest and are laid down around the posterior elements in the area of intended fusion (Fig. 4–51E). The wound is carefully irrigated, and the intermuscular septum is closed in multiple layers with interrupted absorbable suture material. The subcutaneous tissue and skin are closed cosmetically, the wound is dressed, and the neck is splinted. The patient is turned onto his bed, the headrest is removed, and the patient is extubated. External support with a cervicothoracic brace is recommended to prevent extremes of motion until the fusion is established radiographically in four to six months.

COMPLICATIONS

Wound complications are somewhat more common in our experience with the posterior approaches than with anterior approaches. Most problems, however, are encountered after long procedures in which decompression by one surgical team is combined with fusion by another.

Care is required in making the drill holes and in passing the wires to prevent injury to the spinal cord or dura. Posterior fusion without decompressive laminectomy tends to constrict the spinal canal. Because of this we recommend a delay of three to six weeks following trauma before fusion is attempted. This permits the hemorrhage and edema of trauma to subside before constrictive fusion is attempted.

Laminectomy and Facet Fusion

Cervical laminectomy is generally used to decompress the spinal canal posteriorly. It is primarily indicated to relieve the spinal cord and nerve roots from pressure or encroachment arising from the posterior elements, as may occur with certain fractures, dislocation, tumor, infection, and degenerative joint disease. Although laminectomy is not frequently indicated, it is useful to decompress multiple spinal levels, to provide wide surgical exposure, and may be helpful when the level of the pathologic condition is not well localized. Laminectomy also provides effective decompression of the stenotic spinal canal that is narrowed in the anteroposterior plane at multiple levels (Callahan et al., 1977). On the other hand, laminectomy is less effective when the focus of compression is anterior to the spinal cord or nerve roots. In these situations, anterior decompression and fusion will yield equal if not better results with less surgical morbidity (Crandall, 1966; Fager, 1973; Gregorius et al., 1976; and Mayfield, 1966).

In the traumatized cervical spine with fractures, dislocations, and associated complete quadriplegia, there is little hope of recovery if no clinical improvement has occurred within 24 hours. Decompressive laminectomy under these circumstances rarely improves neurologic function and often adds to the patient's preexisting instability. However, decompression may be considered when there is an incomplete neurologic deficit, particularly when there is evidence of progressive neurologic deterioration. A salvage attempt at decompression may be justified under these circumstances, but the decompression should be directed at the primary focus of impingement. For example, if the vertebral body is displaced posteriorly into the canal, anterior vertebral body resection and fusion would be indicated, whereas if the posterior elements are primarily involved, laminectomy could be useful.

Although cervical laminectomy may not cause obvious immediate instability, progressive deformity can occur and has been reported both clinically (Bailey and Badgley, 1960; Cattell and Clark, 1967; Fairbank, 1971; Hall et al., 1977; Mayfield, 1966; Morgan et al., 1975; Sim, 1974; Tachdjian and Matson, 1965) and experimentally (Johnson, 1973; Munechika, 1973; Panjabi et al., 1975; White et al., 1975). In a recent review (Callahan et al., 1977), the authors found that three groups of patients appeared to have a high risk of developing deformity following wide laminectomy. These were children and adults under 25 years of age; patients whose stability was already compromised by fracture-dislocation with primary involvement of the intervertebral ligaments; and those who had foraminotomy or extensive resection of the facets. Fusion is

indicated in these higher-risk groups at the time of laminectomy. We as well as others (Fager, 1973; Jenkins, 1973; Rogers, 1961; Scoville, 1961) have found that older patients with spondylosis and advanced degenerative changes have a lower incidence of acquired structural complications, but fusion may be beneficial in these patients to eliminate motion, continuing nerve root irritation, and associated spondylotic changes. Although laminectomy at multiple levels does influence the amount of deformity, the extent of resection at any one level appears to be of primary importance, and stabilization should be considered whether one or more segments have been resected (Callahan et al., 1977).

Fusion can be performed lateral to the area of laminectomy by passing wires through drill holes in the facets and binding two longitudinal struts of corticocancellous iliac bone graft to the facet pillars at each segment. This technique provides a secure fusion, which may be performed at the same time as laminectomy, does not interfere with decompression, adds significantly to the strength of the spine, and allows early mobilization of the patient with external support. When the procedure is performed correctly, it yields a high rate of fusion (96 per cent) and provides long-term structural stability without the development of progressive deformity (Callahan et al., 1977). On the other hand, facet fusion is a complicated surgical technique, and the risks of complications are great. For this reason, we reserve this procedure for situations in which the spinous processes and lamina are deficient or have been removed and use the simpler interspinous wiring and fusion techniques when the spinous processes are available.

The authors have found that in most cases facet fusion adds enough immediate strength that a precariously unstable spine may be converted to a stable one in which only a simple cervicothoracic brace is required for protection until the fusion is established. Biomechanical studies of this facet fusion technique performed on human cadaver spines in the laboratory have demonstrated that a mean of 467 newtons are added to the strength of the spine by the bone struts and wires (Johnson et al., 1980). The strength of the construct appears to be proportional to the strength of the graft material and not to the wires or drill holes in the facet pillars. Therefore, in very unstable situations, the choice of a strong bone graft, such as the iliac crest with its outer and inner tables, tibia, or fibula, might be preferable to corticocancellous struts of iliac crest, using a single cortex.

Facet fusion is only one of many means of stabilizing the spine following laminectomy. A number of posterior fusion techniques, such as strut grafts (Sim et al., 1974), H-grafts (Fairbank, 1971), and check-rein fusions (Robinson and Southwick, 1960), have been reported, but each has inherent limitations. In most cases, anterior fusions provide an optimal bed for bone grafting, are rapidly incorporated with fewer surgical complications, and may be used in addition to posterior fusion when stability is uncertain. The major disadvantage to the anterior techniques is that no immediate strength is added by the graft, and some may be lost, as Stauffer and Kelly (1977) have reported. Casts, traction, or a halo brace may be required in very unstable situations until the anterior fusion is established. Facet fusion, on the other hand, adds immediate strength and serves as a posterior hinge to prevent horizontal movement between vertebrae.

TECHNIQUE

Decompressive laminectomy and facet fusion may be performed in one surgical procedure using a neurosurgical and orthopedic team. The patient is anesthetized using endotracheal anesthesia, and the spine is stabilized intraoperatively with a three-point pin headrest (Figs. 4–34, 4–35, 4–36). The spine is approached posteriorly, through a generous midlongitudinal incision. The posterior elements are cleared of soft tissues by subperiosteal dissection, including the capsular ligaments over the facets. The spinous processes and laminae are removed over the area of intended decompression and exploration. To do this, the ligamentum flavum is cleared from the superior surface of the lamina below with a sharp curet. The free end is retracted upward with a clamp, and a cottonoid patty is inserted between the lamina and dura to protect the dura during further dissection. Oblique or right-angled punch rongeurs are used to resect the lamina, from the facet pillar on one side to the facet on the other. The spinous processes, lamina, and ligamentum flavum are resected until the cord and dura are fully exposed and decompressed. The cord itself may be exposed through a longitudinal incision in the dura, but the dura should be closed with fine sutures in a nonconstrictive fashion. At this time, the nerve roots may also be unroofed as they enter the neural foramina by removing the medial side of the superior articular facet. To do this, a significant portion of the inferior articular facet must also be removed. The nerve root is located at the level of this articulation and should be protected with a cottonoid patty inserted into the foramen anterior to the superior facet. Bone is carefully removed from the overlying facets using a high-speed burr or angled rongeur until the nerve root is clearly visible and free of encroachment.

After exploration and decompression are complete, fusion is performed posterolaterally at the level of the facets, using the technique described by Robinson and Southwick (1959, 1960) and Callahan and colleagues (1977). The facet surfaces are fused from the upper level of laminectomy to the first intact spinous process below, using corticocancellous bone graft wired to the facets at each level. The soft tissues and capsular ligaments are stripped from the facets and posterior pillars, and the facet joints are pried open using a small, curved elevator. The elevator is rotated to open the joint, and the articular cartilage is removed using a small angled curet. Drill holes 3 mm. in diameter are made in the posterior pillars (Fig. 4–52A and B) at a right angle to the plane of the facet joints. These holes are made somewhat eccentrically toward the midline, so that the grafts may rest on a large area of the posterior pillar. A flat elevator is held within the facet joint to protect the facet below and the vertebral artery and nerve roots in front. Two strands of #24 gauge wire are twisted together using a hand drill. The twisted wire is inserted into each hole, and the tip of the wire is grasped within the joint space, using a fine, curved clamp. One clamp is used to feed the wire into the hole in the posterior pillar while a second clamp is simultaneously used to advance the wire from the facet joint space. Wires are placed at each level of intended fusion bilaterally.

A bone graft that is curved in two planes and is long enough to cover the entire area of intended fusion is taken from the posterior iliac crest (Fig. 4–52C and D). This double curve conforms with the normal cervical lordosis and prevents the graft from impinging on the exposed dura and spinal cord. The graft is composed of the outer table of the iliac crest and subjacent cancellous bone, but to increase its strength, the superior cortical surface of the iliac crest is included. Two biconcave

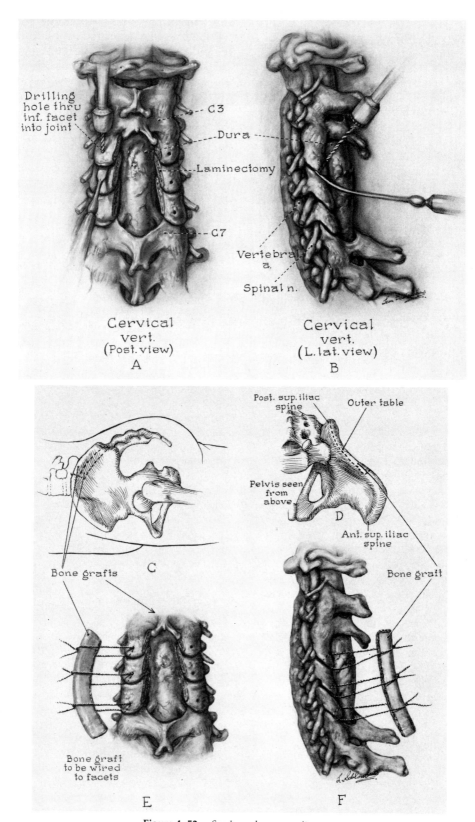

Figure 4–52. *See legend on opposite page.*

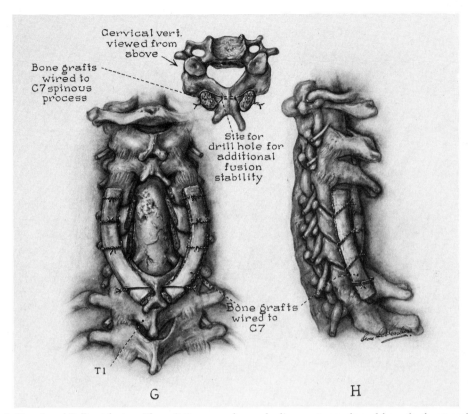

Figure 4–52. *A* and *B*, Facet fusion: The soft tissues and capsular ligaments are cleared from the facets and posterior pillars, and the facet joints are pried open using a small curved elevator. Drill holes are made in the posterior pillars, using a 3 mm. drill, at a right angle to the plane of the facet joints *(B)*. These holes are made eccentrically toward the midline so that the grafts ultimately may rest on a large area of the posterior pillar. During the drilling, a flat elevator is left between the facets to protect the facet below and the vertebral artery and nerve roots to the front.

C and *D*, Bone graft that is curved in two planes is taken from the posterior iliac crest. The posterior ilium is normally curved in two planes. One of these curves (*C* and *E*) keeps the graft from impinging on the exposed dura and spinal cord; the other (*D* and *F*) conforms with the normal cervical lordosis. Two biconcave grafts are taken from the outer table of the ilium. These are notched laterally at their upper and lower poles to keep the wires from slipping off the grafts. *E* and *F*, Twisted 24-gauge stainless steel wire is then inserted into each hole, and the tip of the wire is grasped within the joint space using a fine, curved clamp. Wires are placed at each level of intended fusion bilaterally. The grafts are then placed along the posterior facet pillars, and the wires are tightened and twisted around the grafts. This is usually started at the midpoint of the fusion so the graft will rest snugly against the apex of the lordotic curve. The wire that extends through the hole in the facet pillar is passed medially about the graft *(E)* while the wire that emerges from the facet joint is passed laterally. This prevents the graft from drifting medially toward the exposed spinal canal.

G and *H*, To secure the graft to the spinous process below the laminectomy, a 4 mm. hole is drilled in the outer cortex on either side of the base of the spinous process at its junction with the lamina. These holes are connected using a towel clip or sharp bone clamp, and two additional twisted wires are passed through this hole. The wires are passed around each bone graft and twisted on the lateral aspect of each graft, first on one side and then on the other *(G)*. By using two separate wires, they may be twisted around one graft and then advanced through the hole in the spinous process to bring this graft in close apposition with the posterior elements. The other graft is then secured by twisting the wires on its lateral side. The fusion should extend cranially to the inferior articular processes at the upper end of the laminectomy. If there is doubt about stability at this level, the fusion should be extended further to the spinous process of the vertebra above. Distally, the fusion should extend to the spinous process of the first intact vertebra below the laminectomy. Interspinous wiring to the thoracic vertebrae is indicated only when the stability at the cervicothoracic junction is in doubt or if there is a significant kyphosis at this level. (From Callahan, R. A., Johnson, R. M., Margolis, R. N., et al.: Cervical facet fusion for control of instability following laminectomy. J. Bone Joint Surg., *59A*:991–1002, 1977.)

corticocancellous struts are obtained and applied to the facets with the cancellous surfaces facing the facet pillars (Fig. 4–52E and F). Notches are made in the lateral sides of the graft for the wires at the upper and lower ends of the fusion to improve fixation of the wires to the graft. The wires at each facet are then passed around the graft and tightened by twisting the wire at each segmental level. This is ordinarily started at the midpoint of the fusion so the graft may be closely applied to the facet at the apex of the lordotic curve. The wire that extends through the hole in the facet pillar is passed medially about the graft (Fig. 4–52E), while the wire that emerges from the facet joint is passed laterally. This prevents the graft from drifting medially toward the exposed spinal cord.

To secure the graft to the spinous process, a 4 mm. hole is drilled in the outer cortex on either side of the base of the spinous process at its junction with the lamina (Fig. 4–52G and H). These holes are connected with a towel clip or sharp bone clamp, and two twisted wires are passed through this hole. These two wires are passed around the bone graft and twisted laterally to secure the graft, first on one side and then the other (Fig. 4–52G). By using two separate strands, the wires may be twisted around one graft and advanced through the spinous process to bring the graft in close apposition with the posterior elements. The second side is then secured by twisting the wires laterally on the opposite side.

The fusion should extend cranially to the facet at the upper level of the laminectomy (Fig. 4–52H). If there is any doubt about stability at this level, the fusion should be extended further, to the facet or spinous process of the intact vertebra above. Distally, the fusion should extend to the first intact spinous process below the laminectomy. Interspinous wiring to the thoracic vertebrae is only indicated when the stability at these segments is in doubt.

The wound is irrigated and closed, approximating the intermuscular septum in multiple layers to eliminate dead space and strengthen the closure. A drain is inserted in the deep subcutaneous layer and removed 48 hours postoperatively. The patient is nursed supine for several days until pain and muscular spasm have subsided. The patient is then mobilized, and the neck is protected with a cervicothoracic brace for six to twelve months until fusion is well established radiographically along the facet pillars and there is no motion across the fused segments on flexion-extension roentgenograms. Fusion was established in our series at a mean of 6.5 months (Callahan et al., 1977).

COMPLICATIONS

We have experienced a number of surgical complications, but all but four of these have been minor or temporary and did not result in a permanent deficit (Callahan et al., 1977). Wound complications, such as hematoma, seroma, dehiscence, or infection, were encountered, particularly in association with long procedures involving multiple surgical teams. We have found that prolonged retraction of soft tissues leads to ischemia of the paraspinal muscles and adjacent soft tissues. For this reason, we recommend releasing the retraction of these structures periodically throughout the procedure to permit vascular filling. The intermuscular septum should be closed carefully to prevent wound separation or dehiscence when the shoulders are flexed or when the trapezius muscles contract.

Care is required throughout dissection about the dura and spinal cord to prevent injury to these structures. The wires should be passed carefully to avoid inadvertent puncture of the dura or cord. Although posterolateral facet fusion adds considerable stability to the spine in the immediate postoperative period, extremes of motion may dislodge the bone graft or fixation wires. For this reason, we recommend protection with a cervicothoracic brace until the fusion is well established radiographically. When this procedure is performed correctly and the grafts have been wired at each involved segmental level, facet fusion will yield a high rate of fusion with long-term structural stability.

Interfacet Wiring

We have found that stabilization of the injured spine may be particularly troublesome when the facet joints are damaged or when they have been removed. In these situations, the standard posterior fusion techniques, such as interspinous wiring or facet fusion, have often failed to prevent anterior horizontal displacements, and progressive drifting of one vertebral body forward on another has occurred. To control this problem, we have tried

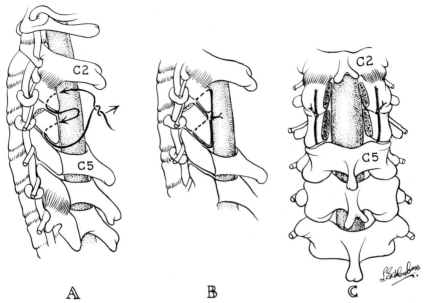

A   B   C

Figure 4–53.   Drill holes are made in the posterior pillars of the involved facets using a 3 mm. drill directed at right angles to the plane of the facet joint. A curved elevator is placed within the facet joint to protect the lower facet and the vertebral artery and nerve roots to the front. Holes are made in the facets at the level of instability and the facet below. A single strand of 18-gauge wire is passed through the hole in the upper facet pillar (A) and is retrieved within the joint using a fine-angled clamp. The wire is advanced by a combination of pushing the wire into the hole within the facet pillar with one hand while pulling the wire from the facet joint with a clamp. When sufficient wire has been retrieved, the free end is introduced into the hole within the next lower facet pillar, and the wire is retrieved from that joint. The wire is pulled snugly, and the facet joints are reduced in a fully apposed position. (B and C). The wire is then tightened and twisted. A lateral roentgenogram is obtained in the operating room to insure that satisfactory stabilization is provided and that there is not too much extension or posterior overriding of the facets. Excessive overriding will compromise the spinal canal and the neural foramina. The wire that leaves the facet joint and is then passed posteriorly to the next lower facet pillar provides a horizontal buttress (B) that effectively prevents anterior translation of one vertebra forward on the next.

a number of technical modifications but have found that a simple wiring technique between the facets is most effective (Figs. 4–53 and 4–54). To date, we have used this technique on eight patients with instability and deficiencies of the facet joints and have found that it controlled anterior horizontal displacements well in most cases. This technique has proved to be effective in controlling shear instability caused by fractures through the facets or the instability that occurs following bilateral facet dislocation when the superior articular facets have been removed to facilitate reduction. Because of the importance of recognizing fractures through the facet surfaces and controlling the resultant instability, we now obtain lateral laminograms, which cut through the plane of the facets in all patients with serious spinal injury to clearly visualize these structures. In addition to identifying facet fractures, these studies may also localize frag-

ments of bone driven forward into the neural foramen compressing the nerve root (Fig. 4–55). These fragments may be removed at the time of stabilization. In several such cases we have been able to gain functional return of the involved nerve root with significant improvement in the patient's level of rehabilitative function.

In previous biomechanical studies on human cadaver spines (Johnson, 1973; Panjabi, 1975), we found that the facets contribute to the angular rotation of the spine in flexion. When the facet joints were removed experimentally, a significant drop in angular rotation was observed in flexion. In addition, the facets were found to limit anterior horizontal translation of one vertebral body on the other, and when the facets were removed, a large increase in horizontal displacement was observed. We have also tested the interfacet wiring technique in human cadaver spines

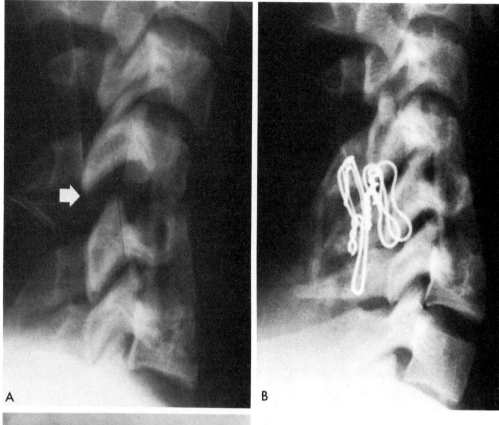

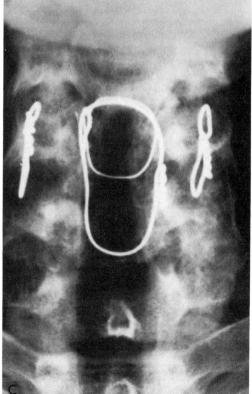

Figure 4–54. Twenty-year-old male with posterior displacement of a fibular graft into the spinal canal, presented in Figure 4–28. The fibular graft was removed and replaced with a graft taken from the iliac crest, which was "keyed" in place (see Fig. 4–47). *A*, Note the wide separation of the spinous processes and facet joints posteriorly, suggesting extensive injury to the posterior ligaments. Because of this posterior instability, interfacet as well as interspinous wiring and fusion was performed (*B* and *C*) to increase the immediate strength of the spine and to speed this patient's rehabilitation without a halo-cast. The interfacet wires are seen in front of the interspinous wires on the lateral roentgenogram (*B*) and are seen laterally on the anteroposterior roentgenogram (*C*).

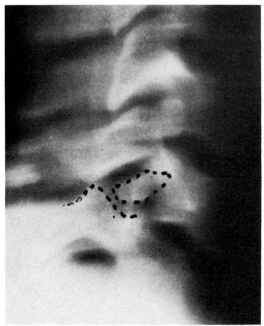

Figure 4–55. Lateral laminogram C6 and C7: This 19-year-old college student was in an automobile accident while vacationing in the West and sustained a bilateral facet dislocation of the sixth on seventh cervical vertebrae. He had complete spinal cord injury at this level, with almost complete loss of his triceps muscle function. He was treated acutely with closed reduction and maintained in skeletal traction. He was transferred to the East three weeks later, at which time continued anterior subluxation of the sixth vertebra on the seventh was noted, despite continued traction. Lateral laminograms revealed bilateral fractures of the superior articular processes of the facets with these fragments driven forward into the neural foramina. These fractures, as well as the associated ligamentous injury at this level, created a remarkably unstable situation and left almost no support against shear forces forward. As a result, the spine continued to sublux forward and could not be adequately held with any form of external support, including a halo-cast. It was hoped that we could stabilize these segments surgically and provide enough immediate strength to prevent this forward drift. In addition, we felt that by removing the fragments driven into the seventh nerve root, we might improve the function of his triceps and increase his overall level of function. The spine was explored posteriorly and the bone fragments were removed, which appeared to alleviate the pressure on the nerve roots. Interfacet wires and bone grafts were installed. This provided enough immediate strength that we could mobilize this patient in a cervicothoracic brace four days after surgery and could begin his therapy in an erect position. The patient has ultimately acquired antigravity strength of his triceps and has been able to use these effectively in his transfers. He has returned to college in a wheelchair without residual vertebral deformity.

(Johnson et al., 1980) and have found that a mean of 753 newtons are added to the strength of the spine when tested in flexion. This technique provides the greatest strength of any wiring method tested in flexion.

TECHNIQUE

Interfacet wiring is normally performed as an adjunct to other posterior fusion techniques. The posterior elements of the spine are approached through a longitudinal midline incision, and the soft tissues are cleared laterally to expose the facets by subperiosteal dissection. The capsular ligaments are removed from the facet surfaces, and the involved facet joints are pried open using a curved Joseph periosteal elevator. At this point, resection of bone fragments or the superior facet, foraminotomy, or reduction of a locked dislocation may be performed. Drill holes are then made in the posterior pillars of the involved facets using a 3 mm. drill directed at right angles to the plane of the facet joint (Fig. 4–52A and B). A flat elevator is placed within the facet to protect the opposing surface from injury when the drill enters the joint. Holes are made in the facets at the level of instability and at the facet below. A single strand of #18 gauge wire is passed through the hole in the upper facet pillar (Fig. 4–53A) and is retrieved within the joint using a fine-angled clamp. The wire is advanced by a combination of pushing the wire into the hole within the facet pillar with one hand while pulling the wire from the facet joint with a clamp. When sufficient wire has been retrieved, this free end is introduced into the hole in the next lower facet pillar, and the wire is retrieved from that joint. The wire is pulled snugly, and the facet joints are reduced in a fully apposed position (Fig. 4–53B and C). The wire is then tightened and twisted using a Shifrin wire tightener. The twisted end is cut short and turned into the bone to prevent irritation of adjacent soft tissues. When completed, the wiring should be inspected, and a lateral roentgenogram should be obtained to insure that satisfactory stabilization is provided and that too much extension or posterior overriding of the facets has not occurred. Excessive overriding will compromise the spinal canal and neural foramina and, therefore, should be avoided.

The wire that leaves the facet joint and is then passed posteriorly to the next lower facet pillar provides a horizontal buttress (Fig. 4–53B), which effectively prevents anterior translation of one vertebra forward on the next. This buttress is effective even when the superior articular surface or part of the upper facet are missing and has been used to control shear displacements when an entire facet pillar has been lost (Fig. 4–56A, B, and C).

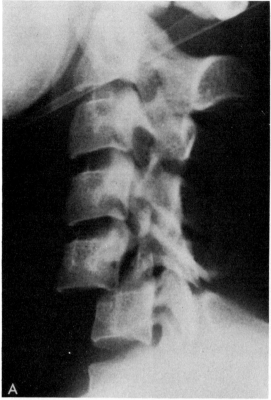

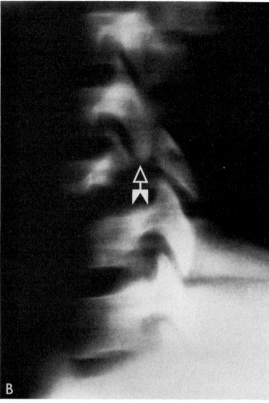

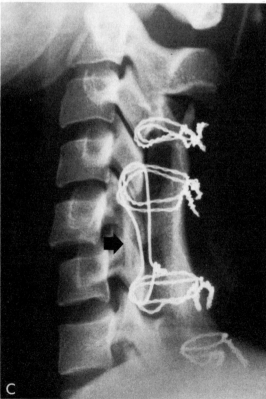

Figure 4–56. This 28-year-old woman was a passenger in the front seat of a car involved in a head-on collision. She sustained a bilateral facet dislocation of the fifth on the sixth cervical vertebrae (A) with complete spinal cord injury at this level. Laminograms (B) revealed a fracture through the middle of the facets. This was easily reduced with longitudinal traction, but there was no resistance against shear displacements anteriorly. As a result, she continued to drift forward at the C5-C6 level. It has been our experience that no external support, including the halo, will prevent these kinds of shear displacement. Therefore, surgical stabilization was attempted to provide enough integral strength so that rehabilitation could be started out of bed and fusion could be performed to prevent late deformity. At surgery, the whole posterior neural arch of the fifth vertebra was found floating freely. This was removed to protect the spinal canal. As a result, the whole posterior pillar of the facets on one side was missing, and even with reduction, she tended to angulate backward. To correct this, a longitudinal graft (C, arrow) was made to replace this facet pillar and was notched into the fourth and sixth facets. This provided a fulcrum that helped to maintain the longitudinal alignment of the vertebrae. An interfacet wire was then installed between the fourth and sixth facets (C) bridging the fifth vertebra but forcing the facet pillar graft forward and snugly into its notches. This was supplemented by two struts of corticocancellous iliac bone, which were wired to the intact facets on either side as described in Facet Fusion (Fig. 4–52). This technique provided enough immediate rigidity that we were able to mobilize this patient shortly after surgery in a cervicothoracic brace. She went on to fuse without significant deformity in four and one half months.

Posterior Laminotomy-Foraminotomy

Nerve root decompression may be performed through the posterior laminotomy-foraminotomy approach described by Scoville (1958, 1961). This "key-hole" exposure of the neural foramen is most conserving of the bone of the posterior elements and facets (Fig. 4–57). The exposure is limited but is most useful to excise a soft disc protruding into the neural foramen, causing unilateral, single nerve root irritation. A hole is burred at the junction of the lamina and facet, and a portion of the superior facet is removed. This decompresses the entrance to the neural foramen by removing its posterior wall without jeopardizing the integrity of the posterior ring or the facet joint.

TECHNIQUE

Scoville (1971) describes the procedure performed under local anesthetic block with the patient sitting upright to reduce venous bleeding. The exposure is through a midlongitudinal incision, and the posterior elements on the involved side are stripped of soft tissues by subperiosteal dissection as far laterally as the facets. A lateral roentgenogram should be obtained with a towel clip fixed to the appropriate spinous process to verify the correct segmental level. A hand-held Meyerding or self-retaining blade and hook retractor are inserted. The posterior wall of the neural foramen is opened lateral to the dural sleeve at the junction of the lamina and facet using a large burr on a low-speed drill. A diamond burr on a high-speed drill and Cloward oblique rongeurs are used to complete the exposure. The nerve root and epidural vein ventral to the root are packed off and protected until the exposure through the bone is completed. Hemostasis of the epidural vessels is obtained by packing with Gelfoam or with "bipolar" coagulation forceps. The exposure may be extended medially by resecting a portion of the lamina with angled rongeurs and excising a part of the ligamentum flavum.

The sensory and motor nerve roots are seen within their separate dural sleeves as they enter the neural foramen. The motor nerve root is one fourth the size of the sensory root and is located anterior and caudal to the larger sensory root. Both roots are freed of adherent tissue and the protruding disc and are retracted carefully upward. The extruded

Figure 4–57. Posterior laminotomy-foraminotomy exposure of the cervical nerve root. (From Robinson, R. A., and Southwick, W. O.: Surgical Approaches to the Cervical Spine. *In* the American Academy of Orthopaedic Surgeons: Instructional Course Lectures, Vol. XVII. St. Louis, 1960, The C. V. Mosby Co., drawing modified after "keyhole" exposure of Scoville, W. B.: Discussion. J. Neurosurg., *15*:614, 1958.)

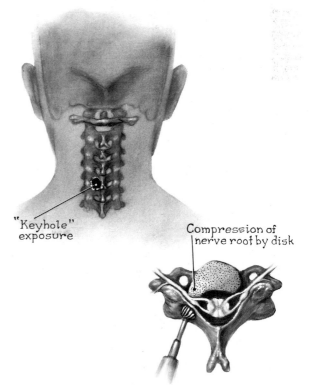

"Keyhole" exposure

Compression of nerve root by disk

disc is then excised with fine pituitary rongeurs and is teased out from beneath the roots
with the assistance of a dental spatula.

Scoville (1971) reports a large series with
few complications, although the upright position has been implicated as an occasional
cause of air embolism. On completing the
procedure, the spinal column should be tested
for stability. If stability is in doubt or if an
entire facet has been removed, we recommend
interfacet wiring and fusion to avoid the complication of late spinal deformity. Care is
required in removing bone around the nerve
roots to protect them from injury. The use of a
diamond burr or angled rongeurs reduces this
risk.

References

Alonso, W. A., Black, P, Connor, G. H., and Vematsu,
S.: Transoral, transpalatal approach for resection of
clival chordoma. Laryngoscope *81*:1626–1631, 1971.

Anderson, L. D., and D'Alonzo, R. T.: Fractures of the
odontoid process of the axis. J. Bone Joint Surg. *56-
A*:1663–1674, 1974.

Aymes, E. W., and Anderson, F. M.: Fracture of the
odontoid process. Arch. Surg. *72*:377–393, 1956.

Bailey, R. W., and Badgley, C. E.: Stabilization of the
cervical spine by anterior fusion. J. Bone Joint Surg.
42-A:565–594, 1960.

Bailey, R. W.: Surgical techniques. *In* Bailey, R. W.
(Ed.): The Cervical Spine. Philadelphia, Lea and Febiger, 1974, pp. 146–156.

Braakman, R., and Penning, L.: Injuries of the cervical
spine. Amsterdam, Excerpta Medica, 1971, pp. 193–
213.

Brooks, A. L., and Jenkins, E. B.: Atlanto-axial arthrodesis by the wedge compression method. J. Bone Joint
Surg. *60-A*:279–284, 1978.

Callahan, R. A., Johnson, R. M., Margolis, R. N., Keggi,
K. J., Albright, J. A., and Southwick, W. O.: Cervical
facet fusion for control of instability following laminectomy. J. Bone Joint Surg. *59-A*:991–1002, 1977.

Cattell, H. S., and Clark, G. L.: Cervical kyphosis and
instability following multiple laminectomies in children.
J. Bone Joint Surg., *49-A*:713–720, 1967.

Crandall, P. H., and Batzdorf, U.: Cervical spondylotic
myelopathy. J. Neurosurg. *25*:57–66, 1966.

Crutchfield, W. G.: Skeletal traction in the treatment of
injuries to the cervical spine. J.A.M.A. *155*:29–32,
1954.

DeAndrade, J. R., and MacNab, I.: Anterior occipitocervical fusion using an extra-pharyngeal exposure. J.
Bone Joint Surg. *51-A*:1621–1626, 1969.

DeWald, R. L.: Halo traction systems. *In* American
Academy of Orthopaedic Surgeons: Atlas of Orthotics,
Biomechanical Principles and Application. St. Louis,
The C. V. Mosby Co., 1975, pp. 407–417.

Fager, C. A.: Results of adequate posterior decompression in the relief of spondylotic cervical myelopathy. J.
Neurosurg. *38*:684–692, 1973.

Fairbank, T. J.: Spinal fusion after laminectomy for cervical myelopathy. Proc. R. Soc. Med. *64*:634–636, 1971.

Fang, H. S. Y., and Ong, G. B.: Direct anterior approach

to the upper cervical spine. J. Bone Joint Surg., *44-
A*:1588–1604, 1962.

Fielding, J. W., Hawkins, R. J., and Ratzan, S. A.: Spine
fusion for atlanto-axial instability. J. Bone Joint Surg.
58-A:400–407, 1976.

Gallie, W. E.: Skeletal traction in the treatment of fractures and dislocations of the cervical spine. Ann. Surg.
106:770–776, 1937.

Gregorius, F. K., Estrin, T., and Crandall, P. H.: Cervical
spondylotic radiculopathy and myelopathy, a long term
follow-up study. Arch. Neurol. *33*:618–625, 1976.

Griswold, D. M., Albright, J. A., Schiffman, E., Johnson,
R. M., and Southwick, W. O.: Atlanto-axial fusion for
instability. J. Bone Joint Surg. *60-A*:285–292, 1978.

Hall, J. E., Denis, F., and Murray, J.: Exposure of the
upper cervical spine for spinal decompression. J. Bone
Joint Surg. *59-A*:121–123, 1977.

Henry, A. K.: Extensile Exposure, 2nd ed. Edinburg, E.
and S. Livingstone, Ltd., 1957, pp. 53–80.

Jefferson, G.: Fracture of the atlas vertebra. Report of
four cases, and a review of those previously recorded.
Br. J. Surg. *7*:407–422, 1920.

Jenkins, D. H. R.: Extensive cervical laminectomy. Br. J.
Surg. *60*:852–854, 1973.

Johnson, R. M.: Biomechanical stability of the lower cervical spine. Thesis, Yale University School of Medicine, Section of Orthopaedic Surgery, pp. 1–58, 1973.

Johnson, R. M., Hart, D. L., Simmons, E. F., Ramsby,
G. R., and Southwick, W. O.: Cervical orthoses: A
study in normal subjects comparing their effectiveness
in restricting cervical motion. J. Bone Joint Surg. *59-
A*:332–339, 1977.

Johnson, R. M., Owen, J. R., Panjabi, M. M., Bucholz,
R. W., and Southwick, W. O.: Immediate strength of
certain cervical fusion techniques. Orthop. Trans.
4:42, 1980.

Kopits, S. E., and Steingass, M. H.: Experience with the
"halo-cast" in small children. Surg. Clin. North Am.
50:935–943, 1970.

Lahey, F. H., and Warren, K. W.: Esophageal diverticula. Surg. Gynecol. Obstet. *98*:1–28, 1954.

Leider, L. L., and Ferlic, F.: Odontoid fractures treated
by halo cast immobilization. Presented at the American
Academy of Orthopaedic Surgeons Annual Meeting,
Las Vegas, Nevada, 1977.

Light, T. R., Wagner, F. C., Johnson, R. M., and Southwick, W. O.: Correction of spinal instability and recovery of neurologic loss following cervical vertebral body
replacement: Case report. Spine, in press.

Lindskog, G. E., Liebow, A. A., and Glenn, W. W. L.:
Thoracic and Cardiovascular Surgery with Related Pathology. New York, Appleton-Century-Crofts, 1962,
pp. 439–440.

Mayfield, F. H.: Cervical spondylosis: A comparison of
the anterior and posterior approaches. Clin. Neurosurg.
13:181–188, 1966.

Mixter, S. J., and Osgood, R. B.: Traumatic lesions of the
atlas and axis. Ann. Surg. *51*:193–207, 1910.

Morgan, R. C., Brown, J. C., and Bonnett, C. A.: The
effect of laminectomy on the pediatric spinal cord injured patient. J. Bone Joint Surg. *57-A*:1025–1026,
1975.

Munechika, Y.: Influence of laminectomy on stability of
the spine. J. Jap. Orthop. Assoc. *47*:111–126, 1973.

Nanson, E. M.: The anterior approach to upper dorsal
sympathectomy. Surg. Gynecol. Obstet. *104*:118–120,
1957.

Panjabi, M. M., White, A. A., and Johnson, R. M.: Cervical spine mechanics as a function of transection of
components. J. Biomech. *8*:327–336, 1975.

Perry, J., and Nickel, V. L.: Total cervical spine fusion for neck paralysis. J. Bone Joint Surg. *41-A*:37–60, 1959.

Perry, J.: The halo in spinal abnormalities, practical factors and avoidance of complications. Orthop. Clin. North Am. *3*:69–80, 1972.

Roberts, A., and Wickstrom, J.: Prognosis of odontoid fractures. *In* Proceedings of the American Academy of Orthopaedic Surgeons. J. Bone Joint Surg. *54-A*:1353, 1972.

Robinson, R. A., and Smith, G. W.: Anterolateral cervical disc removal and interbody fusion for cervical disc syndrome. Bull. Johns Hopkins Hosp. *96*:223–224, 1955.

Robinson, R. A.: Fusions of the cervical spine. J. Bone Joint Surg. *41-A*:1–6, 1959.

Robinson, R. A., and Southwick, W. O.: Indications and technics for early stabilization of the neck in some fracture dislocations of the cervical spine. South. Med. J. *53*:565–579, 1960.

Robinson, R. A., and Southwick, W. O.: Surgical approaches to the cervical spine. Instructional course lectures. The American Academy of Orthopaedic Surgeons, Vol. 17. St. Louis, The C. V. Mosby Co., 1960, pp. 299–330.

Robinson, R. A., and Riley, L. H.: Techniques of exposure and fusion of the cervical spine. Clin. Orthop. *109*:78–84, 1975.

Rogers, W. A.: Treatment of fracture dislocation of the cervical spine. J. Bone Joint Surg. *24*:245–258, 1942.

Rogers, W. A.: Fractures and dislocations of the cervical spine. An end result study. J. Bone Joint Surg. *39-A*:341–376, 1957.

Rogers, L.: The surgical treatment for cervical spondylotic myelopathy. J. Bone Joint Surg. *43-B*:3–6, 1961.

Schatzker, J., Rorabeck, C. H., and Waddell, J. P.: Fractures of the dens (odontoid process), an analysis of thirty-seven cases. J. Bone Joint Surg. *53-B*:392–405, 1971.

Scoville, W. B.: Discussion. J. Neurosurg. *15*:615, 1958.

Scoville, W. B.: Cervical spondylosis — operative treatment. J. Neurosurg. *18*:423–428, 1961.

Scoville, W. B.: Cervical disc lesions treated by posterior operations. *In* Rob, C., Smith, R., and Logue, V. (Eds.): 2nd ed., Vol. 14. Operative Surgery, Neurosurgery. Philadelphia, J. B. Lippincott Co., 1971, pp. 250–258.

Sim, F. H., Svien, H. J., Bickel, W. H., and Janes, J. M.:

Swan-neck deformity following extensive cervical laminectomy. J. Bone Joint Surg. *56-A*:564–580, 1974.

Smith, G. W., and Robinson, R. A.: The treatment of certain cervical spine disorders by anterior removal of the intervertebral disc and interbody fusion. J. Bone Joint Surg. *40-A*:607–624, 1958.

Southwick, W. O., and Robinson, R. A.: Surgical approaches to the vertebral bodies in the cervical and lumbar regions. J. Bone Joint Surg. *39-A*:631–644, 1957.

Southwick, W. O., and Robinson, R. A.: Recent advances in surgery of the cervical spine. Surg. Clin. North Am. *41*:1661–1683, 1961.

Spence, K. F., Decker, S., and Sell, K. W.: Bursting atlantal fracture associated with rupture of the transverse ligament. J. Bone Joint Surg. *52-A*:543–549, 1970.

Stauffer, E. S., and Kelly, E. G.: Fracture-dislocations of the cervical spine. Instability and recurrent deformity following treatment by anterior interbody fusion. J. Bone Joint Surg. *59-A*:45–48, 1977.

Tachdjian, M. O., and Matson, D. D.: Orthopaedic aspects of intraspinal tumors in infants and children. J. Bone Joint Surg. *47-A*:223–248, 1965.

Thomson, S. C., and Negus, V. E.: Diseases of the nose and throat. A Textbook for Students and Practitioners, 5th ed. London, Cassell and Co., Ltd., 1947, pp. 489–509.

Verbiest, H.: Anterolateral operations for fractures and dislocations in the middle and lower parts of the cervical spine. J. Bone Joint Surg. *51-A*:1489–1530, 1969.

White, A. A., Southwick, W. O., DePonte, R. J., Gainor, J. W., and Hardy, R.: Relief of pain by anterior cervical spine fusion for spondylosis: A report of sixty-five patients. J. Bone Joint Surg. *55-A*:525–534, 1973.

White, A. A., Johnson, R. M., Panjabi, M. M., and Southwick, W. O.: Biomechanical analysis of clinical stability in the cervical spine. Clin. Orthop. *109*:85–96, 1975.

Whitecloud, T. S., and LaRocca, H.: Fibular strut graft in reconstructive surgery of the cervical spine. Spine *1*:33–43, 1976.

Whitesides, T. E., Jr., and Kelly, R. P.: Lateral approach to the upper cervical spine for anterior fusion. South. Med. J. *59*:879–883, 1966.

Williams, J. L., Allen, M. B., Jr., and Harkess, J. W.: Late results of cervical discectomy and interbody fusion: Some factors influencing the results. J. Bone Joint Surg. *50-A*:277–286, 1968.

SURGICAL APPROACHES
TO THE THORACIC SPINE

APPROACH TO THE THORACIC SPINE — ANTERIOR VERSUS POSTERIOR

Under most circumstances, the choice of approach to the thoracic spine should be dictated by the site of the primary pathologic condition. Disease or deformity that primarily involves the vertebral bodies anteriorly may be approached directly through the chest or through a posterolateral costotransversectomy, whereas lesions of the posterior elements may be readily reached through the posterior exposures. There are, however, certain indications for and limitations to each approach.

Anterior

The anterior transthoracic approach provides direct access to most of the thoracic vertebral bodies. It should be considered for extensive resection, debridement, and fusion of the vertebral bodies, particularly when multiple levels are involved. The disadvantages to thoracotomy are that it presents a greater operative risk than any of the posterior approaches incur, and it does not yield as effective exposure at the extreme upper and lower levels of the thoracic spine.

The anterior transthoracic approach should be considered in certain specific circumstances. Severe, rigid kyphosis of the thoracic spine is often best controlled by anterior interbody fusion, as posterior fusions tend to attenuate over a severe kyphos (Johnson and Robinson, 1968; Winter, 1973). Scoliosis with associated absence of the posterior elements or severe anterior deformity may be effectively treated with anterior instrumentation and fusion (Dwyer, 1973, 1974; Riseborough, 1973). Spinal cord compression caused by lesions of the vertebral bodies protruding posteriorly into the canal should be decompressed anteriorly in most cases.

Posterolateral

Posterolateral costotransversectomy provides direct access to the transverse processes and pedicles of the thoracic spine and limited access to the vertebral bodies. Exposure at all levels of the thoracic spine is possible without restriction about the thoracic inlet or diaphragm. Costotransversectomy should be considered for simple biopsy or local debridement. However, it does not provide the operative working area or length of exposure to the thoracic vertebral bodies that thoracotomy affords.

Posterior

The midlongitudinal posterior approach provides direct access to the posterior elements of the thoracic spine at all levels. It should be considered for biopsy or debridement of lesions of the posterior elements, decompressive laminectomy, or posterior fu-

sion. Spinal cord compression caused by lesions of the posterior elements impinging on the cord are rare but may be relieved by laminectomy. However, cord compression caused by lesions arising from the anterior elements is rarely improved with laminectomy alone (Brice and McKisseck, 1965; Cook, 1971; Hodgson et al., 1960; Winter et al., 1973). Idiopathic scoliosis may be corrected and fused posteriorly with satisfactory results, and the injured spine may be stabilized and fused with rods or wires through this exposure.

SELECTION OF APPROACH AND VERTEBRAL LEVEL OF INVOLVEMENT

The posterior and posterolateral approaches provide direct access to the posterior elements and limited access to the vertebral bodies at all levels of the thoracic spine. The anterior approaches may be required to provide wide access to the vertebral bodies at multiple levels. However, the exposure is restricted anteriorly at the upper and lower extremes of the thoracic spine by the thoracic inlet and diaphragm. Therefore, modifications in the anterior approach must be made at these levels.

Upper Thoracic Level

The most direct access to the lower cervical and upper thoracic vertebral bodies is provided by the supraclavicular approach described in Part II (p. 118). This approach provides access as low as the level of the third thoracic vertebral body in some patients. The exposure is reasonably unencumbered to the first and often the second thoracic vertebrae, but working area to the third vertebral body becomes restricted by the thoracic inlet.

An alternative approach to the upper thoracic spine is via a left posterolateral thoracotomy at a level as high as the third rib. This requires resection of the dorsal scapular muscles and elevation of the scapula. Working area is limited by the converging rib cage and thoracic inlet. In addition, reversal of the thoracic kyphos in the upper thoracic spine makes resection of the vertebral bodies technically more difficult. Thoracotomy above the level of the third rib is impractical, as the shorter first and second ribs limit the scope of the incision, and the scapula interferes with the exposure posteriorly.

Hodgson (1960, 1969) discusses the sternum-splitting approach to the upper thoracic anterior elements first described by Cauchoix and Binet (1957). Theoretically, this provides direct access to the vertebral bodies and continuity of exposure from the cervical to the thoracic vertebrae. In fact, Hodgson found this to be an unusually complex procedure, with a high operative mortality (40 per cent in 10 cases). The thymus, great vessels, trachea, and esophagus need to be retracted, and the spine appears at the bottom of a deep hole with limited operative working area. The restricted working area over the vertebral bodies is complicated by the fact that one must dissect directly back, toward the spinal canal, from the anterior aspect of the vertebral bodies and not from the side. In Hodgson's opinion, this increases the risk of injuring the spinal cord during decompression. Hodgson found that resection and bone grafting of the upper thoracic spine was easier through a thoracotomy at the level of the third rib than through this sternum-splitting approach.

Lower Thoracic Level

A left posterolateral thoracotomy provides access to the lower thoracic vertebral bodies as far as the twelfth vertebra. As one approaches the diaphragm, the working area becomes more restricted, so that exposures of the twelfth and sometimes the eleventh vertebral bodies become difficult without dividing the medial diaphragmatic insertion. To provide wide exposure across the lower thoracic and upper lumbar vertebral bodies in continuity, a transdiaphragmatic, thoracoabdominal approach is required. This significantly increases the operative risk and should only be considered in reasonably healthy candidates. Limited access to the lower thoracic vertebrae in continuity with the lumbar spine is possible via the retroperitoneal approach through a left flank incision (p. 173). The operative morbidity is lower with this retroperitoneal approach than with the thoracoabdominal exposure, but the visibility and working area within the thorax are restricted.

Anterior Transthoracic Approach to the Thoracic Spine

The transthoracic approach to the spine has only become widely used in the past 20 years and had to await the development of the sophisticated techniques and support systems required to reduce the risks of thoracic surgery. There were reports of successful thoracotomy in the early literature (Robinson, 1917; Nissen, 1931), but these were attended by high risks. In 1933, Reinhoff reported on two successful pneumonectomies, beginning the era of reliable intrathoracic surgery. However, it was not until Hodgson (1956, 1960, 1965) demonstrated the effectiveness of the transthoracic approach to the spine that thoracotomy was accepted as an exposure to the vertebral bodies. Since his first report in 1956, thoracotomy has been used with increasing frequency in treating diseases that primarily involve the thoracic vertebral bodies.

Hodgson first used thoracotomy to debride and bone graft tuberculous abscesses of the spine (1956). In 1960, he noted that tuberculosis of the spine usally involved the anterior elements and that the involvement was often more extensive than was apparent radiographically. He found the best results of treatment occurred after extensive and complete debridement of all involved tissue and that spinal canal decompression and stabilizing fusion were often required. Such extensive procedures are hard to perform effectively through the more limited exposure offered by posterolateral costotransversectomy; therefore, Hodgson (1960) recommended the transthoracic approach. He reported a relatively low complication rate and an operative mortality of only 2.9 per cent in his large series.

The anterior approach to the spine is useful in resecting tumors of the vertebral bodies and in providing bone graft replacement. It may be used to debride osteomyelitis of the vertebral bodies or disc space infections. It has been used to correct certain scoliotic deformities (Dwyer, 1973, 1974; Riseborough, 1973), particularly when the posterior elements of the spine are deficient as in myelomeningocele. It has been used to resect certain fixed anterior deformities and to correct severe, fixed kyphoses.

Winter (1973) found that fixed thoracic kyphoses measuring over 50 degrees in patients over three years of age often require correction and stabilization through the chest. In these situations, osteotomy may be necessary, and if there is associated neurologic involvement, decompression may be performed effectively from the front. Anteriorly placed bone grafts across a kyphos have a higher incidence of stable fusion than posterior grafts (Winter, 1973). Johnson and Robinson (1968) pointed out that anterior grafts are subject to compressive forces in the thoracic spine and are fixed to the large area of corticocancellous bone between the vertebral bodies. These factors appear to increase the incidence of stable fusion. On the other hand, they noted that posterior grafts are subject to tensile forces and may attenuate with time. They illustrated the resorption of a posterior graft across a kyphos in one case.

A major indication for the transthoracic approach is to decompress the spinal canal in those conditions in which the cord is compromised by lesions protruding from the anterior elements. These include tumor or infection of the anterior spine extending into the spinal canal, fixed thoracic kyphosis with associated neurologic involvement, and fractures of the vertebral body with fragments displaced posteriorly into the spinal canal. In all these situations, the cord may be tethered to or tented over these lesions and may have to traverse a longer arc. Laminectomy will only decompress the spinal canal but cannot remove the source of irritation, whereas anterior resection can do both effectively. In these conditions, anterior decompression has proved to be more effective than laminectomy (Brice, 1965; Cook, 1971; Hodgson and Stock, 1956, 1960; Hodgson, 1965; Johnson and Robinson, 1968; Martin and Williamson, 1970; Winter et al., 1973) and does not remove any remaining support provided by the posterior elements.

Posterolateral costotransversectomy permits effective decompression of the anterior spinal canal; however, the exposure is limited, control of bleeding may be difficult, and application of a large anterior bone graft may be impossible. The transthoracic approach adds a significant operative risk and is certainly more hazardous than posterior or even posterolateral approaches. In most cases, however, the increased operative risk of thoracotomy must be weighed against the more limited exposure provided by alternative routes.

The transthoracic approach to the spine provides direct access to the vertebral bodies from the second to the twelfth thoracic segments. The midthoracic vertebral bodies are best exposed, while the upper and lower extremes yield a more limited view. In general, we recommend an approach through a left posterolateral thoracotomy incision. Some surgeons prefer a right thoracotomy for approaches to the upper thoracic spine to avoid the subclavian and carotid arteries in the left superior mediastinum. In our experience, these vessels arise far enough anterior to the vertebral bodies to not affect dissection over the vertebrae. In the lower thoracic spine, a left thoracotomy is definitely preferred. The heart, on the left, may be retracted anteriorly with ease, whereas the liver, on the right, may present a significant obstacle to exposure. The level of the incision should be varied to meet the level of exposure required. We recommend directing the incision as far posteriorly as possible and resecting the rib just beyond its posterior angle to improve the vertebral body exposure. Ordinarily, an intercostal space is selected at or just above the involved segment. When only one segment is involved, the rib at that level should be removed. If multiple levels are involved, however, the rib at the upper level of the proposed dissection should be removed. Because of the natural thoracic kyphosis, dissection is easier from above downward for most surgeons. Although resection of a rib is not always necessary, it does improve the intrathoracic exposure and provides a suitable bone graft for fusion.

TECHNIQUE

The patient is placed on the operating table in a lateral decubitus position. The arm on the operated side is fixed above the head, and an axillary pad is placed in the dependent axilla to prevent neurovascular damage of the dependent extremity. A curvilinear incision is made from the anterior axillary line to the border of the paraspinal muscles, posteriorly over the rib to be resected (Fig. 4–58, insert). The latissimus dorsi muscle is mobilized by blunt dissection and transected over the line of the incision (Fig. 4–58). The posterior border of the subjacent serratus anterior muscle is mobilized, and the space between the serratus anterior muscle and the underlying rib cage is developed (Fig. 4–59). The lateral margin of the trapezius muscle is identified and transected, if necessary. Approaches as high as the third rib may be required to reach the upper thoracic spine. In such cases, the trapezius and rhomboid major and minor muscles may be sectioned adjacent to their scapular insertions to mobilize and elevate the scapula.

The appropriate rib level is selected, and the fibers of the overlying serratus anterior muscle are severed (Fig. 4–59). To verify the correct rib level, the surgeon may palpate

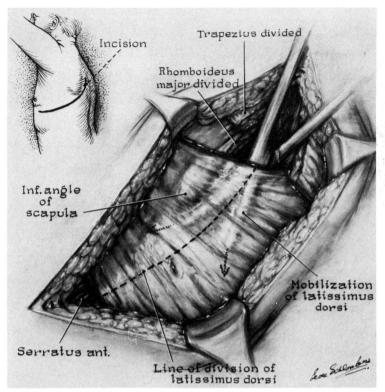

Figure 4–58. A curvilinear incision is made from the anterior axillary line to the paraspinal muscles posteriorly over the rib to be resected (insert). The latissimus dorsi muscle is mobilized from the subjacent serratus anterior muscle and is transected. In approaches through the upper thorax, the lateral margin of the trapezius and rhomboid major may be divided as well.

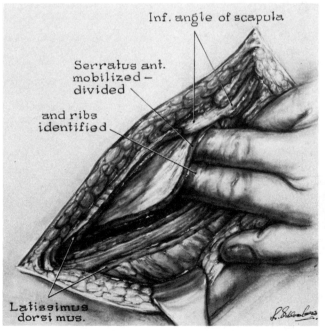

Figure 4–59. The serratus anterior muscle is mobilized and opened in line with its fibers. The surgeon may palpate superiorly within the space between the serratus anterior and the rib cage. The second rib is the uppermost rib, which may be reached within this plane and may be used to identify the level of the incision.

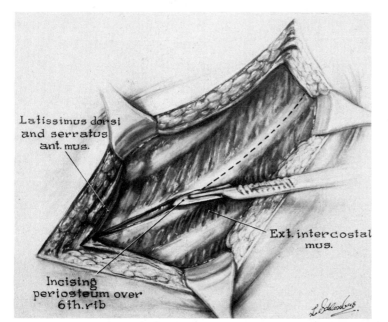

Latissimus dorsi
and serratus
ant. mus.

Ext. intercostal
mus.

Incising
periosteum over
6th. rib

Figure 4–60. The periosteum over the anterior surface of the rib is incised sharply to the bone.

superiorly within this space between the serratus anterior muscle and the rib cage. The second rib is the uppermost rib that may be reached within this plane. The periosteum over the anterior surface of the rib is incised longitudinally (Fig. 4–60) and elevated, using curved periosteal elevators. Care is required to avoid injury to the neurovascular bundle lying within the subcostal groove on the inferior surface of the rib (Fig. 4–61). The subjacent endothoracic fascia and parietal pleura are left intact. The rib should be resected from the costochondral junction anteriorly to the angle of the rib posteriorly, using rib cutters (Fig. 4–62). The paraspinal muscles should be retracted to visualize the posterior angle of the rib during its resection. The rib is removed or rotated upward, and the parietal pleura is opened using scissors. The ribs are spread using a large, self-retaining thoracotomy retractor. The lung is then manually deflated and retracted anteriorly with padded retractors to expose the aorta and vertebral bodies behind (Fig. 4–63A). Adhesions between the visceral and parietal pleura will ordinarily yield to gentle finger dissection, but sharp dissection occasionally may be required. Unless grossly diseased, the vertebral bodies are covered by the glistening parietal pleura. The intervertebral discs protrude prominently, and the vertebral bodies between are relatively concave. The aortic arch reaches to the level of the fourth thoracic vertebra and is closely applied to the anterior aspect of the vertebral bodies

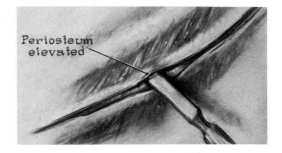

Periosteum
elevated

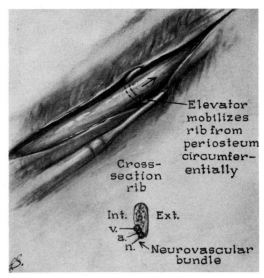

Elevator
mobilizes
rib from
periosteum
circumfer-
entially

Cross-
section
rib

Int.   Ext.
v.
a.
n.   Neurovascular
bundle

Figure 4–61. The periosteum is elevated from the rib circumferentially using straight and curved elevators. Note the neurovascular bundle lying within the subcostal groove on the deep and inferior surface of the rib. This should be elevated freely along with the periosteum.

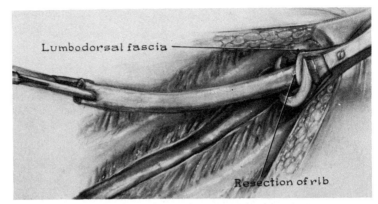

Lumbodorsal fascia

Resection of rib

Figure 4–62. The rib is resected from the costochondral junction anteriorly to the posterior angle behind. To improve the exposure later, after the thorax is opened, the posterior remnant of this rib may be resected back to the transverse process using box rongeurs. The endothoracic fascia and parietal pleura are opened through the bed of the rib.

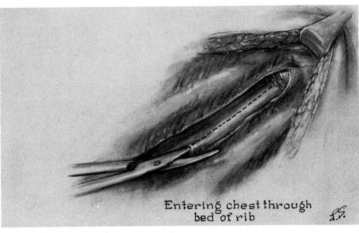

Entering chest through bed of rib

to the left of midline. Above the level of the aortic arch, the esophagus, thoracic duct, and subclavian artery are in close proximity to the vertebral body in this order, posterior to anterior. In the lower thorax, the aorta lies to the left of midline and the azygos vein and thoracic duct to the right of midline, immediately anterior to the vertebral bodies (Fig. 4–64). The aorta leaves the thorax at the level of the twelfth thoracic vertebra. The aorta and azygos system are tethered to the vertebral bodies by the intercostal vessels. These are draped over the vertebral bodies between the disc spaces (Fig. 4–63B) and join the intercostal nerve lateral to the sympathetic trunk. Together they proceed to the costal groove on the undersurface of the rib.

The correct vertebral level may be identified within the thorax by counting downward from the thoracic inlet. The first rib articulates with the superior aspect of the first thoracic vertebral body, and the second rib articulates with the first and second vertebrae. Because the thoracic vertebrae are so similar, we recommend radiographic confirmation of the ver-

tebral level in the operating room, using a radiopaque marker fixed at the level of intended dissection.

An incision is made through the parietal pleura over the posterior rib and is extended to the lateral aspect of the vertebral body (Fig. 4–63B). The pleura is cleared by blunt dissection, sparing the intercostal bundle and sympathetic trunk. A generous space is cleared over the involved vertebra and costovertebral articulations. The intercostal vessels may be ligated and transected to permit greater exposure or to mobilize the aorta. We have found that the intercostal vessels may be easily ligated using metal vascular clips and a long-handled holder. The segmental blood supply to the lower thoracic spinal cord is sparse, and for this reason we recommend that the intercostal arteries be spared when possible.

The transthoracic approach provides a generous exposure to the vertebral bodies anteriorly. It will permit complete excisional biopsy of the bodies and bone grafting at multiple levels. The intrathoracic correction of scoliotic deformities has been well perfect-

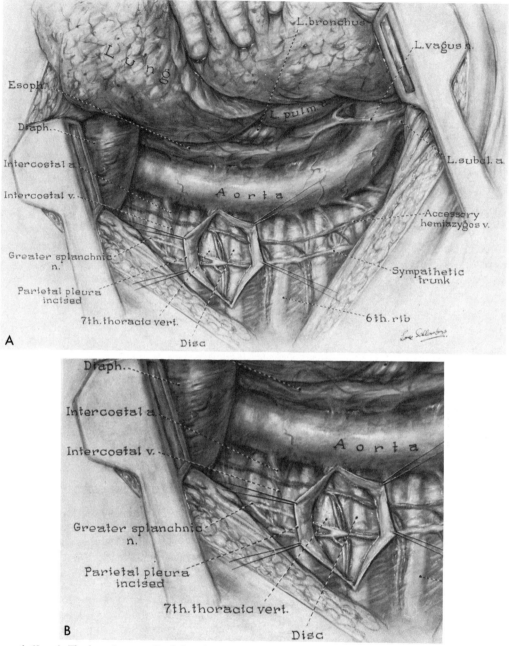

Figure 4–63. *A,* The lung is manually deflated and retracted anteriorly, revealing the aorta lying over the vertebral bodies. The vertebrae are covered by the normally translucent parietal pleura. Note that the intervertebral discs protrude prominently, and the vertebral bodies are relatively concave. The sympathetic trunk lies over the costovertebral articulations. *B,* Detail of the segmental vessels draped over the waist or midportion of the concave vertebral bodies. Lateral to the sympathetic trunk, these are joined by the intercostal nerve, and together they proceed to the subcostal groove on the lower surface of the rib.

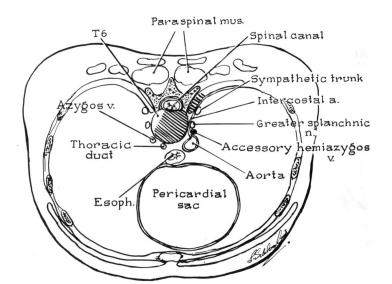

Figure 4–64. Cross-section of the thorax at the level of the sixth thoracic vertebra showing the relationship of the most significant perivertebral structures.

ed, and the spinal cord may be effectively decompressed even when the body and posterior longitudinal ligament are destroyed. In these situations, the segmental nerve is identified and is followed into the canal, and only the bone and ligament anterior to it are removed. In this way, the dura and cord are protected from injury.

The vertebral bodies protrude prominently within the thoracic cavity and are not encumbered laterally by the transverse processes as they are at the cervical levels. This facilitates keying or locking an anterior intervertebral graft in place, as troughs may be prepared and the graft may be inserted from the side (Fig. 4–65).

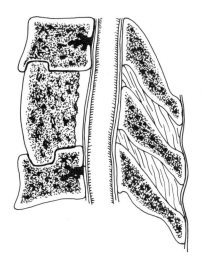

Figure 4–65. Sagittal section of a vertebral body replacement graft.

Chest tubes are inserted to evacuate blood and air. Ordinarily, these are placed one or two intercostal spaces above and below the incision, and the tubes are tunneled beneath the skin to create an air seal and to prevent leakage about the tube (Fig. 4–66). One tube is directed superiorly within the thorax toward the apex of the lung to collect air, and the other is placed below, at the posterior corner of the diaphragm, to evacuate blood. A purse-string suture is installed in the skin around each tube and is then tied to the tube to hold it in place during turning or transfer of the patient. The ribs are reapproximated and held in place with heavy absorbable sutures (Fig. 4–66). The periosteum and intercostal muscles are approximated, using a running suture, to effect an airtight closure. The serratus anterior, trapezius, latissimus dorsi, and rhomboid muscles are approximated in separate layers (Fig. 4–67). The subcutaneous tissue and skin are closed (Fig. 4–68), and the chest tubes are attached to water-seal, constant suction.

Anterior exposures of the upper thoracic vertebral bodies pose one of the great surgical challenges. Ordinarily, the third rib is the highest level through which effective intrathoracic exposure can be gained, as the first and second ribs are too short to provide reasonable room within the chest. To expose the upper thoracic vertebrae through the bed of the third rib, the scapula must be mobilized and retracted laterally and superiorly. To do this, the rhomboid muscles may be detached from their insertion on the vertebral border of

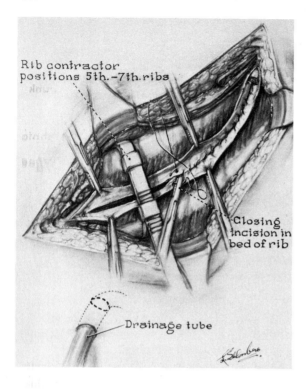

Figure 4–66. The ribs are reapproximated and held in place with heavy absorbable pericostal sutures placed around the ribs above and below the thoracotomy site. The intercostal muscles and periosteum are closed with a running suture to create an airtight closure. Prior to closure, chest tubes are placed at the apex of the lung to collect air and at the posterior base of the thoracic cavity to evacuate blood. The tubes are placed one or two intercostal spaces away from the incision and are tunneled beneath the skin to create an air seal.

the scapula. This may be done by subperiosteally stripping them from the scapula, leaving a layer of periosteum and tendon for later repair. At closure, holes may be made in the scapula, sutures are inserted through these holes, and the rhomboids are repaired through this periosteal-tendon sheath.

If spinal stability is in doubt, plaster of Paris turning shells, similar to a bivalved body cast, are made for the patient, extending from the upper thorax to the pelvis. The front and back components are secured with a circumferential binder, and the patient is transferred to a bed or turning frame.

The patient is nursed supine but is rolled like a log from side to side at two-hour intervals. When drainage of air and blood has stopped, the chest tubes are removed, and

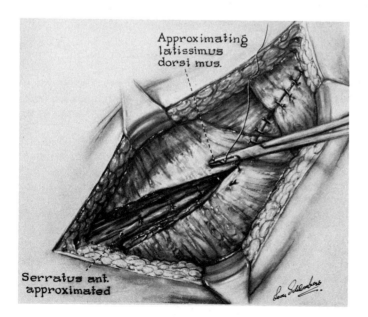

Figure 4–67. Closure of the serratus anterior, trapezius, and latissimus dorsi muscles.

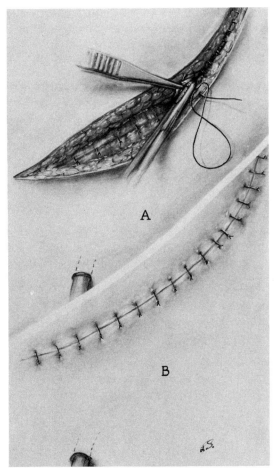

Figure 4–68. Closure of the subcutaneous layer *(A)* and skin *(B)*. Note the chest tubes tunneled beneath the skin away from the incision to create an air seal.

and back components and is made of a "high-temperature," light weight plastic. The front and back components are connected with velcro closures and may be removed to inspect the skin. If the level of instability is in the upper thorax, above the sixth vertebra, we add a chin-occipit extension, or if the instability extends into the lumbar spine, we add a hip spica to the thigh to improve external control. The patient is then mobilized, and roentgenograms are obtained with the patient erect to insure that appropriate control of the spine is maintained and that the vertebrae remain well aligned. Roentgenograms are made at regular intervals until osseous fusion is established, and the patient is then weaned from the brace or cast.

COMPLICATIONS

The transthoracic approach to the spine adds the considerable risk of thoracotomy to the risks of spinal surgery. Postoperatively, these patients require intensive nursing care and close supervision by the surgical team. Many of these patients are debilitated, are poor operative risks, and require heroic efforts to carry them through their postoperative course.

All the complications of major thoracic surgery may occur, such as atelectasis, pneumonia, and airway obstruction. Congestive heart failure and pulmonary edema may occur if fluid replacement is excessive and if venous pressures are not closely monitored.

On resecting the vertebral bodies, considerable bleeding may be encountered from the posterior nutrient vessels. These must be controlled with bone wax, Gelfoam, and thrombin, as it is often unsafe to cauterize these vessels adjacent to the dura.

Injury to the spinal cord is always possible, particularly with extensive anterior decompression, if the operative field is covered with blood or if the normal landmarks are distorted by disease. For this reason, we recommend meticulous control of hemorrhage. When the anatomic landmarks are severely distorted, one can identify a nerve root and follow it centrally until the dura and cord are safely identified. An alternative approach is to initiate the decompression over an uninvolved area and proceed to the involved area following the plane of the dura. Perhaps the greatest neurologic threat is associated with correction

when the patient's condition has stabilized and the wounds are healed, a body cast or brace is made to protect the spine. Ordinarily, we use a hyperextension body cast made on a fracture table using Goldthwaite irons. The cast is padded over the entire posterior thorax and pelvis with a single large sheet of felt, and additional pads are placed anteriorly over the manubrium, lower ribs, iliac crests, and pubic symphysis. The cast extends from the manubrium to the pubic symphysis and is well molded about the pelvis and thorax. A hole is made in the front of the cast about 10 cm. high and 15 cm. wide over the upper abdomen just below the rib cage to facilitate respiration.

If the patient has insensate skin, we avoid using circumferential plaster and usually employ a molded plastic body brace. This is similar to a body cast but has separate front of a severe fixed kyphos by osteotomy, and because of this, patients and their families should be advised preoperatively that paraplegia may complicate this procedure.

Spinal cord ischemia secondary to ligation of the segmental intercostal vessels is a potential threat (p. 179). Anterior spinal artery syndromes with paraplegia, loss of pain and temperature sense, and sphincter disturbance have occasionally been reported following scoliosis correction (Dommisse, 1974; Kiem and Sadek, 1971) or circumferential spinal osteotomy (Dommisse, 1970). On the other hand, no complications have been reported by a number of authors following unilateral resection of multiple segmental vessels in the lower thoracic spine (Burrington et al., 1976; Chou, 1973; Cook, 1971; Hodgson et al., 1960; Winter, 1973). Burrington and colleagues (1976) recommend that the segmental arteries be ligated close to the aorta on one side only, maintaining the collateral circulation through the intercostals described by Lazorthes et al. (1971).

Although pseudarthrosis following anterior fusion is rare, it has been reported (Winter, 1973). Wound infections are rare but do occur, and pressure sores have been a problem, particularly over a prominent gibbus. Hodgson and coworkers (1960) reported the development of a cerebrospinal fluid fistula into the pleural cavity in four cases following resection of a tuberculous spinal abscess, one of which resulted in death.

Thoracoabdominal Approach to the Lower Thoracic and Upper Lumbar Vertebral Bodies

It is occasionally necessary to expose the lower thoracic and upper lumbar vertebral bodies in continuity. This presents a problem in exposure because of the presence of the diaphragm and adds to the risk of surgery if two major body cavities are opened. A number of different approaches are available, beginning from above with a posterolateral thoracotomy at the left seventh intercostal space and dividing the diaphragm peripherally within the thorax. At the inferior extreme, the thorax may be left intact and the vertebrae may be approached through a long, oblique flank incision made below the rib cage, and the diaphragm may be detached posteriorly and medially from below (p. 160). The approach selected should depend upon the level of ver-

tebral involvement and the patient's ability to tolerate major surgery. Ordinarily, thoracic lesions should be approached through the chest, whereas lesions that primarily involve the upper lumbar vertebrae may be approached through a flank incision with less operative risk.

The diaphragm is a dome-shaped organ that is muscular around its periphery and tendinous centrally (Fig. 4–69). Anteriorly and laterally, it originates from the cartilaginous ends of the lower six ribs and xyphoid. Posteriorly, it originates from the upper lumbar vertebrae through the crura, the aponeurotic arcuate ligaments, and the twelfth ribs. The crura are musculotendinous structures that arise from the anterior longitudinal ligament of the lumbar vertebrae and extend superiorly to surround the aortic and esophageal hiatus. The medial arcuate ligaments arise from the crura on their respective sides, cross over the psoas muscles like a bridge, and insert on the transverse processes of the first lumbar vertebrae. The lateral arcuate ligaments arise from the transverse process of the first lumbar vertebra and extend over the quadratus lumborum muscles to the tips of the twelfth ribs.

The diaphragm is innervated by the phrenic nerve, which descends through the thorax on the pericardium. The phrenic nerve joins the diaphragm adjacent to the fibrous pericardium, dividing into three major branches that extend peripherally in an anterior, lateral, and posterior direction. In addition, there are numerous interconnections that loop between these branches (Scott, 1965). Cutting many of these major branches or intercommunications will interfere with diaphragmatic function and will reduce respiratory reserves. An incision around the periphery of the diaphragm will least interfere with diaphragmatic function and is recommended for thoracoabdominal approaches to the spine. A short, radiate incision through the central tendon will spare most major nerve fibers but does not provide direct access to the vertebral bodies posteriorly. To provide wide exposure of the thoracic and lumbar vertebrae in continuity, an incision is made through the periphery of the diaphragm, extending posteriorly through the lateral arcuate ligament. A second incision is then required through the insertions of the medial and lateral arcuate ligaments adjacent to the first lumbar transverse process to open the diaphragm posteriorly and to provide continuity of exposure between the thoracic and lumbar spine.

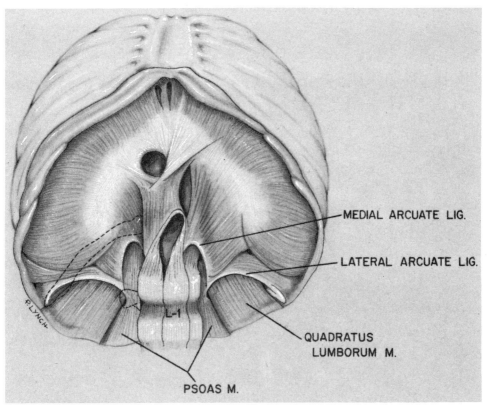

Figure 4–69. The diaphragm, viewed from below within the peritoneal cavity and retroperitoneal space. The medial arcuate ligament arises from the crura along the vertebral bodies, crosses the psoas muscle, and inserts on the first lumbar transverse process. The lateral arcuate ligament arises from the tip of the first lumbar transverse process, crosses over the quadratus lumborum muscle, and inserts on the tip of the twelfth rib.

The eleventh and twelfth thoracic vertebrae may be approached from above or below the diaphragm, but each route provides certain advantages and limitations. For example, in the subdiaphragmatic approach, the surgeon may reflect the left aortic crus and divide the arcuate ligament insertion but leave the muscular diaphragm intact. In addition, he may avoid entering the pleural cavity by limiting the dissection to the retropleural plane around the vertebral bodies. This yields an excellent view of the upper lumbar vertebrae but allows a more limited exposure as high as the eleventh thoracic vertebral body. On the other hand, the transthoracic route through the diaphragm offers a much larger working area over the lower thoracic vertebrae but obligates a more extensive dissection, opening two major body cavities.

Most general surgical approaches to the abdominal viscera are directed anteriorly and laterally. Because the vertebral bodies are posterior to the abdominal viscera, the ap-

proach should be modified in a posterolateral direction to bring the vertebrae as close to the incision as possible and to reduce the depth of the wound. We recommend an approach to the left of midline, as the vena cava on the right may complicate surgery with troublesome hemorrhage, and the liver may be hard to retract.

The anterior approaches are only required when extensive resection and bone grafts are planned. Simple excisional biopsy, drainage, or debridement of the vertebral bodies may be effectively handled through a posterolateral costotransversectomy (see next section) with less operative morbidity.

TECHNIQUE

To approach the lower thoracic spine through the chest, the patient is positioned on the operating table in a lateral decubitus position. An axillary pad is placed in the dependent axilla, and the left arm is fixed above the

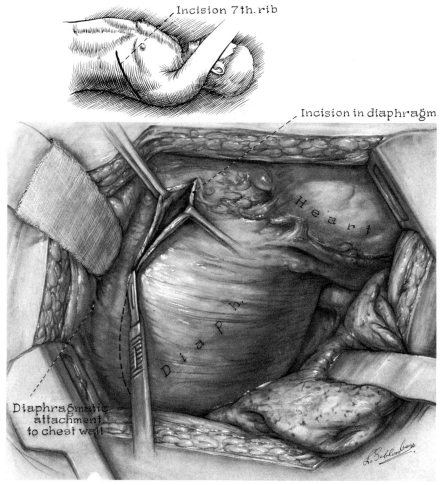

Figure 4–70. Thoracotomy incision (insert). Circumferential incision in the muscular portion of the diaphragm adjacent to the costal margin.

head. A left lateral or posterolateral incision is made at the level of the seventh to eleventh ribs, depending upon the desired level of dissection (Fig. 4–70). The incision extends from the paraspinal muscles posteriorly to the anterior margin of the rib cage. The incision is deepened through the subcutaneous tissues to the thoracic musculature. The latissimus dorsi muscle is transected across the plane of its fibers, and the serratus anterior muscle is divided and spread over the intended rib level. The external and internal intercostal muscles are divided in the intercostal space using scalpel dissection. The endothoracic fascia and parietal pleura are opened, the ribs are spread with a large self-retaining rib retractor, and the lung is deflated and retracted anteriorly. If

bone grafting is planned, the rib may be removed. A circumferential incision is made in the muscular portion of the diaphragm adjacent to the costal margin (Figure 4–70) and extended posteriorly to the lateral arcuate ligament. This incision is extended through the peritoneal reflection of the diaphragm, and the spleen and contents of the left upper quadrant of the abdomen are exposed. The retroperitoneal space is opened either by blunt dissection of the peritoneum at the level of the diaphragmatic incision or through a separate incision adjacent to the spleen (Fig. 4–71). The retroperitoneal space is developed by blunt dissection posterior to the renal fascia. The spleen, kidney, and stomach are gently retracted medially, using a broad, padded Dever

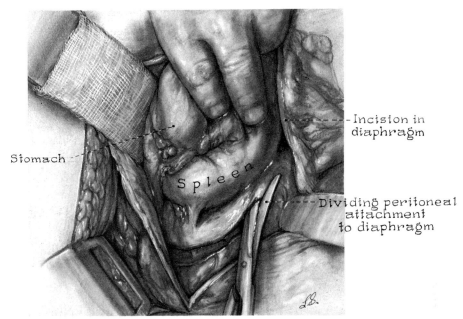

Stomach

Spleen

Incision in diaphragm

Dividing peritoneal attachment to diaphragm

Figure 4–71. The abdominal contents are retracted medially and inferiorly, and the retroperitoneal space is opened through a peritoneal incision adjacent to the diaphragm.

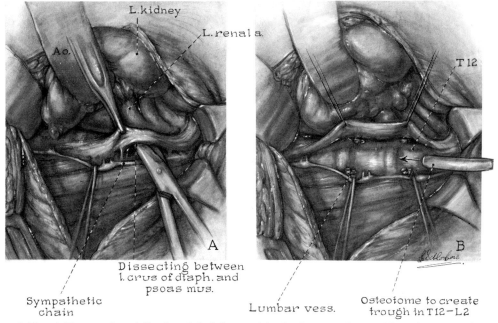

L. kidney

L. renal a.

Ao.

T 12

A

B

Sympathetic chain

Dissecting between l. crus of diaph. and psoas mus.

Lumbar vess.

Osteotome to create trough in T 12–L 2

Figure 4–72. *A,* The aorta is mobilized, and the left crus of the diaphragm is dissected from the anterior longitudinal ligament over the vertebral bodies. *B,* A longitudinal incision is made in the anterior longitudinal ligament, and the vertebral bodies are exposed.

retractor. The psoas muscle, vertebral bodies, and aorta are exposed. The aorta is carefully mobilized by a combination of sharp and blunt dissection, and the segmental vessels are ligated with metal vascular clips and divided at only those levels required for satisfactory exposure. The sympathetic trunk extends over the anterolateral aspect of the vertebral bodies adjacent to the psoas muscle. It is recognized by its periodic ganglionic enlargements and should be spared. The left crus of the diaphragm is dissected from the anterior longitudinal ligament over the upper lumbar vertebral bodies (Fig. 4–72A). The insertion of the arcuate ligament is divided at the first lumbar transverse process. The incision in the diaphragm is extended through the lateral arcuate ligament, providing continuity of exposure from the thoracic to the lumbar vertebrae. A longitudinal incision is made in the anterior longitudinal ligament, and the ligament is reflected laterally to expose the vertebral bodies (Fig. 4–72B). At this point, drainage, resection of a lesion, osteotomy, decompression, or bone grafting may be performed with excellent visibility throughout the thoracic and upper lumbar spine. Fusion and inlay bone grafting in a trough created in the twelfth thoracic and first two lumbar vertebrae is illustrated in Figure 4–73A and B.

The anterior longitudinal ligament may be repaired over the vertebral bodies. The diaphragmatic crus is sutured to the anterior longitudinal ligament to close the defect in the aortic hiatus. The arcuate ligament is repaired at the transverse process of the first lumbar vertebra. The diaphragm is closed with interrupted sutures in an airtight fashion (Fig. 4–74). Chest tubes are inserted for drainage of fluid and air, and the ribs are reapproximated.

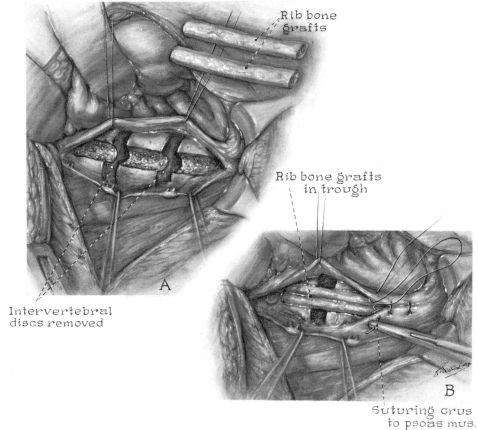

Figure 4–73. *A,* A trough is created in the 12th thoracic and upper two lumbar vertebrae, and the intervertebral disc spaces are excised. *B,* Bone plugs are installed in the disc spaces, rib grafts are laid in the trough, and the anterior longitudinal ligament and left crus are repaired.

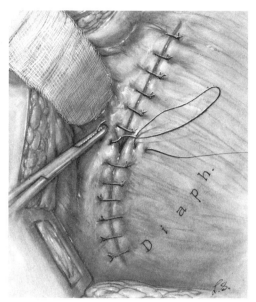

Figure 4–74. The diaphragm is closed in an airtight fashion.

The pleura and intercostal muscles are repaired with running absorbable suture material, and the serratus anterior and latissimus dorsi muscles are reapproximated with separate layers of running suture. The subcutaneous tissue and skin are closed, and the chest tubes are attached to water-seal suction.

Postoperatively, the patient is usually nursed in plaster of Paris shells or a turning frame to protect the integrity of the spine. At about two weeks following surgery, the patient may be placed in a localizer cast or brace, depending upon the intrinsic stability of the spine (see previous section).

COMPLICATIONS

The thoracoabdominal exposure of the thoracic and lumbar spine adds significantly to the risks of surgery, as two major body cavities are exposed. The specific complications encountered are similar to those of thoracotomy alone, as described in the previous section. In addition, injury to the spleen, kidney, or ureters may occur without gentle retraction or cautious dissection. Gastrointestinal complications such as prolonged ileus may be anticipated. Injury to the sympathetic chain may induce a sympathectomy effect with asymmetric warmth of the involved extremity, but this is rarely a problem. The peritoneum

and diaphragm should be closed carefully to restore their continuity and to prevent herniation of visceral structures.

As a rule, these patients are exceedingly sick in the first week postoperatively and require intensive nursing care for much of this period. For this reason, the combined thoracoabdominal exposure should be reserved for those patients with satisfactory cardiopulmonary reserves who are likely to tolerate such surgical risks. In the case of a poor operative risk, the exposure through the flank with retroperitoneal dissection should be considered if limited exposure over the thoracic vertebrae is acceptable.

Posterolateral Costotransversectomy Approach to the Thoracic Vertebral Bodies

The costotransversectomy approach provides access to the anterior and lateral elements of the thoracic vertebrae through a posterolateral incision. With careful dissection in the retropleural space, the vertebral bodies may be reached without entering the pleural cavity. The approach is ideally suited to a poor risk or elderly patient who cannot tolerate formal thoracotomy and provides access for biopsy, drainage of an abscess, and limited resection of the vertebral bodies. In addition, the spinal cord may be decompressed anterolaterally, and a limited anterior fusion may be performed. The posterolateral approach is a less extensive procedure and affords less operative risk than formal thoracotomy imposes. On the other hand, costotransversectomy provides less satisfactory exposure of the midthoracic vertebral bodies, and extensive vertebral resection or fusion at multiple levels may not be technically feasible.

Costotransversectomy was first used by Haidenhaim and described by Menard in 1894. As originally described, it provides limited exposure of the lateral vertebral bodies through a midline posterior longitudinal incision. The transverse process of the vertebra and medial two inches of rib are resected at one of several levels. The vertebral bodies can be palpated within the retropleural space, but because the incision is made in midline and only a short segment of rib is removed, visualization of the vertebral body is limited, and the anterior aspect cannot be reached directly.

Seddon (1956) augmented this exposure

by approaching the spine through a more lateral, curvilinear incision. He recommended resecting longer segments of rib over at least three levels, permitting more extensive exposure and direct visualization of the anterolateral aspect of the vertebral bodies. In 1933, Capener (reported in 1954) made a major addition to this approach by including anterolateral decompression of the cord. He referred to this as lateral rhachotomy. The spine is approached through a curvilinear incision lateral to the midline. The trapezius muscle is detached medially and retracted laterally, and the paraspinal muscles are divided transversely. The transverse processes of the vertebrae and a generous length of rib are resected at several levels. The cord is decompressed laterally and anteriorly by resecting the pedicles and posterior aspect of the vertebral bodies. Until Hodgson popularized transthoracic resection and decompression of the tuberculous spine, this approach was frequently used to resect tuberculous lesions of the thoracic spine (Johnson et al., 1953).

The authors use a minor modification of this approach through a straight, longitudinal incision lateral to the paraspinal muscle mass. The paraspinal muscles are retracted medially, and the transverse process and a generous section of rib are removed. Through this exposure, biopsy or drainage of an abscess, limited resection, anterolateral decompression, and fusion are possible, and it may be the safest approach to excise a herniated intervertebral disc at the thoracic level (Benson and Byrnes, 1975). When a kyphos is present, exposure of the vertebral body is improved and may be increased by removing the ribs and transverse processes at three or four levels, but visualization of the anterior aspect of the vertebral bodies remains limited. Some surgeons have successfully performed extensive decompression and fusion using this exposure (Bohlman, 1976), but we have found this approach more limiting and prefer thoracotomy when extensive resection and grafting are planned at multiple levels. We have also been reluctant to remove more than four ribs posteriorly for fear of removing the lateral stability they provide and allowing a scoliosis to develop.

ANATOMIC CONSIDERATIONS

Certain superficial muscles of the posterior thorax must be divided in the costotransversectomy approach, lateral to the paraspinal muscle mass. The trapezius muscle (Fig. 4–75) extends from the head to the twelfth thoracic spinous process, its fibers running obliquely and laterally to the scapular spine. Beneath this lie the rhomboid muscles, arising from the spinous processes of the seventh cervical and upper five thoracic vertebrae. In the lower thorax, the latissimus dorsi muscle arises beneath the trapezius muscle from the lower six thoracic vertebrae and extends as a broad sheet across the back to the axilla. The serratus posterior inferior muscle is the most characteristic muscle found in the lower thorax beneath the latissimus. It arises as separate, short muscular bundles from the lower four ribs, becomes tendinous, and descends obliquely downward to insert on the lumbar fascia. In posterolateral approaches to the upper five thoracic vertebrae, the trapezius and rhomboid muscles must be divided. These may be sectioned medially about their tendinous origins. Over the lower thorax, the latissimus dorsi as well as the trapezius muscles must be sectioned, and the serratus posterior inferior muscle is found over the lowest three vertebrae.

EXTRINSIC LIGAMENTS

Unique to the thoracic spine are a group of ligaments that bind the ribs to their respective transverse processes and the vertebral bodies. This is an additional ligament system that through the ribs increases the stability over the thoracic spine. These must be divided in a costotransversectomy exposure before the posterior and medial aspect of the ribs may be mobilized and removed.

The costotransverse ligaments are divided into a number of named individual components. The most significant of these is the superior costotransverse ligament (Fig. 4–76), which extends from the inferior aspect of one transverse process to the superior aspect of the rib beneath. Medial to this ligament is a space through which the dorsal rami of the segmental nerves and vessels course posteriorly toward the erector spinae muscle mass (Fig. 4–80, insert). In dissections beneath the transverse processes, these vessels should be identified and ligated to prevent persistent hemorrhage. The posterior costotransverse ligament extends from the inferior aspect of the base of the transverse process to the superior aspect of the rib beneath.

Anterior to the transverse process is the capsular ligament, which secures the neck of the rib to the front of the transverse process.

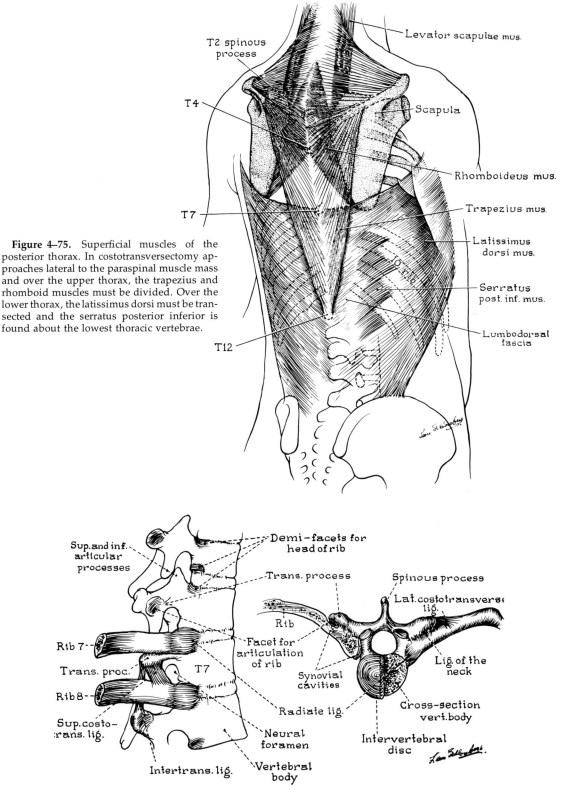

Figure 4–75. Superficial muscles of the posterior thorax. In costotransversectomy approaches lateral to the paraspinal muscle mass and over the upper thorax, the trapezius and rhomboid muscles must be divided. Over the lower thorax, the latissimus dorsi must be transected and the serratus posterior inferior is found about the lowest thoracic vertebrae.

Figure 4–76. Extrinsic ligaments of the thoracic spine and detail of the thoracic vertebrae. Unique to the thoracic spine are a group of ligaments that bind the ribs to the vertebral bodies and transverse processes. This ligament system is additional to the intrinsic ligaments between vertebrae and increases the inherent stability of the thoracic spine.

Laterally, the lateral costotransverse ligaments extend from the tip of the transverse process to the posterior tubercle of the same rib (Fig. 4–76). Finally, the costovertebral or radiate ligaments bind the head of each rib to its respective vertebral body articulations. The sympathetic trunk courses over the heads of the ribs within the thorax just lateral to the radiate ligament insertions on the ribs (Fig. 4–80).

The transverse processes extend like wings from the upper and lateral aspects of the laminae, arching superiorly and posteriorly in their lateral course (Fig. 4–76). Laterally, these widen into a prominent tubercle, which articulates with the rib at the same level on its anterior surface. The pedicle lies directly in front of the base of each transverse process, a fact that is helpful in locating the pedicle and avoiding the nerve root, which emerges from the foramina beneath, during costotransversectomy.

TECHNIQUE

Endotracheal anesthesia is recommended to provide positive pressure ventilation in case the pleura is opened during the surgical dissection. The patient is placed on the operating table, either in a lateral position with an axillary pad in the dependent axilla or in the prone position with chest rolls on either side of the thorax.

A straight, longitudinal incision is made about 2.5 inches lateral to the spinous processes, centered over the level of the desired vertebral dissection (Fig. 4–77). At this location a slight depression is palpable between

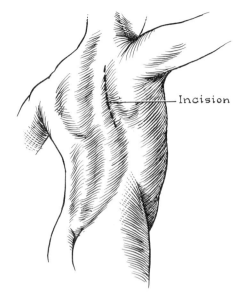

Figure 4–77. A longitudinal incision is made lateral to the paraspinal muscle mass over the posterior angle of the ribs. A depression is normally visible here, and the prominent posterior angles can be palpated beneath this depression.

the dorsal paraspinal muscle mass and the prominent posterior angle of the rib (Fig. 4–78). The incision should be centered over this groove, lateral to the spinous processes. The incision is extended deeply through the subcutaneous tissues; and the trapezius and latissimus dorsi muscles (Fig. 4–75), as well as the lumbodorsal fascia, are divided longitudinally. The paraspinal muscles are dissected sharply from their insertions on the ribs and transverse processes and are retracted medially. In a muscular patient, it may be impossi-

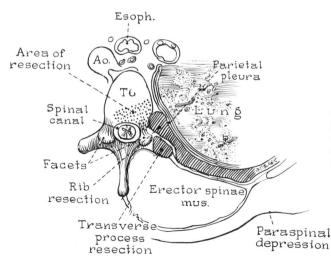

Figure 4–78. Cross-section of the thoracic vertebrae and ribs. The hatched area indicates the bony structures that are normally removed to provide adequate exposure. The stippled area over the vertebral body and pedicle may be removed to decompress the spinal canal.

ble to effectively retract these muscles medially, and one may need to divide the paraspinal muscles transversely; however, subsequent closure may be difficult.

If simple drainage of a small abscess or biopsy of a lesion of the pedicle or vertebral body is contemplated, the rib and transverse process are resected at one or two levels only. Roentgenographic control films should be taken in the operating room with a needle or towel clip attached to the vertebra in question to insure that the proper spinal level is selected. The costotransverse ligaments (Fig. 4–76) are divided sharply, and the transverse process is generously resected at its junction with the lamina (Fig. 4–78) using bone rongeurs or osteotomes. An incision is made through the periosteum into the rib, from the costovertebral articulation to the angle of the rib. The rib is exposed by careful subperiosteal dissection, leaving the pleura and intercostal neurovascular bundles intact (Fig. 4–79). The rib is transected with rib cutters about 3.5 inches lateral to the vertebra at its prominent posterior angle. The cut end of the rib is grasped with a clamp and rotated with one hand while the costovertebral ligaments are separated with a sharp periosteal elevator, dissecting along the rib toward the vertebral articulation. If a porotic rib breaks at its neck, the medial end should be resected cleanly with rongeurs.

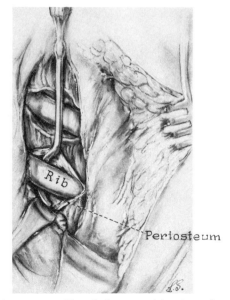

Figure 4–79. The rib is exposed by circumferential subperiosteal dissection from its posterior angle to the transverse process of the vertebra.

Anterior to the stump of the amputated transverse process is the vertebral pedicle, and above and below the pedicle lie the neural foramina (Figs. 4–76 and 4–80). The nerve roots emerge from the inferior pole of the foramina, giving off a dorsal and ventral ramus. The dorsal ramus sweeps posteriorly, with its accompanying vessels, below the transverse process and medial to the superior costotransverse ligaments (Fig. 4–80, insert). The artery and veins should be identified and ligated or they will bleed continually throughout the procedure. The ventral ramus becomes the intercostal nerve and is joined by the intercostal vessels. These travel laterally and meet the ribs at their posterior angle and then enter the subcostal groove. Anteriorly, the intercostal vessels sweep around the waist or midportion of the vertebral body before dividing into the ventral and dorsal branches at the outlet of the neural foramen (Fig. 4–80).

Once the pedicles, neural foramina, and these neurovascular structures have been identified, the dissection should proceed directly anteriorly, on the pedicle, to the vertebral body along a path that is relatively free of major vessels or nerves (Fig. 4–81). We generally use a Cobb elevator beginning at the pedicle, raising the sympathetic trunk and parietal pleura before it and advancing forward to the anterolateral aspect of the body (Fig. 4–82). Once this path is clear, we then extend the dissection inferiorly and superiorly along the vertebral body and disc space, being careful not to injure the segmental vessels draped over the vertebral body. The parietal pleura is then teased from the vertebral body by gentle finger dissection. If the pleura is perforated, the defect should be sealed and repaired.

At this stage, an abscess may be drained, and necrotic debris may be removed over a limited area. If a biopsy of the vertebral body is planned, the pleura is retracted, using a padded Dever retractor, and the vertebral body is biopsied, using curets or rongeurs. If the exposure is not adequate, the transverse processes and ribs should be resected at one or two additional levels.

If a relatively extensive resection, decompression, and bone grafting are planned, at least three and no more than four transverse processes and ribs should be resected. Ordinarily, the intercostal vessels may be retracted sufficiently to provide adequate exposure; however, the vessels may be ligated and divid-

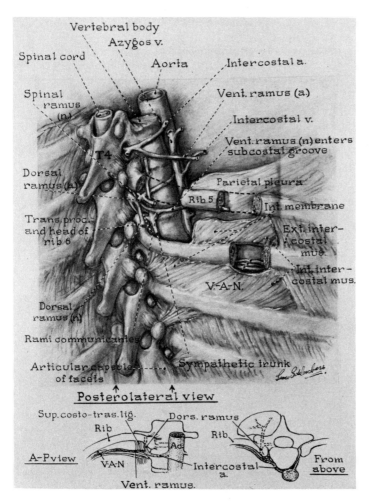

Figure 4–80. Anatomic detail of the deep structures of the posterior thorax showing the relationship of the dorsal and ventral neurovascular structures. *Insert*, The dorsal nerve and artery course beneath the transverse processes and medial to the superior costotransverse ligament. These vessels should be identified and ligated in approaches through the transverse processes.

ed if necessary. The intercostal nerves are isolated from adjacent tissue, and the pleura is depressed, leaving the nerves suspended across the wound (Fig. 4–83).

If decompression is required, the pedicles and posterior aspect of the vertebral bodies may be removed (Figs. 4–78 and 4–83). De-

compression is started at the pedicles adjacent to a nerve root in an area that is least involved with disease. The nerve root is followed centrally as a guide, and the dura and spinal cord are identified and protected. Bone is removed using rongeurs and a high-speed drill and diamond burr to remove dense cortical bone.

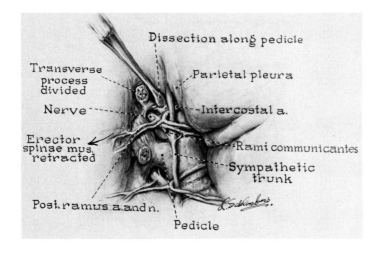

Figure 4–81. The pedicles lie directly in front of the transverse processes. To expose the vertebral body, the dissection should proceed anterior to the stump of the transected transverse process, along the pedicles, to the vertebral body. By restricting the dissection to this plane, one can avoid the nerve roots leaving their foramina above and below the pedicles as well as the segmental vessels draped over the midportion of the vertebral body. We find that a 0.5 in. Cobb periosteal elevator is most useful for this part of the dissection. Once an initial path has been cleared, dissection can proceed inferiorly and superiorly along the vertebral body to widen the exposure, using the periosteal elevator to raise these tissues.

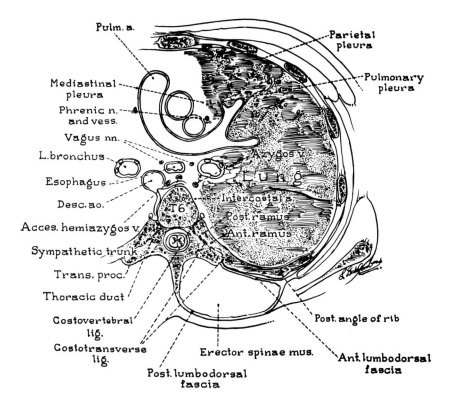

Figure 4–82. Cross-section of the thorax at the level of the sixth thoracic vertebra.

One should be able to see the dura throughout the procedure, and the dura should be used as a guide to protect the cord as bone is resected around the spinal canal. The pedicles may be removed anterior to the facets, but the facets should be left intact to maintain anterior and lateral stability.

If decompression of a kyphos is required, resection of relatively large amounts of the posterior vertebral body may be necessary. The posterior longitudinal ligament and the posterior aspect of the vertebral body may be removed. An alternative method is to enter the cancellous bone anterior to the posterior

Figure 4–83. For relatively extensive decompression and bone grafting, three or four ribs and transverse processes may be transected, leaving the neurovascular structures at each level suspended across the wound. The spinal canal may then be decompressed laterally and anteriorly by removing the pedicles to the side and a portion of the vertebral bodies in front of the spinal canal. The parietal pleura is retracted away from the vertebra with hand-held retractors.

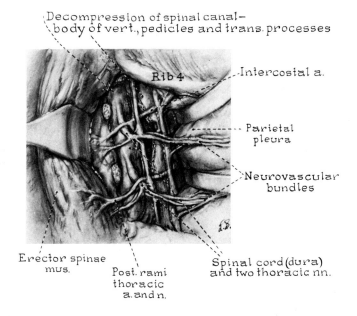

cortex of the vertebral body. Sufficient bone is removed to provide effective decompression. Using a flat elevator, the posterior cortex is broken and depressed anteriorly, relieving the spinal obstruction. This leaves the posterior longitudinal ligament and a veneer of cortical bone between the spinal cord and any sharp subcortical bone fragments. Following this, the cord should be inspected to insure that it is well decompressed and that there are no sharp projections into the canal. Throughout this dissection, it is best to avoid traction or manipulation of the dura or cord.

At the time of closure, the wound is filled with saline, and the lungs are inflated to check for air leaks. The paraspinal muscles, lumbodorsal fascia, and trapezius and latissimus dorsi muscles are repaired in separate layers. The wound is closed with a drain at the lower pole to prevent hematoma collection. The patient is generally nursed in plaster of Paris body shells or a turning frame until a body cast or brace may be applied (see previous section on thoracotomy).

COMPLICATIONS

Although costotransversectomy is a less formidable approach than thoracotomy, there are significant surgical risks. Decompression of the spinal canal is potentially hazardous, and neurologic complications have occurred. Tears in the dura should be identified and repaired to prevent cerebrospinal fluid fistula. Throughout the procedure, bleeding should be meticulously controlled so the operative field is not obscured and the spinal cord is not inadvertently injured. Bleeding about the open vertebral body may be troublesome and can be controlled by cautery away from the cord or by packing and bone wax. Prior to closure, the pleura should be inspected for air leaks, and repairs should be made as required. If a pneumothorax is suspected, roentgenograms of the chest should be obtained in the operating room prior to extubation, and a chest tube should be installed in the upper anterior thorax.

Extensive decompression may induce significant spinal instability. Stability should be assessed at surgery by manipulation of the vertebral elements. If there is any doubt about spinal stability, instrumentation of fusion should be performed, and the spine should be carefully protected postoperatively with traction, a brace, or a cast until fusion is established.

References

Benson, M. K. D., and Byrnes, D. P.: The clinical syndromes and surgical treatment of thoracic intervertebral disc prolapse. J. Bone Joint Surg. 57-B:471–477, 1975.

Bohlman, H. H.: Late, progressive paralysis and pain following fractures of the thoracolumbar spine. J. Bone Joint Surg. 58-A:728, 1976.

Brice, J., and McKissock, W.: Surgical treatment of malignant extradural spinal tumors. Br. Med. J. 1:1341–1344, 1965.

Burrington, J. D., Brown, C., Wayne, E. R., and Odom, J.: Anterior approach to the thoraco lumbar spine — technical considerations. Arch. Surg. 111:456–463, 1976.

Capener, N.: The evolution of lateral rhachotomy. J. Bone Joint Surg. 36-B:173–179, 1954.

Cauchoix, J., and Binet, J.: Anterior surgical approaches to spine. Ann. R. Coll. Surg. Engl. 27:237–243, 1957.

Chou, S. N., and Seljeskog, E. L.: Alternative surgical approaches to the thoracic spine. Clin. Neurosurg. 20:306–321, 1973.

Cook, W. A.: Trans-thoracic vertebral surgery. Ann. Thorac. Surg. 12:54–68, 1971.

Dommisse, G. F., and Enslin, T. E.: Hodgson's circumferential osteotomy in the correction of spinal deformities. J. Bone Joint Surg., 52-B:778, 1970.

Dommisse, G. F.: The blood supply of the spinal cord. A critical vascular zone in spinal surgery. J. Bone Joint Surg., 56-B:225–235, 1974.

Dwyer, A. F.: Experience of anterior correction of scoliosis. Clin. Orthop. 93:191–206, 1973.

Dwyer, A. F., and Schafer, M. F.: Anterior approach to scoliosis: Results of treatment in fifty-one cases. J. Bone Joint Surg. 56-B:218–224, 1974.

Hodgson, A. R., and Stock, F. E.: Anterior spinal fusion, a preliminary communication on the radical treatment of Pott's disease and Pott's paraplegia. Br. J. Surg. 44:266–275, 1956.

Hodgson, A. R., Stock, F. E., Fang, H. S. Y., and Ong, G. B.: Anterior spinal fusion: The operative approach and pathologic findings in 412 patients with Pott's disease of the spine. Br. J. Surg. 48:172–178, 1960.

Hodgson, A. R.: Correction of fixed spinal curves. A preliminary communication. J. Bone Joint Surg. 47-A:1221–1227, 1965.

Hodgson, A. R., and Yao, A. C. M. C.: Anterior approaches to the spinal column. In Apley, A. G. (ed): Recent advances in orthopaedics. London, Longman Group, 1969, pp. 289–323.

Johnson, R. W., Jr., Hillman, J. W., and Southwick, W. O.: The importance of direct surgical attack upon lesions of the vertebral bodies, particularly in Pott's disease. J. Bone Joint Surg. 35-A:17–25, 1953.

Johnson, J. T. H., and Robinson, R. A.: Anterior strut grafts for severe kyphosis. Clin. Orthop. 56:25–36, 1968.

Kiem, H. A., and Sadek, K. H.: Spinal angiography in scoliosis patients. J. Bone Joint Surg., 53-A:904–912, 1971.

Lazorthes, G., Gouaze, A., Zadeh, J. O., Santini, J. J., Lazorthes, Y., and Burdin, P.: Arterial vascularization of the spinal cord: Recent studies of the anastomotic substitution pathways. J. Neurosurg. 35:253–262, 1970.

Martin, N. S., and Williamson, J.: The role of surgery in

the treatment of malignant tumors of the spine. J. Bone Joint Surg. *52-B*:227–237, 1970.

Menard, V.: Causes de la paraplegie dans le mal de Pott. Rev. Orthop. *5*:47–64, 1894.

Nissen, R.: Exstirpation eines Ganzen Lungenflügels. Zentralbl. Chir. *58*:3003–3006, 1931.

Reinhoff, W. J.: Pneumonectomy. Preliminary report of the operative technique in two successful cases. Bull. Johns Hopkins Hosp. *53*:390–393, 1933.

Riseborough, E. J.: The anterior approach to the spine for the correction of deformities of the axial skeleton. Clin. Orthop. *93*:207–214, 1973.

Robinson, S.: The surgery of bronchiectasis: Including a

report of five complete resections of the lower lobe of the lung with one death. Surg. Gynecol. Obstet. *24*:194–215, 1917.

Scott, R.: Innervation of the diaphragm and its practical aspects in surgery. Thorax *20*:357–361, 1965.

Seddon, H. J.: Pott's paraplegia. *In* Platt, H. (ed.): Modern Trends in Orthopaedics. London, Butterworth and Co., Ltd., 1956, pp. 220–245.

Winter, R. B., Moe, J. H., and Wang, J. F.: Congenital kyphosis, its natural history and treatment as observed in a study of 130 patients. J. Bone Joint Surg. *55-A*:223–256, 1973.

SURGICAL APPROACHES TO THE LUMBOSACRAL SPINE

APPROACH TO THE LUMBAR SPINE, ANTERIOR VERSUS POSTERIOR

Under most circumstances, the choice of approach to the lumbar spine should be dictated by the site of the primary pathologic condition. Disease or deformity that primarily involves the vertebral bodies may be approached directly through the abdomen or flank. The posterior elements may be approached directly through a vertical, posterior incision in midline. The spinous processes, laminae, and facets are directly accessible through this approach, and the transverse processes and pedicles may be reached with somewhat more difficulty. The posterolateral approach provides direct access to the transverse processes and pedicles as well as limited exposure of the vertebral bodies themselves.

Anterior

The anterolateral approach to the lumbar vertebral bodies through a long, oblique flank incision provides direct access to all the upper lumbar vertebral bodies in continuity. It should be considered for extensive resection, debridement, or grafting at multiple levels. If access to the lower lumbar vertebrae is desired, the incision may be directed more anteriorly and inferiorly, beginning midway between the symphysis pubis and iliac crest. This incision is extended laterally and obliquely along the iliac crest to the midflank (Hodg-

son and Wong, 1968). A short, transverse flank incision may be used to provide less extensive exposure of the midlumbar spine (Madden, 1964). Longitudinal left paramedian incisions with retroperitoneal or transperitoneal dissections have also been used (Sacks, 1966; Stauffer and Coventry, 1972). The theoretical advantage of the transperitoneal approach is that the abdominal viscera may be more easily retracted than with a retroperitoneal dissection; however, the viscera and the hypogastric nerve plexus are more vulnerable in this line of dissection from the front.

Posterior

The posterior approach through a posterior longitudinal incision in midline provides direct access to the spinous processes, laminae, and facets at all levels of the lumbar spine. The transverse processes and even the pedicles may be reached with some difficulty by retracting the paraspinal muscles laterally. The posterior aspect of the vertebral body and disc space over the lower lumbar levels may be reached following laminectomy by retracting the dura, but the exposure is limited.

Posterolateral

The posterolateral approach through a longitudinal paraspinal incision, retracting the erector spinae muscles medially, provides direct access to the transverse processes and the mamillary processes of the facets (Watkins, 1953; 1959). This area provides an excellent bed for posterolateral lumbosacral fusion even in the face of preexisting pseudarthrosis, laminar defects, or spondylolisthesis. Through this approach, the transverse process may be removed, and the pedicle and vertebral body may be exposed in a limited fashion, as described later in this section. Wiltsie and colleagues (1968) described a similar approach, dividing the erector spinae muscles using a muscle-splitting dissection. They note that with this approach there is less muscle mass to retract medially, that the facets are more directly reached, and that operative hemorrhage may be less significant.

Anterolateral Approach to the Bodies of the Lumbar Vertebrae

The anterolateral approach to the lumbar vertebrae is an extension of the standard flank incision used by general surgeons for years for lumbar sympathectomy (Royle, 1924; Pearl, 1937; Madden, 1964). The transverse flank approach to the sympathetics provides limited access to the bodies of the lower three lumbar vertebrae. By extending this exposure through a long oblique incision from the twelfth rib posteriorly to the lower abdomen in front, broad access to all the lumbar vertebrae in continuity and particularly the upper lumbar levels is gained (Francioli, 1951; Lilly et al., 1954). The lateral half of the twelfth rib is resected subperiosteally, and the anterior abdominal muscles are divided. The major dissection is behind the kidney in the potential space between the renal or Gerota's fascia and the quadratus lumborum and psoas muscles. A chest retractor is used, which provides direct exposure of most lumbar vertebral bodies and allows sufficient room for extensive excision and bone grafting.

This approach to the lumbar spine is useful for drainage of a psoas abscess on the operated side. It provides exposure for complete debridement and reconstructive bone grafting over the upper four lumbar vertebral bodies and should be considered when extensive resection or grafting at these levels is planned. By dividing the insertion of the arcuate ligaments on the first lumbar transverse process (Fig. 4–69), limited access as high as the eleventh thoracic vertebral body may be gained. The working area within the thorax is restricted, however, and if extensive resection

or grafting is planned over the eleventh thoracic vertebral body, we recommend considering the thoraco-abdominal approach described in Part III. To provide access to the lower lumbar vertebral bodies and sacrum, alternative anterior exposures are available, which will be discussed later (p. 175).

The authors recommend the left lateral approach if all other considerations are equal and if the pathologic condition is not assymmetrical. The liver, on the right side, is large and difficult to retract. The vena cava, also on the right, is a capricious structure which, in the presence of infection, may be hard to locate. In addition, the vena cava is injured easily, and bleeding from it may be hard to control. The spleen, on the left, is fragile but smaller than the liver and is more easily retracted. The aorta, owing to its pulsations, is easier to locate than the vena cava, is less susceptible to injury, and bleeding from it is easier to control.

TECHNIQUE

The patient is placed on the operating table with the side to be operated upon tilted upward, at an angle of 60 degrees, by supporting the shoulder and hip on sandbags. This tends to shift the abdominal and retroperitoneal contents toward the nonoperated side and facilitates retraction. The arm on the operated side is held across the chest and supported.

The incision is begun over the lateral half of the twelfth rib and extends obliquely downward and anteriorly to the lateral margin of the rectus fascia, at the level of the anterosuperior iliac spine (Fig. 4–84). The lateral and inferior fibers of the latissimus dorsi and serratus posterior inferior muscles lie over the medial aspect of the twelfth rib and may be partially transected. The distal half of the twelfth rib is resected subperiosteally, and the external oblique muscle is split in line with its fibers to the lower pole of the incision, at the lateral border of the rectus fascia. The internal oblique and transversus abdominis muscles are cut across their fibers in the same oblique line as the skin incision.

Deep to the transversus abdominis muscle is the peritoneum. Continuous with the peritoneum and extending posteriorly behind the kidney is the renal fascia (Fig. 4–85). This fascia surrounds the kidney, ureters, adrenals, and peritoneal fat and is loosely applied to the quadratus lumborum and psoas muscles posteriorly. This layer blends loosely with the

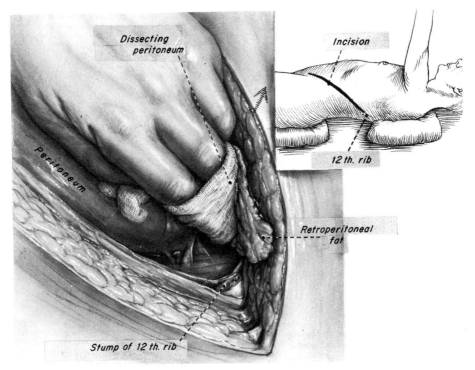

Figure 4–84. Anterolateral approach to the bodies of the lumbar vertebrae. The peritoneum is exposed through an oblique flank incision beginning over the 12th rib. (From Southwick, W. O., and Robinson, R. A.: Surgical approaches to the vertebral bodies in the cervical and lumbar regions. J. Bone Joint Surg., *39A*:638, 1957. Reproduced with permission.)

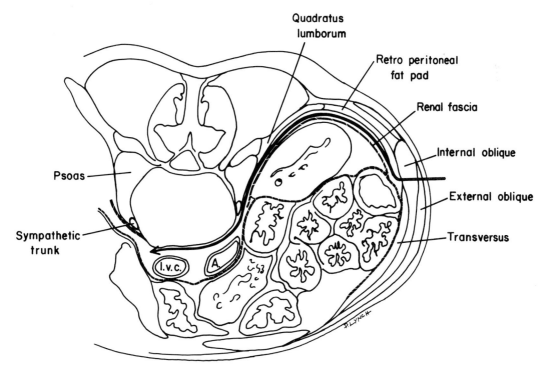

Figure 4–85. Transverse section through the midlumbar vertebrae illustrating the plane of dissection to the vertebral bodies between the renal fascia anteriorly and the retrorenal fat pad, quadratus lumborum, and psoas muscles posteriorly.

psoas fascia and is attached to the vertebral
column, anterior to the medial margin of the
psoas. Dissection proceeds along the peritoneum and renal fascia posterior to the kidney.
This is best accomplished by finger dissection,
as there is a natural plane of cleavage immediately posterior to the fascia. A common mistake is to dissect within or posterior to the fat
pad, which lies behind the renal fascia. This
leads to a blind space posterior to the quadratus lumborum and psoas muscles. The anterior surfaces of the quadratus lumborum and
psoas muscles are fully exposed (Fig. 4–86). A
self-retaining chest retractor is used to open
the wound longitudinally. A padded Dever
retractor is used to retract the kidney and
peritoneal contents medially. Care should be
taken not to tract hard on the aorta and vena
cava, which lie immediately anterior to the
vertebral bodies.

The lumbar veins and arteries effectively
tether the aorta and vena cava to the vertebrae. In order to provide access to the anterior
aspect of the vertebral bodies, these should be
isolated, ligated, or clipped with silver clips
and cut at the level of the desired dissection.

All the lumbar vertebral bodies are easily
palpated, and the anterolateral aspects of the
third, fourth, and fifth vertebral bodies are
easily seen. The left diaphragmatic crus ex-

tends to the second vertebral body, and if
exposure at this level or above is desired, the
left crus may be separated from the anterior
longitudinal ligament. If exposures of the
lower thoracic vertebrae in continuity are desired, the arcuate ligament insertions on the
first lumbar transverse process may be divided
(Fig. 4–69), and the arcuate ligaments may be
retracted upward, anteriorly. Working beneath the diaphragm and by blunt dissection,
the posterior parietal pleura is elevated from
the vertebral bodies and posterior ribs. Ordinarily, this may be done without violating the
integrity of the parietal pleura or entering the
pleural cavity. In this way, limited exposure
as high as the eleventh thoracic vertebral body
is possible. The working area from below is
limited, however, and if extensive resection or
grafting is planned within the thorax, we recommend considering the thoracoabdominal
approach described in Part III (p. 158).

Two nerves are in close proximity with
this level of the dissection and should be
spared. The genitofemoral nerve is a small-
calibered, white structure lying on the muscle
belly of the psoas. The sympathetic chain is
closely applied to the vertebral bodies medial
to the psoas muscle. It may be distinguished
by its yellow-white color and periodic ganglionic enlargements. The sympathetic chain

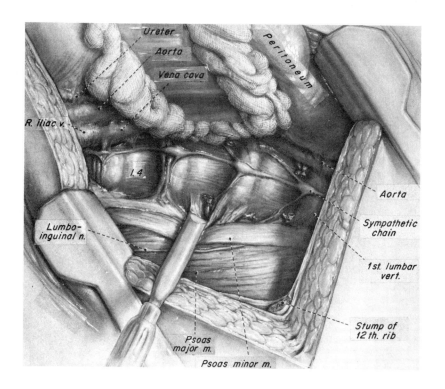

Figure 4–86. A chest retractor opens the wound longitudinally. The peritoneal contents are retracted medially, exposing the vertebral bodies. (From Southwick, W. O., and Robinson, R. A.: Surgical approaches to the vertebral bodies in the cervical and lumbar regions. J. Bone Joint Surg., *39A*:639, 1957. Reproduced with permission.)

and psoas may be displaced posteriorly by careful blunt dissection to reveal the lateral aspect of the vertebral bodies.

The bodies of the vertebrae, unless grossly diseased, are covered in front by the thick, anterior longitudinal ligament and small slips of the psoas muscle laterally. The intervertebral bodies between are relatively concave. The fifth lumbar vertebra is usually most prominent, and using this as a reference point, the vertebral level may be accurately identified. Despite this, we strongly recommend obtaining a lateral roentgenogram of the spine on the operating table, with a radiopaque marker embedded at the desired level to verify anatomic position.

The anterior longitudinal ligament may be elevated from the midportion of the vertebral body at the desired level, and the vertebral body may be entered with drills, probes, or curets as the clinical situation dictates. This flap of ligament may be restored anatomically with sutures after a limited resection to provide continuity and stability.

Anterior Approaches to the Lower Lumbar Spine and Sacrum

The anterolateral approach to the lumbar vertebral bodies just described is best suited to expose the upper and midlumbar vertebral bodies. A long, oblique incision is used, two abdominal wall muscle layers are divided across their fibers, and considerable dissection behind the renal fascia is needed. Such an extensive exposure may not be required for relatively direct biopsy or drainage procedures and may not be tolerated by the elderly or critically ill patient. In addition, in the presence of overt sepsis or when draining an abscess, there may be an advantage to limit the dissection, using muscle splitting techniques, rather than divide muscle groups. The transverse flank approach used for lumbar sympathectomy may be ideally suited for this kind of limited exposure, particularly in the high-risk patient.

Anterior Approach to the Lumbar Spine Through a Transverse Flank Incision

This approach has been used for years by general and vascular surgeons for lumbar sympathectomy (Royle, 1924; Pearl, 1937; Mad-

den, 1964). It employs a muscle splitting dissection and provides limited but direct access to the third and fourth lumbar vertebral bodies, as well as the sympathetic chain and psoas muscle on one side. The upper lumbar vertebrae and the lumbosacral junction can be reached by extending the dissection behind the renal or Gerota's fascia, but the working area is small and crowded. In addition to unilateral lumbar sympathectomy, it is ideally suited to drain a psoas abscess on one side, as the approach is direct and the dissection is limited, so there is less chance of spreading an infection. The muscle splitting approach through the three layers of the abdominal wall tends to reduce the incidence of wound dehiscence or herniations, as the three layers tend to close on themselves.

An incision 12 to 15 cm. in length is made over the lateral flank, midway between the iliac crest and the lower ribs. The first layer of the abdominal wall, the external oblique muscle, is divided in line with its fibers, obliquely downward and medially. The internal oblique fibers course at right angles to the external oblique fibers and are opened in a muscle splitting fashion. The deepest layer, the transversus abdominis, is directed medially and laterally and is spread in line with its fibers. Retractors are placed in the wound, and the peritoneum is identified. By blunt dissection, the peritoneum and the renal fascia behind it are separated from the abdominal wall. The dissection proceeds below the kidney, behind the ureter, along the quadratus lumborum and psoas muscles to the vertebral bodies (Fig. 4–85). The genitofemoral and sympathetic nerves should be identified, and the vertebral bodies should be exposed as described in the preceding section. The third and fourth lumbar vertebral bodies are directly accessible within the base of the wound. The upper lumbar vertebrae and lumbosacral junction can be reached but are relatively distant, and the working area is confined.

Anterior Approach to the Lower Lumbar and Lumbosacral Spine Through an Anterior Oblique Incision

This approach is identical to the anterolateral exposure described first; however, the incision is directed more anteriorly and inferiorly over the lower lumbar elements (Hodgson and Wong, 1968). The incision begins in the lower abdomen lateral to the rectus muscle and extends laterally and superiorly above the iliac crest to the midflank. The external oblique muscle is divided in line with its fibers, and the internal oblique and transversus abdominis muscles are divided across their fibers in line with the incision. Dissection proceeds posterior to the renal fascia, below the kidney and behind the ureter, to the vertebral bodies, as described before.

Through this route, broad exposure of the lower lumbar vertebrae and upper sacrum is obtained. This is suitable for extensive resection and bone grafting as well as anterior lumbosacral fusion. The aorta, iliac vessels, and hypogastric nerve plexus lie anterior to the vertebral bodies and are not in direct line with the dissection. These may be elevated in a block away from the anterior vertebral bodies with less likelihood of disturbing genitourinary function (see Urogenital Complications, p. 180).

Anterior Approach to the Lumbosacral Spine Through a Paramedian Incision Around the Rectus Muscle

The paramedian approach provides direct access to the anterior elements of the lumbosacral spine in continuity with the upper lumbar segments. Once the initial exposure is made through the anterior abdominal wall, the vertebrae may be reached through a transperitoneal or retroperitoneal route. The advantage to the transperitoneal route is that somewhat more extensive exposure is provided, and the abdominal viscera may be packed neatly away from the spine. The disadvantage is that one approaches the spine directly from the front, and one has to mobilize the great vessels and hypogastric nerve plexus before the spine can be reached. This introduces potential urogenital complications, particularly in the male. These may be avoided by careful dissection about the aortic bifurcation, to be described later, or by approaching the spine from the side, behind these structures.

A paramedian incision is made over the lower abdomen, extending from the umbilicus to the pubis. The rectus fascia beneath is identified and opened longitudinally in line with the incision. The rectus muscle is mobilized laterally, taking care to isolate and ligate these segmental vessels, which reach it from behind. The rectus abdominis muscle is retracted medially, and the posterior rectus fas-

cia is opened longitudinally. On closing the wound, this provides a two-layer fascial closure with an intervening muscle layer between. At this stage, the peritoneum may be opened, or dissection may proceed around it laterally, depending upon the surgeon's needs.

TRANSPERITONEAL

In the transperitoneal approach, the peritoneum is opened longitudinally in line with the skin incision, protecting the bowel beneath from injury. The intra-abdominal contents are packed away from the incision to expose the posterior peritoneal layer, draped over the great vessels and vertebral bodies.

The superior hypogastric plexus provides the sympathetic innervation of the urogenital system. It is a direct extension of the thoracolumbar sympathetic chain (Fig. 4–87), which ramifies about the inferior mesenteric artery at the level of the third and fourth lumbar vertebrae. Caudal to this, these fibers ramify as a fine and extensive network that lies primarily anterior to the aorta on the left side. These extend across the left iliac vessels, the fifth lumbar vertebral body, and the lumbosacral junction and will be injured unless special precautions are made in the dissection. To avoid this sympathetic, superior hypogastric plexus, Duncan and Jonck (1965) recommend an approach through this plane eccentric to the right side to avoid the majority of these hypogastric fibers.

A longitudinal incision is made in the posterior peritoneum in the midline about the aortic bifurcation. This peritoneal incision is extended distally and to the right, along the right common iliac artery to its bifurcation at the external and internal iliac arteries. At this point, the right ureter should be identified, crossing the right external iliac artery, and the incision should be curved medially to avoid this structure. The dissection proceeds at the lower pole of the posterior peritoneal incision, directly posteriorly, through the prevertebral tissues to the right and lateral side of the sacrum. This is extended superiorly to the lateral edge of the fifth lumbar vertebra by spreading the tissues longitudinally away from this plane. Dissection continues on to the anterior longitudinal ligament of the spine. By continued blunt dissection along the spine, the iliac vessels and aorta may be mobilized from the vertebrae. In this way, the left side of the peritoneum and all the structures subjacent to it (including the prevertebral tissues, vessels,

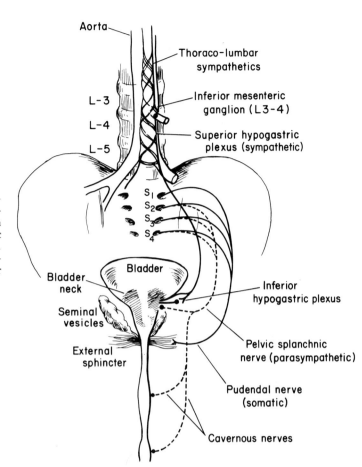

Figure 4–87. Innervation of the urogenital system. Sympathetic via the superior hypogastric plexus, parasympathetic via the pelvic splanchnic nerve, and somatic via the pudendal nerve. (From Johnson, R. M., and McGuire, E. J.: Urogenital complications of anterior approaches to the lumbar spine. Clin. Orthop., in press).

and hypogastric plexus) may be mobilized as a block away from the vertebrae, anteriorly and to the left. By displacing these structures from the side and en bloc and not dissecting through them, there is less risk of injuring the hypogastric nerve fibers, particularly those on the left side, which are responsible for normal urogenital function.

The middle sacral artery may be adherent to the vertebral bodies, and some difficulties may be encountered in mobilizing it. Vascular clips may be used to ligate this artery while sparing the hypogastric plexus. If cautery is to be used in this area, we recommend the bipolar rather than the unipolar machine, as the spark gap or area of thermal injury is confined to the space between the bipolar cautery forcep tips, and there is less likelihood of injuring these nerves with a propagated current or thermal burn.

RETROPERITONEAL

As mentioned previously, once the exposure through the anterior abdominal wall is complete, the spine may be approached using a retroperitoneal plane of dissection. This should proceed laterally, and we prefer dissection to the left side, posteriorly along the renal fascial plane behind the ureter. The hypogastric nerve plexus lies anterior to the great vessels. These and the vessels may be mobilized from the side and behind, en bloc, sparing the ramifying fibers of the hypogastric plexus over the spine. The retroperitoneal dissection provides a less direct route to the spine, but if the tissue planes are well developed by blunt dissection and if the abdominal contents are packed away, satisfactory exposure is obtained with less risk to the viscera and hypogastric nerve plexus.

Anterior Lumbosacral Fusion

Anterior fusion at the lumbosacral junction is useful in certain specific conditions, such as in myelodysplasia, when the posterior elements are deficient, or when the posterior elements have been extensively removed to decompress a stenotic spinal canal. Some authors have found the anterior route useful for the treatment of spondylolisthesis (Burns, 1933; Jenkins, 1936; Mercer, 1936; Speed, 1938; Sacks, 1966) and to reduce and stabilize severe spondylolisthetic displacements (Bradford, 1979). A number have used this route for intervertebral disc excision and interbody fusion, either as a primary treatment modality or as a salvage procedure after failure of previous posterior approaches (Goldner et al., 1969; Harmon, 1948; 1963; Humphries et al., 1961; Lane and Moore, 1948; Sacks, 1966; Stauffer and Coventry, 1972a).

The authors have found that anterior lumbosacral fusion is rarely required. The posterolateral fusion technique described by Watkins (1953; 1959), in which cancellous bone grafts are laid over the facets and transverse processes, is so effective, if done properly, that the anterior route is rarely needed. Furthermore, there is no evidence available that anterior lumbosacral fusions are more reliable or that they have a higher incidence of fusion or better overall clinical results. In fact, Stauffer and Coventry (1972a and 1972b), in their articles contrasting their experience with anterior and posterolateral fusions, found that anterior fusions had a lower incidence of stable fusion and a less satisfactory clinical outcome. Despite this, a few circumstances remain in which anterior lumbosacral fusion is needed. Instability with associated deficiency or absence of the posterior elements, or pathologic conditions of the vertebral bodies anteriorly requiring resection and grafting will be best served using anterior approaches. In addition, infection or extensive scarring posteriorly may make posterior or posterolateral approaches impractical.

TECHNIQUE

The fusion techniques at the lumbosacral junction are similar to those used elsewhere in the spine and vary from simple disc excision and interbody fusion to an extensive resection and replacement grafting. The only modifications are that because of the size of the vertebrae and forces across these, larger or duplicate grafts are usually required with cortical margins around their periphery. The intervertebral lumbosacral disc is excised using rongeurs and curets. We favor leaving the vertebral end plates intact to support the graft and to prevent subsequent collapse of the disc space, which could occur if the softer cancel-

lous portion of the body is entered. Two or more horseshoe-shaped plugs of bone are obtained from the iliac crest, which have their cortical margins intact on three sides (as described for anterior cervical interbody fusion p. 104). These should be thick enough to completely fill the defect and should be under a significant compressive force, holding the graft in place. The disc space is distracted with an intervertebral spreader, and the first graft is tamped in place. The second graft is turned around 180 degrees from the orientation of the first and is tamped in place. Additional graft material is added to fill the defect, and control roentgenograms are obtained to be certain the grafts are not displaced posteriorly into the spinal canal. The grafts are tested for stability, and if they are satisfactory, the soft tissues are repaired about the vertebrae. Postoperatively, when the patient's condition is fully stabilized, we prefer to protect the spine and limit lumbosacral motion using a body cast until the fusion is established roentgenographically. Thereafter, we use a Norton-Brown lumbosacral brace for an additional three to six months. We prefer the Norton-Brown (1957) brace, as this appears to control lumbosacral motion best of any of the conventional and readily available orthoses and is well tolerated by most patients.

In some circumstances, more extensive resection and grafting is required. Longer struts of cortical or corticocancellous graft material may be used. We recommend supporting these on the vertebral body end plates to limit collapse of vertebral height. These struts should be locked into slots previously made in the vertebrae, above and below the levels of intended fusion, to prevent displacement of the grafts. The grafts may be driven in from the lateral side of the vertebral body.

If extensive resection and bone grafts are required over the lumbosacral spine, special care will be required to protect the spine in the postoperative period until osseous fusion is established to prevent collapse of the vertebrae and loss of longitudinal height. These patients may be nursed on a turning frame, or the spine may be protected with plaster of Paris turning shells. Most often when the wounds have healed, a plaster of Paris body cast will be required. Occasionally, supplementary stabilization using Harrington or Knodt rods and hooks or a sacral bar may be required to protect the lumbosacral vertebrae from the large forces and torque across them.

COMPLICATIONS

Perforation of the vena cava or iliac veins may produce dangerous hemorrhage that is difficult to control. Openings into the peritoneal cavity should be avoided, especially in the presence of infection. Irritation of the crus of the diaphragm was considered the cause of prolonged hiccups in one patient. Postoperative ileus is relatively common, but none has been severe or prolonged.

Because one or more major anterior abdominal wall muscles are divided, wound dehiscence or herniation is a potential problem. For this reason, when drainage of an abscess of the lower vertebral bodies is anticipated, the muscle splitting sympathectomy approach, leaving the peritoneum intact, should be considered.

Two rare but potential complications of anterior approaches to the thoracolumbar and lumbosacral spine have been reported. These are (1) The anterior spinal artery ischemic syndrome following extensive dissections about the thoracolumbar spine or scoliosis correction; and (2) the urogenital complications, particularly sterility in males, which may follow anterior exposures of the lumbosacral spine. Some controversy remains as to whether these complications do occur, how they are produced, and how they may be avoided. Because of this, both of these potential complications will be discussed in greater detail and the information currently available in the literature will be summarized.

ANTERIOR SPINAL ARTERY ISCHEMIC SYNDROME

Anterior spinal artery ischemic syndromes with paraplegia, loss of pain and temperature sense, and sphincter disturbance have been reported, particularly following resection and grafting of the aorta. This syndrome has been reported to occur with a frequency as high as 4 per cent when the aorta is cross-clamped proximal to the renal vessels (Kiem and Sadek, 1971). It has also been reported occasionally following spinal surgery for scoliosis correction (Dommisse, 1974; Kiem and Sadek, 1971) or circumferential spinal osteotomy (Dommisse and Enslin, 1970). However, no complications have been reported by a number of authors following unilateral ligation of multiple segmental vessels over the lower thoracic spine (Burrington et al., 1976; Chou and Seljeskog, 1973; Cook, 1971; Hodgson et al., 1960; Winter et al., 1973).

The blood supply of the spinal column is derived from segmental vessels at most levels of the spine. These supply two general networks: an outer network, which feeds the bony elements of the vertebrae, the paraspinal muscles, and the extradural space, and an inner network, which nourishes the spinal cord itself.

The segmental arteries of the thoracic and lumbar spine hug the vertebral bodies, giving off a main dorsal branch as they approach the neural foramina. This main dorsal branch continues posteriorly beneath the transverse process and supplies the bone of the posterior elements and paraspinal muscles. Shortly after its origin, the dorsal branch gives off one or more intraspinal branches, which enter the spinal canal through the neural foramina and feed the nerve roots, vertebral bodies, and dura. This outer network is fed by segmental vessels at most levels of the spine and has extensive anastomotic communications within itself and with the extraspinal system (Gillilan, 1958; Wiley and Trueta, 1959).

At certain segmental levels, separate branches arise from the dorsal segmental artery that feed the anterior two thirds of the spinal cord. These are known as the anterior segmental medullary arteries. These most commonly occur over the upper and lower cervical levels, the upper thoracic spine, and one at the lower thoracic or upper lumbar level. The latter is known as the great anterior medullary artery and is one of the larger and better known segmental feeders. The anterior medullary arteries normally join the anterior median spinal artery directly without branching. The anterior median spinal artery usually occurs as a single channel that meanders along the anterior median fissure of the spinal cord. This varies considerably in size along its course but becomes narrowest over the mid-thoracic spine and only widens after it is joined by the great anterior medullary artery around the thoracolumbar level. The anterior median spinal artery gives off numerous central perforating arteries, which supply the anterior two thirds of the spinal cord. Although there are extensive anastomotic communications in the outer network and about the cord, the arterioles and capillaries within the spinal cord appear to function as end arteries with few significant collateral channels (Gillilan, 1958). This leaves the spinal cord, particularly its anterior two thirds, vulnerable to ischemia.

The posterior third of the spinal cord is

supplied by two posterior spinal arteries and appears to be less vulnerable to vascular ischemia. In part, this is due to the rather extensive anastomoses between the posterior spinal arteries and a well-developed arterial plexus posteriorly. In addition, the posterior segmental medullary feeders are relatively large and numerous (10 to 20 per spine; Dommisse, 1974).

The source of the great anterior medullary artery is variously described by different authors (Dommisse, 1974; Gillilan, 1958; Kiem and Sakek, 1971; Lazorthes et al., 1964; 1971); however, there is a consensus that it most frequently arises on the left side over the lower thoracic or upper lumbar spine. Occasionally, the great anterior medullary artery originates on the right side, and less frequently no single dominant feeder is present and a number of smaller vessels are found. When present, the great anterior medullary artery enters the spinal canal through the neural foramen and courses proximally along the nerve root. It then divides into a small ascending branch and turns at an acute angle to descend as the anterior median spinal artery, which suddenly enlarges. When the great anterior medullary artery is present, it supplies a significant volume of blood to the anterior two thirds of the lower spinal cord.

There is evidence that the functional integrity of the lower spinal cord is not solely dependent upon the great anterior medullary artery. No complications have been reported by several authors following unilateral resection of multiple segmental vessels in the lower thoracic spine (Burrington et al., 1976; Chou and Seljeskog, 1973; Cook, 1971; Hodgson et al., 1960; Winter et al., 1973). DiChiro and colleagues (1970) ligated the great anterior medullary artery in a number of rhesus monkeys without complication, but when the anterior spinal artery was ligated distal to this, paraplegia occurred. This suggests that the anterior median spinal artery and its collaterals are more important than any single feeder, including the great anterior medullary artery.

Lazorthes and others (1971) found extensive anastomotic pathways within the segmental arterial system, such as through the dorsal muscular branches and through the nutrient arteries within the vertebral bodies. This would provide collateral pathways from one side to the other or from above or below when an artery at one level was ligated. He concluded that the closer to the aorta and the further from the spinal cord an artery was interrupted,

the greater the possibility of collateral flow through these anastomoses. This prompted Burrington and others (1976) to recommend that the segmental artery should be ligated close to the aorta to protect this collateral circulation to the cord.

The one factor that appears instrumental in jeopardizing the blood supply to the lower thoracic spinal cord is interruption or compromise of the anterior median spinal artery. This could be interrupted by ligating the great anterior medullary artery as well as a number of smaller medullary feeders, but collateral pathways could maintain the circulation to the cord. Aggressive correction of scoliotic or kyphotic deformities could stretch and narrow the anterior spinal artery and compromise it, even though none of the segmental medullary arteries were injured. This would account for the reports of anterior spinal artery syndromes occurring after scoliosis correction (Dommisse, 1974; Kiem and Sadek, 1971), even when no major segmental arteries were ligated.

It would seem that the most hazardous manipulation of the circulation to the lower spinal cord would include a combination of ligating the medullary feeders and stretching the spinal artery by aggressive correction of spinal deformity. Therefore, in anterior approaches to the lower thoracic and upper lumbar spine, it would seem most prudent to ligate as few intercostal or segmental arteries as possible, to restrict ligation to one side only, and to ligate these arteries as close to the aorta as possible. If bilateral ligation were absolutely necessary, particularly at multiple levels, correction of spinal deformity should be minimized. On the other hand, if correction of deformity were primarily required, the segmental arteries should be spared, and the surgeon should be prepared to reduce this correction if there were evidence of spinal ischemia in the early postoperative period.

UROGENITAL COMPLICATIONS AND STERILITY IN MALES FOLLOWING ANTERIOR EXPOSURES OF THE LUMBOSACRAL SPINE

Sexual impotence or sterility has been reported following anterior surgical approaches to the lumbosacral spine in males (Duncan and Jonck; 1965; Goldner et al., 1969; Sacks, 1966; Stauffer and Coventry, 1972a). These reports are rare, and there is uncertainty as to whether the problem seen is a physiologic failure of normal penile erection, a failure of normal ejaculation, or a psychologically based problem.

The anatomic nerve supply to the urogenital system has been known for many years, but the function of these nerve systems remains controversial. Most of our current knowledge about the neurophysiology of the urogenital system is derived from clinical studies of patients with specific nerve damage following spinal cord and cauda equina injuries or following surgical dissections about the pelvis and lower lumbar spine (Kedia et al., 1975; McGuire, 1975, McGuire et al., 1977). These have been reinforced by a number of neurophysiologic laboratory studies using animal models (Albert et al., 1977; Awad and Downie, 1976; Tulloch, 1975).

The urogenital system is innervated by three basic nerve complexes — the sympathetic, parasympathetic, and the somatic — through the pudendal nerve. Sexual function is directly influenced by these systems. In the normal male, sperm are continuously created in the testes and are passed on to the epididymis, where the sperm flagella become mobile and are then referred to as spermatozoa. These spermatozoa are carried along the vas deferens via peristaltic action to the seminal vesicles, where they are stored and where certain essential nutrients are added, such as fructose. With ejaculation, the smooth muscle of the seminal vesicles contracts, delivering a bolus of sperm into the prostatic urethra. At the same time, the bladder neck closes by reflex, directing the spermatozoa out the tip of the penis (Kedia et al., 1975).

SYMPATHETIC. The sympathetic nerve supply to the urogenital system is a direct continuation of the thoracolumbar sympathetic nerves (Duncan and Jonck, 1965; Elaut, 1932; LaBate, 1938), coursing along the anterolateral aspects of the lumbar vertebral bodies (Fig. 4–87). At the level of the third and fourth lumbar vertebrae, these ramify about the inferior mesenteric artery at the inferior mesenteric ganglion. Almost 80 per cent of these ramifications occur on the left side of the aorta; the remainder are found centrally or to the right. Once ramified, these fibers are referred to as the superior hypogastric plexus as they course distally. Most commonly, the superior hypogastric fibers are found within the retroperitoneal space lying along the left side of the aorta. These cross the left common iliac artery and vein and below this are closely applied to the fifth lumbar vertebral body and lumbosacral disc space within the prevertebral

tissues. At the level of the pelvic brim, the plexus normally separates into two complexes, one on the right, the other on the left, each extending distally to reach the bladder, vas deferens, and seminal vesicles.

The sympathetic nervous system, through the superior hypogastric plexus, appears to have a direct effect upon normal ejaculation. The sympathetic nerves control the transfer of spermatozoa from the epididymis to the seminal vesicles by affecting the motility of the vas deferens. They appear to affect seminal function by controlling the storage of sperm and secretion of seminal fluid. With ejaculation, they control the emission of spermatozoa and properly direct the delivery of sperm by closing the bladder neck, where a specialized area rich in alpha receptors is found (Kedia et al., 1975).

PARASYMPATHETIC. The parasympathetic innervation of the urogenital system is derived from the second, third, and fourth sacral segments (Bradley et al., 1974). These leave the anterior foramina of the sacrum (Fig. 4–87) well below the pelvic brim and course along the side of the rectum as the pelvic splanchnic nerve (Winkler, 1967). These fibers ramify at the inferior hypogastric plexus and extend to the prostate, posterior bladder, and to the base of the penis as the cavernous nerves.

The parasympathetic system, through the pelvic splanchnic nerves, appears to influence penile errection by regulating the venous plexus at the base of the penis. In addition, with voiding, they contract the bladder and open the urethra through an intrinsic reflux.

SOMATIC. The somatic innervation of the urogenital system is through the pudendal nerves (Fig. 4–87). These are derived from the first, second, third, and fourth sacral segments below the pelvic brim and provide both motor and sensory innervation of the pelvic floor and external genitalia. The pudendal nerves control the external urethral sphincter and the muscles of the pelvic floor. With ejaculation, the muscles of the pelvic floor contract, providing the force to emit a bolus of spermatozoa under pressure. In addition, the pudendal nerves provide sensation over the urethra and penis.

COMPLICATIONS. In anterior exposures of the lower lumbar spine, it appears that the only nerve complex to the urogenital system that is normally at risk is the sympathetic (superior hypogastric plexus). Only if the dissection is carried well below the pelvic brim could the parasympathetic (pelvic splanchnic nerve) or the pudendal nerve be injured. Therefore, if the surgical dissection is restricted to the lumbar spine above the pelvic brim, one should only see impairment of sympathetically mediated urogenital function.

Theoretically, if the superior hypogastric plexus is completely divided at the pelvic brim, a normal male could develop sterility, through the loss of normal spermatozoa transport from the testicles, and retrograde ejaculation into the bladder. Sterility would occur because of the loss of normal spermatozoa transport along the vas deferens to the seminal vesicles and failure of the seminal vesicles to store spermatozoa or secrete seminal fluid. Dry or retrograde ejaculation would occur because the seminal vesicles would fail to contract, and any spermatozoa delivered to the prostatic urethra would be misdirected in a retrograde manner to the bladder, as the bladder neck would not close as part of its normal reflex.

Following dissections about the pelvic brim, dry or retrograde ejaculation is more likely to occur than sterility, as the control of muscle contraction at the bladder neck and seminal vesicles appears to be more sensitive to denervation (Johnson and McGuire, 1980). Furthermore, retrograde ejaculation is most difficult to correct, whereas sterility caused by the loss of normal spermatozoa transport along the vas deferens or storage within the seminal vesicles may be reversed by certain alpha adrenergic agents (Kelly and Needle, 1979; McGuire, 1978).

In general, one would not expect failure of penile erection or impotence to follow sympathectomy at any level in normal males. On the contrary, there is evidence that suggests that the normal, young male may be afflicted with prolonged penile erection or priapism as the normal sympathetic control of the arteriovenous sphincter complex at the penis would be lost, leaving the parasympathetic control of venous egress unopposed (Appell et al., 1977). While this is true in young and otherwise healthy males, in older males with advanced peripheral vascular disease, erectile impotence has been reported following extensive lumbar sympathectomy (Whitelaw and Smithwick, 1951).

In women there is a possibility that sympathectomy would effect normal bladder control, resulting in inappropriate urine leakage due to the loss of the normal smooth muscle control at the internal urethral sphincter. Clin-

ically, this is more likely to occur in patients subjected to radical pelvic surgery, where a more complete sympathetic neural transection could occur than with surgery at the pelvic brim. Females do not have a genital sphincter, so the influence of sympathectomy on genital function is less striking.

Surgical Approach. Because the superior hypogastric plexus is situated directly anterior to the fifth lumbar vertebral body and lumbosacral disc space, it lies in jeopardy in midline exposures to the lumbosacral spine from the front. To avoid injuring this plexus, the vertebral bodies may be exposed from the side using a retroperitoneal dissection or by careful dissection from the right side as described earlier (p. 172). (Duncan and Jonck, 1965).

Posterolateral Approach to the Lumbar Vertebrae

The posterolateral approach to the lumbar vertebrae was developed as a means of providing direct access through the transverse processes to the pedicles and vertebral bodies with less extensive surgical dissection and operative risk than the anterior approaches require (Southwick and Robinson, 1957). It is an extension of the costotransversectomy approach to the thoracic vertebrae described in the preceding section and in the Watkins (1953, 1959) posterolateral approach to the lumbosacral spine. The posterolateral approach provides limited exposure of the lumbar vertebral bodies and is suitable for open surgical biopsy or drainage of small lesions. It is ideally suited for high-risk surgical candidates who could not tolerate more extensive procedures.

The direct posterior approach to the lumbar vertebrae through a midline incision provides direct access to the posterior elements but is limited in exposing the pedicles or vertebral bodies. The vertebral bodies may be approached around the posterior elements, but this requires retraction of the erector spinae muscles laterally, which may be difficult in obese or muscular individuals. Laminectomy provides access to the posterior vertebral body and disc through a confined working area. It does not permit thorough inspection or curettage, particularly of the anterior and lateral aspects of the vertebral bodies. In addition, there is always the risk of injuring the dura, inducing hemorrhage from the epidural vessels, or of spreading infection from the anterior elements into the spinal canal.

Open biopsy has been demonstrated to improve the accuracy of diagnosis in obscure lesions of the spine (Johnson et al., 1953; Nagel et al., 1965). The direct surgical approach may be safer than needle biopsy even under fluoroscopic control and provides more material for culture and pathologic examination. In addition, open biopsy may provide an opportunity to remove a small tumor or focus of infection and maintain drainage. The posterolateral approach provides limited access to the vertebral bodies and is primarily useful for biopsy, curettage, and debridement of small lesions. The anterior approach provides more direct access to the anterior vertebral bodies and may be required for more extensive resection and grafting.

TECHNIQUE

General endotracheal anesthesia is recommended for this procedure. The patient is placed on the operating table in a lateral decubitus position with an axillary pad in the dependent axilla or in the prone position with chest rolls on either side of the thorax to protect ventilation. A roentgenogram cassette holder should be placed beneath the patient so that localizing roentgenograms may be made during surgery in the anteroposterior and lateral planes. A control roentgenogram is obtained with a radiopaque skin marker at the proposed level to verify position and standardize radiographic technique.

A four- to six-inch longitudinal incision is made at the lateral border of the erector spinae muscles centered over the vertebral level to be biopsied (Fig. 4–88, insert). The incision is extended through the lumbar fascia, and the erector spinae muscles are identified. The lateral border of the erector spinae is found, and dissection proceeds between these muscles and the anterior layer of the lumbar fascia to the transverse processes of the vertebrae (Figs. 4–88 and 4–89). The paraspinal muscles are retracted medially, the transverse process at the desired level is tagged with a radiopaque marker, and roentgenograms are made to confirm the vertebral level. The transverse process is divided with an osteotome and is retracted laterally with its musculotendinous attachments. The vertebral pedicle is palpated, and the lumbar nerves are identified and protected as they leave their foramina above and below the pedicle (Fig. 4–90). The psoas

muscle is carefully separated from the vertebra using a periosteal elevator. The lumbar vessels lie on the waist or midportion of the vertebral body posterior to the psoas muscle and should be separated from the body during this portion of the dissection. They may be clamped and cauterized if necessary. An opening may be made in the lateral aspect of the vertebral body anterior to the pedicle, using a curet or drill (Fig. 4–91). The lesion may be identified grossly at this time but should be verified radiographically with a curet placed within the lesion.

Through this approach, specimens may be obtained from the lateral, central, or anterior aspect of the vertebral body or pedicle. The lesion may be curetted, and small chips of cancellous bone graft may be installed to stimulate osteogenesis within a sterile defect. The wound is copiously irrigated with saline and inspected for hemorrhage. The margins are allowed to fall together, and the lumbar fascia is closed with interrupted sutures. The skin is repaired, and the patient is nursed with some form of external spinal support, depending upon the postoperative stability of the spine.

If wider exposure is required, two transverse processes may be divided, and the intervening nerve root may be retracted. If the lower lumbar vertebrae are to be approached, the distal end of the skin incision should be curved medially over the posterior crest of the ilium to the sacrum. The iliac attachment of the sacrospinalis may be released by dividing the superior aspect of the posterior ilium with an osteotome, separating the remaining attachments with a periosteal elevator. In this fashion, the posterior sacrum may be exposed in continuity with the lumbar vertebrae, and the transverse process of the fifth lumbar vertebra may be more easily approached.

COMPLICATIONS

In our experience there have been few serious complications. Some of the most likely potential complications are injury to the lumbar nerves or vessels with ensuing troublesome hemorrhage. Dissection within the anterior aspect of the vertebral body is often performed under limited direct vision. Care is required to prevent injury to the inferior vena cava or aorta immediately anterior to the vertebral body. To ensure that the spinal lesion is accurately identified, control roentgenograms are required with a radiopaque marker within the lesion.

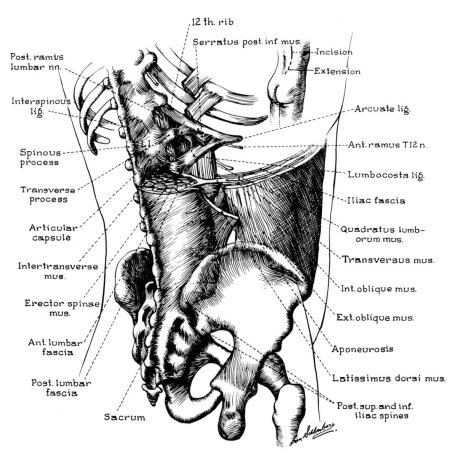

Figure 4–88. *Insert,* Longitudinal skin incision over the lateral border of the erector spinae muscles. Anatomy of the lumbosacral spine and paraspinal muscles viewed from the side and posteriorly.

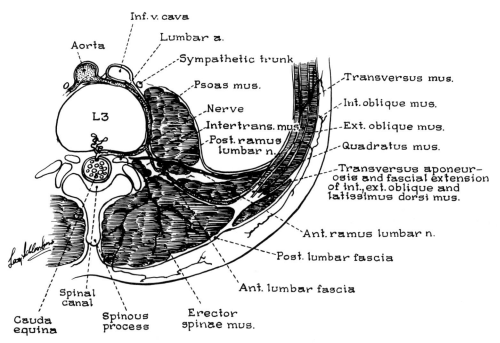

Figure 4–89. Cross-section of the lumbar spine and paraspinal structures at the level of the third lumbar vertebra.

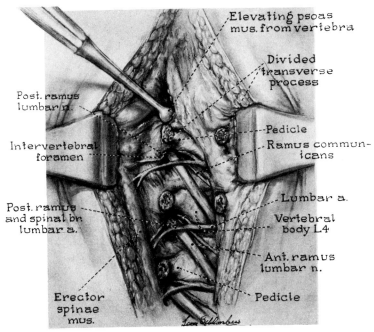

Figure 4–90. Lumbar vertebrae as viewed from the posterolateral approach. The transverse processes have been divided at their junctions with the pedicles and retracted laterally. The dissection proceeds directly anterior to the stump of the transverse process, along the pedicle, to the vertebral body in front. Note the lumbar segmental vessels draped over the waist or midportion of the vertebral bodies. By dissecting directly anterior to the pedicles, one can avoid these vessels as well as the lumbar nerves leaving the neural foramina below the pedicles.

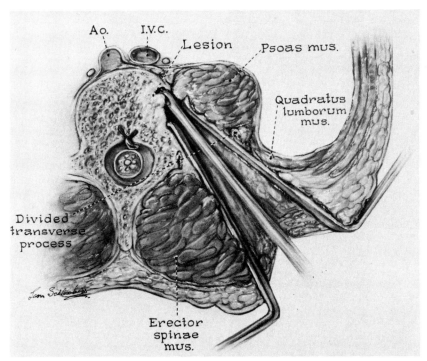

Figure 4–91. Posterolateral approach to the lumbar vertebrae, lateral to the erector spinae muscle mass and behind the psoas. The transverse process is divided and retracted laterally with its musculotendinous insertions to gain access to the lateral aspect of the vertebral body.

References

Albert N. E., Sparks, F. C., and McGuire, E. J.: Effect of pelvic and retroperitoneal surgery on the urethral pressure profile and perineal floor electromyogram in dogs. Invest. Urol. *15*:140–142, 1977.

Appell, R. A., Shield, D. E., and McGuire, E. J.: Thoridiazine induced priapism. Br. J. Urol. *49*:160, 1977.

Awad, S. A., and Downie, J. W.: The effect of adrenergic drugs and hypogastric nerve stimulation on the canine urethra. A radiologic and urethral pressure study. Invest. Urol. *13*:298, 1976.

Bradford, D. S.: Management of severe spondylolisthesis by the combined anterior and posterior approach. Presented at University of Miami symposium, Surgery of the Spine — Indications and Techniques, April, 1979.

Bradley, W. E., Timm, G. W., and Scott, F. B.: Innervation of the detrusor muscle and urethra. Urol. Clin. North Am. *1*:3, 1974.

Burns, B. H.: An operation for spondylolisthesis. Lancet *1*:1233, 1933.

Burrington, J. O., Brown, C., Wayne, E. R., and Odom, J.: Anterior approach to the thoraco lumbar spine — technical considerations. Arch. Surg. *111*:456–463, 1976.

Chou, S. N., and Seljeskog, E. L.: Alternative surgical approaches to the thoracic spine. Clin. Neurosurg. *20*:306–321, 1973.

Cook, W. A.: Trans-thoracic vertebral surgery. Ann. Thorac. Surg. *12*:54–68, 1971.

DiChiro, G., Fried, L. C., and Doppman, J. L.: Experimental spinal cord angiograph. Br. J. Radiol. *43*:19, 1970.

Dommisse, G. F., and Enslin, T. E.: Hodgson's circumferential osteotomy in the correction of spinal deformity. J. Bone Joint Surg. *52-B*:778, 1970.

Dommisse, G. F.: The blood supply of the spinal cord. A critical vascular zone in spinal surgery. J. Bone Joint Surg. *56-B*:225–235, 1974.

Duncan, H. J. M., and Jonck, L. M.: The presacral plexus in anterior fusion of the lumbar spine. Suid-Afrikaanse Tydskrif Vir Chirurgie *3*:93–96, 1965.

Elaut, L.: The surgical anatomy of the so called presacral nerve. Surg. Gynecol. Obstet. *53*:581–589, 1932.

Francioli, P.: Voies d'acces dans les sympathectomies lumbaire et lumbothoracique. Helv. Chir. Acta *18*:536–543, 1951.

Gillilan, L. A.: The arterial blood supply of the human spinal cord. J. Comp. Neurol. *110*:75–103, 1958.

Goldner, J. L., McCollum, D. E., and Urbaniak, J. R.: Anterior disc excision and interbody spine fusion for chronic low back pain. *In* American Academy of Orthopaedic Surgeons, Symposium on the Spine. St. Louis, The C. V. Mosby Co., 1969, pp. 111–131.

Harmon, P. H.: The removal of lower lumbar intervertebral discs by the transabdominal extraperitoneal route. Permanente Found. Med. Bull. *6*:169, 1948.

Harmon, P. H.: Anterior excision and vertebral body fusion operation for intervertebral disc syndromes of the lower lumbar spine: Three to five year results in 244 cases. Clin. Orthop. *26*:107–127, 1963.

Hodgson, A. R., Stock, F. E., Fang, H. S. Y., and Ong, G. B.: Anterior spinal fusion: The operative approach and pathologic findings in 412 patients with Pott's disease of the spine. Br. J. Surg. *48*:172–178, 1960.

Hodgson, M. B., and Wong, S. K.: A description of a technic and evaluation of results in anterior spinal fusion for deranged intervertebral disc and spondylolisthesis. Clin. Orthop. *56*:133–162, 1968.

Humphries, A. W., Hawk, W. A., and Berndt, A. L.: Anterior interbody fusion of lumbar vertebrae: Surgical technique. Surg. Clin. North Am. *41*:1685–1700, 1961.

Jenkins, J. A.: Spondylolisthesis. Br. J. Surg. *24*:80–85, 1936.

Johnson, R. W., Jr., Hillman, J. W., and Southwick, W. O.: The importance of direct surgical attack upon lesions of the vertebral bodies, particularly in Pott's disease. J. Bone Joint Surg. *35-A*:17–24, 1953.

Johnson, R. M., and McGuire, E. J.: Urogenital complications of anterior approaches to the lumbar spine. Clin. Orthop. in press.

Kedia, K. R., Markland, C., and Fraley, E. E.: Sexual function following high retroperitoneal lymphadenectomy. J. Urol. *114*:237, 1975.

Kelly, M. E., and Needle, M. A.: Imipramine for aspermia after lymphadenectomy. Urology *13*:414, 1979.

Kiem, H. A., and Sadek, K. H.: Spinal angiography in scoliosis patients. J. Bone Joint Surg. *53-A*:904–912, 1971.

LaBate, J. S.: The surgical anatomy of the superior hypogastric plexus — "presacral nerve." Surg. Gynecol. Obstet. *67*:199–211, 1938.

Lane, J. D., Jr., and Moore, E. S., Jr.: Transperitoneal approach to the intervertebral disc in the lumbar Area. Ann. Surg. *127*:537–551, 1948.

Lazorthes, G., Bastide, G., and Chancholle, A.: Etude anatomique de l'artere du renflement lombaire. C. R. Ass. Anat. *120*:883–886, 1964.

Lazorthes, G., Gouaze, A., Zadeh, J. O., Santini, J. J., Lazorthes, Y., and Burdin, P.: Arterial vascularization of the spinal cord: Recent studies of the anastomotic substitution pathways. J. Neurosurg. *35*:253–262, 1971.

Lilly, G. D., Smith, D. W., and Biggane, C. F.: An evaluation of "high" lumbar sympathectomy in arteriosclerotic circulatory insufficiency of the lower extremities. Surgery *35*:1–8, 1954.

Madden, J. L.: Atlas of Techniques in Surgery, 2nd ed. New York, Appleton-Century-Crofts, 1964, pp. 398–405.

McGuire, E. J.: Urodynamic observations after abdominoperineal resection and lumbar intervertebral disc herniation. Urology *6*:63, 1975.

McGuire, E. J., Wagner, F. C., and Diddel, G.: Balanced bladder function in spinal cord injury. J. Urol. *118*:626, 1977.

McGuire, E. J.: Neurogenic male incontinence. Urol. Clin. North Am. *5*:335, 1978.

Mercer, W.: Spondylolisthesis, with a description of a new method of operative treatment and notes on ten cases. Edin. Med. J. *43*:545–572, 1936.

Nagel, D. A., Albright, J. A., Keggi, K. J., and Southwick, W. O.: A closer look at spinal lesions. Open biopsy of vertebral lesions. J.A.M.A. *191*:975–978, 1965.

Norton, P. L., and Brown, T.: The immobilizing efficiency of back braces. J. Bone Joint Surg. *39-A*:111–138, 1957.

Pearl, F. L.: Muscle splitting extraperitoneal lumbar ganglionectomy. Surg. Gynecol. Obstet. *65*:107–112, 1937.

Royle, N. D.: The treatment of spastic paralysis by sympathetic rami-section. Surg. Gynecol. Obstet. *39*:701–720, 1924.

Sacks, S.: Anterior interbody fusion of the lumbar spine. Indications and results in 200 cases. Clin. Orthop. *44*:163–170, 1966.

Southwick, W. O., and Robinson, R. A.: Surgical approaches to the vertebral bodies in the cervical and lumbar regions. J. Bone Joint Surg. *39-A*:631–643, 1957.

Speed, K.: Spondylolisthesis: Treatment by anterior bone graft. Arch. Surg. *37*:175–189, 1938.

Stauffer, R. N., and Coventry, M. B.: Anterior interbody lumbar spine fusion, analysis of Mayo Clinic series. J. Bone Joint Surg. *54-A*:756–768, 1972a.

Stauffer, R. N., and Coventry, M. B.: Posterolateral lumbar-spine fusion. Analysis of Mayo Clinic series. J. Bone Joint Surg. *54-A*:1195–1204, 1972b.

Tulloch, A. G. S.: Sympathetic activity of internal urethral sphincter. Urol. *5*:353, 1975.

Watkins, M. B.: Posterolateral fusion of the lumbar and lumbosacral spine. J. Bone Joint Surg. *35-A*:1014–1018, 1953.

Watkins, M. B.: Posterolateral bone grafting for fusion of the lumbar and lumbosacral spine. J. Bone Joint Surg. *41-A*:388–396, 1959.

Whitelaw, G. P., and Smithwick, R. H.: Some secondary effects of sympathectomy with particular reference to disturbance of sexual function. N. Engl. J. Med. *245*:121, 1951.

Wiley, A. M., and Trueta, J.: The vascular anatomy of the spine and its relationship to pyogenic vertebral osteomyelitis. J. Bone Joint Surg. *41-B*:796–809, 1959.

Wiltsie, L. L., Bateman, J. G., Hutchinson, R. H., and Nelson, W. E.: Paraspinal sacrospinalis-splitting approach to the lumbar spine. J. Bone Joint Surg. *50-A*:919–926, 1968.

Winkler, G.: Contribucion al estudio de la inervacion de las visceras pelvianas. Archivos Espanoles de Urologia *20*:295, 1967.

Winter, R. B., Moe, J. H., and Wang, J. F.: Congenital kyphosis, its natural history and treatment as observed in a study of 130 patients. J. Bone Joint Surg. *55-A* 223–256, 1973.

CHAPTER 5

Congenital Anomalies of the Spine

ROBERT N. HENSINGER, M.D.
G. DEAN MAC EWEN, M.D.
Alfred J. DuPont Institute

INTRODUCTION

Congenital anomalies of the spine occur infrequently and receive little attention when pathologic conditions of the spine are considered. Yet, these spinal abnormalities have great impact on the afflicted individuals, and physicians who deal with problems of the spine should be familiar with their diagnosis and management. These structural defects originate early in fetal development and, when discovered in childhood, appear to be static and unchanging. This appearance is deceptive, as with further growth the majority prove to be capable of dramatic change and progressive deformity, and a few, particularly in the cervical spine, may be life-threatening. An excellent example is the spinal deformity so common to myelodysplasia. The dysraphic posterior elements are obvious at birth, yet frequently we fail to recognize the slow and subtle progression of spine curvature until it is completely out of control. Many spinal anomalies are not discovered until a complication occurs. Diastematomyelia, anomalies of the occipitocervical junction, and spondylolisthesis often remain undetected until late childhood or adolescence, and some remain hidden well into adult life.

Other anomalies of the spine, although recognized in early life, may not become clinically significant until adulthood. During the growing years, a delicate balance is struck between the congenitally distorted bony elements of the vertebral column and the neurologic elements. Later, in adult life, factors such as aging or intercurrent trauma may alter this relationship. The patient with an os odontoideum may gradually develop laxity of the supporting structures after countless flexion-extension movements of the neck or, following a seemingly trivial injury, may develop serious instability of the atlantoaxial joint and spinal cord compression. Those afflicted with the Klippel-Feil syndrome may gradually develop symptoms of degenerative arthritis at the hypermobile articulations adjacent to the cervical synostosis. Late onset of paraplegia in the adult achondroplast may be precipitated by progressive deterioration of a dorsal kyphosis or spurring from degenerative osteoarthritis.

Diagnosis and assessment of these congenital spinal problems is hampered by the difficulties encountered during roentgenographic evaluation. In the normal child, the pattern of vertebral growth and ossification has wide variation and often is not complete until late in the second decade. As a result, a congenital anomaly of the odontoid or a primary bone disease, such as spondyloepiphyseal dysplasia or mucopolysaccharidosis, may be difficult or impossible to recognize roentgenographically in the child. Fixed bony deformities often prevent proper positioning for standard views. Nonstandard views and oblique projections add to diagnostic confusion and hinder complete assessment of the patient. Laminagraphy, cineradiography, myelography, and arteriography will be helpful at times in the evaluation of these conditions and should be available to the physician engaged in treating the more complex problems.

In this chapter, we will be particularly concerned with the treatment of these spinal anomalies. Too frequently a policy of observation is adopted, whereas more vigorous management could control, ameliorate, and even on occasion correct the deformity. Sufficient information is available concerning the natural history of these anomalies, and now our attention must be directed to the results of treatment. The severe spinal malalignment of the adolescent myelodysplastic is an excellent example. Many of these children should have been controlled by earlier use of spinal orthoses or spinal fusion. Early application of a brace for control of the kyphosis found in achondroplasia or mucopolysaccharidosis may prevent the late onset of paraplegia. Similarly, operative stabilization of the patient with chronic atlantoaxial instability may prevent a neurologic disaster.

Physicians who treat these children must be concerned with their total care. It is tempting to focus one's attention on the problems of the spine to the exclusion of all others. However, it is imperative that the physician be aware of the high incidence of associated anomalies found with vertebral malformations. Recognition of a vertebral abnormality should stimulate a thorough and intensive search for associated anomalies. Poor management of these related problems, particularly urinary complications, may nullify a well planned and executed orthopaedic program for the spinal deformity. Particular emphasis is placed on related anomalies of the central nervous system, which may be subtle in their manifestation yet have great impact on the patient's social and educational adjustment to life. A hearing deficit may be unrecognized until well into the school years. Mirror motions of the upper extremities may limit effective two-handed activity, such as playing a piano or climbing a ladder. These and other learning disabilities can be an important part of the condition and yet may not be appreciated by the physician, teacher, or parent. Early recognition and appropriate treatment of these problems can be of substantial benefit to the general well-being of the child.

CONGENITAL ANOMALIES OF THE CERVICAL SPINE

Basilar Impression

Basilar impression (or basilar invagination) is a deformity of the osseous structures that form the base of the skull at the margin of the foramen magnum. The floor of the skull appears to be indented by the upper cervical spine. The tip of the odontoid is more cephalad in its position and may protrude into the foramen magnum. As a consequence, the odontoid may encroach upon the brain stem, increasing the risks of neurologic damage from injury, circulatory embarrassment, or impairment of cerebrospinal fluid flow. Chamberlain[4] was first to call attention to the clinical significance of this anomaly, and his vivid description of the morphologic features is worth repeating: "The changes shown by the roentgenogram give the impression of softening of the base of the skull and moulding through the force of gravity. It is as though the weight of the head has caused the ears to approach the shoulders, while the cervical spine, refusing to be shortened, has pushed the floor of the posterior fossa upward into the brain space."

This condition is rare and difficult to assess both clinically and roentgenographically. (For detailed discussion, the reader is referred to several excellent articles on the subject by Dolan,[8] McGregor,[16] McRae,[17] and Spillane.[21] It is important that physicians dealing with spinal deformity be familiar with this anomaly, as the symptoms may closely resemble those of many acquired neurologic diseases. Frequently, these are not manifested in the child but are found later in adult life, and often the presence of basilar impression is unrecognized. The symptoms have been confused with tumors of the posterior fossa, bulbar palsy of polio, syringomyelia, amyotrophic lateral sclerosis, spinal cord tumor, spastic paraplegia, and multiple sclerosis.

The terms platybasia and basilar impression are often used as synonyms, but the two are not related anatomically or pathologically. Platybasia has no clinical significance and is rather an anthropologic term used to denote flattening of the angle formed by the intersection of the plane of the anterior fossa with the plane of the clivus, as opposed to invagination in the region of the foramen magnum, basilar impression. Patients with symptomatic basilar impression are seldom found to have an asso-

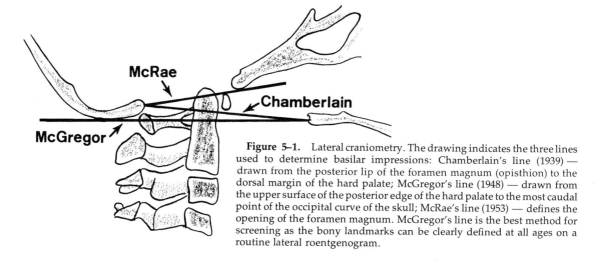

Figure 5–1. Lateral craniometry. The drawing indicates the three lines used to determine basilar impressions: Chamberlain's line (1939) — drawn from the posterior lip of the foramen magnum (opisthion) to the dorsal margin of the hard palate; McGregor's line (1948) — drawn from the upper surface of the posterior edge of the hard palate to the most caudal point of the occipital curve of the skull; McRae's line (1953) — defines the opening of the foramen magnum. McGregor's line is the best method for screening as the bony landmarks can be clearly defined at all ages on a routine lateral roentgenogram.

ciated platybasia.[18, 21] Chamberlain's article, "Basilar Impression (Platybasia)," is a classic and is first to call attention to the clinical aspects of this anomaly. Unfortunately, he also used the term platybasia and initiated the subsequent confusion between the two conditions.

There are two types of basilar impression: (1) primary basilar impression, a congenital abnormality often associated with a variety of vertebral defects, such as atlanto-occipital fusion, hypoplasia of the atlas, bifid posterior arch of the atlas, odontoid abnormalities, and the Klippel-Feil syndrome, or skeletal dysplasias, such as achondroplasia;[8, 15] and (2) secondary basilar impression, a developmental condition usually attributed to softening of the

osseous structures at the base of the skull with the deformity developing later in life. This is occasionally seen in conditions such as severe osteoporosis,[8] osteomalacia,[3] rickets, renal osteodystrophy, Paget's disease,[9] osteogenesis imperfecta,[7] or following trauma.[8]

ROENTGENOGRAPHIC FINDINGS. Basilar impression is difficult to evaluate roentgenographically, and many measurement techniques have been proposed. Those most frequently referred to are Chamberlain's,[4] McGregor's,[16] and McRae's[18] line in the lateral roentgenogram (Fig. 5–1) and in the anterior-posterior projection, Fischgold-Metzger's line (Fig. 5–2).[10] Chamberlain's line is drawn on the lateral roentgenograms of the skull from the posterior lip of the foramen magnum to the

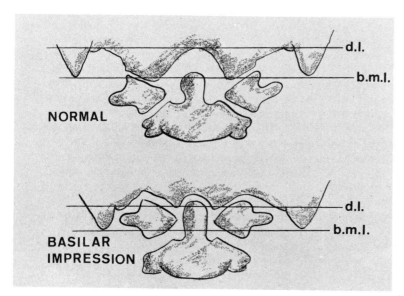

Figure 5–2. Anterior craniometry. Fischgold and Metzger (1953) noted that in the normal skull a line joining the lower poles of the mastoid processes (b.m.l.) passes through the tip of the odontoid. Owing to the variability in the size of mastoid processes, this was further refined to a line drawn between the digastric grooves (d.l.). These lines are best visualized on an anterior-posterior transoral tomogram. Although this is the most accurate method for assessing basilar impression, routine use is impractical and expensive.

dorsal margin of the hard palate (Fig. 5–1). He considered any projection of the odontoid process and the body of the first cervical vertebra above this line as constituting a basilar impression. There are, however, two drawbacks to Chamberlain's line. The posterior lip of the foramen magnum (opisthion), a key point of reference, is difficult to define on a standard lateral roentgenogram (Fig. 5–3A), and in certain types of basilar impression, the opisthion is often itself invaginated. Consequently, McGregor[16] suggested that "a line be drawn from the upper surface of the posterior edge of the hard palate to the most caudal point of the occipital curve in the true lateral roentgenogram" (Fig. 5–1). McGregor's line is more useful than Chamberlain's, as the posterior point is consistent and much easier to define, and flexion and extension do not significantly alter the measurement. The position of the tip of the odontoid is measured in relation to this base line, and a distance of 4.5 mm. above McGregor's line was considered to be on the extreme edge of normality. However, Hinck's study of normal variations demonstrated a wide range of normality, as well as a

difference between males and females.[14] McRae's line[18] is not based on anatomic measurement; instead, it defines the opening of the foramen magnum (Fig. 5–1). It was derived from his clinical observation that if the tip of the odontoid lies below the opening of the foramen magnum, the patient probably will be asymptomatic (Fig. 5–3B). McRae's line is rather a rule of thumb or a guide in the clinical assessment of patients with basilar impression, and the accuracy of his observation has since been substantiated by several authors.[14, 21]

A common criticism of the lateral lines (McGregor's and Chamberlain's) is that the hard palate (the anterior reference point) is not actually a part of the skull and may be distorted by an abnormal facial configuration or a high arch palate quite independent of a craniovertebral anomaly. In addition, the patient may have an abnormally long or short odontoid or an abnormality of the axis or occipital facets, which can diminish the value of the measurements.[11] To avoid these problems, Fischgold and Metzger[10] described a more accurate method to assess basilar impression

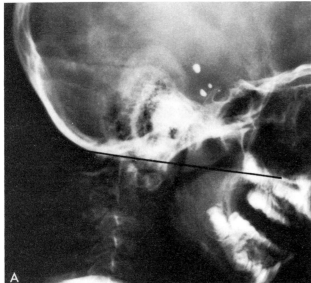
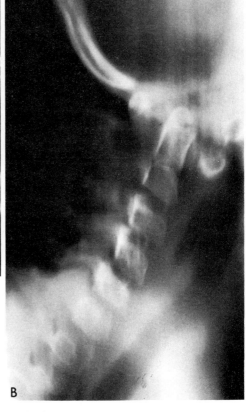

Figure 5–3. A six-year-old female with history of an unusual gait and a recent episode of unconsciousness after mild head trauma. *A*, Routine lateral roentgenogram suggests that the odontoid is displaced proximally into the opening of the foramen magnum. McGregor's line has been drawn from the most caudal portion of the occiput to the hard palate. The tip of the odontoid is more than 5 mm. above this line, indicating basilar impression. *B*, Lateral laminagram demonstrates subluxation of C1 on C2 and that the tip of the odontoid is above the opening of the foramen magnum (McRae's line).

based on a line drawn between the two digastric grooves (junction of the medial aspect of the mastoid process at the base of the skull) on an anterior-posterior laminagraphic view of the skull (Fig. 5–2). In the normal skull, the digastric line will pass well above the odontoid tip (10.7 mm.) and the atlanto-occipital joints (11.6 mm.).[14]

In summary, McGregor's line is the best method for routine screening, as the landmarks can be defined clearly at all ages on a routine lateral roentgenogram. More elaborate measurements (Fischgold-Metzger's digastric line) are generally reserved for the patient whose routine examination or clinical findings may suggest the presence of an occipitocervical anomaly. McRae's line is a helpful guide in assessing the clinical significance of basilar impression.

CLINICAL FINDINGS.   It is interesting to note that the majority of patients with basilar impression have a clinical deformity of the skull or neck, such as a short neck (78 per cent), asymmetry of the face or skull, or torticollis (68 per cent).[5] However, these physical findings are commonly found in patients with congenital vertebral anomalies (the Klippel-Feil syndrome, occipitalization) often unaccompanied by basilar impression and are not considered pathognomonic of basilar impression.

The symptoms (or lack of them) in basilar impression are difficult to explain. Many patients have been discovered with severe basilar impression and no neurologic complaints or findings.[5] In addition, the condition is frequently associated with other anomalies of the craniovertebral area, which may form part or all of the symptoms presented by the patient, such as atlanto-occipital fusion or abnormalities of the odontoid. Similarly, basilar impression is frequently associated with anomalous neurologic conditions, such as the Arnold-Chiari malformation,[5, 21] and syringomyelia.[13, 21] Symptoms are generally due to crowding of the neural structures at the level of the foramen magnum, particularly the medulla oblongata.[18, 21] There is an unusually high incidence of basilar impression in northeast Brazil, and the work of DeBarros[5] has been helpful in delineating the symptoms and signs common to basilar impression. He found that patients who were symptomatic with pure basilar impression had the dominant complaints of motor and sensory disturbances, specifically weakness and paresthesia of the limbs (85 per cent). In contrast, those patients who are symptomatic with the Arnold-Chiari malformation alone are more likely to have cerebellar and vestibular disturbances leading to unsteadiness of gait (ataxia), dizziness, and nystagmus. In both conditions, there may be impingement of the lower cranial nerves as they emerge from the medulla oblongata, particularly the trigeminal (fifth), glossopharyngeal (ninth), vagus (tenth), and hypoglossal (twelfth),[5] and the majority of patients report sexual disturbances ranging from reduction to complete loss of sexual potency.[6]

Autopsies have revealed flattening, softening, and atrophy of the medulla at the point of the impingement by the abnormally located, hypermobile odontoid process (Fig. 5–3B).[17, 21] In some, an indentation of the medulla oblongata was found that exactly matched the shape of the odontoid.[17, 21] Headache in the greater occipital nerve distribution is a common finding, but the patient may complain of pain over the entire head and neck.[5]

If the posterior encroachment predominates, the presenting symptoms may be those of raised intracranial pressure and hydrocephalus due to a block of the aqueduct of Sylvius.[5, 16] Compression of the cerebellum or herniation of the cerebral tonsils (the Arnold-Chiari malformation) is a frequent finding.[5, 21] Nystagmus, either vertical or lateral, seems peculiarly common in patients with basilar impression (65 per cent) and is due to cerebellar or vestibular involvement.[5, 21] Impingement on the posterior columns and pyramidal tracts will be associated with weakness, hyperreflexia, and spasticity.[5] It is important to note that these symptoms may not be due to direct pressure from the posterior rim of the foramen magnum but rather from a thickened band of dura not visible on plain roentgenograms. The possibility of this dural band has prompted several authors to recommend routine myelographic evaluation.[17, 21] If this situation is unrecognized, bony decompression alone (without opening the dura) will be unsuccessful in obtaining remission of symptoms or halting progression of the neurologic injury.[5]

Compression of the vertebral arteries as they pass through the stenotic foramen is another source of symptoms.[16, 20] In addition, there is a higher than normal incidence of vertebral artery anomalies associated with basilar impression and atlanto-occipital fusion.[2] These factors may account for symptoms suggestive of vertebral arterial insufficiency, such as dizziness, seizures, mental deterioration, and syncope, which have been found to occur alone or in combination with those of spinal cord compression.[5, 12, 16] Michie[19] and Bachs[1] have suggested that one explanation for the frequent association of syringomyelia or syringobulbia[21] and basilar impression is that the vertebral arteries and the anterior spinal artery are compromised in the region of the foramen magnum with subsequent degeneration of the spinal cord and medulla. Unfortunately, arteriographic studies are not available to confirm this interesting hypothesis. Children with occipitocervical anomalies may be more susceptible to vertebral artery injury and brainstem ischemia, particularly those who undergo skull traction for correction of scoliosis. Even moderate amounts of traction (less than 15 lbs.) that normally would be well tolerated may compromise these abnormal vessels. Careful roentgenographic evaluation of the occipitocervical junction should precede any use of skull traction even if only minimal traction forces are planned.

Although this condition is congenital, many patients do not develop symptoms until the second or third decade of life.[4, 5] This may be due to a gradually increasing degree of ligamentous laxity and instability with aging, similar to the delayed myelopathies reported following atlantoaxial dislocations or the increasing instability of C1-C2 in patients who have odontoid agenesis.[11] Also, these individuals are more prone to the early development of cervical osteoarthritis; this finding is noted in the family studies by Gunderson.[12] Chamberlain[4] and others[17, 21] have theorized that the young developing brain might be more tolerant to compressive effects that later prove to be deleterious to older tissues. Similarly, arteriosclerotic changes in the vertebral arteries may make these vessels more susceptible to minor or temporary constrictions that would go unnoticed and may later cause ischemia or infarction. The symptoms frequently occur in older patients in whom a congenital anomaly would not ordinarily be considered. Patients with this malformation have been mistakenly diagnosed as having multiple sclerosis, posterior fossa tumors, amyotrophic lateral sclerosis, or traumatic injury. It is therefore important to survey this area whenever such diagnoses are considered.

TREATMENT. Treatment depends on the cause of the symptoms and often requires the combined talents of the orthopaedist, neurosurgeon, neurologist, and radiologist. It is quite possible to have a severe basilar impression without neurologic symptoms, and careful search for associated conditions must be conducted. If the symptoms are predominantly due to anterior impingement from a hypermobile odontoid, stabilization of the occipitocervical junction in extension may be required. If the odontoid cannot be reduced, an anterior excision can be considered but should be preceded by stabilization in extension. Posterior impingement usually requires suboccipital craniectomy and decompression of the posterior ring of C1 and possibly C2 coupled with posterior stabilization. Most authors suggest opening the dura to avoid overlooking a tight posterior dural band.[5] These are not recommendations but are merely generalizations regarding treatment, and appropriate references should be consulted in the evaluation of individual patients.

References

1. Bachs, A., Barraquer-Bordas, L., Barraquer-Ferre, L, Canadell, J. M., and Modolell, A.: Delayed myelopathy following atlantoaxial dislocation by separated odontoid process. Brain 78:537–553, 1955.
2. Bernini, F., Elefante, R., Smaltino, F., and Tedeschi, G.: Angiographic study on the vertebral artery in cases of deformities of the occipito-cervical joint. Am. J. Roentgenol. 107:526–529, 1969.
3. Chakrabarti, A. K., Johnson, S. C., Smantray, S. K., and Ajaram-Reddy, E.: Osteomalacia, myopathy and basilar impression. J. Neurol. Sci. 23:227–235, 1974.
4. Chamberlain, W. E.: Basilar impression (platybasia): A bizarre developmental anomaly of the occipital bone and upper cervical spine with striking and misleading neurologic manifestations. Yale J. Biol. Med. 11:487–496, 1939.
5. DeBarros, M. C., Farias, W., Ataide, L., and Lins, S.: Basilar impression and Arnold-Chiari malformation: A study of 66 cases. J. Neurol. Neurosurg. Psychiatry 31:596–605, 1968.
6. DeBarros, M. C., daSilva, W. F., DeAzevado-Filho, H. D., and Spinelli, C.: Disturbances of sexual potency in patients with basilar impression and Arnold-Chiari malformation. J. Neurol. Neurosurg. Psychiatry 38:598–600, 1975.
7. DirHeimeri, Y., and Babin, E.: Basilar impression and hereditary fragility of the bones. Neuroradiology 3:41–43, 1971.
8. Dolan, K. D.: Cervico-basilar relationships. Radiol. Clin. North Am. 15:155–166, 1977.
9. Epstein, B. S., and Epstein, J. A.: The association of cerebellar tonsillar herniation with basilar impression incident to Paget's disease. Am. J. Roentgenol. 107:535–542, 1969.
10. Fischgold, H., and Metzger, J.: Etude radiotomographique de l'impression basilaire. Rev. Rheum. 19:261–264, 1952.
11. Fromm, G. H., and Pitner, S. E.: Late progressive quadriparesis due to odontoid agenesis. Arch. Neurol. 9:291–296, 1963.
12. Gunderson, C. H., Greenspan, R. H., Glaser, G. H., and Lubs, H. A.: Klippel-Feil syndrome: Genetic

and clinical reevaluation of cervical fusion. Medicine *46*:491–512, 1967.

13. Hertel, G., Nadjmi, M., and Kunze, J.: A statistical comparative study of the basilar impression in syringomyelia. Eur. Neurol. *11*:363–372, 1974.

14. Hinck, V. C., Hopkins, C. E., and Savara, B. S.: Diagnostic criteria of basilar impression. Radiology *76*:572–585, 1961.

15. Luyendijk, W., Matricoli, B., and Thomeer, R. T.: Basilar impression in an achondroplastic dwarf. Causative role in tetraparesis. Acta Neurochir. *41*:243–253, 1978.

16. McGregor, M.: The significance of certain measurements of the skull in the diagnosis of basilar impression. Br. J. Radiol. *21*:171–181, 1948.

17. McRae, D. L.: The significance of abnormalities of the cervical spine. Am. J. Roentgenol. *84*:3–25, 1960.

18. McRae, D. L., and Barnum, A. S.: Occipitalization of the atlas. Am. J. Roentgenol. *70*:23–46, 1953.

19. Michie, I., and Clark, M.: Neurological syndromes associated with cervical and cranio-cervical anomalies. Arch. Neurol. *18*:241–247, 1968.

20. Nagashima, C.: Atlanto-axial dislocation due to agenesis of the os odontoideum or odontoid. J. Neurosurg. *33*:270–280, 1970.

21. Spillane, J. D., Pallis, C., and Jones, A. M.: Developmental abnormalities in the region of the foramen magnum. Brain *80*:11–48, 1957.

Congenital Atlantoaxial Instability

The clinical significance of a bony anomaly in the region of the atlantoaxial joint is primarily related to its influence on the stability of this articulation. The precipitating factor may be an abnormal odontoid, atlanto-occipital fusion, or laxity of the transverse atlantal ligament, but the end result is narrowing of the spinal canal and impingement on the neural elements. It is important not to lose sight of this basic problem, but frequently it becomes obscured in roentgenographic detail, conflicting reports, and unusual clinical symptoms and signs. Therefore, it is important to review atlantoaxial instability prior to a detailed discussion of the individual anomalies that may be contributory.

PATHOMECHANICS. The articulation between the first and second cervical vertebrae is the most mobile part of the vertebral column and normally has the least stability of any of the vertebral articulations. The normal cervical spine permits about 90 degrees of rotatory motion. Fifty per cent of this motion occurs in the atlantoaxial joint. Considerable shifting from side to side (lateral slide) also occurs as a component of this rotatory motion. Flexion and extension are permitted to a limited degree (normally about 10 degrees of extension and 5 degrees of forward flexion), and more than 10 degrees of flexion indicates subluxation.[16] The odontoid acts as a bony buttress to prevent hyperextension, but the remainder of the normal range of motion is maintained and is solely dependent on the integrity of the surrounding ligaments and capsular structures.

The articulation between the condyles of the skull and the atlas (atlanto-occipital joint) normally allows only a few degrees of flexion-extension, slight nodding motion of the head. In rotation, the atlas and head turn as a unit. The articulation between the axis and the third cervical vertebra permits some flexion-extension but is similarly restricted in rotation. Thus, the atlantoaxial joint is extremely mobile but structurally weak and is located between two relatively fixed points, the atlanto-occipital and C2-C3 joints.

Motion of the atlantoaxial articulation is usually accentuated in patients with bony anomalies of the occipitocervical junction. An excellent example is the patient with atlanto-occipital fusion, who is frequently found to have compensatory hypermobility of the atlantoaxial joint. If this same patient has an associated synostosis of C2-C3, it is reasonable to expect that this additional stress on the atlantoaxial articulation may eventually lead to significant instability.[28] This assumption has clinical support, in that 60 per cent of patients with symptomatic atlanto-occipital fusion have associated fusion of C2-C3.[18]

Still, it is unusual for patients to become symptomatic prior to the third decade. What accounts for this delay? We must assume that at least initially, a delicate balance is struck between the hypermobile articulation and the adjacent spinal cord. Motion is maintained without neurologic compromise. This relationship must be altered prior to the development of symptoms. In the symptomatic patient, trauma is an immediate suspect, but statistically, it is not often associated or is of a minor nature. More likely, the degenerative changes of aging cause the lower cervical articulations to become more rigid. This gradual restriction of motion below places an increased demand on the ligaments and capsular structures of the atlantoaxial articulation with the development of instability.[11] With aging, the central nervous system itself becomes less tolerant to intermittent compression, and its ability to recover is diminished. There is evidence to suggest that intermittent compression is more harmful or irritating to the spinal cord than static, constant compression.[25] Arteriosclerosis and loss of elasticity from aging affect the vertebral arteries, making them more sensitive to compression at the foramen magnum.[20]

As a consequence, the symptomatic patient often presents with a puzzling clinical picture. Only a few patients present initially with a history of head or neck trauma, neck pain, torticollis, quadriparesis, or signs of high spinal cord compression, any of which would facilitate the diagnosis. A changing, intermittent pattern of symptoms is more typical than the localized pattern suggested by the roentgenograms alone. Many are mistakenly diagnosed as having a diffuse demyelinating disease, such as multiple sclerosis or amyotrophic lateral sclerosis.

In patients with basilar impression or atlanto-occipital fusion, the clinical findings suggest that the major damage is occurring anteriorly from the odontoid. The symptoms and signs of pyramidal tract irritation, muscle weakness and wasting, ataxia, spasticity, hyperreflexia, and pathologic reflexes are commonly found.[1, 18] Autopsy findings consistently demonstrate that the brain stem is indented by the abnormal odontoid.[1, 19] Other less common complaints include diplopia, tinnitus, earaches, dysphasia, and poor phonation, all of which are due to cranial nerve or bulbar irritation from direct pressure of the odontoid on the medulla. If the primary area of impingement is posterior from the rim of the foramen magnum, dural band, or the posterior ring of the atlas (typical of odontoid anomalies), there will be symptoms referable to the posterior columns with alterations in deep pain and vibratory responses and proprioception. If, in addition, there is an associated cerebellar herniation, nystagmus, ataxia, and incoordination can be observed. Symptoms referable to vertebral artery compression — dizziness, seizures, mental deterioration, and syncope — may occur alone or in combination with those of spinal cord compression.[11]

In children, the presenting symptoms may be quite subtle and nonspecific. Kopits reports that in the majority of his patients, the only presenting symptom was generalized weakness manifested as lack of physical endurance, history of frequent falling, or asking to be carried.[22] Pyramidal tract signs appeared later, and posterior column signs and sphincter disturbances were less frequently encountered.[22] Similarly, in achondroplasia, retardation of motor skills and increasing hydrocephalus may be the only clinical manifestation of impending quadriparesis.

Atlantoaxial instability is commonly associated with other anomalies of the spine, many of which lead to scoliosis. Patients with congenital scoliosis, Down's syndrome, bone dysplasias, such as Morquio's syndrome, spondyloepiphyseal dysplasia, osteogenesis imperfecta, and neurofibromatosis, all are capable of having significant atlantoaxial instability, which may be unrecognized. Radiologic surveys, particularly flexion-extension views of C1-C2 articulation, should be obtained prior to administration of general anesthesia or preliminary spinal traction in the management of their scoliosis.

ROENTGENOGRAPHIC FINDINGS. The atlas-dens interval (ADI) is the space seen on the lateral roentgenogram between the anterior aspect of the dens and the posterior aspect of the anterior ring of the atlas (Fig. 5–4). There is general agreement that in children the ADI should be no greater than 4 mm.,[16] particularly in flexion where the greatest distance can be noted. The upper limit of normal in adults is less than 3 mm.[14] A subtle increase in the ADI in the neutral position may indicate disruption of the transverse atlantal ligament. This is a valuable aid in evaluation of acute injury, when standard flexion-extension views would be potentially hazardous.[16] Fielding notes that the shift of C1-C2 will not exceed 3 mm. in the adult if the transverse ligament is intact.[5] The transverse ligament ruptures within the range of 5 mm.[5]

The ADI is of limited value in evaluating chronic atlantoaxial instability due to congenital anomalies, rheumatoid arthritis, or Down's syndrome. In these conditions the odontoid is frequently found to be hypermobile with a widened ADI, particularly in flexion (Fig. 5–5), yet not all are symptomatic nor do all require surgical stabilization. In this situation, attention should be directed to the amount of space available for the spinal cord (SAC). This is accomplished by measuring the distance from the posterior aspect of the odontoid or axis to the nearest posterior structure (foramen magnum or posterior ring of the atlas). This measurement is particularly helpful when evaluating a patient with nonunion of the odontoid or os odontoideum, as in both conditions the ADI may be normal, yet in flexion or extension there may be considerable reduction in the space available for the spinal cord (Fig. 5–6). Lateral flexion-extension stress views should be conducted voluntarily by the patient, particularly those with a neurologic deficit. The majority of symptomatic patients

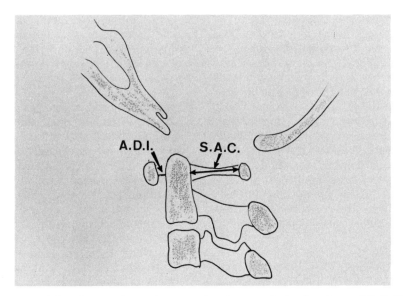

Figure 5–4.   Drawing of the atlantoaxial joint demonstrating the normal atlas-dens interval (A.D.I.) and the normal space available for the spinal cord (S.A.C.), the distance between the posterior aspect of the odontoid or axis and the nearest posterior structure.

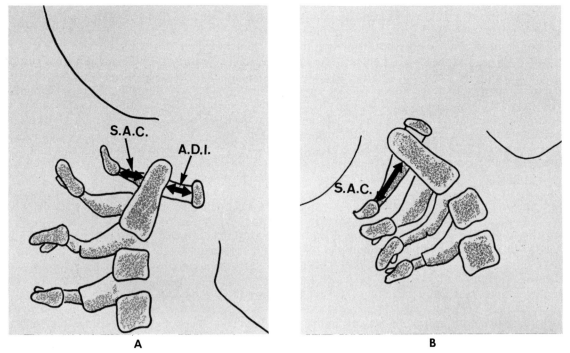

A   B

Figure 5–5.   Atlantoaxial instability with intact odontoid. *A*, Flexion — forward sliding of the atlas with an increased A.D.I. and decreased S.A.C. *B*, Extension — the A.D.I. and S.A.C. return to normal as the intact odontoid provides a bony block to subluxation in hyperextension.

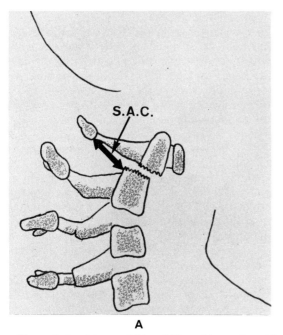 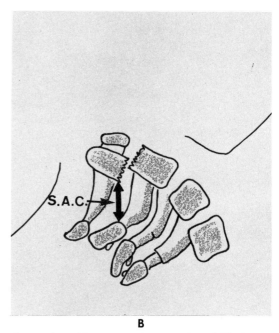

A   **B**

Figure 5–6. Atlantoaxial instability with os odontoideum, absent odontoid, or traumatic non-union. *A*, Flexion — forward sliding of the atlas with reduction of the S.A.C., but no change in A.D.I. *B*, Extension — posterior subluxation with reduction in S.A.C. and no change in the A.D.I.

exhibit significant instability. In a large series of patients with os odontoideum reported by Fielding, the average was 1 cm., the majority either anterior or posterior, but some were unstable in all directions.[4]

Patients with an intact or normal odontoid process are particularly at risk; with anterior shift of the atlas over the axis, the spinal cord is more easily damaged by direct impingement against the odontoid process, such as atlanto-occipital fusion. The situation is less dangerous if the odontoid process is absent or fractured and is carried forward with the atlas (os odontoideum).[5]

In patients with multiple anomalies, the usual roentgenographic views are not always reliable in confirming the presence or absence of an odontoid.[22] Similarly, in patients with abnormal bone, such as Morquio's syndrome or spondyloepiphyseal dysplasia, the odontoid may be present but dysplastic, blending with the surrounding abnormal bone, and cannot be differentiated (Fig. 5–8A). In these situations, adequate visualization can be obtained by using lateral laminagraphic techniques (Fig. 5–3). When the exact cut at the level of the odontoid is determined, it is repeated in flexion-extension to ascertain the stability of the atlantoaxial articulation. Extension views

should not be ignored. Many patients have been found to have significant posterior subluxation.[4, 9] Cineradiography is quite valuable in understanding the pathomechanics of odontoid anomalies, particularly those with atlantoaxial instability.

Steel[26] has called attention to the checkrein effect of the alar ligaments and how they form the second line of defense after disruption of the transverse atlantal ligament (Fig. 5–7). This secondary stability no doubt plays an important role in patients with chronic atlantoaxial instability.[6] Steele's anatomic studies provide a simple rule that is helpful to physicians evaluating this area. He defined the "rule of thirds" in that the area of the vertebral canal at the first cervical vertebra can be divided into one third cord, one third odontoid, and one third "space." The one third "space" represents a safe zone in which displacement can occur without neurologic impingement and is roughly equivalent to the full transverse diameter of the odontoid (usually 1 cm.).[5] In chronic atlantoaxial instability, it is of prime importance to recognize when the patient has exceeded the "safe zone" of Steele and enters the area of impending spinal cord compression. At this point the second line of defense, the alar ligaments, has failed,

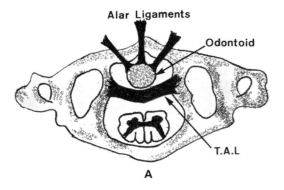

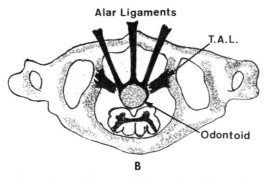

Figure 5–7. Atlantoaxial joint as viewed from above. *A,* Normal. *B,* Disruption of transverse atlantal ligament (T.A.L.): odontoid now occupies the "safe zone of Steel." The intact alar ligaments (second line of defense) prevent spinal cord compression.

and there is no longer a margin of safety (Fig. 5–7). Experimentally, Fielding[5] found that following rupture of the transverse ligament, the alar ligaments are usually inadequate to prevent further displacement of C1-C2 when a force similar to that which ruptured the transverse ligament is applied. Although the alar ligaments appear thick and strong, they stretch with relative ease and permit significant displacement.[5]

McRae[18] was first to call attention to the relationship of neurologic symptoms and the sagittal diameter of the spinal canal (SAC). He noted that in his patients with atlanto-occipital fusion, those with less than 10 mm. of available space behind the odontoid or atlas were always symptomatic. However, with the availability of more clinical data, this measurement has been more specifically defined. Greenberg, after an extensive review of the literature, has determined that in adults, spinal cord compression always occurs if the sagittal diameter of the cervical canal behind the dens is 14 mm. or less.[11] Cord compression is possible between 15 and 17 mm. and never

occurs if the distance is 18 mm. or more.[11] However, variations in patient size and the presence or absence of soft tissue elements will affect the clinical significance of the measurement. Myelography has demonstrated in some patients a ventral impingement due to a thick wad of radiolucent soft tissue posterior to the dysplastic odontoid and the body of the axis.[22]

Information on normal variations in sagittal and transverse diameter of the cervical spine has been collected for infants, children, and young adults.[12, 14, 21] As might be expected, these measurements in general are smaller than those found in adults and follow a predictable growth curve. Clinical significance is determined using two parameters: (1) comparison of the absolute diameter to the known norms for that vertebral level and age; and (2) comparison of successive vertebral levels within the same individual. Variations in the latter are more sensitive in determining an abnormality involving a single vertebra, as there is good correlation between adjacent levels in the same child. These tables should be readily available when evaluating the growing spine both for pathologic narrowing and expansion.[3] The transparencies developed by Haworth and Keillor[12] are particularly helpful in this regard and provide an efficient screening test for assessing the transverse diameter of the spinal canal in the growing child. The sagittal diameter of the cervical canal is largest at C1 and gradually narrows in size until C5-C7. The appearance is similar to a funnel, and enlargement in the outline suggests an intraspinal mass, even if the absolute measurements do not exceed upper limits of normal.[3]

Children have several normal variations in cervical spine mobility that can be alarming to physicians who are unaware of them. Cattel[2] has called attention to the frequent (20 per cent) finding of overriding of the anterior arch of the atlas on the odontoid with extension of the neck. This is due to normal elasticity of ligaments and diminishes with growth, as it is not present after age seven. Pseudosubluxation of C2 on C3 of 3 mm. can be found in more than one half of the children under age eight (Fig. 5–8).[2, 7] Less frequently, hypermobility occurs at the C3-C4 interspace. Recognition becomes important particularly when evaluating a young child with the Klippel-Feil syndrome or those with recent trauma.

In children, the normal pattern of ossification of the cervical spine can pose problems

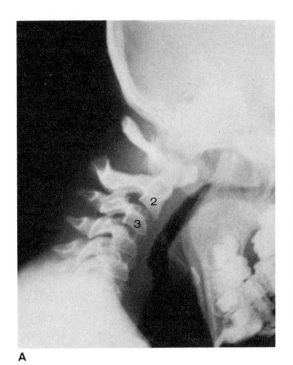
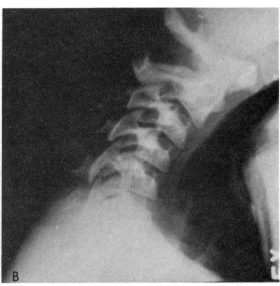

A

Figure 5–8. *A*, Pseudosubluxation of C2 on C3 occurring in a child at age five. *B*, Same patient at age 10 — flexion view of cervical spine demonstrating normal motion without pseudosubluxation. This normal variation can be found in over one half of children under the age of eight.

in roentgenographic interpretation. At birth the odontoid is separated from the body of the axis by a wide cartilaginous band, which represents the vestigial disc space, referred to as the neurocentral synchondrosis (Fig. 5–5*B*). On the lateral radiograph, this lucent line is similar in appearance to an epiphyseal growth plate (Fig. 5–5*A*). This may be confused with the jointlike articulation between the odontoid and the body of the atlas found in os odontoideum. This is present in nearly all children at age three and absent in most by age six. Consequently, the diagnosis of os odontoideum in children must be confirmed by demonstrating motion between the odontoid and the body of the axis. Atlantoaxial fusion may be difficult to diagnose in the young child, as a significant portion of the ring of C1 is unossified at birth. There is usually a 5 to 9 mm. gap posteriorly, which ossifies by age four.[28] The anterior arch of the atlas is not visible in 80 per cent of infants, and the entire ring may not be completely ossified until age ten.[28]

Myelographic evaluation can be of great help in defining an area of constriction. In this regard, gas or a water-soluble contrast agent (Metrizamide) myelography should be used in preference to oil contrast media (Fig. 5–9).[8, 17, 18, 22, 23] Recent reports indicate computerized tomography in conjunction with Metrizamide myelography is particularly helpful when evaluating children with rotational deformities or compromise of the neural canal in the upper cervical spine.[8, 23] These advances will allow a more complete and accurate examination of the brain stem, an area of considerable importance in the patient with occipitocervical anomalies.[8, 23] Vertebral arteriography is helpful in evaluating patients who exhibit symptoms of transient brain stem ischemia. If cerebellar herniation (Arnold-Chiari malformation) is suspected, arteriography combined with myelography can demonstrate the anomaly (Fig. 5–10).[23]

TREATMENT OF ATLANTOAXIAL INSTABILITY

In general, effective treatment can be provided only if the exact cause of symptoms has been determined. This must be accomplished by a careful correlation of the clinical and radiologic findings. Prior to surgical intervention, reduction of the atlantoaxial articula-

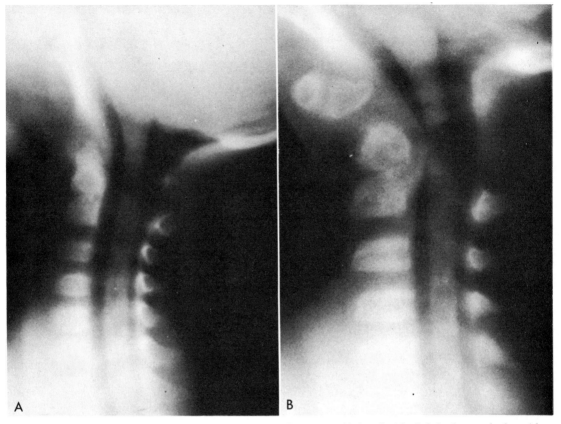

Figure 5–9. Normal gas myelogram-polytomograms. *A*, Three-year-old dwarf with slightly abnormal odontoid, no atlantoaxial instability and no neurological signs or symptoms. *B*, Atlantoaxial instability without cord compression and myelopathy. Seven-year-old dwarf with a congenitally detached odontoid which dislocates forward with the anterior arch of the atlas. The posterior ring of the atlas is absent, and therefore posterior impingement of the spinal cord against the axis is avoided. (Roentgenograms provided courtesy of Steven E. Kopits, M.D., Division of Orthopaedics, Johns Hopkins University; and Milos Perovic, M.D., Department of Radiology, University of Connecticut.)

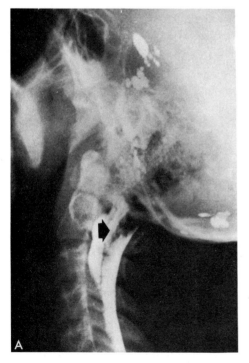

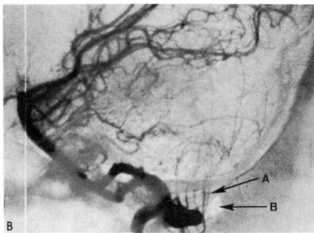

Figure 5–10. Twelve-year-old with nystagmus and cerebellar ataxia. *A*, Myelogram demonstrates the Arnold-Chiari malformation with herniation of the cerebellar tonsils through the foramen magnum. The arrow indicates the distal migration of the tonsils. *B*, Same patient — vertebral arteriography demonstrates inferior cerebellar vessels looping down to the spinal canal. A (arrow), inferior cerebellar vessels. B (arrow), posterior ring of the atlas. (Roentgenograms courtesy of Frank Lee, M.D., Department of Radiology, Jefferson Medical College, Philadelphia, Pennsylvania.)

tion should be achieved either by positioning or traction.[6, 7] Operative reduction should never be attempted, as it is associated with an increased morbidity and mortality.[24, 29] The patient should be maintained in the reduced position preoperatively until spinal cord edema and local irritation resolve. This is usually accompanied by improvement of the neurologic status and often remission of symptoms. If neurologic symptoms are unchanged with reduction and rest, the physician should carefully search for other causes.

Too little attention has been paid in the past to occult respiratory dysfunction in these patients.[10, 15] Many have an unrecognized decrease in vital capacity and chronic alveolar hypoventilation as a result of the neurologic injury to the brain stem. Similarly, the gag and cough reflexes are often depressed,[10] and the patient may not be able to clear pulmonary secretion adequately in the postoperative period. Periods of apnea and respiratory distress either during surgery or in the immediate postoperative period have frequently resulted in death or have required prolonged respiratory support. Preoperative pulmonary evaluation can be of help in limiting the severity of respiratory complications. If pulmonary function is significantly reduced or if the gag and cough reflexes are depressed, consideration should be given to preoperative tracheostomy.[10] Equipment for mechanical respiratory support must be immediately available during the postoperative period.

References

1. Bharucha, E. P., and Dastur, H. M.: Craniovertebral anomalies (a report on 40 cases). Brain 87:469–480, 1964.
2. Cattell, H. S., and Filtzer, D. L.: Pseudosubluxation and other normal variations in the cervical spine in children. J. Bone Joint Surg. 47A:1295–1309, 1965.
3. Dolan, K. D.: Expanding lesions of the cervical spinal canal. Radiol. Clin. North Am. 15:203–214, 1977.
4. Fielding, J. W., Hensinger, R. N., and Hawkins, R. J.: Os odontoideum. J. Bone Joint Surg. 62A:376–383, 1980.
5. Fielding, J. W., Cochran, G. V., Lawsing, J. F., III, and Hohl, M.: Tears of the transverse ligament of the atlas. J. Bone Joint Surg. 56A:1683–1691, 1974.
6. Fielding, J. W., Hawkins, R. J., and Ratzan, S. A.: Spine fusion for atlanto-axial instability. J. Bone Joint Surg. 58A:400–407, 1976.
7. Garber, J. N.: Abnormalities of the atlas and axis vertebrae; Congenital and traumatic. J. Bone Joint Surg. 46A:1782–1791, 1964.
8. Geehr, R. B., Rothman, S. L. G., and Kier, E. L.: The role of computed tomography in the evaluation of upper cervical spine pathology. 2:79–97, 1978.
9. Giannestras, N. J., Mayfield, F. H., Provencio, F. P., and Maurer, J.: Congenital absence of the odontoid process. A case report. J. Bone Joint Surg. 46A:839–843, 1964.
10. Grantham, S. A., Dick, H. M., Thompson, R. C., Jr., and Stinchfield, F. E.: Occipito-cervical arthrodesis. Indications, technic and results. Clin. Orthop. 65:118–129, 1969.
11. Greenberg, A. D.: Atlanto-axial dislocations. Brain 91:655–684, 1968.
12. Haworth, J. B., and Keillor, G. W.: Use of transparencies in evaluating the width of the spinal canal in infants, children and adults. Radiology 79:109–114, 1962.
13. Hinck, V. C., and Hopkins, C. E.: Measurement of the atlantodental interval in the adult. Am. J. Roentgenol. 84:945–951, 1960.
14. Hinck, V. C., Hopkins, C. E., and Savara, B. S.: Sagittal diameter of the cervical spinal canal in children. Radiology 79:97–108, 1962.
15. Krieger, A. J., Rosomoff, H. L., Kuperman, A. S., and Zingesser, L. H.: Occult respiratory dysfunction in a craniovertebral anomaly. J. Neurosurg. 31:15–20, 1969.
16. Locke, G. R., Gardner, J. I., and Van Epps, E. F.: Atlas-dens interval (ADI) in children: A survey based on 200 normal cervical spines. Am. J. Roentgenol. 97:135–140, 1966.
17. Lowman, R. M., and Finkelstein, A.: Air myelography for demonstration of the cervical spinal cord. Radiology 39:700–706, 1942.
18. McRae, D. L.: Bony abnormalities in the region of the foramen magnum: Correlation of the anatomic and neurologic findings. Acta Radiol. 40:335–354, 1953.
19. McRae, D. L.: The significance of abnormalities of the cervical spine. Am. J. Roentgenol. 84:3–25, 1960.
20. Nagashima, C.: Atlanto-axial dislocation due to agenesis of the os odontoideum or odontoid. J. Neurosurg. 33:270–280, 1970.
21. Naik, D. R.: Cervical spinal canal in normal infants. Clin. Radiol. 21:323–326, 1970.
22. Perovic, N. M., Kopits, S. E., and Thompson, R. C.: Radiologic evaluation of the spinal cord in congenital atlanto-axial dislocations. Radiology 109:713–716, 1973.
23. Resjo, M., Harwood-Nash, D. C., and Fitz, C. R.: Normal cord in infants and children examined with computed tomographic metrizamide myelography. Radiology 130:691–696, 1979.
24. Sinh, G., and Pandya, S. K.: Treatment of congenital atlanto-axial dislocations. Proc. Aust. Assoc. Neurol. 5:507–514, 1968.
25. Spillane, J. D., Pallis, C., and Jones, A. M.: Developmental abnormalities in the region of the foramen magnum. Brain 80:11–48, 1957.
26. Steel, H. H.: Anatomical and mechanical considerations of the atlanto-axial articulations. J. Bone Joint Surg. 50:1481–1482, 1968.
27. Sullivan, C. R., Bruwer, A. J., and Harris, L. E.: Hypermobility of the cervical spine in children. A pitfall in the diagnosis of cervical dislocation. Am. J. Surg. 95:636–670, 1958.
28. von Torklus, D., and Gehle, W.: The Upper Cervical Spine. New York, Grune and Stratton, 1972.
29. Wadia, N. H.: Myelopathy complicating congenital atlanto-axial dislocation (a study of 28 cases). Brain 90:449–472, 1967.

ATLANTO-OCCIPITAL FUSION

(Occipitalization; Assimilation of the Atlas)

This condition is characterized by partial or complete congenital fusion of the bony ring of the atlas to the base of the occiput. Atlanto-occipital fusion is the most commonly recognized anomaly of the craniovertebral junction[14] and as a consequence has been the subject of numerous reports in the literature, including autopsy findings and detailed clinicopathologic correlations. These studies demonstrate common agreement in findings and provide adequate information on which to plan a treatment program.

CLINICAL FINDINGS. Spillane[12] noted that none of his patients with atlanto-occipital fusion had a normal-appearing neck, which is in contradistinction to other bony anomalies of the craniovertebral junction. This finding is remarkably consistent,[1, 8, 12] and the patients are commonly found to have low hairline, torticollis, short neck, and restricted neck movements not unlike those in patients with the Klippel-Feil syndrome. Twenty per cent have associated congenital abnormalities, including anomalies of the jaw, incomplete cleft of the nasal cartilage, cleft palate, congenital deformities of the external ear, cervical ribs, hypospadias, and anomalies of the urinary tract.[1, 8, 12]

Symptoms are characteristic of those conditions that lead to chronic atlantoaxial instability and may have wide variation depending upon the area of spinal cord impingement. McRae[8] is supported by other authors[1, 4, 15] in his impression that the most significant finding in the symptomatic patient with atlanto-occipital fusion is an odontoid process of abnormal size, position, or mobility. In this regard, he has suggested a simple rule: "If the dens lies below the foramen magnum (Fig. 5–1), the patient probably will be asymptomatic." If the dens lies in the foramen magnum or is angled posteriorly, there is likely to be crowding of the anterior neurologic elements, particularly in the region of the medulla oblongata (Fig. 5–11). The clinical findings support McRae's observation that the major damage is occurring anteriorly from the odontoid, as symptoms and signs of pyramidal tract irritation, muscle weakness and wasting, ataxia, spasticity, hyperreflexia, and pathologic reflexes are commonly found in atlanto-occipital fusion.[1, 8] Autopsy findings consistently demonstrate that the brain stem is indented by the abnormal odontoid.[1, 7] Other less common complaints include diplopia, tinnitus, earaches, dysphagia, and poor phonation, all of which are probably due to cranial nerve or bulbar irritation anteriorly.

Compression posteriorly by the posterior lip of the foramen magnum or a dural band is less common and results in symptoms and signs referable to the posterior columns. Thus, loss of deep pain sensation, light touch, pro-

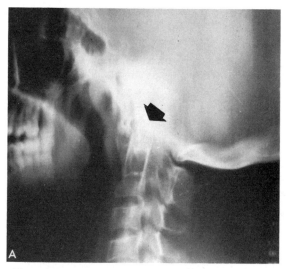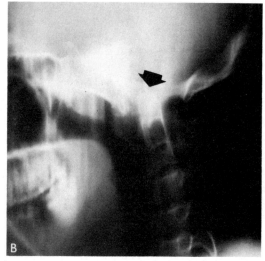

Figure 5–11. Twenty-two-year-old with symptomatic atlanto-occipital fusion and hypermobile odontoid. Lateral laminagraphic views in *A,* extension; *B,* flexion. The odontoid extends well into the opening of the foramen magnum (McRae's line), and with flexion the odontoid moves posteriorly with impingement of the brain stem. (Roentgenograms courtesy of Donald L. McRae, M.D., Department of Radiology, University of Toronto, Canada. Reproduced by permission from the Am. J. Roentgenol. *84*:3–25, 1960.)

prioception, or vibration sensation are less common complaints. As in basilar impression, nystagmus is a prominent finding and when present generally indicates herniation of the cerebellar tonsils. Headache is a frequent complaint, characterized as dull and aching, never a shooting pain, located over the posterior two thirds of the cranium (greater occipital nerve) and sometimes initiated by coughing or neck movements. Tenderness of the scalp in the same distribution may be noted.

The onset of symptoms is usually in the third or fourth decade. Symptoms usually begin insidiously and progress slowly, but sudden onset and instant death have been reported.[5] Trauma has been implicated as a precipitating factor in about one half of the patients but is usually not severe, nor does it often result in immediate onset of symptoms.[1, 8, 15] Local swelling from infection of the pharynx or nasopharynx has initiated symptoms.[1] Occasionally, patients present with suddon onset of symptoms without any precipitating cause, and in this situation, an error in diagnosis may result; multiple sclerosis or amyotrophic lateral sclerosis may be suspected wrongly.

Several explanations have been advanced to account for late onset of symptoms. Gradual laxity of the ligaments about the odontoid from repeated flexion and extension of the neck, particularly if the vertebral segments below are fixed (synostosis of C2-C3), requires compensatory motion of the atlantoaxial joint.[1, 4, 8, 15] With aging, the central nervous system itself may become less tolerant to repeated blows from the odontoid similar to a hearing deficit from repeated noise injury. Symptoms are more likely due to intermittent narrowing of the spinal canal rather than static situations to which the central nervous system has adapted.[12] Bony spurs secondary to degenerative arthritis or swelling from infection of the nasopharynx may compromise a marginally adequate space. Finally, arteriosclerotic changes in the vertebral arteries may render these vessels more susceptible to transient compression with diminished blood supply to the brain stem.

ROENTGENOGRAPHIC FINDINGS. Standard roentgenographic views of the craniovertebral junction can be difficult to interpret, and the condition may range from total incorporation of the atlas into the occipital bone to a bony or even fibrous band uniting one small area of the atlas to the occiput. Laminagrams are often necessary to demonstrate bony continuity of the anterior arch of the atlas with the occiput. Posterior fusion is not usually evident, as this portion of the ring may be represented only by a short bony fringe on the edge of the foramen magnum. Despite its innocuous radiologic appearance, this fringe is frequently directed downward and inward and can compromise the spinal canal posteriorly and has been found to create a groove in the spinal cord. It is usually assumed that the assimilated atlas is fused symmetrically to the occipital opening, but several autopsy specimens have demonstrated a posterior positioning of the atlas.[8] This in effect pushes the odontoid posteriorly, narrowing the spinal canal and the space available for the spinal cord. Computerized tomography, myelography,[2, 10] or both may be necessary to further delineate the degree and site of impingement.

In the young child, roentgenographic interpretation may be difficult, as a significant portion of the ring of C1 is unossified at birth. Ossification of the atlas begins in the paired lateral masses and progresses posteriorly into the cartilaginous neural arches. At birth there is a 5 to 9 mm. radiolucent gap in the posterior neural arch. This gap is usually ossified by age four.[14] At birth, the anterior arch of the atlas is not yet ossified in 80 per cent of children.[13] Ossification of this area is variable but usually develops from a single midline center that appears during the first year and gradually extends to the facets (lateral masses) by the third year. Ossification of the atlas is usually completed between ages seven and ten.[14]

Approximately half of the patients have "relative" basilar impression due to the diminished vertical height of the ring of the atlas. This brings the tip of the odontoid closer to the opening of the foramen magnum and the medulla oblongata (Fig. 5–11). McRae[8] suggests the position of the dens is the key to the development of neurologic problems. If the odontoid projects into the opening of the foramen magnum (Fig. 5–12), the patient probably will be symptomatic, and if it projects below the foramen magnum, the patient probably will be asymptomatic. The odontoid itself often has an abnormal shape and direction; it frequently is longer, and its angle with the body of the axis is directed more posteriorly.[8, 15] McRae[8] noted that in 60 per cent of patients with atlanto-occipital fusion, the odontoid was displaced behind the anterior arch of the atlas greater than 3 mm. and occasionally as much as 12 mm. Equally important is the width of the spinal canal be-

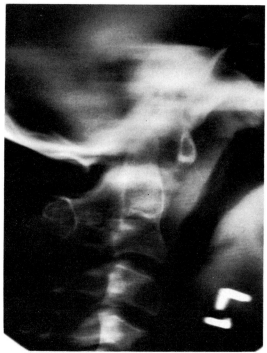

Figure 5–12. Twenty-three-year-old male with the Klippel-Feil syndrome, ataxic gait, hyperreflexia, and a history of several episodes of unconsciousness. Lateral laminagraphic view of the cervical spine and base of the skull demonstrates a C2-C3 fusion and fusion of the ring of C1 to the opening of the foramen magnum (occipitalization). The odontoid is hypermobile. Patients with this pattern of fusion are at great risk. With aging, the odontoid may become hypermobile, and the space available for the spinal cord posteriorly may be compromised.

tween the odontoid and the posterior lip of the foramen magnum (Fig. 5–12). McRae[6, 8] noted that a neurologic deficit is usually present if this distance is less than 19 mm. This measurement should be done with the neck in flexion, as this is where maximal narrowing due to an abnormal dens will occur.

The superior facets of the atlas are generally absorbed in the fusion, and the inferior facets, though present, are often asymmetrical. The transverse processes are usually abnormal, either missing or fused with the occiput, and the foramen for the vertebral artery may be absent.

McRae[6] was first to note the frequent occurrence of congenital fusion of C2-C3 (70 per cent) in patients with atlanto-occipital fusion. This suggests that greater demands are placed on the atlantoaxial articulation, particularly in flexion and extension when the joints above and below are fused.[1, 8] von Torklus notes that approximately 50 per cent of patients will develop the late onset of atlantoax-

ial instability and the resultant potential for compromise of the spinal cord.[14]

Another commonly associated abnormality is the presence of a constricting band of dura posteriorly. This has been found to create a groove in the spinal cord and may be the primary cause of symptoms. The band cannot be visualized on routine roentgenograms, nor does it correlate with the presence or absence of the posterior bony fringe of the atlas. Consequently, myelography should be an integral part of the evaluation. The water-soluble contrast material (metrizamide) alone or in conjunction with computed tomography can provide excellent visualization of the lumen of the spinal canal and its contents.[2, 10] A properly performed study will yield valuable information regarding the presence of a dural band, tonsillar herniation, and the size, shape, and position of the spinal cord in the spinal canal (Fig. 5–9A-B). Spillane[12] has demonstrated that a block of the myelographic material at the foramen magnum frequently indicates cerebellar herniation. Vertebral angiography has been helpful with the demonstration of the posterior inferior cerebellar arteries looped down into the cervical canal (Fig. 5–10).

TREATMENT.   Some patients will respond to nonoperative measures. Immobilization in plaster, traction, and cervical collars has been reported as helpful in management, particularly in patients who become symptomatic following minor trauma or infection.[1, 9, 15] An adequate trial of conservative measures is preferred, as surgical intervention represents a serious risk of morbidity and mortality to the patient.

If anterior symptoms predominate, usually this stems from hypermobility of the odontoid (Fig. 5–11) and can be controlled by posterior spinal fusion from the occiput to C2. Success of this procedure can be predicted if during preliminary traction the odontoid can be reduced and the patient's symptoms remit. Operative reduction should be avoided, as this has frequently resulted in death.[11, 15] No satisfactory solution for the unreducible odontoid has been determined, and the reader is referred to the work of Bharucha and Dastur,[1] Greenberg,[4] and Wadia.[15]

If the majority of symptoms originate from posterior spinal cord compression, then suboccipital craniectomy, excision of the posterior arch of the atlas, and removal of the dural band, if present, are suggested. Several patients have had full recovery following posterior decompression. However, many have remained unchanged, and a few have died during or shortly after this procedure.[1, 9, 15]

References

1. Bharucha, E. P., and Dastur, H. M.: Cranioverte-bral anomalies (a report of 40 cases). Brain 87:469–480, 1964.
2. Geehr, R. B., Rothman, L. G., and Kier, E. L.: The role of computed tomography in the evaluation of the upper cervical spine pathology. Comput. Tomog. 2:79–97, 1977.
3. Grantham, S. A., Dick, H. M., Thompson, R. C., Jr., and Stinchfield, F. E.: Occipito-cervical arthrodesis: Indications, technic and results. Clin. Orthop. 65:118–129, 1969.
4. Greenberg, A. D.: Atlanto-axial dislocations. Brain 91:655–684, 1968.
5. Hadley, L. A.: The Spine. Springfield, Charles C Thomas, 1956.
6. McRae, D. L.: Bony abnormalities in the region of the foramen magnum: Correlation of the anatomic and neurologic findings. Acta Radiol. 40:335–354, 1953.
7. McRae, D. L.: The significance of abnormalities of the cervical spine. Am. J. Roentgenol. 84:3–25, 1960.
8. McRae, D. L., and Barnum, A. S.: Occipitalization of the atlas. Am. J. Roentgenol. 70:23–46, 1953.
9. Nicholson, J. T., and Sherk, H. H.: Anomalies of the occipito-cervical articulation. J. Bone Joint Surg. 50A:295–304, 1968.
10. Resjo, M., Harwood-Nash, D. C., Fitz, C. R., and Chuang, S.: Normal cord in infants and children examined with computed tomographic metrizamide myelography. Radiology 130:691–696, 1979.
11. Sinh, G., and Pandya, S. K.: Treatment of congenital atlanto-axial dislocations. Proc. Aust. Assoc. Neurol. 5:507–514, 1968.
12. Spillane, J. D., Pallis, C., and Jones, A. M.: Developmental abnormalities in the region of the foramen magnum. Brain 80:11–48, 1957.
13. Tompsett, A. C., and Donaldsen, S. W.: The anterior tubercle of the first cervical vertebra and the hyoid bone. Their occurrence in newborn infants. Am. J. Roentgenol. 65:582, 1951.
14. von Torklus, D., and Gehle, W.: The Upper Cervical Spine. New York, Grune and Stratton, 1972.
15. Wadia, N. H.: Myelopathy complicating congenital atlanto-axial dislocation. Brain 90:449–472, 1967.

CONGENITAL ANOMALIES OF THE ODONTOID

(Congenital Agenesis, Hypoplasia, and Os Odontoideum)

Congenital anomalies of the odontoid are uncommon[34] and are usually discovered on roentgenograms of patients following trauma to the neck. This trauma may initiate atlantoaxial instability or may precipitate symptoms in an already compromised, previously asymptomatic atlantoaxial joint.[22] Knowledge of these deformities is important, as they have great potential for neurologic sequelae, even death, from spinal cord pressure due to abnormal atlantoaxial shift.

Three variations of odontoid anomalies have been described: aplasia (complete absence) (Fig. 5–13A), hypoplasia (partial absence), and the most common, os odontoideum (Fig. 5–13B and C).[20, 24, 37, 44, 54] Aplasia is an extremely rare anomaly and is associated with complete absence of the base of the odontoid. The commonest form of hypoplasia presents as a short, stubby peg of odontoid projecting just above the C1-C2 facet articulation. Os odontoideum is a radiolucent oval or round ossicle with a smooth, dense border of bone, separate from the axis and suggesting a congenital nonunion. The ossicle may be of variable size, located usually in the position of the normal odontoid tip (orthotopic) or near the basal occiput in the area of the foramen magnum, where it may fuse with the clivus (dystopic).[50] Separating aplasia or hypoplasia from os odontoideum is of limited importance, as they usually lead to atlantoaxial instability, and clinical signs, symptoms, and treatment are identical. The only distinctive features are roentgenographic.

The frequency of odontoid anomalies is unknown. As with many conditions that may be asymptomatic, the frequency is probably more common than appreciated. The majority are discovered following trauma to the head or neck or the spontaneous onset of symptoms sufficient to require roentgenographic investigation.[15] Rarely, the lesion is found as an incidental finding. Aplasia is extremely rare. McRae[34] noted that there was no proved case of odontoid aplasia at the Montreal Neurological Institute up to 1960. Many previous reports have confused aplasia for hypoplasia. Aplasia probably has been a misnomer, since it almost never describes an associated absence of the odontoid below the articular facets, which contributes to the body of the axis. Hypoplasia and os odontoideum are infrequently reported and can be considered rare.[20, 24, 37, 44, 54] With increased awareness, however, these lesions are being recognized more commonly than the previous literature might indicate. In a large series reported by Wollin, the average age of diagnosis was 30 years,[54] but in a recent series it was 18.9 years, suggesting earlier recognition.[15] An increasing number of children with these anomalies are being discovered. In conditions such as Down's syndrome,[16] the Klippel-Feil syndrome, and certain skeletal dysplasias, such as Morquio's syndrome[4, 28, 35] and spondylo-epiphyseal dysplasia,[27, 52] odontoid anomalies are more common than in the general population.[4, 7, 9, 26, 27, 31, 35, 42, 47, 50, 52] It is interesting

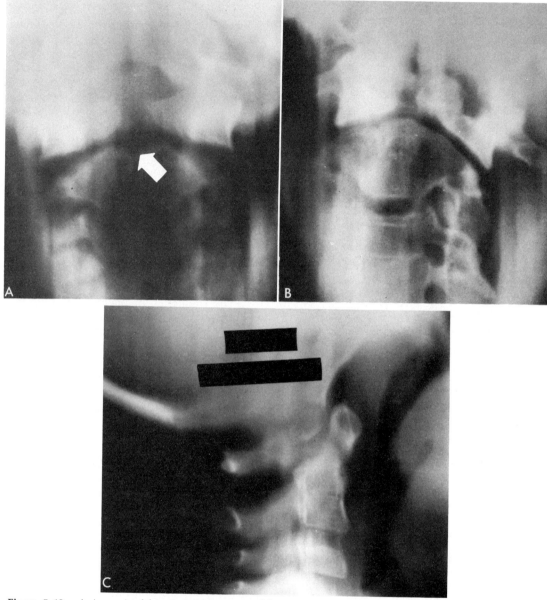

Figure 5–13. *A,* Agenesis of the odontoid (open mouth laminagraphic view). Note the slight depression between the superior articular facets of the axis (arrow). A short bony remnant in this position is termed odontoid hypoplasia. *B,* Os odontoideum (open mouth laminagraphic view). The os odontoideum is an oval or round ossicle, usually approximately one half the normal size of the odontoid, with a smooth cortical border of uniform thickness. There is a jointlike articulation between the os odontoideum and the body of the axis, which appears radiologically as a wide radiolucent gap and usually extends above the level of the superior facets. *C,* Lateral roentgenogram of an os odontoideum. The odontoid ossicle is fixed to the anterior ring of the atlas and moves with it in flexion and extension and lateral slide. There is usually a short, bony remnant projecting superiorly from the body of C2.

to note the relative infrequency of associated regional malformations with os odontoideum.[3, 15, 44, 50] One would expect that with such a fundamental congenital anomaly, it would be more frequently associated with other anomalies, similar to those described in the Klippel-Feil syndrome.[26]

EMBRYOLOGY AND NORMAL ANATOMY. The body of the odontoid is derived from the mesenchyme of the first cervical sclerotome and is actually the centrum of the first cervical vertebra. During development, the odontoid becomes separated from the atlas to fuse with the superior portion of the axis.[30, 42, 45, 50, 54] Between the first and fifth prenatal month, the dens begins to ossify from two centers, one on each side of the midline and by birth has fused into a single mass.[2, 5, 12] Occasionally, in the infant the right and left halves of the odontoid are not fused, and a longitudinal midline cleft may be seen.

At birth, the odontoid is separated from the body of the axis by a wide cartilaginous band that represents the vestigial disc space and is referred to as the neurocentral synchondrosis. On the lateral radiograph it resembles an epiphyseal growth plate (Fig. 5–14A). It is not at the anatomic base of the dens at the level of the superior articular facets of the axis

but lies well below this level within the body of the axis (Fig. 5–14B). Therefore, the embryologic base of the odontoid contributes a substantial portion of the body of the axis. On the open mouth view, the odontoid fits like a cork in a bottle, lying sandwiched between the neural arches (Fig. 5–14B). The neurocentral synchondrosis is present in nearly all children at age three, 50 per cent of children by age four, and is absent in most by age six.[6, 12] It rarely persists into adolescence or adult life. If present, it is not seen at the base of the dens where a fracture would be anticipated but lies below the level of the superior articular facets within the body of the axis.

The apex or tip of the odontoid process is derived from the mesenchyme of the most caudal occipital sclerotome or proatlas. At birth, the tip of the odontoid is not ossified and roentgenographically appears as a "V"-shaped depression known as the dens bicornuis. A separate ossification center or ossiculum terminale usually appears at age three and fuses with the body of the dens by age twelve.[2, 5, 40, 50] Cattell and Filtzer[6] found an ossiculum terminale to be present in 26 per cent of 70 normal children between ages five and eleven. It may never appear, or it may occasionally fail to fuse with the odontoid and

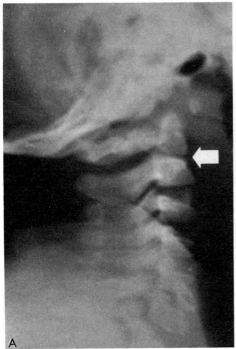

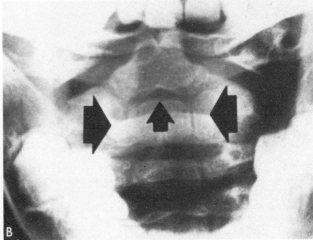

Figure 5–14. *A,* Six-month-old infant. The odontoid is normally formed and recognizable on routine roentgenograms at birth but is separated from the body of the axis by a broad cartilaginous band (arrow), similar in appearance to an epiphyseal plate. It represents the vestigial disc space and is referred to as the neurocentral synchondrosis. *B,* The neurocentral synchondrosis is not at the anatomic base of the dens, at the level of the superior articular facets of the axis. This open mouth view demonstrates that the embryologic base of the odontoid is below the articular facets and contributes a substantial portion to the body of the axis. The odontoid appears to fit like a cork in a bottle, lying sandwiched between the neural arches. This radiolucent line is present in nearly all children at age three, 50 per cent by age four, and is absent in most by age six.

is then called ossiculum terminale persistens. Anomalies of this terminal portion are rarely of clinical significance,[10, 42, 50] as it is usually firmly bound to the main body of the odontoid by fibrous tissue. In the young child, the unossified portions of the odontoid may give the false impression of odontoid hypoplasia. Similarly, one may erroneously conclude that the child has C1-C2 instability, as commonly the anterior arch of the atlas may slide upwards and actually may protrude beyond the ossified portion of the odontoid[6] on the lateral extension roentgenogram (Fig. 5–26C).

The blood supply to the odontoid, delineated by Schiff and Parke (Chap. 2), is from two sources:[42] (1) the vertebral arteries provide both an anterior and posterior ascending artery that arise at the level of C3 and pass ventral and dorsal to the body of the axis, and the odontoid, anastomosing in an apical arcade in the region of the alar ligaments. These arteries supply small penetrating branches to the body of the axis and the odontoid. (2) Lateral to the apex of the odontoid, the anterior ascending arteries and apical arcade receive anastomotic derivatives from the carotids by way of the base of the skull and the alar ligaments. This curious arrangement of the blood supply is necessary because of the embryologic development and anatomic function of the odontoid. The transient neurocentral synchondrosis between the odontoid and the axis prevents the development of any significant vascular channels between the two structures. The body of the odontoid is surrounded entirely by synovial joint cavities, and its fixed position relative to the rotation of the atlas precludes vascularization by direct branches from the vertebral arteries at the C1 segmental level.

ETIOLOGY AND PATHOGENESIS. A congenital etiology of the os odontoideum has been assumed, and two theories have been advanced: (1) Failure of fusion of the apex or ossiculum terminale to the odontoid. This is unlikely, as the fragment is too small and never approximates the size of the os odontoideum.[42] (2) Failure of fusion of the odontoid to the axis. This too is doubtful, as one would expect a crater or depression in the body of C2, since a substantial portion of C2 is derived from the odontoid, and this has not been reported. Rather, there is more often an associated short, stubby projection or hypoplastic odontoid remnant in the area of the odontoid base.[36, 54] Hypoplasia and os odontoideum can be acquired secondary to trauma or, rarely,

infection.[7, 11, 13, 18, 25, 33, 39, 40, 54] Nine cases of os odontoideum have been reported that developed several years after trauma, where a normal odontoid was initially present (Fig. 5–15).[11, 13, 15, 18, 25, 39] The majority of patients have a significant episode of trauma prior to the diagnosis of os odontoideum.[15]

Fielding and associates suggest the great weight of evidence would favor an unrecognized fracture in the region of the base of the odontoid as the most common cause and less often a congenital origin.[15] They postulate that following fracture of the odontoid there may be only slight separation of the fragments, but with time, contracture of the alar ligaments, which attach to the tip of the odontoid, exert a distraction force that pulls the fragment away from the base and closer to their origin at the occiput (Fig. 5–16). The blood supply to the odontoid is precarious, as it passes up along the sides of the odontoid, is easily traumatized, and contributes to poor fracture healing or callus formation that might retard retraction of the fragment. The position of the odontoid adjacent to the ring of C1 is maintained by the intact transverse atlantal ligament. The blood supply to the fragment is maintained by the proximal arterial arcade, from the carotid through the alar ligaments, and may be sufficient only to maintain a portion of the odontoid. Similarly, the blood supply to the proximal portion of the odontoid can be interrupted by excessive traction on these ligaments.[49]

CLINICAL SIGNS AND SYMPTOMS. Patients may present clinically with no symptoms, local neck symptoms, transitory episodes of paresis following trauma, or frank myelopathy secondary to cord compression.[48, 51] Minor trauma is commonly associated with the onset of symptoms, often of sufficient degree to warrant radiologic evaluation of the cervical spine. Symptoms may be mechanical, owing to local irritation of the atlantoaxial articulation, such as neck pain, torticollis, or headache. Neurologic symptoms are due to C1-C2 displacement and spinal cord compression. An important point differentiating os odontoideum from other anomalies of the occipitovertebral junction is that these patients seldom have symptoms referable to cranial nerves,[37] as the area of the spinal cord impingement is below the foramen magnum.

If the clinical manifestations are limited to neck pain and torticollis (local joint irritation) without neurologic involvement (40 per cent of cases),[24] the prognosis is excel-

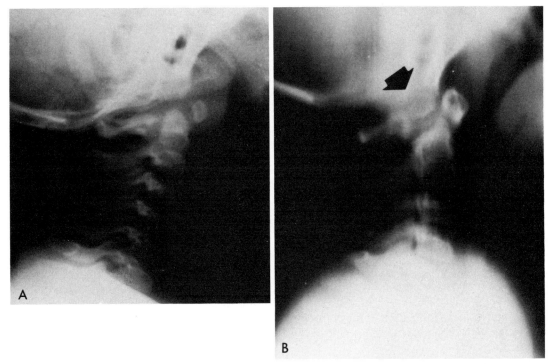

Figure 5–15. *A,* Five-year-old male, who at age two fell from a couch. Lateral roentgenogram demonstrates a normal-appearing odontoid and cervical spine. He complained of pain in the neck and occiput and presented with torticollis. Symptoms and signs gradually resolved over one month. *B,* The child was asymptomatic until age five, when over a period of six months he developed increasing neck pain and stiffness without neurologic complaints or findings. Roentgenograms revealed an os odontoideum and 7 mm. of flexion-extension motion. The patient subsequently underwent C1-2 stabilization.

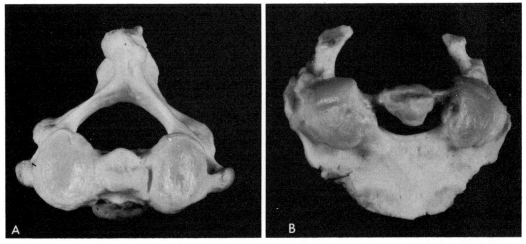

Figure 5–16. *A,* Anatomic specimen of an os odontoideum from a 17-year-old male with multiple congenital anomalies who died from renal disease. The previous bony attachment of the odontoid to the axis was rough and blunted. There was a fibrocartilage pseudarthrosis between the os odontoideum and C2. *B,* The occiput and occipital joints, with the os odontoideum suspended between the facets. The transverse ligament was intact but loosened during the preparation of the specimen. The alar ligaments remain attached to the tip of the os odontoideum. They are shortened and appear to have pulled the residual odontoid tip closer to their origin on the occiput. The os odontoideum was firmly attached by soft tissue to the occiput and ring of C1 and moved freely with these structures on C2. The foramen magnum is incomplete posteriorly. The posterior ring of C1 (not pictured) was intact and otherwise normal in its appearance. The spinal cord was narrowed and attenuated at the level of C1.

lent.[15, 32, 37, 41] Similarly, patients who exhibit only transient weakness of the extremities and dysesthesia following trauma usually have complete return of function. However, those with insidious onset and slowly progressive neurologic impairment have a greater potential for permanent deficit.[15] Damage may be mixed, with involvement of both the anterior and posterior spinal cord structures. Weakness and ataxia are more common complaints than is sensory loss. However, spasticity, increased deep tendon reflexes, clonus, loss of proprioception, and sphincter disturbances in various combinations have all been described.

A small number of patients may have symptoms and signs of cerebral and brain stem ischemia, seizures, mental deterioration, syncope, vertigo, and visual disturbances.[14, 17, 41, 44] These patients typically have a paucity of cervical cord signs and symptoms, and it is presumed that they are experiencing vertebral artery compression at the foramen magnum or just below it.[32] Thus, the diagnosis can be quite confusing, and many patients are misdiagnosed or thought to have progressive neurologic illness. Whenever the diagnosis of Friedreich's ataxia, multiple sclerosis, or other unexplained neurologic complaints is encountered, survey of the occipitocervical junction is suggested.

RADIOLOGIC FINDINGS. *Agenesis or Hypoplasia of the Odontoid* (Fig. 5–13A). The diagnosis of odontoid aplasia can be made with standard roentgenograms at birth. There should be a recognizable odontoid, though not yet fused at its base to the axis. If the odontoid is absent, a slight depression may be noted between the superior articular facets in the open mouth view (Fig. 5–13A). A short, bony remnant in this portion is termed odontoid hypoplasia.

In patients with multiple anomalies, the usual roentgenographic views are not always reliable in confirming the presence or absence of an odontoid. Similarly, in patients with abnormal bone, such as in Morquio's syndrome and spondyloepiphyseal dysplasia,[28] the odontoid may be present but dysplastic, blending with the surrounding abnormal bone, and cannot be differentiated (Fig. 5–17A). In these situations, good results have been obtained by using lateral laminagraphic techniques (Fig. 5—17B and C). When the exact cut at the level of the odontoid is determined, it is repeated in flexion and extension to ascertain the stability of the atlantoaxial artic-

ulation. The extension view should not be ignored. Many patients have been found with significant posterior subluxation.[15, 20] Giannestras reported a youngster who became quadriparetic from prolonged hyperextension while lying prone watching television.[20]

Os Odontoideum. In os odontoideum, there is a jointlike articulation between the odontoid and the body of the axis, which appears radiologically as a wide radiolucent gap (Fig. 5–13B-C). This gap may be confused with the normal neurocentral synchondrosis (Fig. 5–14A) prior to age five. Therefore, in children, the diagnosis of os odontoideum is confirmed by demonstrating motion between the odontoid and the body of the axis. In the adult, the diagnosis of os odontoideum is suggested by observing a radiolucent defect between the dens and the body of the axis. However, the radiologic appearance of the condition may be quite similar to a traumatic nonunion, and frequently they cannot be differentiated.[33, 54] In os odontoideum, the gap between the free ossicle and the axis usually extends above the level of the superior facets and is wide with a smooth edge. The ossicle is usually approximately one half the normal size of the odontoid, is rounded or oval in shape, and the cortex is of uniform thickness. In the traumatic nonunion, the gap between the fragments is characteristically narrow and irregular and frequently extends into the body of the axis below the level of the superior facets of the axis. The bone fragments appear to "match," and there is no marginal cortex at the level of the fracture or the rounded-off appearance that is found with os odontoideum.[39] Laminagrams may be helpful in determining these subtle differences. The odontoid ossicle is fixed firmly to the anterior ring of the atlas and moves with it in flexion, extension, and lateral slide. The anterior portion of the atlas is usually hypertrophied, and the posterior portion of the ring may be hypoplastic or absent.[15, 37]

Recommended roentgenographic views are the open mouth and lateral flexion-extension views. Lateral laminagrams are indicated when routine views are not satisfactory in demonstrating the anomaly. Lateral flexion-extension stress views should be conducted voluntarily by patients, particularly those with a neurologic deficit. The degree of anterior-posterior displacement of the atlas on the axis should be documented (Fig. 5–18). The os odontoideum will move with

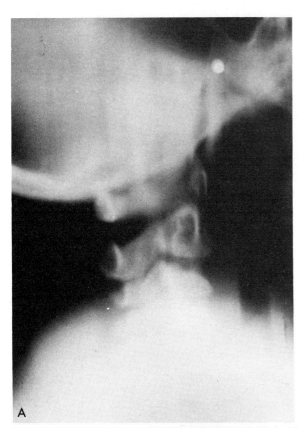

Figure 5–17. Seven-year-old with the diagnosis of spondyloepiphyseal dysplasia. *A*, The patient was discovered to have an absent odontoid. Lateral laminagraphic views demonstrate a stable atlantoaxial articulation in *B*, extension, and *C*, flexion. The patient is neurologically normal.

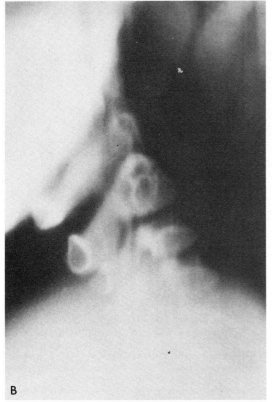

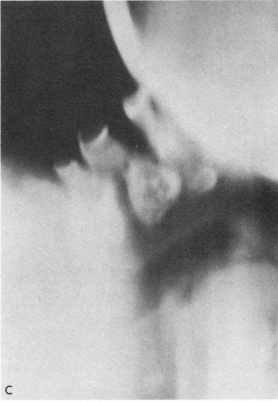

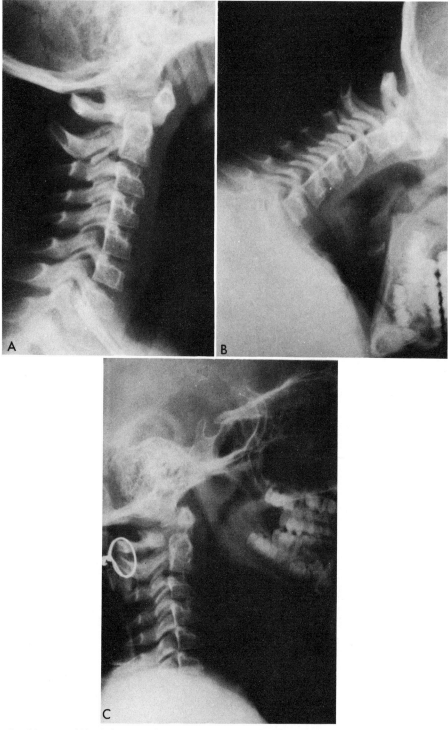

Figure 5–18.   Six-year-old had a history of peculiar posturing and stiffness of the neck beginning at age 11 months and persisting for five years. Subsequent roentgenograms demonstrated *A*, an os odontoideum, and *B*, subluxation of C1-C2 in flexion. The degree of anteroposterior displacement of the atlas on the axis should be documented. The os odontoideum will move with the ring of C1, and consequently measurements of its relationship to C1 are of little value. Measurements can be made using a line projected inferiorly from the posterior border of the anterior arch of the atlas. Measurements greater than 3 mm. should be considered pathologic. *C*, Roentgenographic appearance following posterior stabilization. Reduction must be accomplished prior to surgery, and if wire stabilization is selected, care must be taken to avoid further flexion of the neck during the surgery.

the ring of C1, and consequently measurements of its relationship to C1 are of little value. Measurements can be made using a line projected superiorly from the posterior border of the body of the axis to a line projected inferiorly from the posterior border of the anterior arch of the atlas. Measurements greater than 3 mm. should be considered pathologic. The majority of symptomatic patients exhibit significant instability.[15] In a large series reported by Fielding and associates, the average was 1 cm., the majority were either anterior or posterior, but some were unstable in all directions.[15] Posteriorly, the lumen of the spinal canal or the space available for the spinal cord should be determined (p. 196). Cineradiography is quite valuable in understanding the pathomechanics of odontoid anomalies, particularly those with atlantoaxial instability.

TREATMENT. Patients with congenital anomalies of the odontoid are leading a precarious existence. The concern is that a trivial insult superimposed on an already weakened or compromised structure may be catastrophic. Patients with local symptoms or transient myelopathy can expect recovery at least temporarily.[32, 37, 41] Cervical traction or plaster cast immobilization may be helpful in such circumstances.

There is considerable controversy concerning the role of prophylactic atlantoaxial stabilization in patients who have complete resolution of symptoms or the asymptomatic patient whose anomaly is discovered on routine radiologic examination. Some authors[19, 21, 32, 37] feel that the risk of surgery is significant and recommend the procedure only for those patients who experience recurrent episodes or demonstrate progressive neurologic symptoms. Surgical intervention has been associated with a high mortality and frequent worsening of the neurologic deficit. They recommend the patient avoid all activities that may cause trauma to the head and neck. Shepard[45] feels that such restrictions are impractical and unrealistic for most patients and that the risks of a neurologic catastrophe are so great that all patients with absent odontoid or os odontoideum should have elective stabilization. Obviously, the patient must share in this decision, and the treatment must be tailored to the patient's age, general condition, and attitude toward such restrictions.

There is general agreement that surgical stabilization is indicated with neurologic involvement even if transient, with instability of greater than 5 mm. anterior or posterior, or with progressive instability or persistent neck complaints.[15] If possible, reduction of the atlantoaxial articulation must be accomplished prior to surgery either by careful positioning of the patient or by skull traction. Open reduction during surgery is discouraged, as it has proved extremely hazardous and may result in respiratory distress, apnea, or death.[19] Ideally the patient should be maintained in the reduced position one to two weeks prior to surgery to allow recovery of neurologic function and to lessen spinal cord irritation.

The suggested method of stabilization is posterior cervical fusion of C1-C2, employing wire fixation and an iliac bone graft (Fig. 5-18C). This is not without risk, as slight flexion is often required to pass the wire beneath the posterior ring of the atlas and can have tragic results.[37] In the patient with a marginally functioning neurologic status, it may be wiser to perform an occiput to C2 arthrodesis and plan to maintain immobilization in extension during the postoperative period.[37] In this regard, the halo-cast is helpful. Incomplete development of the posterior ring of C1 is uncommon (3 in 1000 persons) but is reported to occur with increased frequency in patients with an os odontoideum.[15, 29] The completeness of the C1 arch should be evaluated preoperatively, as a large gap may preclude wire fixation. If wire fixation is employed, excessive tightening of the wire should be avoided (Fig. 5-18C). The articulation is frequently unstable both in flexion and extension, and posterior dislocations may occur owing to overcorrection with disastrous results.

Those patients in whom the C1-C2 dislocation is unreducible after an adequate trial of traction pose a difficult management problem.[8] In this situation, posterior decompression by laminectomy has been associated with an increased morbidity and mortality.[37] In addition, posterior decompression alone may potentiate C1-C2 instability and if performed must be accompanied by occiput to C2 arthrodesis.[8, 16] For those patients without a neurologic deficit, a simple in situ posterior fusion will be the least hazardous procedure. If reduction of the C1-C2 dislocation is considered necessary or if the clinical situation precludes posterior stabilization, an anterior approach should be considered.[22, 53] The lateral retropharyngeal approach described by Whitesides has provided anterior exposure of the C1-C2 articulation adequate to perform decompression, reduction, and stabilization.[53] This route is preferred over the transoral or mandibular and tongue-splitting approaches, which are associated with an increased incidence of infection.[53]

A common clinical problem is differentiation between a fractured odontoid and os odontoideum. Discovery is usually made following trauma in both conditions, and an accurate diagnosis may not be possible by roentgenographic techniques alone. In this situation, a period of immobilization (skull traction or cast) is recommended. Overdistraction, particularly in children, should be avoided as it can lead to os odontoideum.[39] If the lesion represents an acute fracture, healing will usually occur. If a congenital or traumatic nonunion is present, surgical stabilization will be necessary if atlantoaxial instability is demonstrated.

CONGENITAL LAXITY OF THE TRANSVERSE ATLANTAL LIGAMENT

This is a diagnosis of exclusion suggested by the clinical occurrence of chronic atlantoaxial dislocation without a predisposing cause.[22] There is no history of trauma, congenital anomaly, infection, or rheumatoid arthritis to account for the radiologic finding. The majority of patients discovered (excluding those with Down's syndrome) have the typical symptoms of atlantoaxial instability and require surgical stabilization.

Laxity of the transverse atlantal ligament is common in Down's syndrome, with a reported incidence of 20 per cent (Fig. 5–19).[31, 47] The lesion may be found in all age groups without a preponderance in any age bracket. It appears that these patients have rupture or attenuation of the transverse atlantal ligament with encroachment of the "safe zone" of Steel (C1-C2 instability, Fig. 5–16B)

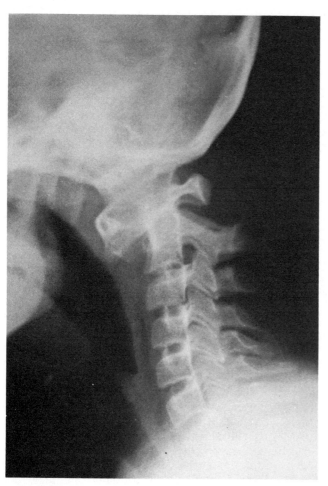

Figure 5–19. Eleven-year-old with Down's syndrome and gross atlantoaxial instability. The patient's gait was clumsy, and physical examination revealed poor coordination of the extremities. There was no other evidence of motor or sensory impairment or pathologic reflexes. The patient has no symptoms referable to the cervical spine two years following surgical stabilization.

but are protected by checkrein action of the alar ligaments from spinal cord compression. In other words, many have excessive motion, but few are symptomatic, and the majority are discovered only by radiologic survey.[7, 9, 31] With our present knowledge, prophylactic stabilization does not seem to be indicated, but more clinical information is required. The C1-C2 articulation should be evaluated in patients with Down's syndrome prior to administration of a general anesthetic.

SUMMARY

Anomalous development of the odontoid is uncommon, and its clinical significance lies in its potential to produce serious neurologic sequelae due to atlantoaxial instability. Although there are several recognized variations (aplasia, hypoplasia, and os odontoideum), clinically they share the same signs and symptoms, and treatment is identical. Symptoms are usually due to instability of the atlantoaxial joint, with compression of the spinal cord anteriorly against the axis or posteriorly from the ring of the atlas. Patients may present with no symptoms, with persistent neck complaints, with transient or permanent neurologic deficits, or may die suddenly. Symptoms from cranial nerve irritation seldom occur, but occasionally symptoms of cerebral and brain stem ischemia are noted owing to compression of the vertebral arteries in the area of the atlas.

If the condition is suspected, the diagnosis can usually be confirmed on lateral flexion-extension roentgenograms. Special techniques are often required, particularly lateral flexion-extension laminagrams. Flexion-extension stress roentgenograms are often necessary to determine the presence and degree of atlantoaxial instability.

The role of prophylactic surgical stabilization is not yet established. If marked instability is demonstrated or if the patient has clinical findings of neurologic compromise, there is general agreement that surgical fusion should be performed. Operative reduction should be avoided, and preoperative correction by traction or positioning is preferred. Posterior surgical stabilization of the first and second cervical vertebrae is sufficient, if it can be accomplished without further flexing the head. In this situation, occiput to C2 stabilization is recommended to avoid all possibility of further neurologic trauma during the procedure.

References

1. Ahlback, S., and Collert, S.: Destruction of the odontoid process due to atlanto-axial pyogenic spondylitis. Acta Radiol. (Diagn.) (Stockh.) 10:394–400, 1970.
2. Bailey, D. K.: The normal cervical spine in infants and children. Radiology 59:712–719, 1952.
3. Bassett, F. H., III, and Goldner, J. L.: Aplasia of the odontoid process. In Proceedings of the American Association of Orthopedic Surgeons. J. Bone Joint Surg. 50A:833–834, 1968.
4. Blaw, M. E., and Langer, L. O.: Spinal cord compression in Morquio-Brailsford's disease. J. Pediatr. 74:593–600, 1969.
5. Caffey, J.: Paediatric X-ray Diagnosis. 5th Ed. Chicago, Yearbook Medical Publishers, Inc., 1967.
6. Cattell, H., and Filtzer, D. L.: Pseudosubluxation and other normal variations in the cervical spine in children. J. Bone Joint Surg. 47A:1295–1309, 1965.
7. Curtis, B. H., Blank, S., and Fisher, R. L.: Atlanto-axial dislocation in Down's syndrome. J.A.M.A. 205:464–465, 1968.
8. Dyck, P.: Os odontoideum in children: Neurological manifestations and surgical management. Neurosurgery 2:93–99, 1978.
9. Dzenitis, A. J.: Spontaneous atlanto-axial dislocation in mongoloid child with spinal cord compression. Case report. J. Neurosurg. 25:458–460, 1966.
10. Evarts, C. M., and Lonsdale, D.: Ossiculum terminale — an anomaly of the odontoid process: Report of a case of atlanto-axial dislocation with cord compression. Cleve. Clin Q. 37:73–76, 1970.
11. Fielding, J. W.: Disappearance of the central portion of the odontoid process. J. Bone Joint Surg. 47A:1228–1230, 1965.
12. Fielding, J. W.: Selected observations on the cervical spine in the child. Curr. Pract. Orthop. Surg. 5:31–35, 1973.
13. Fielding, J. W., and Griffin, P. P.: Os odontoideum: An acquired lesion. J. Bone Joint Surg. 56A:187–190, 1974.
14. Fielding, J. W., Hawkins, R. J., and Ratzan, S. A.: Spine fusion for atlanto-axial instability. J. Bone Joint Surg. 58A:400–407, 1976.
15. Fielding, J. W., Hensinger, R. N., and Hawkins, R. J.: Os odontoideum. J. Bone Joint Surg. 62A:376–383, 1980.
16. Finerman, G. A., Sakai, D., and Weingarten, S.: Atlanto-axial dislocation with spinal cord compression in a mongoloid child. J. Bone Joint Surg. 58A:408–409, 1976.
17. Ford, F. R.: Syncope, vertigo and disturbances of vision resulting from intermittent obstruction of the vertebral arteries due to defect in the odontoid process and excessive mobility of the second cervical vertebra. Bull. Johns Hopkins Hosp. 91:168–173, 1952.
18. Freiberger, R. H., Wilson, P. D., Jr., and Nicholas, J. A.: Acquired absence of the odontoid process. A case report. J. Bone Joint Surg. 47A:1231–1236, 1965.
19. Garber, J. N.: Abnormalities of the atlas and axis vertebrae: Congenital and traumatic. J. Bone Joint Surg. 47A:1782–1791, 1964.
20. Giannestras, N. J., Mayfield, F. H., Provencio, F. P., and Maurer, J.: Congenital absence of the odontoid

process. A case report. J. Bone Joint Surg. 46A:839–843, 1964.

21. Gillman, E. L.: Congenital absence of the odontoid process of the axis: Report of a case. J. Bone Joint Surg. 41A:345–348, 1959.

22. Greenberg, A. D.: Atlanto-axial dislocations. Brain 91:655–684, 1968.

23. Greenberg, A. D., Scoville, W. B., and Davey, L. M.: Transoral decompression of atlanto-axial dislocation due to odontoid hypoplasia: Report of two cases. J. Neurosurg. 28:266–269, 1968.

24. Gwinn, J. L., and Smith, J. L.: Acquired and congenital absence of the odontoid process. Am. J. Roentgenol. 88:424–431, 1962.

25. Hawkins, R. J., Fielding, J. W., and Thompson, W. J.: Os odontoideum: Congenital or acquired. J. Bone Joint Surg. 58A:413–414, 1976.

26. Hensinger, R. N., Lang, J. R., and MacEwen, G. D.: The Klippel-Feil syndrome: A constellation of associated anomalies. J. Bone Joint Surg. 56A:1246–1253, 1974.

27. Langer, L. O., Jr.: Spondyloepiphysial dysplasia tarda. Hereditary chondrodysplasia with characteristic vertebral configuration in the adult. Radiology 82:833–839, 1964.

28. Lipson, S. J.: Dysplasia of the odontoid process in Morquio's syndrome causing quadriparesis. J. Bone Joint Surg. 59A:340–344, 1977.

29. Logan, W. W., and Stuard, I. D.: Absent posterior arch of the atlas. Am. J. Roentgenol. 118:431–434, 1973.

30. Macalister, A.: Notes on the development and variations of the atlas. J. Anat. Physiol. 27:519–542, 1892.

31. Martel, W., and Tishler, J. M.: Observations on the spine in mongoloidism. Am. J. Roentgenol. 97:630–638, 1966.

32. McKeever, F. M.: Atlanto-axoid instability. Surg. Clin. North Am. 48:1375–1390, 1968.

33. McRae, D. L.: Bony abnormalities in the region of the foramen magnum: Correlation of the anatomic and neurologic findings. Acta Radiol. 40:335–354, 1953.

34. McRae, D. L.: The significance of abnormalities of the cervical spine. Am. J. Roentgenol. 84:3–25, 1960.

35. Melzak, J.: Spinal deformities with paraplegia in two sisters with Morquio-Brailsford syndrome. Paraplegia 6:246–258, 1969.

36. Michaels, L., Prevost, M. J., and Crang, D. F.: Pathological changes in a case of os odontoideum (separate odontoid process). J. Bone Joint Surg. 50A:965–972, 1969.

37. Minderhoud, J. M., Braakman, R., and Penning. L.: Os odontoideum: Clinical, radiological, and therapeutic aspects. J. Neurol. Sci. 8:521–544, 1969.

38. Nicholson, J. S., and Sherk, H. H.: Anomalies of the occipito-cervical articulation. J. Bone Joint Surg. 50A:295–304, 1968.

39. Ricciardi, J. E., Kaufer, H., and Louis, D. S.: Acquired os odontoideum following acute ligament injury. J. Bone Joint Surg. 58A:410–412, 1976.

40. Rothman, R. H., and Simeone, F. A.: The Spine, Vol. 1. Philadelphia, W. B. Saunders Co., 1975.

41. Rowland, L. P., Shapiro, J. H., and Jacobson, H. G.: Neurological syndromes associated with congenital absence of the odontoid process. Arch. Neurol. Psychiatry 80:286–291, 1958.

42. Schiff, D. C. M., and Parke, W. W.: Arterial blood supply of the odontoid process (dens). Anat. Rec. 172:399–400, 1972.

43. Schiller, F., and Nieda, I.: Malformations of the odontoid process. Report of a case and clinical survey. Calif. Med. 86:394–398, 1957.

44. Shapiro, R., Youngberg, A. S., and Rothman, S. L. G.: The differential diagnosis of traumatic lesions of the occipito-atlanto-axial segment. Radiol. Clin. North Am. 11:505–526, 1973.

45. Shepard, C. N.: Familial hypoplasia of the odontoid process. J. Bone Joint Surg. 48A:1224, 1966.

46. Sherk, H. H., and Nicholson, J. T.: Rotatory atlanto-axial dislocation associated with ossiculum terminale and mongolism. A case report. J. Bone Joint Surg. 51A:957–964, 1969.

47. Spitzer, R., Rabinowitch, J. Y., and Wybar, K. C.: A study of the abnormalities of the skull, teeth and lenses in mongolism. Can. Med. Assoc. J. 84:567–572, 1961.

48. Stratford, J.: Myelopathy caused by atlanto-axial dislocation. J. Neurosurg. 14:97–104, 1957.

49. Tredwell, S. J., and O'Brien, J. P.: Avascular necrosis of the proximal end of the dens. A complication of halo-pelvic distraction. J. Bone Joint Surg. 57A:332–336, 1975.

50. Von Torklus, D., and Gehle, W.: The Upper Cervical Spine. New York, Grune and Stratton, 1972.

51. Wadia, N. H.: Myelopathy complicating congenital atlanto-axial dislocation (a study of 28 cases). Brain 90:449–472, 1967.

52. Weinfeld, A., Ross, M. W., and Sarasohn, S. H.: Spondyloepiphyseal dysplasia tarda: A cause of premature osteoarthritis. Am. J. Roentgenol. 101:851–859, 1967.

53. Whitesides, T. E., and McDonald A. P.: Lateral retropharyngeal approach to the upper cervical spine. Orthop. Clin. North Am. 9(4):1115–1127, 1978.

54. Wollin, D. G.: The os odontoideum; Separate odontoid process. J. Bone Joint Surg. 45A:1459–1471, 1963.

Klippel-Feil Syndrome

(Congenital Synostosis of the Cervical Vertebrae; Brevicollis)

In 1912, Klippel and Feil[21] published the first complete clinical and pathologic description of this condition. Their attention was attracted to a patient who had the unusual findings of marked shortening of the neck, low posterior hairline, and severe restriction of neck motion. The patient died, and at the postmortem examination they discovered a complete fusion of the cervical vertebrae. Subsequently, Feil was able to collect 13 additional examples and published in 1919 a thesis that included his findings from this larger group and a review of the literature. The term Klippel-Feil syndrome, in its present usage, refers to all individuals with congenital fusion of the cervical vertebrae, whether it be two segments, congenital block vertebrae (Fig. 5–20), or the entire cervical spine (Fig. 5–21).

Feil originally suggested a classification based on the extent and type of the cervical fusion. However, with the exception of the area of genetics,[10, 14] this classification has not proved to be clinically useful. Rather, as additional patients were discovered and radiologic techniques were improved, it became apparent that certain anomalies of the occipitocervical junction (atlanto-occipital fusion, basilar impression, and abnormalities of the odontoid) should be considered separately from the original syndrome. Although these conditions occur commonly in conjunction with fusion of the lower cervical vertebrae, their significance is dependent upon how they influence the atlantoaxial joint. Thus, their prognostic and therapeutic implications are distinctly different, and they occur with sufficient frequency to warrant separate analysis.

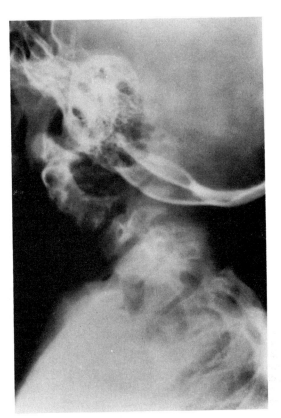

Figure 5–21. Twelve-year-old female with the Klippel-Feil syndrome and iniencephaly: enlarged foramen magnum and absent posterior laminae. Note the fixed hyperextension and the long segment of cervical fusion (C2 to C6) and an abnormal occipitocervical articulation. This pattern could be viewed as a more elaborate variation of the C2-C3 pattern of McRae. Flexion-extension and rotational forces are concentrated in the area of the abnormal occipitocervical junction. These patients may be at risk of developing instability with aging.

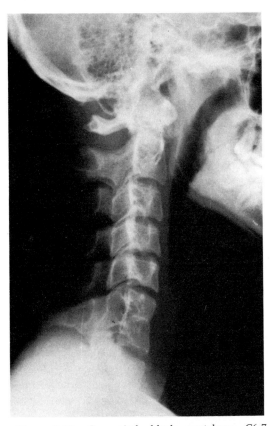

Figure 5–20. Congenital block vertebrae C6-7. Symptoms are directly related to the number and level of involved vertebrae; thus, this represents the most benign form of the Klippel-Feil syndrome.

Congenital cervical fusion is the result of failure of the normal segmentation of the cervical somites during the third to eighth week of life. With the exception of a few patients in whom this condition is inherited,[14, 15] the etiology is as yet undetermined. However, it is important to note that the effect of this embryologic abnormality is not limited to the cervical spine. The entire fetus may be adversely influenced. Patients with the Klippel-Feil syndrome, even those with minor cervical lesions, may have other less apparent or even occult defects in the genitourinary,[17, 24, 35] nervous,[4, 5] and cardiopulmonary systems[3, 29, 32] and even hearing loss.[17, 25, 34, 38] Many of these "hidden" abnormalities may be far more detrimental to the patient's general well-being than the obvious deformity of the neck. In a recent review, we found a high incidence of these related congenital anomalies (Table 5–1).[17] The Klippel-Feil syndrome should be viewed as the tip of the iceberg, and discovery of the cervical lesion should stimulate the physician to probe deeper for less visible abnormalities. This will be rewarding, as early identification and treatment can be of great benefit to the patient.

CLINICAL FINDINGS. *Clinical Appearance.* The classical clinical description of the syndrome is a triad: low posterior hairline, short neck, and limitation of neck motion (Figs. 5–22 and 5–23). Although the nature of the anatomic lesion was not discovered until the 20th century, the characteristic appearance had been recognized for centuries. There are reports in both early medical and lay literature of people "whose head appears to sit on their chest" and mythical people called Acephala (no necks).[6] Numerous art objects

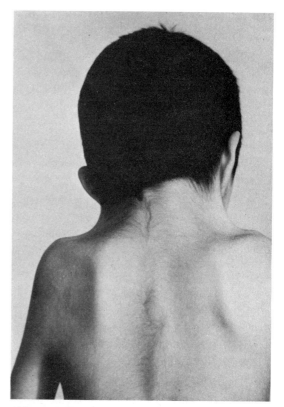

Figure 5–23. Extreme form of webbing of the neck, pterygium colli. Note low posterior hairline.

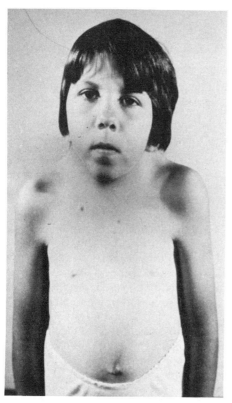

Figure 5–22. Nine-year-old with the Klippel-Feil syndrome, demonstrating short neck with a tendency to webbing, mild torticollis, and symmetry of eye level. The patient clinically has marked restriction of neck motion, impaired hearing, and mirror motions (synkinesia) of the upper extremities.

have been preserved that portray the obvious physical deformities of the Klippel-Feil syndrome.[6] The condition may exist, however, without this classic triad. Fewer than one half of the patients have all three signs.[17] Their presence is directly related to the degree of cervical spine involvement. The deformity may be severe and recognized at birth or mild and discovered as an incidental radiologic finding.

Clinically, the most consistent finding is limitation of neck motion.[14] However, if fewer than three vertebrae are fused or if only the lower cervical segments are fused, the patient will generally have no detectable limitation of neck motion.[14] Many patients with marked cervical involvement are able to maintain a deceptively good range of motion. We discovered several who clinically appeared to have mild restriction of neck motion yet were found to have 90 degrees of flexion-extension, occurring at only one open interspace (Fig. 5–24).[17] In general, flexion-extension of the neck is better preserved than rotation or lateral bending, as it occurs at the atlantoaxial articula-

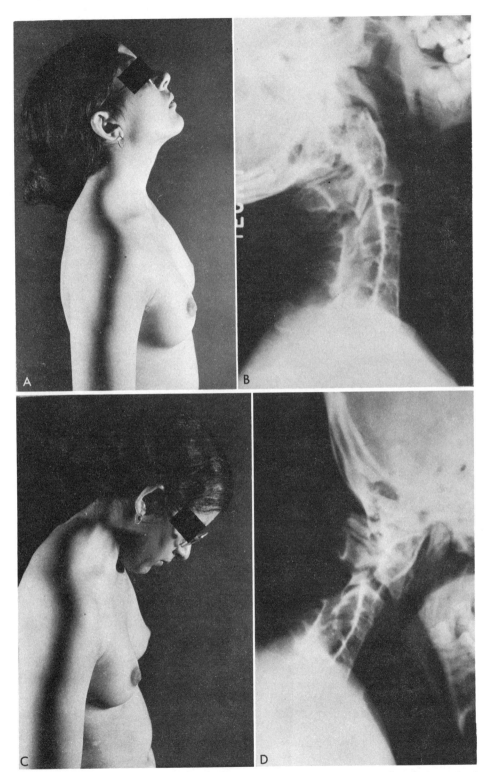

Figure 5–24. Eighteen-year-old female with the Klippel-Feil syndrome demonstrating flexion-extension of the cervical spine, both clinically (A and C) and radiologically (B and D). The majority of the neck motion is occurring at the C3-C4 disc space. Clinically the patient is able to maintain adequate range (90 degrees) of flexion-extension. At present she is asymptomatic, but with aging this hypermobile articulation may become grossly unstable.

tion, which is frequently spared. Rarely, patients will have no detectable motion and fixed hyperextension of the neck; this is usually associated with iniencephaly (absence of the posterior cervical laminae and an enlarged foramen magnum) (Fig. 5–21).[36]

Shortening of the neck, unless extreme, is a subtle finding, and similarly, a low posterior hairline does not naturally attract one's attention (Figs. 5–22 and 5–23). Approximately 20 per cent of patients with the Klippel-Feil syndrome have obvious facial asymmetry, torticollis, or webbing of the neck.[14, 17] Webbing of the neck in the extreme form is called "pterygium colli" (Fig. 5–23) and consists of large skin folds extending from the mastoid process to the acromion.[13] The underlying muscles may be involved and may give the impression of a contracted sternocleidomastoid or trapezius, but surgical release does not generally result in improved neck motion.

Sprengel's deformity is a well-known accompaniment (25 to 35 per cent), and may be unilateral or bilateral (30 per cent) (Fig. 5–25).[10, 14, 17, 24, 37] At the third week of gestation, the scapula develops from mesodermal tissue high in the neck at the level of C4. It descends into its normal thoracic position by the eighth week, or at approximately the same time that the Klippel-Feil lesion is thought to occur.[10, 14] Therefore, it is logical to expect a significant relationship between these two anomalies. Occasionally, there will be a bony bridge between the cervical spine and scapula, an omovertebral bone.

Other clinical findings that are occasionally found include ptosis of the eye, Dwayne's contracture (contracture of the lateral rectus muscle),[14] lateral rectus palsy, facial nerve palsy, and cleft or high arched palate. Abnormalities of the upper extremities include syndactyly, hypoplastic thumb, supernumerary digits, and hypoplasia of the upper extremities. Abnormalities of the lower extremities are infrequent.

Symptoms. With the exception of the anomalies that involve the atlantoaxial joint, there are no symptoms that can be directly attributed to the lower fused cervical vertebrae. All symptoms commonly associated with the Klippel-Feil syndrome originate at the open segments adjacent to the area of synostosis; these remaining free articulations may become compensatorily hypermobile. Owing to the increased demands placed on these joints or in response to trauma, this hypermobility can lead to frank instability, or early degenerative arthritis.[37] Symptoms may then arise from two sources: mechanical symptoms, due to root irritation or spinal cord compression, and neurologic symptoms. Patients having a short segment of fusion are less likely to develop symptoms,[14] as the loss of motion is adequately compensated by the remaining free segments. Patients with synostosis of the lower cervical spine are at less risk, as the limitation is minimal, and can be adequately compensated by the normally more mobile joints above. Very few children are symptomatic. The majority of patients who develop symptoms are in the second or third decade,[14] suggesting that the instability is in part a function of time with increasing ligamentous laxity. Those who have the greatest risk of developing symptoms have the following anatomic characteristics: massive involvement with more than four fused vertebrae (Fig. 5–21), fusion of the occiput to the atlas and C2 to C3, leading to excessive demands on the atlantoaxial articulation (Fig. 5–11), and an open articulation between two zones of vertebral fusion (Fig. 5–24).

Mechanical symptoms are localized to the neck and are due to stretching of the capsular structures and ligaments about the hypermobile joints. This can lead to degenerative changes in both the joint and the open disc space, resulting in the typical pain of cervical osteoarthritis (Fig. 5–33). Gray[14] noted that 39 per cent of the patients had pain; unfortunately, he did not discuss the cause.

Neurologic symptoms are generally localized to the head, neck, and upper extremities and result from direct irritation or impingement of the cervical nerve roots with radicular symptoms in the upper extremities.[27] The symptoms are usually due to constriction of the nerve root at the foramen from osteophytic spurring.[27] If the joint instability is progressive or if trauma has occurred, spinal cord impingement may result with complaints ranging from mild spasticity, hyperreflexia, and muscular weakness to sudden, complete quadriplegia following minor trauma.[14, 15, 18, 27, 37] Fortunately, there are relatively few reports of neurologic injury in the Klippel-Feil syndrome.[14] If the patient's instability is primarily in the area of the occipitocervical junction, cranial nerve symptoms may be present.

ROENTGENOGRAPHIC FEATURES. In the severely involved patient an adequate roentgenographic evaluation can be both frustrating

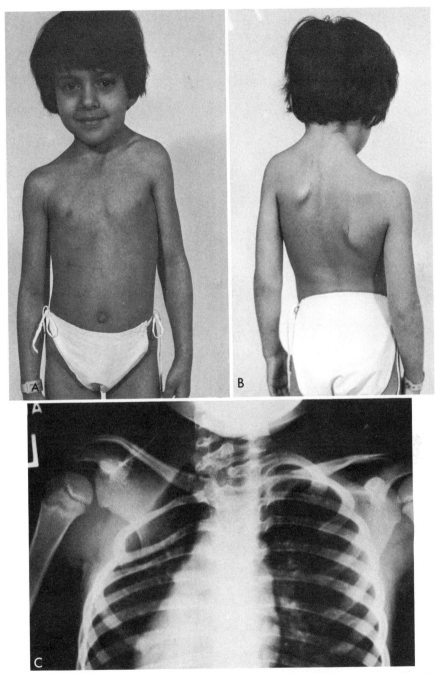

Figure 5–25. Six-year-old with the Klippel-Feil syndrome and Sprengel's deformity on the left. *A,* Frontal view. *B,* Posterior view. *C,* Roentgenographic appearance demonstrating the posterior vertebral anomalies of the cervical spine and the high-riding left scapula. Patient has subsequently had a left scapuloplasty.

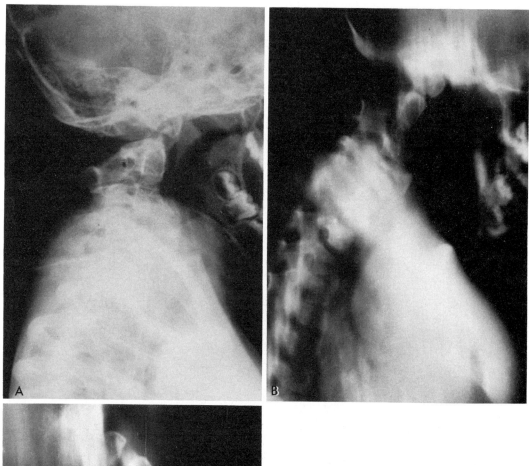

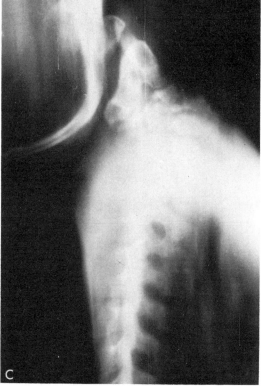

Figure 5–26. Six-year-old male with the Klippel-Feil syndrome. *A,* Routine lateral roentgenogram of the cervical spine. Overlapping shadows from the shoulder and occiput obscure much of the cervical spine. *B,* Lateral laminagram in flexion demonstrates an anterior hemivertebra (arrow), probably C4, and congenital fusion of C2-C3, C6-C7, and T3-T4. *C,* Lateral laminagram in extension demonstrates absence of the posterior ring of C1 and an unstable C1-C2 articulation. Flexion-extension laminagraphic views are helpful in providing the information necessary to evaluate children with severe deformity, particularly if vertebral instability is suspected.

and time-consuming to both the physician and technician. Fixed bony deformities frequently prevent proper positioning for standard views. Overlapping shadows from the mandible, occiput, or foramen magnum may obscure the critical upper vertebrae (Fig. 5–26A). Nonstandard views and oblique projections are frequently obtained but are confusing to interpret. In this situation, flexion-extension laminagraphic views are quite helpful in providing the information necessary to evaluate the deformity (Fig. 5–26 B and C). If vertebral instability is suspected, the study should be augmented by cineradiography. Knowledge of the normal variations in cervical spine mobility, particularly in children, is important when evaluating patients with the Klippel-Feil syndrome.[7, 39] Pseudosubluxation of C2 on C3 with flexion can be observed in 45 per cent of normal children under eight years of age (Fig. 5–8).[7] Marked angulation at a single interspace during flexion rather than a uniform arch of vertebral motion can be observed in normal children (16 per cent)[7] and may be misinterpreted as vertebral fusion below.

Fusion of cervical vertebrae is the hallmark of the Klippel-Feil syndrome. This may be simply synostosis of two bodies (congenital block vertebrae) (Figs. 5–20 and 5–27) or massive fusion of vertebrae, which was found in Klippel and Feil's first patient (Fig. 5–21).[21] Flattening and widening of the involved vertebral bodies and absent disc spaces are the most common findings. Hypoplasia of the disc space or remnants of it can often be seen (Fig. 5–24A). In the young child, narrowing of the cervical disc space cannot always be appreciated. The ossification of the vertebral body will not be complete until adolescence, and

the unossified end plates may give the false impression of a normal disc space (Fig. 5–28). With continued growth, however, the ossification of the vertebral bodies is completed, and the fusion becomes obvious. If fusion is suspected in a child, it may be confirmed by lateral flexion-extension views (Fig. 5–29). Juvenile rheumatoid arthritis (Fig. 5–30), rheumatoid spondylitis, and infection can mimic the radiologic findings, but usually, the clinical history and physical examination will indicate the correct diagnosis.

Hemivertebrae are common (Fig. 5–31); they occurred in 74 per cent of the patients in Gray's review;[14] and the incidence of occurrence increases with the number of segments fused. Fusion of the posterior elements usually parallels that of the vertebral bodies. In the young child, particular attention should be paid to the laminae, as fusion posteriorly is often more apparent than anteriorly in early life (Fig. 5–32).[17] The sagittal and transverse diameters of the spinal canal are usually normal. Narrowing of the spinal canal, if it occurs, usually takes place in adult life and is due to degenerative changes (osteoarthritic spurs) or hypermobility (Fig. 5–33).[9] Enlargement of the cervical canal is uncommon and if found, would suggest the presence of conditions such as syringomyelia, hydromyelia, or the Arnold-Chiari malformation.[8, 31] The intervertebral foramina in the fused area are usually smooth in contour but frequently are smaller than normal and oval rather than circular in shape (Fig. 5–34). Posterior spina bifida is common (45 per cent), but anterior spina bifida is rare. Rarely, there is complete absence of the posterior elements. This is usually accompanied by enlargement of the

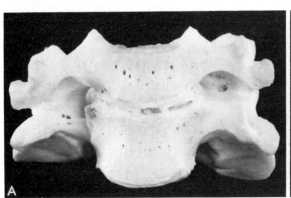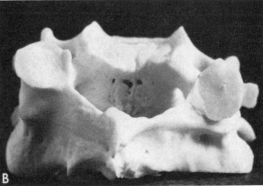

Figure 5–27. Postmortem specimen of a congenital block vertebra of C3-C4. *A*, Anterior view and *B*, posterior view. The specimen demonstrates complete fusion, but remnants of the cartilaginous vertebral endplates can still be seen.

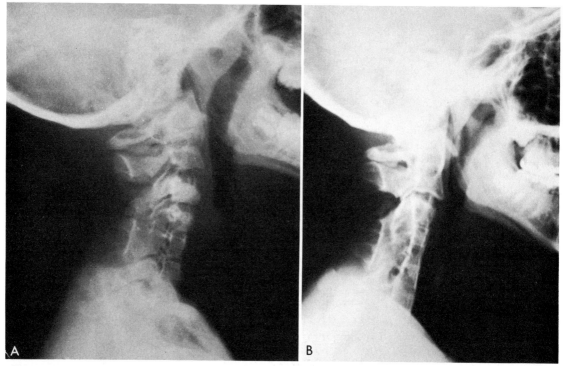

Figure 5–28. *A,* Eight-year-old demonstrating posterior fusion of the laminae and spinous processes but incomplete fusion of the vertebral bodies anteriorly. *B,* Same patient at age 19, now demonstrating complete fusion of the vertebral bodies C2-C3 and C4-C7. In children, narrowing of the cervical disc spaces cannot always be appreciated, as ossification of vertebral bodies is not completed until adolescence. The unossified cartilage end plates can give a false impression of a normal disc space.

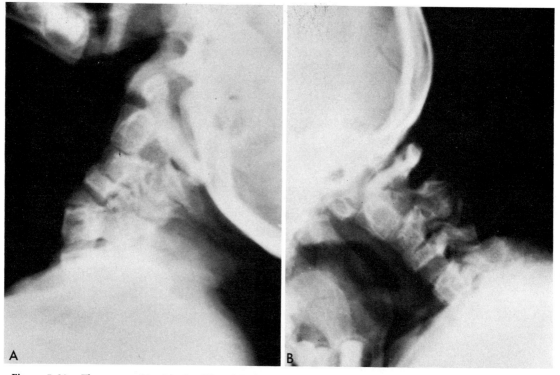

Figure 5–29. Three-year-old with the Klippel-Feil syndrome and congenital scoliosis. Lateral flexion-extension roentgenograms of the cervical spine *(A* and *B)* demonstrate that neck motion occurs predominantly between C4-C5. Flexion-extension views are helpful in determining the type and extent of congenital fusion in the young child.

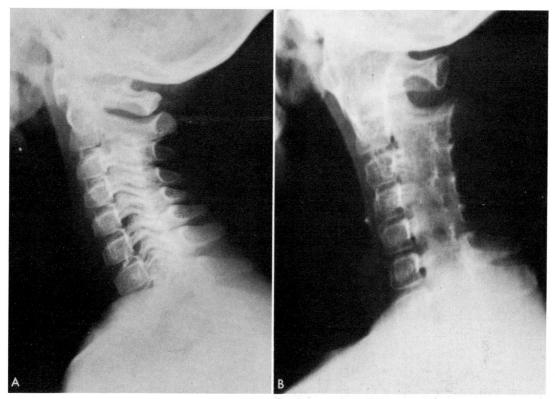

Figure 5–30. Juvenile rheumatoid arthritis. *A,* the roentgenographic appearance of the cervical spine, age five, at the onset of the rheumatoid process. *B,* Same patient at age ten with complete fusion of the laminae posteriorly and severely restricted neck motion. We would expect that with further growth these vertebral bodies will subsequently fuse.

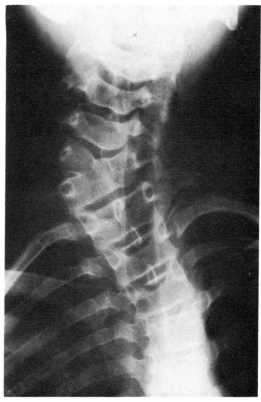

Figure 5–31. Fourteen-year-old with cervical hemivertebrae. Hemivertebrae are common in the Klippel-Feil syndrome but usually are found in the dorsal or lumbar vertebral segments.

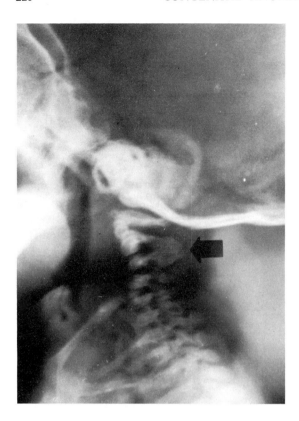

Figure 5–32. Three-month-old with the Klippel-Feil syndrome. The roentgenograms demonstrate posterior fusion of the laminae of C2-C3 (arrow). In the young child, particular attention should be paid to the laminae, as fusion posteriorly is often more apparent than anteriorly in early life.

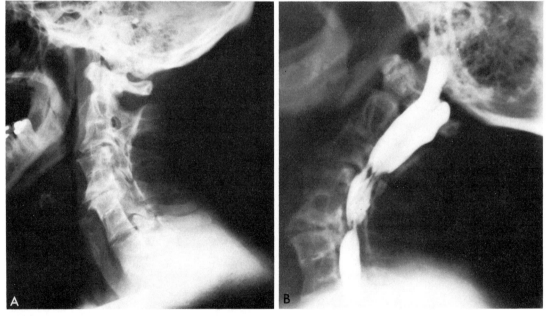

Figure 5–33. Forty-year-old male with a four-month history of persistent neck pain with radiation into upper extremities. He had no previous history of neck complaints but had a long history of occipital headaches. He recently noted paresthesias in the upper and lower extremities. Neurologic examination and EMG were within normal limits. *A,* Lateral roentgenogram of the cervical spine, demonstrating congenital fusion between C2-C3, C4-C5, and C6-C7. Note marked changes of degenerative osteoarthritis with large osteophyte formation at the open interspace of C3-C4 and C5-C6. *B,* Myelogram during extension of the cervical spine demonstrates narrowing of the spinal canal due to the large osteoarthritic spurs at C3-C4 and C5-C6. He subsequently underwent spine stabilization with relief of neck complaints.

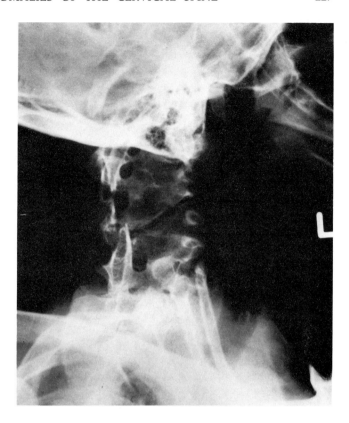

Figure 5–34. Oblique view of the cervical spine demonstrating the smooth contour of the intervertebral foramina, which are frequently smaller than normal and oval rather than circular in shape.

foramen magnum and fixed hyperextension of the neck, referred to as iniencephaly (Fig. 5–21).

All these defects may extend into the upper thoracic spine, particularly in the severely involved patient. A disturbance of the upper thoracic spine on a routine chest roentgenogram may be the first clue to an unrecognized cervical synostosis. Fused, absent, or deformed ribs are present in approximately one third of patients. It should be a routine procedure when evaluating a high thoracic congenital scoliosis that roentgenographic evaluation include lateral views of the cervical spine.

Instability. One can gain insight into the problem of instability by reviewing the lateral flexion-extension views of the Klippel-Feil patient. The type or pattern of cervical motion is dependent upon the location and extent of fused cervical vertebrae. Patients with fusion of the lower cervical vertebrae or with two or more disc spaces between fused segments seem to be at low risk for serious problems. There are, however, three high-risk patterns of cervical spine motion that potentially have a poor prognosis, either from late instability or degenerative osteoarthritis.

Pattern #1: Fusion of C2-C3 with occipitalization of the atlas (Fig. 5–11). Complications associated with this pattern were first reported in 1953 by McRae[26] and have received substantial support in the literature.[15] Flexion-extension is concentrated in the area of C1-C2. With aging, an odontoid can become hypermobile (dislocate posteriorly), narrowing the spinal canal and compromising the spinal cord and brain stem.

Pattern #2: A Long Fusion with an Abnormal Occipitocervical Junction (Fig. 5–21). This is similar to the C2-C3 fusion of McRae and could be viewed as a more elaborate variation. The forces of flexion-extension and rotation are concentrated in the area of the abnormal odontoid or poorly developed ring of C1, which cannot withstand the wear and tear of aging. It is important to differentiate this pattern from the patient with a long fusion and a normal C1-C2 articulation (Fig. 5–35), which is usually compatible with normal life expectancy.

Pattern #3: Single Open Interspace Between Two Fused Segments (Fig. 5–36). In this situation, cervical spine motion is concentrated at the single open articulation. In some patients this hypermobility may lead to frank

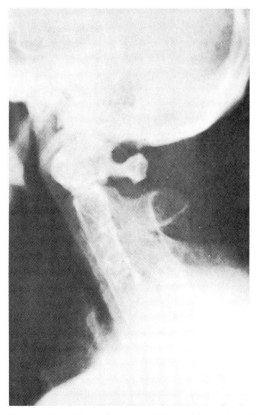

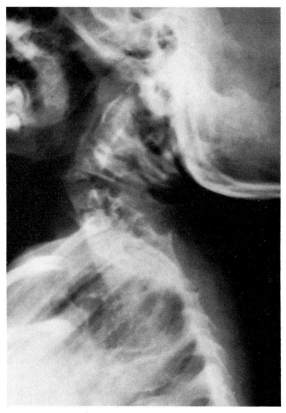

Figure 5–35. Forty-five-year-old male with the Klippel-Feil syndrome and complete fusion of C2-C7. Flexion-extension occurs only at the atlantoaxial articulation. The patient has no symptoms referable to the neck despite two previous serious falls. This pattern appears to be relatively safe, as the normal occipitocervical junction serves as a protection from late instability.

Figure 5–36. Open interspace between two fused segments. Seven-year-old with the Klippel-Feil syndrome; flexion-extension motion of the neck occurs primarily at one interspace. The cervical spine appears to angle or hinge at this point. This is a worrisome pattern, as wear and tear of aging may lead to early degenerative change or instability and narrowing of the spinal canal.

instability or degenerative osteoarthritis (Fig. 5–33).[15, 27, 37] This pattern can be easily recognized, as the cervical spine appears to angle or hinge at the open segment.

ASSOCIATED CONDITIONS (Table 5–1). *Scoliosis.* Scoliosis is the most frequent anomaly found in association with this syndrome.[17, 24] Sixty per cent of these patients have a significant degree of scoliosis (greater than 15 degrees by the Cobb method), kypho-

sis,[17] or both. The majority of these patients will require treatment and should be followed through the growth years. The roentgenographic examinations should include lateral views of the spine, as a progressive kyphosis may make the need for treatment of the scoliosis more urgent. If the deformity is recognized early, many children can be successfully controlled with standard spinal orthoses, such as the Milwaukee brace.[17] At present, the majori-

TABLE 5–1. ABNORMALITIES ASSOCIATED WITH THE KLIPPEL-FEIL SYNDROME

Common	Percentage	Less Common
Scoliosis	60	Ptosis
Renal abnormalities	35	Dwayne's contracture
Sprengel's deformity	30	Lateral rectus palsy
Deafness	30	Facial nerve palsy
Synkinesia	20	Syndactyly
Congenital heart disease	14	Hypoplastic thumb
		Upper extremity hypoplasia

ty of these patients have required posterior spine stabilization, in part owing to the late recognition.[17, 24, 30, 37]

Two types of scoliosis can be identified: congenital scoliosis due to vertebral anomalies and differential growth patterns (Fig. 5–37) and compensatory scoliosis below the area of vertebral involvement. In our series, congenital scoliosis is the most common (55 per cent), and in more than one half of the children, the curvature was progressive and required treatment.[17] The majority (75 per cent) required posterior spinal fusion to arrest an increasing deformity, and the remainder were controlled with a brace or cast.[17]

Of interest is the frequent occurrence of progressive scoliosis in the normal-appearing vertebrae below the primary congenital curve.

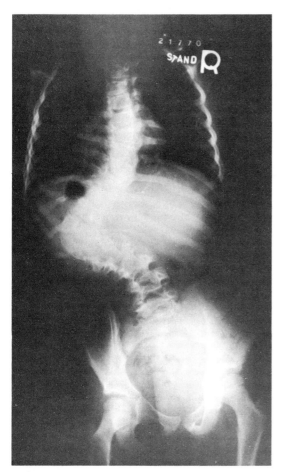

Figure 5–37. Eight-year-old with the Klippel-Feil syndrome. Deafness and severe kyphoscoliosis subsequently required halofemoral traction and posterior spine fusion.

If only the congenitally involved segments are examined in follow-up, an increasing compensatory scoliosis in the lower vertebrae may not be recognized, and its significance might not be appreciated until serious deformity results.

When surgical intervention is required, the same principles apply as discussed in Chapter 6 (Congenital Scoliosis). When spinal fusion is performed, the orthopedist should carefully consider the overall alignment of the patient's spine. The temptation to achieve maximum radiologic correction of the mobile segments must be tempered by careful consideration of the congenitally fixed segments. Failure to observe this principle may result in an unbalanced spine; the patient will have traded one deformity for another that may be even worse than the original.

Documented progression of scoliosis, whether in the congenitally distorted elements or the compensatory curve below, demands immediate and appropriate treatment to prevent serious additional deformity. Scoliosis in the thoracic area should not be allowed to progress beyond 55 degrees by the Cobb method in the erect position, as further increase will seriously compromise pulmonary function.[3, 17] More subtle or occult abnormalities can lead to respiratory difficulty in some Klippel-Feil patients. Abnormal rib spacing, congenital fusion of the ribs, and deformed costovertebral joints may inhibit full expansion of the rib cage during respiration.[2] Although it may not cause an angular deformity, fusion of the thoracic vertebrae may decrease the size of the thoracic cage. The spondylothoracic dwarf may represent a severe form of this problem, leading to early death from respiratory failure.[30] Krieger[22] has recently reported on the relationship of occult respiratory dysfunction and craniovertebral anomalies. He notes that in addition to the obvious problems of bony impingement or traction upon the brain stem, these patients may have intrinsic malformation of the nervous system or disturbances of cerebrospinal fluid that may adversely affect respiratory function.

This information has particular application when cervical distraction devices are contemplated in the treatment of scoliosis (halofemoral or halopelvic traction). When the use of such a device is considered, the physician should be aware that children with the Klippel-Feil syndrome may be more susceptible to neurologic or vascular injury.[17]

Renal Abnormalities. In the Klippel-Feil

syndrome, more than one third of the patients can be expected to have a significant urinary tract anomaly.[17, 28] The condition is often asymptomatic in the young child,[15] and intravenous pyelography should be a routine procedure for these children (Fig. 5–38). This parallels the incidence of renal anomalies associated with congenital scoliosis of 20 per cent.[23] The pronephros, the embryologic tissue destined to become the genitourinary tract, develops between the seventh and fourteenth somites, in the same region and at the same time as the cervical spine,[1, 28] quite similar to the scapulae in Sprengel's deformity.

The most frequent abnormality is unilateral absence of the kidney. Other abnormalities include double-collecting system, renal ectopia, horseshoe kidney, hydronephrosis from ureteropelvic obstruction, and less frequently, anomalies of the vagina and genitalia.[28] We found that two of our 50 patients

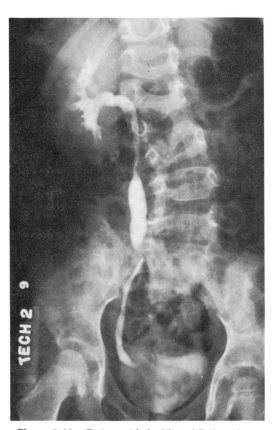

Figure 5–38. Patient with the Klippel-Feil syndrome. Roentgenograms demonstrate multiple vertebral anomalies, unilateral absence of the kidney, and hydroureter. This patient required ureteral reimplantation for ureteral reflux and hydronephrosis.

developed severe pyelonephritis in their remaining kidney, requiring renal transplantation.[17] Indeed, in Klippel and Feil's original case report, the patient died from nephritis, not from the massive cervical fusion that first attracted their attention.[21] Comprehensive follow-up of the patient with the Klippel-Feil syndrome must include renal evaluation. Abnormalities in this area may prove to be life-threatening and of greater consequence to the patient than those of the cervical spine.

Cardiovascular Abnormalities. The literature notes the association of the Klippel-Feil syndrome with congenital heart disease (4.2 to 14 per cent).[12, 17, 29, 32] The most common lesion reported has been an interventricular septal defect occurring alone or in combination with other defects, such as a patent ductus arteriosus or abnormal positioning of the heart and aorta.

Deafness. The association of hearing impairment and even deafness with the Klippel-Feil syndrome (30 per cent) has been reported in the otology literature.[19, 25, 34, 38] It has seldom been mentioned in orthopaedic reports.[17, 24] Other otologic defects include the absence of the auditory canal and microtia. Jalladeau[19] is credited with the first report of deafness associated with the Klippel-Feil syndrome; in his group of 20 patients, 30 per cent were deaf mutes. Stark[38] noted that detailed audiologic data are not yet available, and the precise defect is often not known. There is no characteristic audiologic anomaly, and all types of hearing loss (conductive, sensorineural, and mixed) have been described. Patients with the Klippel-Feil syndrome should have an audiometric test when the diagnosis of this syndrome is first made. The relationship between hearing loss and speech and language retardation is well documented. Early detection of hearing impairment can reduce the retardation by permitting early initiation of speech and language training.[38]

Mirror Motions (Synkinesia). Synkinesia consists of involuntary paired movements of the hands and occasionally the arms. The patient is unable to move one hand without similar reciprocal motion of the opposite hand. Mirror motions were first described by Bauman, who found this phenomenon in four of six patients with the Klippel-Feil syndrome.[5] This condition has been found to occur occasionally in normal preschool children and patients with cerebral palsy or Parkinson's disease. However, the majority of patients afflicted with this problem have the

Klippel-Feil syndrome.[10] Approximately 20 per cent will demonstrate mirror motions clinically.[17] Baird,[4] in examining 13 patients with the Klippel-Feil syndrome using electromyography found 10 patients with electrically detectable paired motion in the opposite extremity. This suggests that many patients may be subclinically affected and more clumsy at two-handed activities. Some authors have suggested it should be included as part of the syndrome.[4, 10]

The etiology of synkinesia is unknown, but it appears to be a separate congenital neurologic defect and not due to bony impingement or irritation of the spinal cord. Examination of two autopsy specimens suggests that the clinical findings are due to inadequate or incomplete decussation of the pyramidal tracts in conjunction with a dysraphic cervical cord.[3, 16] As a consequence, cerebral control over the upper extremities must follow less direct pathways located in the extrapyramidal system, and the afflicted individual requires more extensive practice to disassociate the movements of the individual extremities.

Synkinesia is most pronounced in the young child, particularly under five years of age. Fortunately, the condition tends to improve with age. Occupational therapy has been helpful in teaching the patient individual control over the extremities or at least to disguise the reciprocal motion to a tolerable cosmetic level. Still, many patients may find discriminating two-handed activity difficult,[33] such as playing the piano, typing, sewing, or ladder climbing. The clinician should be aware of this disability, so that he or she can help the patient choose activities and a career that will accommodate this handicap.

TREATMENT. The minimally involved patient with the Klippel-Feil syndrome can be expected to lead a normal, active life with no or only minor restrictions or symptoms. Many of the severely involved patients can enjoy the same good prognosis if early and appropriate treatment is instituted where needed. This is particularly applicable in the area of associated scoliosis and renal abnormalities. Prevention of further deformity or complications can be of great benefit to the patient, both in longevity and quality of life. The actual treatment in the patient with the Klippel-Feil syndrome is confined mostly to the area of associated conditions and has been included under their respective headings.

At present, treatment modalities for the cervical spinal anomalies are quite limited. Those patients with major areas of cervical synostosis or high-risk patterns of cervical spine motion should be strongly advised to avoid activities that place stress on the cervical spine. In these patients, the mobile articulations are under greater mechanical demands and are less capable of protecting the patient against traumatic insults.

Sudden neurologic compromise or death following minor trauma have been reported in the Klippel-Feil syndrome and are usually due to disruption at the hypermobile articulation.[15, 27, 37] The role of prophylactic surgical stabilization in the asymptomatic patient has not yet been defined. There is no satisfactory answer to the questions of when does hypermobility become instability or when does the risk of instability warrant further reduction of neck motion. Some insight can be gained by radiologic examination and cineradiography. The ultimate decision will rest with the physician and the patient. If the instability is found in the region of the occipitocervical junction, more specific data are available.

For the patient with mechanical symptoms, the usual treatment measures for degenerative osteoarthritis are applicable and include traction, use of a cervical collar, and analgesics. Symptoms that suggest neurologic compromise need careful consideration and evaluation by a neurologist, neurosurgeon, and orthopedist (Fig. 5–33). The exact area of irritation must be determined prior to surgical intervention. An attempt should be made preoperatively to obtain reduction of the bony architecture prior to surgical stabilization. Operative reduction has proved extremely hazardous. The physician must be mindful that there may be other associated abnormalities, both in the brain stem and in the spinal cord itself, which may be contributing to the symptoms.

Treatment of cosmetic aspects of this deformity has met with limited success. Occasionally, children with the fixed torticollis posture may be improved with bracing (Fig. 5–39). This, however, requires long-term application and excellent patient cooperation. Surgical correction of the bony deformity by direct means such as wedge osteotomy is not recommended and may have tragic results.[6, 14] Occasionally, carefully selected patients who have cervical congenital scoliosis may obtain some correction and improvement of appearance by use of the halo-cast combined with posterior cervical fusion. Bonola[6] described a

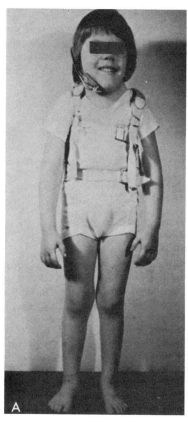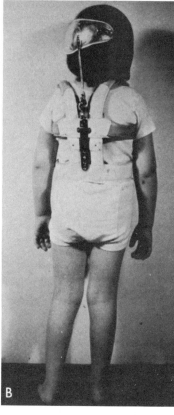

Figure 5–39. Four-year-old with a bony torticollis secondary to the Klippel-Feil syndrome undergoing treatment with a brace. *A*, Frontal view. *B*, Posterior view.

method of rib resection to attain an apparent increase in neck length and motion. This procedure is an extensive surgical experience, however, and is a great risk to the patient. No subsequent reports have appeared in the literature.

Soft tissue procedures, Z-plasty, and muscle resection may achieve cosmetic improvement in properly selected patients.[24] These procedures generally do not increase neck motion, and the scars may be extensive, particularly in the patient with a large skin web. A common problem is implanting hair-bearing skin to the top of the shoulders.

Surgical treatment of Sprengel's deformity in properly selected patients can provide considerable cosmetic brenefit. It can restore a more natural contour to the shoulders and neck as well as an apparent increase in neck length. If an omovertebral bone is present, its removal may permit an increase in neck and shoulder motion. The surgeon should be aware that the risk of brachial plexus injury from traction is higher in patients with the Klippel-Feil syndrome, as they are likely to have anomalous origins of the cervical nerve

roots. Iniencephaly and absence of the posterior cervical elements (Fig. 5–21) may be associated with Sprengel's deformity and must be identified if surgical correction is considered.[36]

SUMMARY

The Klippel-Feil syndrome is an uncommon condition due to congenital fusion of two or more cervical vertebrae. The majority of afflicted individuals are asymptomatic or have a mild restriction of neck motion. If symptoms referable to the cervical spine occur, it is usually in adult life and is due to degenerative arthritis or instability of the hypermobile articulations adjacent to the area of synostosis. The majority respond to conservative treatment measures, and a small percentage will require judicious surgical stabilization. Cosmetic surgery is of limited benefit in treatment of the neck deformity.

The relatively good prognosis of the cervical lesion is overshadowed by the "hidden" or unrecognized associated anomalies. The high incidence of significant scoliosis, renal anomalies, deafness, neurologic malformations, Sprengel's deformity, and cardiac anomalies should be of great concern to the physician. Early recognition and treatment of these problems may be of substantial benefit, sparing the patient further deformity or serious illness.

References

1. Arey, L. B.: Developmental Anatomy. A Textbook and Laboratory Manual of Embryology, 7th ed. Philadelphia, W. B. Saunders Co., 1965, pp. 404–407.

2. Avery, L. W., and Rentfro, C. C.: The Klippel-Feil syndrome: A pathologic report. Arch. Neurol. Psychiatry 36:1068–1076, 1936.

3. Baga, N., Chusid, E. L., and Miller, A.: Pulmonary disability in the Klippel-Feil syndrome. Clin Orthop. 67:105–110, 1969.

4. Baird, P. A., Robinson, C. G., and Buckler, W. St. J.: Klippel-Feil syndrome. Am. J. Dis. Child. 113:546–551, 1967.

5. Bauman, G. I.: Absence of the cervical spine. Klippel-Feil syndrome. J.A.M.A. 98:129–132, 1932.

6. Bonola, A.: Surgical treatment of the Klippel-Feil syndrome. J. Bone Joint Surg. 38B:440–449, 1956.

7. Cattell, H. S., and Filtzer, D. L.: Pseudosubluxation and other normal variations in the cervical spine in children. J. Bone Joint Surg. 47A:1295–1309, 1965.

8. Dolan, K. D.: Expanding lesions of the cervical canal. Radiol. Clin North Am. 15:203–214, 1977.

9. Epstein, J. A., Carras, R., Epstein, B. S., and Levine, L. S.: Myelopathy in cervical spondylosis with vertebral subluxation and hyperlordosis. J. Neurosurg. 32:421–426, 1970.

10. Erskine, C. A.: An analysis of the Klippel-Feil syndrome. Arch. Pathol. 41:269–281, 1946.

11. Feil, A.: L'absence et la diminution des vertebres cervicales (étude clinique et pathogenique): Le syndrome de reduction numerique cervicale. Theses de Paris, 1919.

12. Forney, W. R., Robinson, S. J., and Pascoe, D. J.: Congenital heart disease, deafness, and skeletal malformations: A new syndrome? J. Pediatr. 68:14–26, 1966.

13. Frawley, J. M.: Congenital webbing. Am. J. Dis Child. 29:799–805, 1925.

14. Gray, S. W., Romaine, C. B., and Skandalakis, J. E.: Congenital fusion of the cervical vertebrae. Surg. Gynecol. Obstet. 118:373–385, 1964.

15. Gunderson, C. H., Greenspan, R. H., Glaser, G. H., and Lubs, H. A.: Klippel-Feil syndrome: Genetic and clinical reevaluation of cervical fusion. Medicine 46:491–512, 1967.

16. Gunderson, C. H., and Solitare, B. G.: Mirror movements in patients with the Klippel-Feil syndrome: neuropathic observations. Arch. Neurol. 18:675–679, 1968.

17. Hensinger, R. N., Lang, J. R., and MacEwen, G. D.: Klippel-Feil syndrome: A constellation of associated anomalies. J. Bone Joint Surg. 56A:1246–1253, 1974.

18. Illingsworth, R. S.: Attacks of unconsciousness in association with fused cervical vertebrae. Arch. Dis. Child. 31:8–11, 1956.

19. Jalladeau, J.: Malformations congenitales associées au syndrome de Klippel-Feil. Theses de Paris, 1936.

20. Kirkham, T. J.: Cervico-oculo-acusticus syndrome with pseudopapilloedema. Arch. Dis. Child. 44:504–508, 1969.

21. Klippel, M., and Feil, A.: Un cas d'absence des vertebres cervicales avec cage thoracique remontant jusqu'a la base du craine. Nouv. Icon. Salpetriere 25:223–250, 1912.

22. Krieger, A. J., Rosomoff, H. L., Kuperman, A. S., and Zingesser, L. J.: Occult respiratory dysfunction in a craniovertebral anomaly. J. Neurosurg. 31:15–20, 1969.

23. MacEwen, G. D., Winter, R. B., and Hardy, J. H.: Evaluation of kidney anomalies in congenital scoliosis. J. Bone Joint Surg. 54A:1451–1454, 1972.

24. McElfresh, E., and Winter, R.: Klippel-Feil syndrome. Minn. Med. 56:353–357, 1973.

25. McLay, K., and Maran, A. G.: Deafness and the Klippel-Feil syndrome. J. Laryngol. 83:175–184, 1969.

26. McRae, D. L.: Bony abnormalities in the region of the foramen magnum: Correlation of the anatomic and neurologic findings. Acta Radiol. 40:335–354, 1953.

27. Michie, I., and Clark, M.: Neurological syndromes associated with cervical and craniocervical anomalies. Arch. Neurol. 18:241–247, 1968.

28. Moore, W. B., Matthews, T. J., and Rabinowitz, R.: Genitourinary anomalies associated with Klippel-Feil syndrome. J. Bone Joint Surg. 57A:355–357, 1975.

29. Morrison, S. G., Perry, L. W., and Scott, L. P.: Congenital brevicollis (Klippel-Feil syndrome) and cardiovascular anomalies. Am. J. Dis. Child. 115:614–620, 1968.

30. Moseley, J. E., and Bonforte, R. J.: Spondylothoracic dysplasia — a syndrome of congenital anomalies. Am. J. Roentgenol. 106:166–169, 1969.

31. Naik, D. R.: Cervical spinal canal in normal infants. Clin. Radiol. 21:323–326, 1970.

32. Nora, J. J., Cohen, M., and Maxwell, G. M.: Klippel-Feil syndrome with congenital heart disease. Am. J. Dis. Child. 102:858–864, 1961.

33. Notermans, S. L. H., Go, K. G., and Boonstra, S.: EMG studies of associated movements in a patient with Klippel-Feil syndrome. Psychiatr. Neurol. Neurochir. 73:257–266, 1970.

34. Palant, D. I., and Carter, B. L.: Klippel-Feil syndrome and deafness. Am. J. Dis. Child. 123:218–221, 1972.

35. Ramsey, J., and Bliznak, J.: Klippel-Feil syndrome with renal agenesis and other anomalies. Am. J. Roentgenol. 113:460–463, 1971.

36. Sherk, H. H., Shut, L., and Chung, S.: Iniencephalic deformity of the cervical spine with Klippel-Feil anomalies and congenital elevation of the scapula. J. Bone Joint Surg. 56A:1254–1259, 1974.

37. Shoul, M. I., and Ritvo, M.: Clinical and roentgenological manifestations of the Klippel-Feil syndrome (congenital fusion of the cervical vertebrae, brevicollis): Report of eight additional cases and review of the literature. Am. J. Roentgenol. 68:369–385, 1952.

38. Stark, E. W., and Borton, T. E.: Hearing loss and the Klippel-Feil syndrome. Am. J. Dis. Child. 123:233–235, 1972.

39. Sullivan, C. R., Bruwer, A. J., and Harris, L. E.: Hypermobility of the cervical spine in children: A pitfall in the diagnosis of cervical dislocation. Am. J. Surg. 95:636–640, 1958.

Congenital Muscular Torticollis

(Congenital Wryneck)

This is a common condition usually discovered in the first six to eight weeks of life. The deformity is due to contracture of the sternocleidomastoid muscle, with the head tilted toward the involved side and the chin rotated toward the contralateral shoulder (Fig. 5–40A). If the infant is examined within the first four weeks of life, a mass, or "tumor," is usually palpable in the neck.[9] It is generally a nontender, soft enlargement, which is mobile beneath the skin and attached to or located within the body of the sternocleidomastoid muscle (Fig. 5–41). The mass attains maximum size within the first month of life and then gradually regresses. If the child is examined after four to six months of age, the tumor is usually absent, and the contracture of the sternocleidomastoid muscle and torticollis posture are the only clinical findings (Fig. 5–42). The mass is frequently unrecognized and, as Coventry and Harris noted, was undetected in 80 per cent of their patients.[3] However, only one baby in seven with a sternocleidomastoid tumor subsequently develops congenital muscular torticollis.[11]

If the condition is progressive, deformities of the face and skull can result and are usually apparent within the first year. Flattening of the face on the side of the contracted sternocleidomastoid muscle may be particularly impressive (Fig. 5–40A). This deformity is probably due to the position that is assumed when sleeping (Fig. 5–40B). Children in the United States generally sleep prone,[1] and in this position it is more comfortable for them to have the affected side down. As a consequence, the face remodels to conform to the bed. In children who sleep supine, reverse modeling of the contralateral aspect of the skull (plagiocephaly) will be evident. If the condition remains untreated during the growth years, the level of the eyes and ears becomes distorted and may result in considerable cosmetic deformity, an infrequent finding since most children have come to treatment before that time.

ETIOLOGY. At present, congenital muscular torticollis is believed to be the result of local trauma of the soft tissues of the neck at the time of delivery. Birth records of affected children demonstrate a preponderance of breech or difficult forceps deliveries or primiparous births.[9, 11] However, it should be noted that the deformity has occurred following otherwise normal deliveries and has been reported in infants born by cesarean section.[9, 11] Microscopic examinations of resected surgical specimens[11] and experimental work with dogs[2] suggests that the lesion is due to occlusion of the venous outflow of the sternocleidomastoid muscle. This results in edema, degeneration of

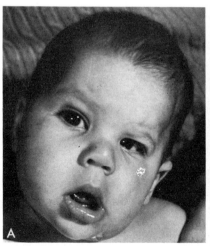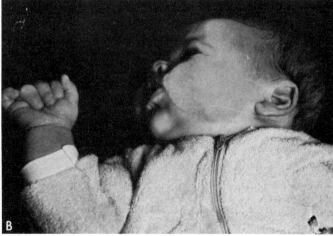

Figure 5–40. Six-month-old infant with right-sided congenital muscular torticollis. *A*, Note the rotation of the skull, asymmetry and flattening of the face, and depression adjacent to the left eye on the side of the contracted sternocleidomastoid. *B*, The patient with the head resting on glass and photographed from below. Note how the face conforms to the surface. When the child sleeps, usually prone, it is more comfortable to have the affected side down, and consequently the face remodels to conform to the bed.

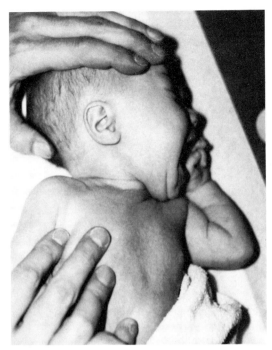

Figure 5–41. Six-week-old infant with swelling in the region of the sternocleodomastoid muscle. The mass is usually soft, nontender, and mobile beneath the skin but is attached to the muscle.

muscle fibers, and eventually fibrosis of the muscle body. Coventry[3] suggests that the clinical deformity is related to the ratio of fibrosis to remaining functional muscle. If sufficient normal muscle is present, the sternocleidomastoid will stretch with growth, and the child will not develop a torticollis posture, whereas if there is a predominance of fibrosis, there is very little elastic potential. There are two additional factors that as yet are not explained. In three of four children, the lesion is on the right side,[9, 11] and 20 per cent of the children with congenital muscular torticollis have congenital dysplasia of the hip (Fig. 5–43).[7] This may be related to uterine malposition as proposed by Coventry[3] or the mode of presentation during breech delivery. Roentgenograms of the cervical spine should be obtained to rule out a congenital anomaly of the cervical spine.

TREATMENT. Excellent results can be obtained in the majority of patients with conservative measures.[3, 9, 11] Coventry[3] found that 90 per cent of his patients responded to stretching exercises alone. We recommend that exercises begin immediately upon recognition of the condition. The exercises should be performed by the parent with guidance from the physical therapist and physician. Standard maneuvers include positioning of the ear opposite the contracted muscle to the shoulder, and positioning of the chin to the shoulder on the affected side. It must be emphasized that when adequate stretching has been obtained in the neutral position, these maneuvers should be repeated with the head hyperextended. This will achieve maximal stretching and prevent residual contractures. Other treatment measures include positioning of the crib and toys so that the neck will be

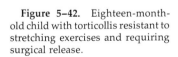

Figure 5–42. Eighteen-month-old child with torticollis resistant to stretching exercises and requiring surgical release.

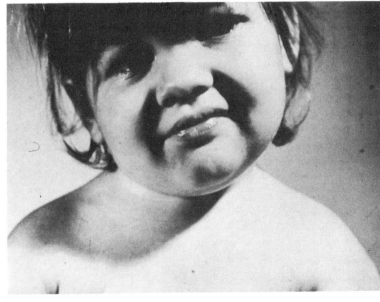

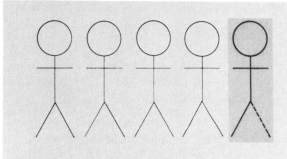

one in five requires treatment

Figure 5–43. Twenty per cent of children with congenital muscular torticollis have congenital dysplasia of the hip.

stretched when trying to reach and grasp. The parent should discourage sleep patterns that perpetuate the deformity and the facial deformation. There is no apparent indication for surgical removal of the mass, as it will spontaneously disappear in early infancy.

If conservative measures are unsuccessful, surgical intervention will be required. The surgery should be performed prior to school age, usually after the patient has achieved adequate size and health to tolerate elective general anesthesia (Fig. 5–43).[10] The timing of such procedures is of little importance, as a good, but not perfect, cosmetic result can be obtained as late as 12 years of age.[3] Asymmetry of the skull and face will correct as long as adequate growth potential remains after the sternocleidomastoid is released.[3, 10]

Surgery consists of resection of a portion of the distal sternocleidomastoid muscle (Fig. 5–44). At least a 1 cm. segment of the tendon should be removed to guard against anomalous reattachment and recurrence of the deformity. A transverse incision is made low in the neck to coincide with a normal skin fold.[14] It is important not to place the incision near or over the clavicle, as scars in this area tend to spread and are cosmetically unacceptable (Fig. 5–45).[10] Similarly, closures with a subcuticular suture is preferred.[10] The most common postoperative complaint is disfiguring scars.[10, 11, 14] The two heads of the sternocleidomastoid are identified, and both are sectioned (Fig. 5–44). It is important to release the investing fascia about the sternocleidomastoid, as this too is frequently contracted.[10]

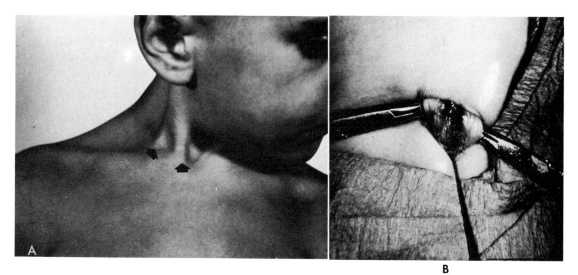

B

Figure 5–44. *A,* Clinical appearance of a six-year-old with congenital muscular torticollis. Note the appearance of the two heads of the sternocleidomastoid (arrows). *B,* Operative exposure of the same patient demonstrating complete replacement with fibrous tissue of the two heads of the sternocleidomastoid.

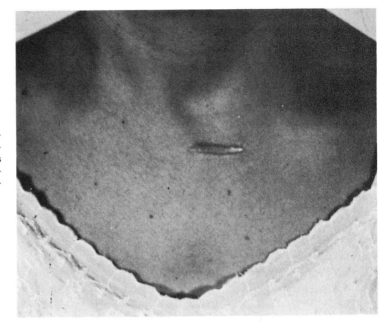

Figure 5–45. Older patient following resection of a portion of the sternocleidomastoid. The incision was placed too near the clavicle and consequently spread, becoming cosmetically unacceptable.

Rotation of the chin and head at this point will generally reveal the adequacy of the surgery, and palpation of the neck will demonstrate any extraneous tight bands that could lead to a partial recurrence or incomplete correction (Fig. 5–46).[8] In the older child, an accessory incision is often required to section the muscle at its origin on the mastoid process. The whole muscle should not be excised, as this may lead to reverse torticollis[11] or additional deformity from asymmetry in the contour of the neck.[10]

The postoperative regimen includes passive stretching exercises in the same manner as preoperatively and should begin as soon as the patient will tolerate manipulation of the neck. Occasionally, head traction at night, particularly with an older child, will be helpful.[10] A brace or cast may be needed following the surgery to maintain the corrected position, particularly in the older child or the young child who has a strong tendency to hold the head in the deformed position.[10] Results of surgery have been uniformly good with a low

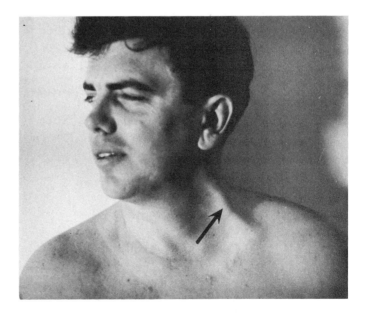

Figure 5–46. Twenty-three-year-old male who has undergone release of the sternocleidomastoid. The patient has a residual fascial band (arrow) and slight restriction of neck motion.

incidence of complications or recurrence, and nearly all patients are pleased with the result.[3, 9, 11] Slight restriction of neck motion and anomalous reattachment occur frequently but generally are unnoticed by the patient.[10, 11, 14] In the young child, facial asymmetry can be expected to resolve unless there is persistence of the torticollis, particularly from residual fascial bands (Fig. 5–46).

DIFFERENTIAL DIAGNOSIS OF TORTICOLLIS (Table 5–2). Torticollis, or wryneck, is a common childhood complaint. The etiology is diverse, and identifying the cause can pose a difficult diagnostic problem. If the posturing of the head and neck is noted at or shortly following birth, congenital anomalies of the cervical spine should be considered. Bony problems, particularly those that involve the occipitocervical junction, are frequently accompanied by torticollis. The clinical finding of torticollis may be present in the Klippel-Feil syndrome (20 per cent, p. 216),[6] basilar impression (68 per cent, p. 189), and nearly all patients with atlanto-occipital fusion (p. 202). Unlike muscular torticollis, the sternocleidomastoid muscle on the short side is not contracted.

If torticollis is noted in the weeks following delivery, the usual cause will be congenital muscular torticollis. If the child is less than two months of age, a palpable lump may be found in the sternocleidomastoid. Congenital muscular torticollis is painless, is associated with a contracted or shortened sternocleidomastoid muscle, and is unaccompanied by any bony abnormalities or neurologic deficit. Soft tissue problems are less common and include abnormal skin webs or folds (pterygium colli), which maintain the torticollis posture (Fig. 5–18). Tumors in the region of the sternocleidomastoid, cystic hygroma, branchial cleft cyst, and thyroid teratoma are rare but should be considered.

In later childhood, bacterial or viral pharyngitis and involvement of cervical nodes is the primary cause of torticollis. Spontaneous atlantoaxial rotatory subluxation may follow acute pharyngitis.[5] Radiographic confirmation is difficult, and the methods for evaluation suggested by Fielding should be used.[5] Early diagnosis and reduction of the displacement is important. If it becomes fixed it poses a considerable treatment problem.

Persistent torticollis may be the first manifestation of rheumatoid arthritis. This may pose a diagnostic problem, as often initially the child presents with normal roentgenograms and laboratory studies. The diagnosis may be suspected if other joints become involved, or a favorable response to a trial of aspirin may provide presumptive evidence of juvenile rheumatoid arthritis.

Traumatic causes should always be considered and carefully excluded early in the evaluation. If unrecognized, they may have serious neurologic consequences. In general, torticollis most commonly follows injury to the C1-C2 articulation. Minor trauma can lead to spontaneous C1-C2 subluxation. Fractures or dislocation of the odontoid may not be apparent in the initial roentgenographic views (Fig. 5–5), and consequently a high index of suspicion and careful follow-up is required. Children with bone dysplasia, Morquio's syndrome (p. 308), spondyloepiphyseal dysplasia (p. 299), and Down's syndrome have a high incidence of C1-C2 instability and should be evaluated routinely.

Neurologic problems, particularly space-occupying lesions of the central nervous system, such as tumors of the posterior fossa or spinal column and syringomyelia, are often accompanied by torticollis. Generally there will be additional neurologic findings, such as long tract signs and weakness in the upper extremities. Uncommon causes include problems of hearing and vision, which have been known to lead to head tilt, and acute calcification of a cervical disc,[12, 13] which can be

---

TABLE 5–2. DIFFERENTIAL DIAGNOSIS OF TORTICOLLIS

Congenital
  Congenital muscular torticollis (p. 234)
  Klippel-Feil syndrome (p. 216)
  Basilar impressions (p. 189)
  Atlanto-occipital fusion (p. 202)
  Pterygium colli (skin webs) (p. 220)
  Odontoid anomalies (p. 205)
Neurologic
  Ocular dysfunction
  Syringomyelia
  Spinal cord or cerebellar tumors (posterior fossa)
  Bulbar palsies
Inflammatory
  Lymphadenitis of the neck
  Spontaneous hyperemic atlantoaxial rotatory subluxation
  Tuberculosis
  Typhoid
  Rheumatoid arthritis
Miscellaneous
  Acute calcification of a cervical disc
  Sandifer's syndrome (hiatal hernia and esophageal reflux)
Trauma
  Fractures, subluxations, dislocations of the cervical spine, particularly C1-C2

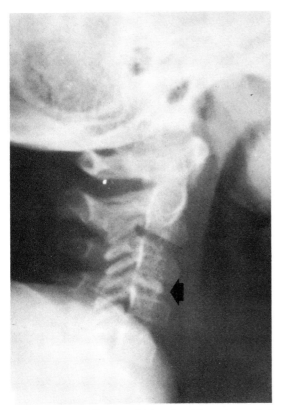

Figure 5–47. Six-year-old female with acute onset of torticollis and neck pain. No history of trauma or recent infection. Lateral roentgenograph of the cervical spine demonstrates acute calcification of the disc between C3 and C4 (arrow). The child was treated conservatively with a neck collar with spontaneous resolution of the torticollis and symptoms over a two-week period. The disc calcification, however, was still radiologically visible at six months following onset of symptoms but not at 12 months.

References

1. Brackbill, Y., Douthitt, T. C., and West, H.: Psychophysiologic effects in the neonate of prone versus supine placement. J. Pediatr. *82*:82–84, 1973.
2. Brooks, B.: Pathologic changes in muscle as a result of disturbances of circulation. Arch. Surg. *5*:188–216, 1922.
3. Coventry, M. B., and Harris, L. E.: Congenital muscular torticollis in infancy. Some observations regarding treatment. J. Bone Joint Surg. *41A*:815–822, 1959.
4. DeBarros, M. C., Farias, W., Ataide, L., and Lins, S.: Basilar impression and Arnold-Chiari malformation. A study of 66 cases. J. Neurol. Neurosurg. Psychiatry *31*:596–605, 1968.
5. Fielding, J. W., and Hawkins, R. J.: Atlanto-axial rotatory fixation (fixed rotatory subluxation of the atlanto-axial joint). J. Bone Joint Surg. *59A*:37–44, 1977.
6. Hensinger, R. N., Lang, J. R., and MacEwen, G. D.: The Klippel-Feil syndrome: A constellation of associated anomalies. J. Bone Joint Surg. *56A*:1246–1253, 1974.
7. Hummer, C. D., Jr., and MacEwen, G. D.: The coexistence of torticollis and congenital dysplasia of the hip. J. Bone Joint Surg. *54A*:1255–1256, 1972.
8. Kaplan, E. B.: Anatomical pitfalls in the surgical treatment of torticollis. Bull. Hosp. Joint Dis. *15*:154–162, 1954.
9. Ling, C. M., and Low, Y. S.: Sternomastoid tumor and muscular torticollis. Clin. Orthop. *86*:144–150, 1972.
10. Ling, C. M.: The influence of age on the results of open sternomastoid tenotomy in muscular torticollis. Clin. Orthop. *116*:142–148, 1976.
11. MacDonald, D.: Sternomastoid tumour and muscular torticollis. J. Bone Joint Surg. *51B*:432–443, 1969.
12. Melnick, J. C., and Silverman, F. N.: Intervertebral disk calcification in childhood. Radiology *80*:399–408, 1963.
13. Schechter, L. S., Smith, A., and Pearl, M.: Intervertebral disk calcification in childhood. Am. J. Dis. Child. *123*:608–611, 1972.
14. Staheli, L. T.: Muscular torticollis: Late results of operative treatment. Surgery *69*:469–473, 1971.
15. Sutcliff, J.: Torsion spasms and abnormal postures in children with hiatus hernia: Sandifer's syndrome. Prog. Pediatr. Radiol. *2*:190–197, 1969.

visualized on routine roentgenographic study of the neck (Fig. 5–47). Hiatal hernia and esophageal reflux in children inexplicably on occasion have been associated with torticollis posture (Sandifer's syndrome).[15]

All children with torticollis should be evaluated with roentgenograms to exclude a bony abnormality or fracture. Roentgenographic evaluation may be difficult in the young child or in those with a painful wry neck. It may be impossible to appropriately position the child for a standard view of the occipitocervical junction. A helpful guide is that the atlas moves with the occiput, and if the x-ray beam is directed 90 degrees to the lateral skull, a satisfactory view of the occipitocervical junction will usually result. Visualization may be further enhanced by obtaining flexion-extension stress views or laminagrams. On occasion, cineradiography is a helpful adjuvant.

SPINAL DEFORMITY IN MYELODYSPLASIA

Only in the past 15 years have pediatricians and orthopedists begun to realize the magnitude and complexity of spinal deformity in the child with myelodysplasia. Previously these severely afflicted children rarely survived infancy or early childhood (Fig. 5–48).[2, 11, 17, 20, 23] With the advent of reliable means of controlling hydrocephalus, early closure of the meningocele, antibiotics to prevent meningitis, and improved postnatal care, an

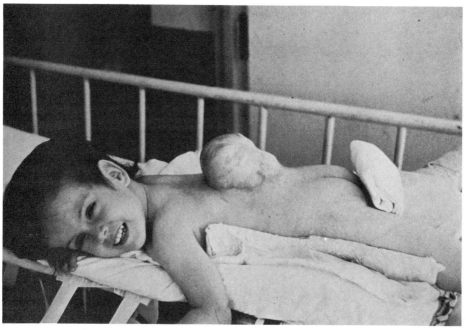

Figure 5–48. Three-year-old with an untreated myelomeningocele and hydrocephalus. The patient died from sepsis following closure of the meningocele.

increasing number of these children are living to adulthood. Although the incidence of 2.4 to 2.8 per thousand live births has not changed, the number surviving infancy has increased dramatically.[2, 26] This advancing wave of children with myelodysplasia has confronted the physician with a vast array of problems that previously did not exist. Initially, orthopedists adapted management principles derived from the previous years of polio surgery, but muscle paralysis is the only similarity between the two conditions.[23] The child with myelodysplasia has additional problems not encountered in polio, the most significant of which are hydrocephalus, absent or diminished sensation, dysfunction of bladder and bowel, and mental retardation.[20, 21]

As clinical experience with the myelodysplastic patient has increased, new principles and treatment techniques have emerged. Yet, we are still in a learning phase, particularly in the area of spinal deformity. Clinical data are limited, and follow-up studies are too short to be confident of the treatment techniques employed at present. Our intent in this chapter is only to summarize current opinion. The reader is forewarned that these recommendations will undoubtedly be altered over the next few years and should be considered more as principles rather than exact techniques.

Etiology and Embryology

Research efforts to discover the etiologic agent or agents of myelodysplasia have not been productive. A variety of exogenous factors have been examined: drugs, viruses, and environmental and social influences, and as yet no consistent pattern has emerged.[13] A small percentage of cases have a multifactorial origin with a positive family history of myelodysplasia (Smith, 7.8 per cent; Ingraham, 6 per cent; and Doron and Gluthkelch, 8 per cent).[26]

Whatever the agent, its influence occurs early in embryonic life, on or before the 19th day when the neural folds meet to form the neural tube (neuralation). Closure of the tube begins first in the cervical region and then proceeds cephalad and caudad like a double-ended zipper.[13, 16] The segmentally formed mesodermal somites arrange themselves about this tube to become the spinal muscles and vertebral bodies. If the neural tube is dysraphic, the adjacent mesodermal structures do not develop normally, and the vertebral laminae fail to fuse posteriorly.[13] This is supported clinically, as there is usually a correlation between the extent of the posterior vertebral defect and the neurologic deficit.[4] Similarly, if tubalization is interrupted in its progress distally, the remaining neural segments will usually fail to fuse.[4] Thus, the more proximal the lesion, the more extensive the neurologic deficit. An important exception is a small number of children, inexplicably, who have short segments of dysraphism in the upper thoracic and cervical area without gross neurologic disturbance.[26]

Pathologic Anatomy and Definitions

There is a wide variation in the extent of the lesion from complete exposure of the neural elements to minor laminar defects of no clinical consequence. Previously, the entire range of posterior defects was included under the general term spina bifida. In present usage, myelodysplasia encompasses all children with neurologic deficit regardless of the extent of the vertebral defect.

SPINA BIFIDA OCCULTA. This term refers to a minor bony defect in the spinous process and laminae without a neurologic deficit. It is frequently found in the lower lumbar and upper sacral segments. It occurs in 5 to 10 per cent of the general population and is usually an incidental finding on routine roentgenograms of the lumbar spine. In the vast majority, it is of no clinical significance, but occasionally it is associated with a neurologic abnormality or tumor, such as lipoma, angioma, or dermoid cyst. The occurrence of spina bifida occulta with spondylolysis and spondylolisthesis is more than chance and may be related to the pathogenesis (p. 203).

DERMAL SINUS. This is a tube or tract lined with stratified squamous epithelium originating at the skin and attaching to or communicating with the dura. The sinus usually opens on the surface in or near the midline in the lumbosacral region, but it may be found at any point along the spinal axis. It is commonly associated with laminar defects and can be an important clue to the presence of diastematomyelia. It may represent a repository for infection and may lead to recurrent episodes of meningitis. A careful search should be conducted for a dermal sinus in children who have a changing neurologic problem or recurrent meningitis.

MENINGOCELE. This is a herniation of the meninges through a defect in the posterior vertebral elements without associated protrusion of spinal cord or nerve roots. The vertebral laminae are incompletely formed, and the spinal canal is widened in the area of the defect. The meninges are covered only with thin, parchment-like skin, and the cyst is filled with cerebrospinal fluid. These patients are usually without significant neurologic impairment, and closure of the sac is performed to decrease the risk of meningitis and improve the appearance of the back.[17, 26]

MYELOMENINGOCELE. This is a herniation of the neural elements through a posterior vertebral defect and is the lesion commonly found in the myelodysplastic child. It usually is not covered with skin but a thin membrane of tissue (arachnoid) filled with cerebrospinal fluid.[26] The dysplastic spinal cord or nerve roots can be seen in the base of the sac. Early closure is recommended if the child is to be protected from meningitis, which inevitably follows rupture of the sac. The laminae and pedicles of the involved vertebrae are usually rudimentary and remain as a bony ridge adjacent to the widened spinal canal. The vertebral bodies are widened in the transverse diameter and narrowed in the anterior-posterior projection. The nerve roots emerge from normally formed foramina, in contrast to the jumble of neurologic tissue in the dysraphic vertebral canal.

RACHISCHISIS OR MYELOSCHISIS. These terms are used to describe an extensive degree of dysraphism with exposure of the entire spinal cord and associated with anencephaly.[13] Fortunately, these infants are usually stillborn or die shortly after birth.

Classification and Incidence of Spine Deformity

In the past decade, orthopedists have begun to appreciate the frequent occurrence of spinal deformity in the myelodysplastic child. More than one half of these patients may be expected to develop a significant spine curvature; in the majority of patients, this starts before age ten (Fig. 5–49).[1, 22] The pattern of curvature is quite varied, combining elements of scoliosis, lordosis, and kyphosis. Factors influencing the development and progression of the spinal deformity are multiple and include congenital structural anomalies, muscle weakness, and imbalance and soft tissue contractures. As yet, the complex interaction of these dynamic and static forces on the spine has defied classification, in part owing to the limited clinical experience. A strict structural classification is of limited application, as it does not include the dynamic

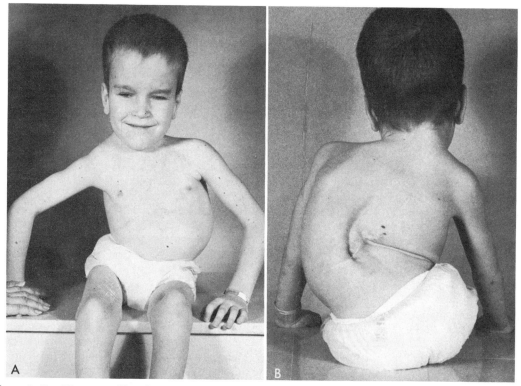

Figure 5–49. Nine-year-old with severe developmental scoliosis secondary to myelodysplasia. *A,* Frontal view. *B,* Posterior view. He is unable to maintain sitting balance, owing to truncal instability, and requires his hands for support. Subsequent surgical stabilization of spine has allowed him to sit unsupported in a wheelchair. He now works as a potter.

aspect of muscle imbalance or soft tissue contracture, nor is grouping on the basis of neurologic deficit completely reliable in planning management or prognosis.

Raycroft and Curtis[1] have suggested a classification for the scoliosis of myelodysplasia, which we have used with some success. They divide the causes of scoliosis into two primary categories, congenital and developmental (Table 5–3). Patients with congenital scoliosis have a primary lateral structural dis-

organization of the vertebral bodies with asymmetrical growth potential. This includes hemivertebrae, unilateral unsegmented bars, or both and can be recognized at or shortly after birth on routine roentgenograms. In the second category, developmental scoliosis, the patient is born with a straight spine and gradually develops a progressive curvature. The factors that contribute to the deformity are further subdivided into suprapelvic, intrapelvic, and infrapelvic causes.[1] The special problems of lordosis and kyphosis have evaded classification and must as yet be viewed apart from scoliosis. It is hoped that with more clinical experience, a scheme that incorporates the interrelations of all the deforming forces will replace this preliminary classification.

Diagnosis of Spinal Deformity in Myelodysplasia

Diagnosis of spinal deformity in the myelodysplastic patient is easily accomplished by

TABLE 5–3. SPINAL DEFORMITIES OF MYELODYSPLASIA

I. Scoliosis
   A. Congenital vertebral anomalies
   B. Developmental
      1. Suprapelvic causes
      2. Intrapelvic causes
      3. Infrapelvic causes
II. Lordosis
III. Kyphosis
   A. Congenital
   B. Developmental

obtaining appropriate roentgenograms. A recurring problem is that the physician does not always appreciate the great potential for spine curvature and fails to obtain the necessary roentgenograms. Frequently, attention is focused on the feet, hips, or urinary tract, and significant spine deformity is allowed to progress.[2] Similarly, while carefully observing for scoliosis with serial anterior-posterior roentgenograms, a significant lordosis or kyphosis can be totally overlooked.

To avoid these errors, certain guidelines should be established for routine follow-up study. Roentgenograms should be obtained at regular intervals in both the anterior-posterior and lateral projections beginning shortly after birth. If congenital vertebral anomalies are discovered, they should be carefully evaluated for potential deformity and appropriate measures should be taken. If the spine is straight and the deformity is limited to the dysraphic posterior elements, then these views should

be repeated when the child first begins to sit, again when standing in braces or parapodium, and at least yearly thereafter.

The importance of obtaining roentgenograms of the patient upright, either standing or sitting, cannot be overemphasized. Many early curves are of the collapsing type or are related to pelvic obliquity and soft tissue contractures and tend to correct in the supine position (Fig. 5–50).[5] The physician must remember that nearly 100 per cent of the myelodysplastic patients with congenital vertebral body anomalies and 50 per cent of those born initially with a straight spine can be expected to develop a significant deformity.[1, 2, 22] The onset of spine curvature is usually before age five and seldom occurs after age ten (Fig. 5–49); therefore, observation during the first years will be most beneficial to the patient.[22, 27] Further, this will provide the physician with some insight into the natural history of the curve in this particular patient and will

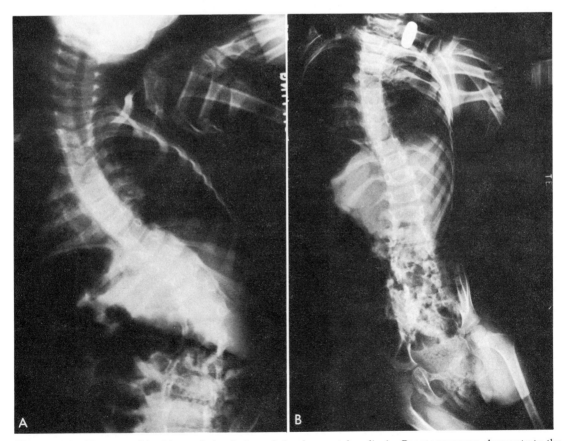

Figure 5–50. Two-year-old with myelodysplasia and developmental scoliosis. Roentgenograms demonstrate the extent of spine curvature while sitting. *A,* Curvature is supple and *B,* can be nearly corrected by positioning alone.

permit the institution of corrective measures prior to severe deformity.

The level of neurologic deficit should be carefully evaluated. In general, those with lesions above L3-L4 are most prone to developmental scoliosis.[1, 2, 22, 27] Asymmetry of the neurologic level is of particular concern, as muscle imbalance about the pelvis is a prime cause of pelvic obliquity and possibly scoliosis. Recently Hall[9] has called attention to an alarming cause of developmental scoliosis, communicating hydrosyringomyelia. In these children, the onset of curvature was between five to eight years of age and rapidly progressive. More than one half of the patients had associated progressive extremity paralysis and spasticity, particularly those with a low-level myelodysplasia. In each patient the hydrocephalus was thought to be clinically arrested. Several had never been shunted, and the remainder had a nonfunctioning ventricular shunt. Neurologic deficit was improved, and the milder curves were stabilized with ventricular shunting; however, those who had severe curves showed continued progression.[9]

Abduction or adduction contractures of the hips can lead to pelvic tilt. Hip flexion contractures, dislocation, or limited range of motion have all been implicated as factors influencing scoliosis and lordosis, and a thorough evaluation of these parameters should be conducted at each follow-up visit. Pathologic fractures of the lower extremities are a common occurrence in patients with myelodysplasia and may lead to unilateral shortening and pelvic obliquity.

Gait and sitting patterns have been implicated by Kilfoyle[15] as a cause of progressive spine deformity, particularly lordosis. The child stands with the crutches thrust out (tripod stance) and the trunk sloped forward, allowing the center of gravity to pass anterior to the lumbar spine and increasing the normal lumbar lordosis. This can result in a fixed lordosis and flexion contractures of the hip in the child who is capable of standing and walking (Fig. 5–56). In the same manner, the sitting posture of the patient with congenital lumbar kyphosis accentuates the preexisting deformity (Fig. 5–58).[15] If there is an extension contracture of the hips, when the child sits the lumbar spine is forced into kyphosis. A helpful guideline: Those who can stand and walk are likely to develop lordosis; those who must sit are prone to kyphosis.

Chronic positioning because of a fixed deformity, decubitus care, or poor brace fit may directly or indirectly establish a vicious cycle that eventually leads to progressive spinal deformity. As Hibbs[10] noted in the treatment of paralytic scoliosis over 50 years ago, prevention of deformity is far easier than correction once it is established. This recommendation applies to all children with myelodysplasia, and early detection of the spinal deformity is mandatory.

Evaluation of Developmental Scoliosis

The majority of patients in this group have a neurologic deficit of L3-L4 or above.[1] Although emphasis is placed on the more proximal lesions, all myelodysplastics, regardless of neurologic level, should be carefully observed for spinal deformity. Developmental scoliosis has been viewed as compensatory to a pelvic obliquity, but it is quite possible that for many patients the spine curvature precedes the pelvic obliquity. Later, once the deformity is established, it is often impossible to determine the primary offender. The curvature is usually discovered first in the lumbar spine, and if it is not controlled, a compensatory thoracic curve will ensue. The factors that cause pelvic obliquity and can lead to developmental scoliosis have been divided by Raycroft and Curtis[1] into suprapelvic, transpelvic, and infrapelvic.

SUPRAPELVIC FACTORS. It is frequently assumed that the neurologic deficit of the myelodysplastic is symmetrical, but often it is not, and significant muscle imbalance can occur. This may result from several causes: an asymmetric primary lesion, inadvertent injury to nerve roots during closure of the sac, or meningitis. Even minor differences in the flank and deep back muscles can eventually lead to a significant spine deformity.[16] The effects of soft tissue contractures are similar but of slower onset, occurring with growth of the patient.

TRANSPELVIC FACTORS. Here the psoas muscle is the primary offender, originating at the transverse process of the lumbar spine and passing through the pelvis to insert at the lesser trochanter. It is innervated by the L1-L2 nerve roots, which are frequently spared except in the most severely involved patient. If the hip flexion function of the psoas is unopposed, flexion contractures will quickly ensue. When the child stands, the lumbar spine is forced into lordosis, both from the dynamic pull of the iliopsoas and the static forward tilt of the pelvis imposed by the hip flexion contracture. This deformity is further aggravated by the tripod stance and "swing to" gait of the paraplegic[15] (Fig. 5–56C). Unilateral contracture of the iliopsoas can lead to flexion-adduction contracture of the hip and pelvic obliquity.

INFRAPELVIC FACTORS. Hip abduction and adduction contracture are the most frequent causes of pelvic obliquity in the myelodysplastic child. This may result from muscle imbalance or soft tissue contractures and may be present in the neonatal period or may develop with growth. A common finding is the "windblown" appearance of the pelvis and hips. This term is applied to the patient who presents an abduction contracture of one hip, usually the iliotibial band, and adduction contracture of the opposite hip. If the deformity is not recognized, physical therapy and bracing efforts to align the extremities will only serve to increase the obliquity. The pelvis will be pulled down on the abducted side and elevated on the side of the adducted hip, increasing its potential to dislocate.

Hip dislocation on the high side of the pelvis and its relationship to scoliosis is well known to the orthopedist.[15] Patients with cerebral palsy and polio are subject to the identical clinical problem, and experience with these conditions indicates that once the dislocation occurs, control of the scoliosis is considerably more difficult. So, too, with myelodysplasia, prevention is obviously more satisfactory but depends on early recognition. Patients with sparing of the L3 nerve root (strong hip flexors and adductors) are more susceptible, but all should be carefully observed.

Treatment Principles in Developmental Scoliosis

Early recognition of potentially hazardous situations is essential in the management of developmental scoliosis. Many can be recognized soon after sitting balance is established and before five years of age (Fig. 5–50).[1, 22] Careful attention must be paid to any contractures about the hip, and the efforts by the physical therapist and parents should be directed at keeping a full and supple range of hip motion. Sleeping braces and splints may be helpful in preventing contractures or maintaining proper position. Dislocation of the hip can be avoided to some extent by aligning the long leg braces in abduction and maintaining the hips reduced in the acetabulum. Frequently, with the moderately involved patient, we are tempted to use short leg braces, ignoring the weak or absent abductors and allowing hip subluxation and dislocation to proceed unrecognized.

If conservative efforts to align the pelvis fail, surgical correction may be necessary. Iliotibial band release can be helpful in correcting hip abduction contracture and should be performed prior to application of full control braces. Iliopsoas transfer to strengthen hip abduction is not effective in preventing dislocation and can rob the patient of a strong hip flexor.[12] Varus osteotomy of the hips has been helpful in controlling hip subluxation, as it positions the femoral head more deeply into the acetabulum.[12] The innominate osteotomy of Salter is not recommended, as it does not provide sufficient buttress to the typical paralytic posterior dislocation.[12] Severe (greater than 18 degrees) fixed pelvic obliquity can be improved using a posterior iliac osteotomy as described by Lindseth.[18] He noted improvement in sitting and standing balance following the procedure but recommended it be considered after the spinal deformity is stabilized (Figs. 5–51 and 5–52).[18]

Spinal orthoses have been used sparingly in myelodysplastic children, as the anesthetic skin about the pelvis easily develops pressure sores.[27] Total contact lightweight corrective plastic orthoses have been used with good results if carefully fitted in children with mild to moderate curvatures. The brace must be carefully molded to the patient and applied for short periods until skin tolerance has increased. The patient is closely observed for areas of increased pressure or friction, and appropriate alterations are made. With time, most children will be able to wear the brace for all activities throughout the day. (Refer to Chapter 6 for further discussion on orthotic management of scoliosis.)

If progression of the developmental curve is not halted by bracing, surgical stabilization is required. At present, many patients have been allowed to develop severe scoliosis that precludes adequate standing balance, and in some cases, even sitting unsupported is impossible.[2, 5, 27] It is hoped that in the future, early surgical intervention will gain greater acceptance and less extensive procedures will be required (Fig. 5–53).[22, 27] (Refer to Chapter 6 for further discussion of surgical management.)

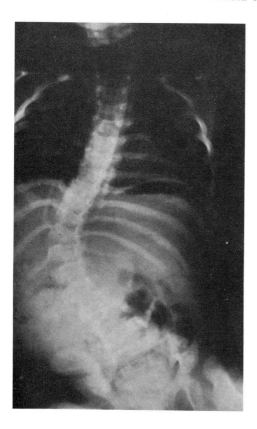

Figure 5–51. Six-year-old with myelodysplasia and developmental scoliosis and associated subluxation of the left hip.

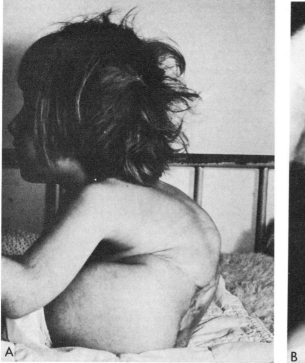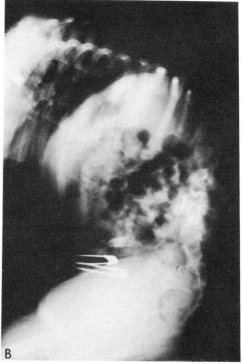

Figure 5–52. Eight-year-old with myelodysplasia and a severe collapsing kyphosis. *A*, Clinical appearance. *B*, Lateral roentgenographic appearance.

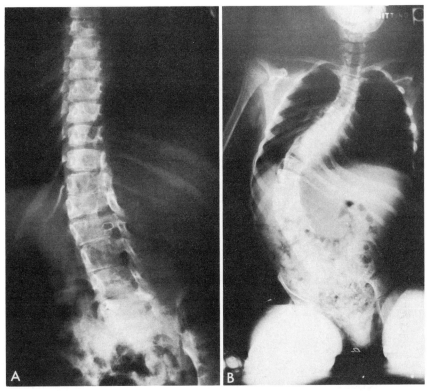

Figure 5–53. Patient with myelodysplasia demonstrating progression of her developmental scoliosis over a four-year period. *A,* Age six. *B,* Sitting roentgenogram at age 10 demonstrating marked deformity of spine.

Congenital Scoliosis

Obviously, patients with severe dysraphism of the posterior spinal elements will have a high incidence of anomalous vertebral bodies.[1, 6] In Raycroft and Curtis'[1] series, approximately 30 per cent had congenital distortion of the vertebral bodies, and all eventually developed significant spinal malalignment. The deformity may not be limited to the dysraphic area alone, and significant curvature can occur in the relatively normal thoracic spine even though the lumbar anomalies remain stable. The management of unilateral bars and hemivertebrae is discussed in Chapter 6. Conservative treatment measures — spinal orthoses and plaster casts — often used for children with congenital scoliosis will be less effective in the myelodysplastic child. The problems due to anesthetic skin and pressure sores severely limit the effectiveness of these corrective or stabilizing devices.[27]

Urinary collection devices, fecal incontinence, full control braces, and crutches compound the problem and fatigue even the most conscientious parent. In summary, we strongly recommend surgical intervention earlier than would ordinarily be done if the deformity occurred in an otherwise normal individual. Early evaluation, therefore, becomes of utmost importance to obtain proper appreciation of the curve's progress (Fig. 5–54). Linear spine growth is limited in these children,[6] and an early, timely fusion is less hazardous with a more satisfactory end result than allowing the curve to progress. If progression occurs, correction of these severely distorted and rigid curves is a major surgical procedure with considerable risk to the patient and a prolonged investment of time in traction and at bedrest.[27] Further, the results (degree of correction) that can be obtained by these heroic maneuvers are limited and much less satisfactory than those following early spinal fusion.

Lordosis

The most common spinal deformity in the myelodysplastic child is lordosis, irrespective

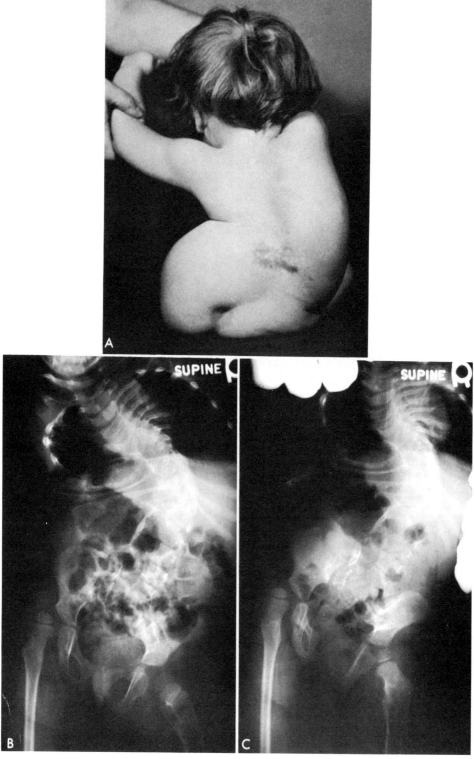

Figure 5–54. Myelodysplasia and congenital scoliosis. *A,* Clinical appearance at age three, unable to sit without support owing to severe scoliosis. *B,* Roentgenogram demonstrating the spine curvature and dislocation of the left hip on the side of the high pelvis. *C,* The curvature is quite rigid and very little correction can be obtained with forced bending.

of the presence or absence of scoliosis.[28] The deformity is usually confined to the lumbar spine but may develop in the thoracic vertebrae to compensate for a severe lumbar kyphosis (Fig. 5–57) or a high neurologic deficit (Fig. 5–55). Lordosis is not usually present at birth and is compensatory to fixed distal deformities. If the factors that influence its development are not controlled, the lordosis quickly becomes resistant to passive correction.

Muscle imbalance about the pelvis is the

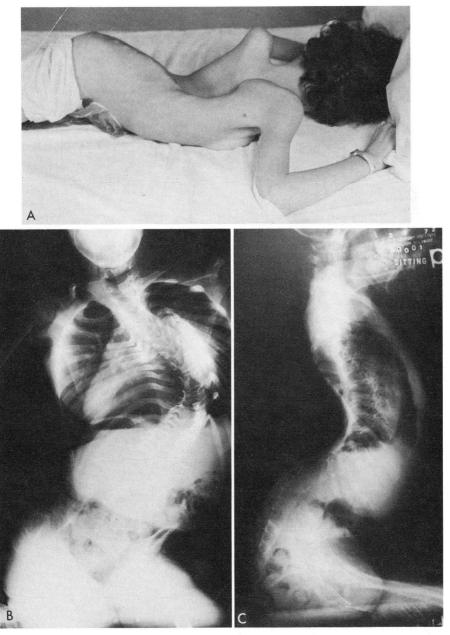

Figure 5–55. Thirteen-year-old with a high level myelodysplasia. The patient has a thoracic lordosis which is compensatory to lumbar kyphosis; both curves are resistant to passive correction. *A*, Clinical appearance with marked deformity of the dorsal vertebrae and thorax. *B*, Roentgenogram demonstrating the marked degree of scoliosis. *C*, Lateral of spine. The patient's pulmonary function was markedly impaired with a decrease in vital capacity, such that she was unable to ventilate adequately while prone.

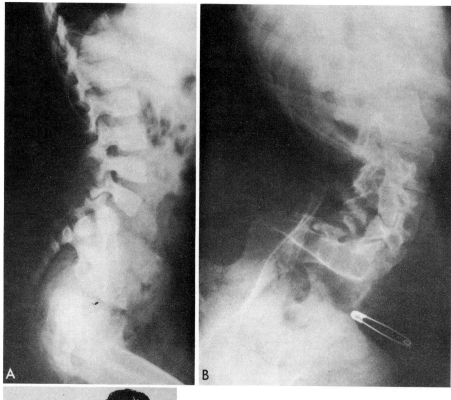

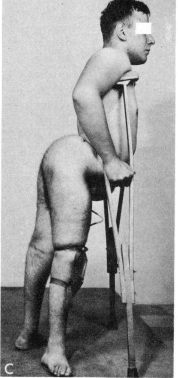

Figure 5–56. Low-level myelodysplastic, ambulatory with crutches. *A*, Roentgenogram of the lumbar spine at age three, with a normal lumbar lordosis. *B*, Age 19, severe lumbar lordosis with bilateral dislocation of the hips. Lordosis has increased, owing in part to flexion contractures of the hip and the tripod stance and "swing to" gait of the paraplegic. *C*, Clinical appearance demonstrating a severe lumbar lordosis accentuated by the tripod crutch stance.

most common cause of lordosis; the imbalance usually is due to unopposed hip flexors.[12] This is a common pattern in the myelodysplastic child, as the innervation of hip flexion (L2, L3) is more often spared than hip extension (L5, S1). Soft tissue contractures about the hip, particularly the iliopsoas and iliotibial band, are a frequent predisposing cause; their role already has been discussed. There are several situations that commonly accentuate lordosis: the tripod stance of the paraplegic, the "swing-to" or "swing-through" gait, or an improperly positioned pelvic band of full control braces. Paralytic calcaneal deformity of the feet and posterior dislocation of the hips are aggravating causes but are seldom the primary cause. Sharrard[25] has suggested the scarring and fibrosis secondary to surgical closure of the myelomeningocele may lead to tight posterior structures, and with growth, the child can develop a progressive lumbar lordosis.

To determine the presence of increased lumbar lordosis, the patient should be examined in the standing position. If during standing the pelvis is inclined forward, to maintain trunk balance, the patient must increase the normal lumbar lordosis. When the spine is balanced, the center of gravity should fall immediately in front of the ankle. Using these guidelines, it is easy to see that a small degree of hip flexion or calcaneal deformity of the feet may unbalance the lumbar spine. In the non-ambulatory patient, lumbar lordosis is best examined in the supine position. With extension of the hips, the lumbar spine should remain flat to the table. Lordosis is less of a problem in the patient who is wheelchair bound, as the deforming forces are normally relaxed when the hips are flexed in the sitting position.

If the lordosis is allowed to progress and become a structural curve, it is very difficult to control (Fig. 5–56).[6] Passive stretching of the hips or lumbar spine are good preventive measures but seldom correct a fixed contracture. Release of the iliotibial band and hip flexion contractures can be helpful if done early, preferably prior to fitting of the full control orthosis or parapodium. Extension osteotomy of the hips may be considered to control lordosis due to hip flexion contractures. Release of the iliopsoas seldom reduces lordosis, and transfer of this muscle to function as a hip abductor will fail to correct lordosis if the deformity is rigid, and it will not alter the hip flexion contracture.[12]

If fixed lordosis requires correction, surgical spine stabilization will be necessary (Chap. 6). The fusion must include the sacrum, and careful attention must be paid to the position of the pelvis during the period of postoperative immobilization.

Congenital Lumbar Kyphosis

The problem of congenital lumbar kyphosis is unique to myelodysplasia and warrants separate discussion. It should be differentiated from the short, one or two segment gibbus due to a congenitally wedged or absent vertebra. Congenital lumbar kyphosis involves the entire lumbar spine from the thoracolumbar junction and includes the sacrum with an apex at L2 or L3. It is usually accompanied by complete paralysis below the level of the lesion and a large myelomeningocele. The condition is common among myelodysplastic patients, with a reported incidence of 12.5 per cent[11] to 29 per cent,[4] is extremely rigid even at birth,[7, 8] and portends a poor prognosis.[20, 21] Many of these infants do not survive owing to the severity of the neurologic lesion and associated anomalies.

ETIOLOGY. This deformity is believed to represent a more profound error in development than that which leads to the typical dysraphism found in the majority of children with myelodysplasia. Barson[3] has suggested that the deformity is due to retention or persistence of the primitive tailfold and is analogous to the proximal Arnold-Chiari malformation or persistence of the headfold. Other authors speculate that the deformity results from differential rates of growth between the neural ectoderm and the vertebral mesoderm. Patten[24] demonstrated that if closure of the neural tube is prevented, the neural plate is stimulated to grow faster and in greater volume. As a consequence, the enlarging mass of neural tissue forces the lumbar spine into kyphosis in the same manner as expansion of two dissimilar metals bolted together results in buckling.

PATHOLOGIC ANATOMY. Autopsy specimens have been extensively studied and have provided some insight into the pathomechanics of this deformity.[3, 4, 7, 10] The most impressive finding is the rigidity of the deformity and its resistance to passive correction even in the newborn (Fig. 5–59A and B). The pedicles, as expected, are widely separated and protrude posterolaterally to accentuate the kyphotic appearance.[11] The splayed pedicles and lamin-

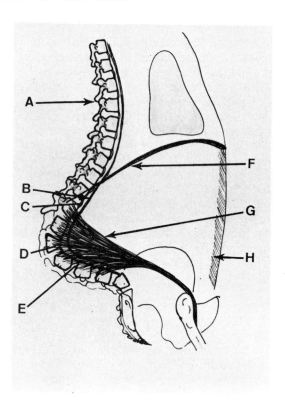

Figure 5–57. Drawing illustrating the deforming forces found in congenital lumbar kyphosis. *A,* Compensatory dorsal lordosis. *B,* Contracted anterior longitudinal ligament. *C,* Contracted anulus fibrosus. *D,* Wedge-shaped vertebral bodies. *E,* Intervertebral discs narrowed anteriorly with the nucleus pulposus shifted posteriorly. *F,* Diaphragm attached to the apex of the deformity. *G,* Psoas muscle is hypertrophied and bowstrings across the curve. *H,* Anterior abdominal musculature.

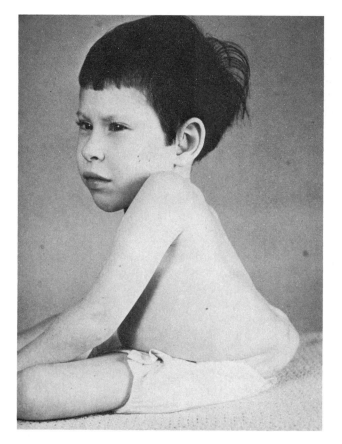

Figure 5–58. Nine-year-old with a congenital lumbar kyphosis. Typical sitting posture serves to accentuate the kyphosis. The child is sitting directly on the sacrum and lower portion of the lumbar spine.

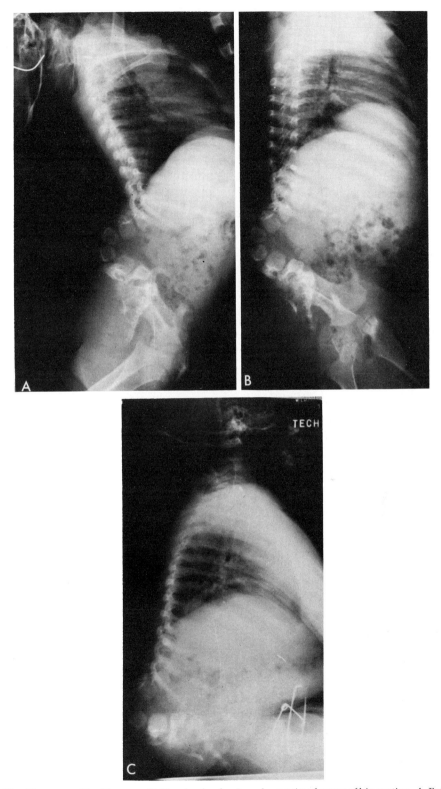

Figure 5–59. Five-year-old with congenital lumbar kyphosis and a restricted range of hip motion. *A*, Extension of the hips and spine. *B*, Flexion. The roentgenograms demonstrate very little motion of the hips and a rigid lumbar kyphosis. *C*, Roentgenogram of the patient sitting on the sacrum and lower portion of the lumbar spine.

ae push the deep back muscles to a more anterior position, and if innervated, they may function as pathologic flexors of the lumbar spine and serve to increase the deformity. Drennan[7] found that the psoas muscle is frequently hypertrophied and arises from the roof of the kyphos to bowstring across the curve (Fig. 5–57). The crura of the diaphragm usually attach at the apex of the deformity (thoracolumbar junction) and further enhance the strength of the psoas by providing a fixed point to pull against. The anterior abdominal muscles and quadratus lumborum are usually innervated and also aggravate the deformity. The vertebral bodies are wedge-shaped, and the intervertebral discs are narrowed anteriorly with the nucleus pulposus shifted posteriorly.[11] The anulus fibrosus is contracted as well as the anterior longitudinal ligament, which is occasionally found to be a cordlike thickening.[11] Hoppenfeld[11] found that release of the anterior longitudinal ligament permitted limited correction, but only with sectioning of the anulus fibrosus could the deformity be corrected.

CLINICAL FINDINGS. Congenital lumbar kyphosis is easily recognized at birth by clinical and radiologic examination. The size of the cutaneous defect and the rigidity of the curve often combine to pose a difficult problem in skin closure. Extensive mobilization of skin flaps is often required, and it is not unusual for the initial attempt at skin coverage to fail or be impossible.[8, 26] This situation has prompted Sharrard to recommend immediate resection of the kyphosis to facilitate closure.[25] Recurrent skin breakdown over the kyphos is common and healing of these trophic ulcerations is often impossible.[1, 8, 19] In the older untreated patient, squamous cell carcinoma has developed at the site of chronic skin ulceration and has resulted in death by metastasis.[14]

If the infant survives the newborn period, the kyphosis remains relatively static until the child begins to sit. Then, gravity in conjunction with the deforming muscles causes progression of the curve. The child is forced to sit with the trunk well forward, using the hands for support (Fig. 5–58). If the hips are stiff in extension, the child appears to sit directly on the sacrum and a portion of the lumbar spine (Fig. 5–59). A compensatory lordosis of the thoracic spine often develops in an effort to improve sitting posture (Fig. 5–57, drawing).[11] The anterior rib cage soon comes to lie on the pelvic brim and may be a source of irritation and pain. The abdominal contents are forced against the diaphragm, restricting its excursion and ultimately respiratory function.[16, 19]

TREATMENT. Bracing for ambulation is frequently impossible owing to irritation of the skin over the kyphos.[1, 19] Functional ambulation is probably not a realistic goal for these severely paralyzed children, but the same problems are encountered when the child is braced for the wheelchair. We have had only limited success with spinal orthoses and cannot recommend their application. Physical therapy and soft tissue stretching have been totally unsuccessful in achieving correction or even halting progression.[1] Owing to frequent failure of conservative measures, surgery is often required to control progression and achieve reduction of the curve.[19] For a detailed discussion of surgical management, refer to Chapter 6.

References

1. American Academy of Orthopaedic Surgeons: Symposium on myelomeningocele. St. Louis, C. V. Mosby Co., 1972.
2. Barden, G. A., Meyer, L. C., and Stelling, F. H., III.: Myelodysplastics—fate of those followed for twenty years or more. J. Bone Joint Surg. *57A*:643–647, 1975.
3. Barson, A. J.: Radiological studies of spina bifida cystica; the phenomenon of congenital lumbar kyphosis. Br. J. Radiol. *38*:294–300, 1965.
4. Barson, A. J.: Spina bifida: The significance of the level and extent of the defect to the morphogenesis. Dev. Med. Child. Neurol. *12*:129–144, 1970.
5. Bonnett, C. A., Brown, J. C., Perry, J., Nichel, V. L., Walinski, T., Brooks, T., Hoffor, M., Stiles, C., and Brooks, R.: Evolution of treatment of paralytic scoliosis. At the Rancho Los Amigos Hospital. J. Bone Joint Surg. *57A*:206–215, 1975.
6. Bunch, W. H., et al.: Modern management of myelomeningocele. St. Louis, Warren H. Green, Inc., 1972.
7. Drennan, J. C.: The role of muscles in the development of human lumbar kyphosis. Dev. Med. Child. Neurol. (Suppl.) *22*:33–38, 1970.
8. Eckstein, H. B., and Vora, R. M.: Spinal osteotomy for severe kyphosis in children with myelomeningocele. J. Bone Joint Surg. *54B*:328–333, 1972.
9. Hall, P. V., Lindseth, R. E., Campbell, R. L., and Kalsbeck, J. E.: Myelodysplasia and developmental scoliosis. Spine *1*:48–56, 1976.
10. Hibbs, R. A.: A report of fifty-nine cases of scoliosis treated by the fusion operation. J. Bone Joint Surg. *6*:3–15, 1924.
11. Hoppenfeld, S.: Congenital kyphosis in myelomeningocele. J. Bone Joint Surg. *49B*:276–280, 1967.
12. Huff, C. W., and Ramsey, P. L.: Myelodysplasia: The influence of the quadriceps and hip abductor muscles on ambulatory function and stability of the hip. J. Bone Joint Surg. *60A*:432–443, 1978.
13. Källen, B.: Early embryogenesis of the central nervous system with special reference to closure defects. Dev. Med. Child. Neurol. (Suppl.) *16*:44–53, 1968.

14. Kaufer, H.: Personal communication.
15. Kilfoyle, R. M., Foley, J. J., and Norton, P. L.: Spine and pelvic deformity in childhood and adolescent paraplegia. J. Bone Joint Surg. *47A*:659–682, 1965.
16. Kilfoyle, R. M.: Myelodysplasia. Pediatr. Clin North Am. *14*:419–438, 1967.
17. Laurence, K. M.: The natural history of spina bifida cystica. Detailed analysis of 407 cases. Arch. Dis. Child. *39*:41–57, 1964.
18. Lindseth, R. E.: Posterior iliac osteotomy for fixed pelvic obliquity. J. Bone Joint Surg. *60A*:17–22, 1978.
19. Lindseth, R. E., and Stelzer, L., Jr.: Vertebral excision for kyphosis in children with myelomeningocele. J. Bone Joint Surg. *61A*:699–704, 1979.
20. Lorber, J.: Results of treatment of myelomeningocele: An analysis of 524 unselected cases, with special reference to possible selection for treatment. Dev. Med. Child. Neurol. *13*:279–303, 1971.
21. Lorber, J.: Spina bifida cystica: Results of treatment of 270 consecutive cases with criteria for selection for the future. Arch. Dis. Child. *47*:854–873, 1972.
22. Macel, J. L., and Lindseth, R. E.: Scoliosis in myelodysplasia. J. Bone Joint Surg. *57A*:1031, 1975.
23. Norton, P. L., and Foley, J. J.: Paraplegia in children. J. Bone Joint Surg. *41A*:1291–1309, 1959.
24. Patten, B. M.: Embryological stages in the establishing of myeloschisis with spina bifida. Am. J. Anat. *93*:365–395, 1953.
25. Sharrard, W. J. W.: Spinal osteotomy for congenital kyphosis in myelomeningocele. J. Bone Joint Surg. *50B*:466–471, 1968.
26. Smith, E. D.: Spina bifida and the total care of spinal myelomeningocele. Springfield, Ill., Charles C Thomas, 1965.
27. Spiram, K., Bobechko, W. P., and Hall, J. E.: Surgical management of spina bifida. J. Bone Joint Surg. *54B*:666–676, 1972.
28. Tachdjian, M. O.: Pediatric Orthopedics. Philadelphia, W. B. Saunders Co., 1972.

DIASTEMATOMYELIA

Prior to 1950, diastematomyelia was seldom recognized clinically. The majority of observations were based on autopsy findings in infants with multiple vertebral anomalies, and scant information was available regarding the clinical manifestations. This situation changed rapidly with the publication of a report by Matson[20] in which he described the clinical findings, radiologic features, and surgical results in 11 patients. The report stimulated widespread clinical interest and an increased frequency of discovery. At present, over 150 patients have been recorded, and diastematomyelia has assumed a prominent position in the differential diagnosis of lower extremity neurologic impairment in children.

Diastematomyelia means cleft of the spinal cord, and it is to be differentiated from duplication of the spinal cord, diplomyelia, a rare condition.[7] In diastematomyelia, the spinal cord or intraspinal nerve roots are split into two columns by a mass fixed anteriorly to the vertebral body and posteriorly to the dura or lamina. The mass may be an osseous or cartilaginous spicule or a fibrous septum partially or completely dividing the neural canal. The neural elements usually have separate arachnoid sheaths but share a common dura.[7] Diastematomyelia may be localized at one vertebral level or may extend over several segments.[18, 30] It is commonly found in the lumbar region but has been reported as high as the third thoracic vertebra.[14, 18, 31]

Etiology and Pathogenesis

The etiology of diastematomyelia is not known, but currently two embryologic mechanisms are being considered. Bremer[5] has suggested that the division is due to the persistence of the neurenteric canal, a transient connection between the yolk sac (the future intestinal cavity) and the amniotic cavity occurring early in embryonic development. This structure perforates the proliferating primitive knot (Hensen's node), the cells that eventually form the brain and spinal cord. He supports this theory by citing the frequent occurrence of dorsal cutaneous abnormalities, dermoid cysts, and intestinal anomalies (duplications and enterogenous cysts) in association with diastematomyelia. Gardner[12] proposes that after the spinal cord is formed, a transient overdistention of the neural tube causes splitting of the cord and subsequent ingrowth of mesodermal structures from the vertebral body. He points to the widened spinal canal in the region of the diastematomyelia as evidence of previous expansion. All authors reject the theory that a lesion represents a developmental arrest, as the spinal cord is never double during embryonic life.

The bony vertebral column and the spinal cord are of equal length until the third month of embryonic life. Growth then proceeds at a differential rate, with the vertebral column lengthening at a faster pace; and at birth, the conus medullaris is found opposite the lower border of the second lumbar vertebra.[3] Through early childhood, this discrepancy continues, and at age five, the conus comes to lie at the upper border of the body of the second lumbar vertebra.[16] It is presumed that the clinical consequences are due to the "tethering" effect of the diastematomyelia on the normal ascent of the spinal cord. It may act as a "check rein" to the upward migration of the neural elements, with progressive neurologic signs in the lower extremities, or the spicule may resemble the tine of a comb moving through the cauda equina and may remain undetected. It should be emphasized that the greatest change occurs in the last six months of intrauterine skeletal growth. Differential growth during childhood is at a slower pace with more time for adaptive changes in the spinal cord and nerve roots.[3, 16]

Clinical Findings

The majority of patients have a cutaneous abnormality in the midline of the back,[5, 6, 9, 23, 30] which can be an important clue to the diagnosis. The form of the cutaneous defect is extremely varied and may not correspond to the area of the diastematomyelia. It

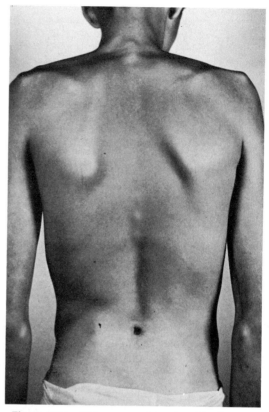

Figure 5–61. Fifteen-year-old male with a large dermal sinus in the midline of the back. Discovery of such cutaneous defects should make one suspect diastematomyelia.

may be an obvious area of hypertrichosis with profuse long, silky hair (Fig. 5–60) or simply a small dimple. Subcutaneous fatty tumors, pigmented nevi, and hemangiomas have all been reported.[7, 8, 9, 23] The association of a dermal sinus is infrequent (Fig. 5–61) but is of particular concern and must be carefully searched for, as it may represent a portal for entry of bacteria into the spinal canal.[1] The orifice may be quite discrete and innocuous in its appearance yet may lead to abscess formation and meningitis or a frank neurocutaneous fistula.[1] Similarly, incidental discovery of such a defect should make one suspect a diastematomyelia.[9]

The majority of patients with diastematomyelia have associated congenital deformities of one or both lower extremities, but commonly they are not recognized as being related to a vertebral anomaly during infancy.[30] As growth proceeds, a progressive neurologic deficit may be seen. The child fails to walk at an appropriate time or walks nor-

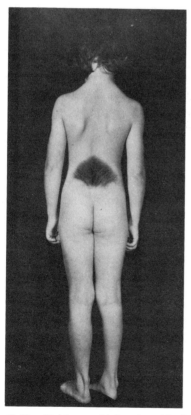

Figure 5–60. Eight-year-old female with diastematomyelia and a large area of hypertrichosis with profuse long silky hair. Note atrophy of the right calf.

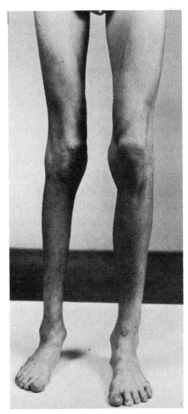

Figure 5–62. Fourteen-year-old male with unilateral atrophy of the thigh and calf secondary to diastematomyelia. Asymmetry of findings in the lower extremities is highly suggestive of diastematomyelia.

mally and then develops a disturbance of gait. Muscle weakness or paralysis, atrophy of the thigh or calf (Figs. 5–60 and 5–62), foot deformities (Fig. 5–63), and skin ulcerations are common presenting complications.[14, 30] Uri-

nary incontinence and poor bowel control are less common than motor and sensory disturbances.[4, 6, 18, 23] Asymmetry of lower extremities is highly suggestive, and discovery of unilateral calf atrophy or club foot should stimulate a thorough examination of the spine.[13] Children with Sprengel's deformity (congenital elevation of the scapula) have an unusually high incidence of diastematomyelia (20 per cent), but other anomalies of the upper extremity are uncommon.[2]

The level of the diastematomyelia influences the clinical signs and symptoms. If the lesion is low in the lumbar spine, involving only the cauda equina, the findings will be those of lower motor neuron compression and commonly will be unilateral. If the diastematomyelia is in the region of the conus medullaris or spinal cord, the findings will be more typical of an upper motor neuron lesion with spasticity, pathologic reflexes, and bilateral involvement. Late onset of symptoms in adult life (back pain and neurologic deficit) is an uncommon occurrence.[9, 11, 18, 27]

Sensory changes usually occur in the saddle area, but ulceration and trophic skin changes, particularly about the foot and toes, are not uncommon findings.[23] Pain is an infrequent complaint, but if a single nerve root is impinged, the clinical picture may mimic a herniated nucleus pulposus.[23, 27] It should be emphasized that the symptoms and signs associated with diastematomyelia are not diagnostic for this condition.[16] There are many diseases that can cause similar clinical findings and that must be ruled out. Spinal cord tumors, congenital transverse bands, taut filum terminale, arachnoid adhesions, and pro-

Figure 5–63. A patient with unilateral clubfoot secondary to diastematomyelia.

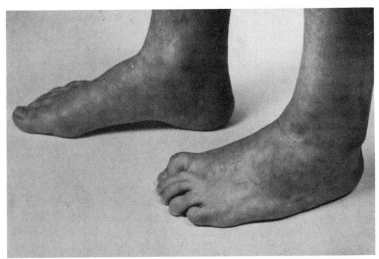

gressive neurologic diseases, such as Friedreich's ataxia or spinal muscular atrophy, are only a few to be considered.[7, 16] Conversely, the patient with diastematomyelia may be symptomatic, and the condition may not be recognized radiographically.[13]

Diastematomyelia is frequently associated with other vertebral anomalies, commonly congenital scoliosis from unilateral bars or hemivertebrae and less often myelomeningocele.[5, 13, 14, 18, 30] The majority can be expected to develop a significant spinal deformity (average 60 degrees) during the growth years, often requiring bracing or early spinal fusion.[14, 18, 30] Winter has reported a 4.9 per cent incidence of diastematomyelia in patients with congenital scoliosis.[30] The lesion may not be visible on routine roentgenographic views of the spine owing to distortion of the bony architecture.[13, 14, 30] This has prompted Keim,[18] Winter,[30] and Gillespie[13] to recommend meylographic examination of all patients with congenital scoliosis prior to surgical treatment, irrespective of the presence or absence of a neurologic deficit.

Roentgenographic Findings

The characteristic roentgenographic appearance of a diastematomyelia is a midline bony mass projecting posteriorly from the vertebral body and accompanied by a fusiform widening of the vertebral canal (Fig. 5–64). Variations from this classic appearance occur regularly, and it is often impossible to visualize this condition on routine roentgenograms of the spine.[13, 14, 30] The midline spicule may not be osseous; rather, it may be cartilaginous or fibrous and thus radiolucent.[18, 30] The bony spicule is best seen on the anterior-posterior roentgenogram, usually in the midline and approximately 1 cm. in length. In the lateral view, the spicule is obscured by the pedicles, and laminagraphic techniques are necessary for visualization.[8]

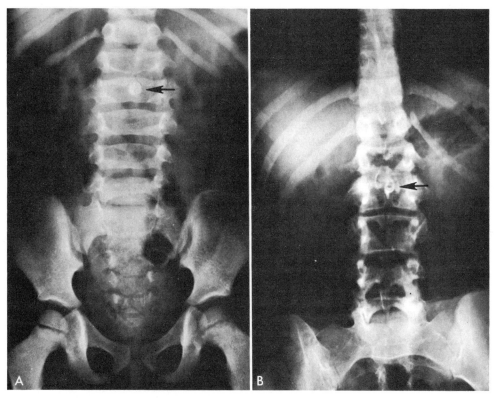

Figure 5–64. A, Roentgenogram of a three-year-old demonstrating the characteristic midline bony mass (arrow) and fusiform widening of the lumbar canal. B, Roentgenologic appearance of the same patient at age 22. She has had no progression of her neurologic findings over the 20-year period and consequently has not required excision of the diastematomyelia (arrow).

The vertebral canal widening is a consistent finding but may be subtle or obscured by associated vertebral anomalies.[13, 14, 26] Winter suggests that widening of the spinal canal should be considered as diastematomyelia until proved otherwise.[30] The interpedicular distance is usually maximal at the level of the lesion but may extend over several adjacent vertebral segments.[14] This widening of the spinal canal can be confused with the pressure erosion accompanying an intraspinal tumor. In this situation, thinning of the pedicles and erosion of the posterior aspect of the vertebral body suggest the presence of an expanding mass rather than a diastematomyelia.[22] The sagittal diameter of the vertebral body may be narrowed (Fig. 5–65). The disc space is absent or narrowed, and occasionally the lesion occurs in conjunction with a hemivertebra.[22] The laminae generally are not fused in the midline (spina bifida). However, the dysraphic area is often not located at the same level as

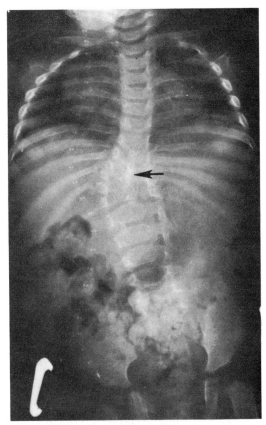

Figure 5–66. One-year-old patient with a midline bony spicule (arrow) in the thoracic region, multiple congenital anomalies, and myelodysplasia.

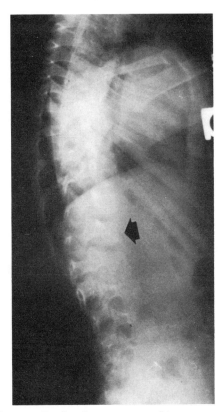

Figure 5–65. Local roentgenographic appearance of diastematomyelia, demonstrating anterior-posterior narrowing of the vertebral body in the area of the bony anomaly (arrow).

the diastematomyelia and may extend over several segments (Fig. 5–66).[30]

Myelographic examination is essential to confirm the diagnosis and often is the only method to demonstrate the presence of a diastematomyelia.[18, 30] The myelographic contrast material should be introduced at a low interspace to avoid damage by the needle to the conus medullaris, which frequently is low in the lumbar spine.[6] Several authors[6, 14, 16, 27] recommend a cisternal route in order to avoid this complication. Recent reports suggest that the use of a water-soluble contrast agent (metrizamide) in conjunction with computed tomography is more sensitive in demonstrating the diastematomyelia than conventional myelography.[24, 25] The contrast medium divides into two columns that flow easily around the midline obstruction. Multiple views in both the supine and prone positions are frequently necessary to completely delineate the lesion.[14, 26, 30] The defect is usually found to be

wider and longer than the bony spur itself
(Fig. 5–67). The spinal canal must be examined carefully in its entirety even if a diastematomyelia is found. The presence of two spi-
cules at different levels is not uncommon.[6, 8, 14,
16, 31] Dermoid cyst, neurofibroma, lipoma,
spinal cord tumors,[6, 23] arachnoid adhesions,
and congenital bands should not be overlooked even if a spicule is found.

Treatment

Matson[20] and many other authors[16, 21, 26]
since have recommended complete surgical
removal whenever a diastematomyelia is discovered. Their recommendation is based on
the assumption that the bony spicule prevents
normal upward migration of the neural elements and if not removed, progressive neurologic deficit will ensue. They view this surgical

procedure as prophylactic rather than cura-
tive. Matson[20] emphasized "that in general,
there is little improvement to be expected
following this type of surgery and that such
improvement should not be promised to the
patient's family nor stressed to them as the
reason why the surgery should be performed."

There are, however, several points that
favor a conservative approach and a longer
period of evaluation prior to surgical intervention. A significant number of patients with
diastematomyelia remain asymptomatic during growth or have a minimal neurologic deficit without evidence of progression (Fig. 5–
64).[2, 4, 7, 17] James[17] has suggested that too
much stress has been placed on the concept of
spinal cord tethering, that perhaps the spinal
cord can accommodate to traction, and the
clinical findings may be due to other causes
not understood, as Gillespie terms a "congeni-

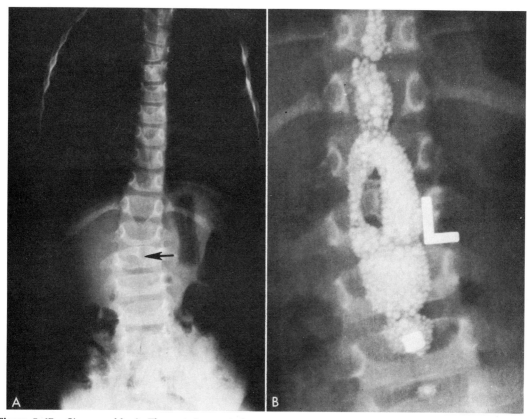

Figure 5–67. Six-year-old. *A,* The anterior-posterior roentgenogram suggests a midline bony mass and slight
widening of the lumbar canal in the region of the second lumbar vertebra. *B,* Myelographic appearance of the same area
demonstrating division of the contrast medium into two columns which flow easily around the midline obstruction. The
defect is usually found to be wider and longer than the bony spur itself.

tal myelopathy" or inadequacy of the cord tissue itself.[13] Patients with vertebral anomalies and congenital scoliosis (Fig. 5–66) cannot be expected to have normal vertical growth of the spine and may not develop stretching sufficient to cause problems.[13] In these patients the risks of extensive surgery would seem to outweigh the small potential gain. Surgery seldom results in dramatic improvement[30] and has on occasion resulted in an increase in neurologic deficit, even paraplegia, particularly when the lesion develops in the thoracic spine.[9, 30]

Preoperatively, the patient should be evaluated carefully for other lesions that could be the source of symptoms. The presence of a second spicule is not uncommon, and it may not be visible on the anterior-posterior myelogram.[6, 8] Spinal cord tumors, dermoid cysts, and lipomas have all been reported in association.[6, 13, 23] The majority of these children have congenital scoliosis, and occasionally symptoms are due to a high thoracic kyphos.[18, 30] If these conditions are unrecognized, the surgical exploration will be of little benefit and may have tragic results.

Surgical intervention is recommended if the patient exhibits a progressive neurologic deficit or if spinal traction or corrective casts are to be used in the treatment of congenital scoliosis.[13, 18, 30] Shorey[29] notes a 12-year-old who became paraplegic during cast treatment for severe kyphoscoliosis and diastematomyelia. Surgical exploration should be done as a separate procedure prior to definitive management of the spinal deformity.[13, 18, 30] Winter[30] further suggests that the patient with congenital scoliosis and widening of the interpedicular distance, neurologic deficit, and foot deformities should undergo exploration even though the myelogram is negative. As yet no confirmatory data are available with which to assess the efficacy of this recommendation.

The procedure described by Matson[20] and amplified by Meachem[21] is commonly employed. The spinal canal is unroofed by laminectomy starting at least one level away from the lesion. The lamina over the lesion is frequently dysraphic, and the septum may be attached to the dorsal structures (Fig. 5–68). The bony spicule is removed by subperiosteal dissecton to minimize bleeding. The dura is

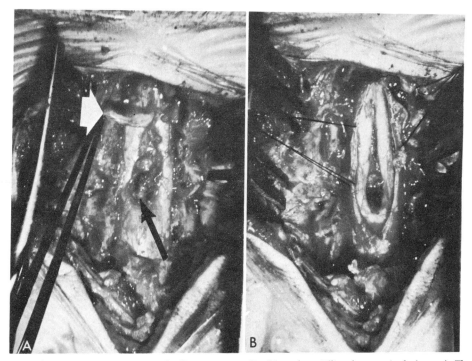

Figure 5–68. *A,* Operative appearance of a diastematomyelia. Note the midline bony spicule (arrow). The adjacent neurologic elements are enclosed within separate arachnoid sheaths. Arrow indicates a dural-cutaneous fistula prior to excision. *B,* Appearance after excision of the spicule, prior to closure of dura.

then opened, and the spinal cord or cauda equina is usually bound by adhesions. These are gently removed, and the neural structures are completely freed. Occasionally a tight filum terminale will be found, and this will require release. The remaining anterior portion of the spicule is then carefully removed. The neural segments will be seen to move closer together and freely in the canal. The dura is closed posteriorly, and no attempt is made to close it anteriorly.

Summary

Diastematomyelia is an uncommon congenital disturbance of vertebral architecture in which a midline mass develops in the spinal canal and splits the neural elements. Its etiology is uncertain, but the clinical findings presumably are due to its restriction, "tethering" of the normal upward migration of the spinal cord. Signs and symptoms are dependent on the level of diastematomyelia. If the spinal cord or conus medullaris is involved, spasticity and pathologic reflexes will be present, whereas low lumbar lesions lead to peripheral nerve signs, muscle weakness, and sensory loss. Congenital anomalies of the spine, of one or both lower extremities, and asymmetry of clinical findings are frequently found with this condition. Dorsal midline cutaneous abnormalities are present in the majority of patients and often provide a valuable clue to the diagnosis.

Roentgenographic features include fusiform widening of the interpedicular distance at the level of the lesion and a midline bony mass projecting from the posterior aspect of the vertebral body. It must be remembered that the mass may be cartilaginous or fibrous and thus radiolucent. Congenital scoliosis is often associated, and the distorted vertebral architecture may obscure the lesion. It is frequently impossible to diagnose diastematomyelia on routine roentgenograms, and myelographic exaination is essential to confirm the presence or absence of the lesion.

Surgical removal should be viewed as prophylactic, as it does not result in improvement of an existing neurologic deficit but can halt progression of neurologic impairment. The role of surgery in the asymptomatic patient or those with minimal complaints is not yet defined. Children with congenital scoliosis who may require spine traction or in whom Harrington instrumentation is being considered should be carefully evaluated for diastematomyelia.

References

1. Amador, L. V., Hankison, J., and Bigler, J. A.: Congenital spinal dermal sinuses. J. Pediatr. *47*:300–310, 1955.
2. Banniza Von Bazan, J.: The association between congenital elevation of the scapula and diastematomyelia. J. Bone Joint Surg. *61B*:59–63, 1979.
3. Barson, A. J.: The vertebral level of termination of the spinal cord during normal and abnormal development. J Anat. *106*:489–497, 1970.
4. Bligh, A. S.: Diastematomyelia. Clin. Radiol. *12*:158–163, 1961.
5. Bremer, J. L.: Congenital Anomalies of the Viscera. Cambridge, MA, Harvard University Press, 1957.
6. Burrows, F. G. G.: Some aspects of occult spinal dysraphism: A study of 90 cases. Br. J. Radiol. *41*:496–507, 1968.
7. Cohen, J., and Sledge, C. B.: Diastematomyelia: An embryological interpretation with report of a case. Am. J. Dis. Child. *100*:257–263, 1960.
8. Cowie, T. N.: Diastematomyelia: Tomography in diagnosis. Br. J. Radiol. *25*:263–266, 1952.
9. Eid, K., Hochberg, J., and Saunders, D.: Skin abnormalities of the back in diastematomyelia. Plast. Reconstr. Surg. *63*:534–539, 1979.
10. English, W. J., and Maltby, G. L.: Diastematomyelia in adults. J. Neurosurg. *27*:260–264, 1967.
11. Freeman, L. L.: Late symptoms from diastematomyelia. J. Neurosurg. *18*:538–541, 1961.
12. Gardner, W. J.: Diastematomyelia and the Klippel-Feil syndrome: Relationship to hydrocephalus, syringomyelia, meningocele, meningomyelocele and iniencephalus. Cleve. Clin. Q. *31*:19–44, 1964.
13. Gillespie, R., Faithfull, D. K., Roth, A., and Hall, J. E.: Intraspinal anomalies in congenital scoliosis. Clin. Orthop. *93*:103–109, 1973.
14. Hilal, S. K., Marton, D., and Pollack, E.: Diastematomyelia in children. Radiographic study of 34 cases. Radiology *112*:609–621, 1974.
15. James, C. C. M., and Lassman, L. P.: Spinal dysraphism: The diagnosis and treatment of progressive lesions in spina bifida occulta. J Bone Joint Surg. *44B*:828–840, 1962.
16. James, C. C. M., and Lassman, L. P.: Diastematomyelia: A critical survey of 24 cases submitted to laminectomy. Arch. Dis. Child. *39*:125–130, 1964.
17. James, C. C. M., and Lassman, L. P.: Diastematomyelia and the tight filum terminale. J. Neurol. Sci. *10*:193–196, 1970.
18. Keim, H. A., and Greene, A. F.: Diastematomyelia and scoliosis. J. Bone Joint Surg. *55A*:1425–1435, 1973.
19. Lourie, H., and Bierny, J. P.: Diastematomyelia with two spurs and intradural neural crest elements. J. Neurosurg. *32*:248–251, 1970.
20. Matson, D. D., Woods, R. P., Campbell, J. B., and Ingraham, F. D.: Diastematomyelia (congenital clefts of the spinal cord): Diagnosis and surgical treatment. Pediatrics *6*:98–112, 1950.
21. Meacham, W. F.: Surgical treatment of diastematomyelia. J. Neurosurg. *27*:78–85, 1967.
22. Neuhauser, E. B. D., Wittenborg, M. H., and Dehlinger, K.: Diastematomyelia: Transfixation of the

cord or cauda equina with congenital anomalies of the spine. Radiology *54*:659–664, 1950.

23. Perret, G.: Symptoms and diagnosis of diastematomyelia. Neurology *10*:51–60, 1960.

24. Resjö, I. M., Harwood-Nash, D. C., Fitz, C. R., and Chuang, S.: Computed tomographic metrizamide myelography in spinal dysraphism in infants and children. J. Comput. Assist. Tomogr. *2*:549–558, 1978.

25. Resjö, I. M., Harwood-Nash, D. C., Fitz, C. R., and Chuang, S.: Normal cord in infants and children examined with computed tomographic metrizamide myelography. Radiology *130*:691–696, 1979.

26. Sands, W. W., and Clark, W. K.: Diastematomyelia. Am. J. Roentgenol. *72*:64–67, 1954.

27. Sarwar, M., and Kelly, P. J.: Adult diastematomyelia. Spine *2*:60–64, 1977.

28. Seaman, W. B., and Schwartz, H. G.: Diastematomyelia in adults. Radiology *70*:692–696, 1958.

29. Shorey, W. D.: Diastematomyelia associated with dorsal kyphosis producing paraplegia. J. Neurosurg. *12*:300–305, 1955.

30. Winter, R. B., Haven, J. J., Moe, J. H., and Lagaard, S. M.: Diastematomyelia and congenital spine deformities. J. Bone Joint Surg. *56A*:27–39, 1974.

31. Zeuge, R. C., Tang, T. T., Dieus, W. T., and Blount, W. P.: A disastrous dysraphism. J. Bone Joint Surg. *55A*:434–435, 1973.

SPONDYLOLYSIS AND SPONDYLOLISTHESIS IN CHILDREN

In 1782, Herbiniaux,[21] a Belgian obstetrician, reported a patient with gross forward displacement of the fifth lumbar vertebra on the first sacral segment with its attendant narrowing of the birth canal. This was followed by several reports of similar findings discovered during anatomic dissections. The popular conclusion was that it represented an acute subluxation. In 1854, Kilian[25] correctly deduced that the displacement occurred gradually and termed the condition spondylolisthesis. He suggested that the slow slipping was due to the superimposed body weight. Robert[49] in 1855 performed an experiment that included removal of all the soft tissue attachments about the lumbosacral junction. He demonstrated that no displacement could occur if the posterior neural arch remained intact. When a defect was created in the arch, however, the vertebra was free to slide forward. Although many investigators had discovered spondylolisthesis at postmortem examinations, it was not always found to be associated with the neural arch defect (spondylolysis). This apparent discrepancy between clinical and experimental data was partially resolved in 1888 by Neugebauer,[42] who concluded that there were two conditions that could lead to spondylolisthesis: (1) a break (spondylolysis) in continuity of the neural arch or (2) elongation of the pars interarticularis. However, with improvements of radiologic techniques, attention was focused on the spondylolysis as the etiologic factor leading to spondylolisthesis,[22] and the work of Neugebauer[42] and others was largely ignored for many years.

More recently, Newman[44] reemphasized that there are several distinct conditions that may lead to displacement of the lumbosacral junction, and subsequently a more comprehensive classification of spondylolysis and spondylolisthesis has been suggested.[62]

1. Dysplastic spondylolisthesis (Fig. 5–69) — congenital deficiency of the superior sacral or inferior fifth lumbar facets (or both) with gradual slipping of the fifth lumbar vertebra;

2. Isthmic (spondylolytic) spondylolisthesis (Fig. 5–70) — the typical spondylolysis defect in the pars interarticularis, permitting forward sliding of the fifth lumbar body. This group is further divided into three types: (a) lytic (fatigue fracture of the pars); (b) elongated (attenuated) but intact pars interarticularis, and (c) acute fracture;

3. Degenerative spondylolisthesis — degeneration of L5-S1 joints, allowing forward displacement;

4. Traumatic spondylolisthesis — acute fracture in areas of the bony hook (pedicle, lamina, or facets) other than the pars interarticularis; and

5. Pathologic spondylolisthesis — attenuation of the pedicle secondary to structural weakness of the bone, such as osteogenesis imperfecta.

In this chapter, we will be concerned with those types that occur in children and adolescents. The onset and pattern of symptoms and clinical presentation of the child with spondylolisthesis are quite different from their adult counterparts.[33, 44, 46] Additional considerations, such as the influence of hormones or lack of degenerative change, suggest that spondylolisthesis as it occurs in the immature patient should be viewed as a distinct clinical entity separate from that found in adults.[11, 17, 20, 29, 43] These same differences should be considered when treatment is required, particularly when surgical intervention is contemplated.

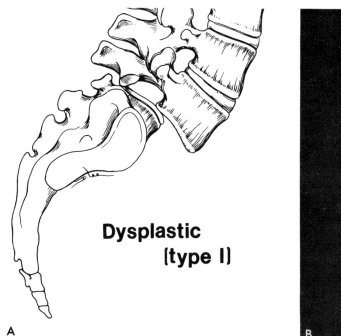

**Dysplastic
(type I)**

A

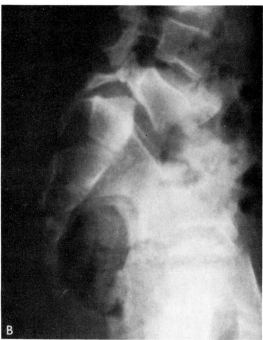

B

Figure 5–69. *A,* Type I — dysplastic (congenital) spondylolisthesis. The drawing of the lumbosacral junction demonstrates forward subluxation of the body of the fifth lumbar vertebra on the sacrum. The facets are subluxed, and the pars interarticularis is elongated. The posterior elements slide forward with the fifth lumbar vertebra. *B,* Roentgenogram of a 14-year-old female with a Grade IV, due to type I dysplastic spondylolisthesis.

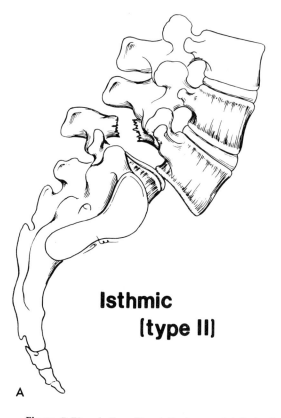

**Isthmic
(type II)**

A

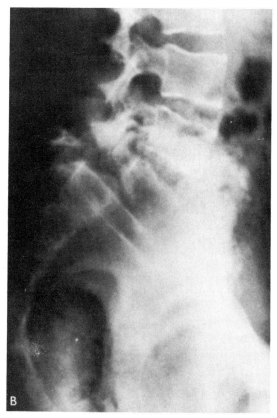

B

Figure 5–70. *A,* Type II — isthmic spondylolisthesis with disruption of the pars interarticularis. The defect in the pars interarticularis allows the body of the fifth lumbar vertebra to slide forward on the sacrum. The spinous process and lamina of L5 remain posterior with the sacral facets. *B,* Roentgenogram of a 13-year-old female with Grade IV spondylolisthesis due to Type II isthmic spondylolysis.

Etiology

Spondylolysis and spondylolisthesis are often referred to as congenital anomalies of the spine, yet there is no supporting embryologic or anatomic evidence for this assumption. Despite an anatomic incidence of 5 per cent in the general population, only one infant has been discovered to have the pars interarticularis defect.[5, 29, 51, 64] Spondylolysis in children occurs after walking age but rarely before five years of age and more commonly at seven or eight years.[2, 51, 61, 63] The incidence of spondylolysis and spondylolisthesis increases with age until 20 and then remains the same as in the general population.[2, 26, 27, 29, 30, 60, 61, 63] This has suggested to some investigators that trauma is a prominent factor in the etiology. However, Rowe[51] was unable to produce the typical pars interarticularis lesion in infant cadavers despite vigorous flexion and extension. Hitchcock[22] could produce spondylolysis only by forced hyperflexion, and laboratory tests indicate that a high degree of force is required. Although the history of minor trauma is common and often initiates the onset of symptoms, seldom would the injury be classified as severe.[6, 11, 20, 35, 58] Rather, the onset of symptoms coincides closely with the adolescent growth spurt.[3, 11, 58]

Wiltse suggests that spondylolysis represents a ''stress'' or fatigue fracture of the pars interarticularis.[63] It is postulated that lumbar lordosis is accentuated by the normal hip flexion contractures of childhood.[43] This posture focuses the force of weight bearing on the pars interarticularis, leading to gradual disruption.[40] Anatomic studies suggest that shear stresses are greater on the pars interarticularis when the spine is extended[40] and are further accentuated by lateral flexion movements on the extended spine, as may occur during a back walk-over in gymnastics.[23] Jackson[23] noted spondylolysis to be four times higher (11 per cent) in female gymnasts than expected, some of whom initially had normal roentgenograms and later developed spondylolysis. Spondylolysis has been documented to occur in soldiers while carrying heavy backpacks or while performing exercises to which they had been unaccustomed.[42, 47, 63] Newman[43] noted that in many the defects healed with conservative treatment and became asymptomatic. Others developed pseudarthrosis with continued symptoms and the radiologic appearance of spondylolysis. Wiltse[63] has reported similar findings even occasionally leading to spondylolisthesis. A similar increased incidence has been noted in weight lifters and in college football linemen.

Further support is found in the examination of resected specimens. The area of the spondylolysis exhibits the same reactive changes and callus formation common to pseudarthrosis in other bones.[40, 43] In a child who has greater plasticity of bone, these same forces may lead to gradual attenuation of the pedicle and stretching like pulled taffy. Wiltse[63] suggests that this is an unusual manifestation of the healing process of a fatigue fracture.

There are several findings that favor a congenital origin. The most significant argument is that of heredity. A high rate of occurrence among family members has been reported by numerous authors with an incidence of 27 per cent to 69 per cent in close relatives versus an expected frequency of 4 to 8 per cent in the general population.[14, 19, 24, 28, 65] Furthermore, Wynne-Davies and Scott[65] in a radiographic family survey found that patients with each type of spondylolisthesis, isthmic and dysplastic, had relatives with the opposite type. Interestingly, those with the dysplastic form had a higher proportion of affected relatives (33 per cent) than those with the isthmic type (15 per cent).[65] A high incidence (45 per cent) has been discovered among certain Eskimo tribes.[24] There is a racial and sex difference, with a 1.1 per cent incidence in black females, 2.3 per cent in white females, 2.8 per cent in black males, and 6.4 per cent in white males.[51]

It has been suggested that the spondylolysis is due to a congenital failure of fusion between two separate centers of ossification. Extensive examination of fetal specimens, however, demonstrate that there is only one ossification center extending across the area of the pars interarticularis. Individuals with spondylolysis have an increased incidence of sacral spina bifida (28 per cent to 42 per cent) and congenital lack of development of the proximal sacrum and superior sacral facets.[11, 23, 24, 65] As might be expected, posterior defects in the fifth lumbar or first sacral arch are almost invariable in the dysplastic (congenital) type (94 per cent) and are more common in the isthmic type (32 per cent) than in the general population.[10, 65] It is theorized that this lack of posterior support may increase the concentration of forces on the pars interarticularis with resultant stress fracture.[63] Similarly, when the superior sacral facets are poorly developed, forward subluxation of the entire posterior neural arch of the fifth lumbar vertebra may occur.[11, 43, 44]

Thus, there are substantial arguments and supporting data in favor of both a developmental and congenital origin for spondylolysis and spondylolisthesis. In order to resolve this conflict, the following summary is offered. Spondylolisthesis (forward slipping of L5 on S1) is due to concentration of the trunk weight on the unstable fifth lumbar vertebral body. There are several lesions that may lead to this instability. Congenital deficiency of the sacrum and lack of integrity of the posterior structures, probably on a genetic basis, may predispose to spondylolysis or subluxation of the lumbosacral facets. Developmental factors, such as trauma, posture, or certain repetitive activities, may lead to a stress fracture of the pars interarticularis. Furthermore, intrinsic weakness of the bone, such as occurs in osteogenesis imperfecta or with the normal bone plasticity of youth, may permit gradual stretching of the pars interarticularis and pedicle.

Clinical Findings

Spondylolysis and spondylolisthesis commonly occur by late childhood or adolescence and seldom after age 20; yet, symptoms are relatively uncommon in children. In La-Fond's[26] series of 415 patients, 23 per cent had the onset of low back or radicular pain before the age of 20, but only 9 per cent of these sought medical attention during childhood or adolescence. For the child who does develop symptoms, the onset usually coincides with the adolescent growth spurt.[7, 11, 20] Although pain is the predominant complaint in adults, a significant number of children do not have pain and seek medical evaluation only because of a postural deformity or abnormality of gait. If the child does complain of pain, it is generally localized to the low back and, to a lesser extent, to the posterior buttocks and thighs.[20] Symptoms are usually initiated or aggravated by strenuous activity and are decreased by rest or limitation of activity.[18] Less commonly, the patient presents with a radicular pattern of pain in the lower extremities and only mild back complaints. This is more typical in frank spondylolisthesis and suggests nerve root irritation. This usually involves the first sacral root with pain radiating to the posterior

thigh. Rarely do adolescents experience pain below the knee or in the foot.[20]

Children, unlike adults, seldom have objective signs of nerve root compression, such as motor weakness, reflex change, or sensory deficit. In Turner and Bianco's[58] report of 173 children with spondylolisthesis and spondylolysis, only four exhibited a neurologic deficit. Examination, however, should include a careful search for sacral anesthesia and bladder dysfunction.

Hamstring tightness (so-called spasm) is commonly found in the symptomatic patient (80 per cent) and is thought by some[58] to be a sign of nerve root irritation; however, there is no evidence to support this contention.[2, 46] Hamstring tightness may be found in patients with spondylolysis or with all grades of spondylolisthesis (Fig. 5–71). It is seldom accompanied by neurologic signs.[2, 7, 20, 54] The hamstring muscles are innervated by several nerve roots (L4 to S3), and an extensive single lesion

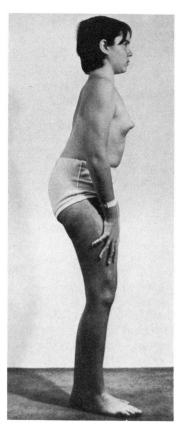

Figure 5–71. Teenager with severe hamstring tightness and the typical posture, flexion of the hips and knees, with the pelvis tilted backward, and flattening of the normal lumbar lordosis.

would be required to cause such massive involvement. The exact mechanism that initiates the tightness is not completely understood but probably involves an attempt to control the unstable L5-S1 junction. It is interesting to note that adolescents with severe hamstring tightness have had complete resolution of the tightness with surgical fusion alone and no accompanying nerve root decompression (Fig. 5–72).[7, 20]

Hamstring tightness has a variable pattern and can be quite impressive. The patient may not be able to flex the hips with the knees extended and may be forced to squat and bend at the knees in order to pick up an object. Frequently, the child prefers to sleep with the knees and hips in marked flexion.[12] During the straight leg raising test, the physician may be able to raise the foot only a few inches off the bed without causing severe pain or tightness. (In normal children, one can expect 70 to 80 degrees of hip flexion without bending the knees.) Occasionally, the patient does not experience actual pain but does have severe limitation of motion and resists attempts at straight leg raising by rolling the pelvis. Hamstring spasm is also found in other conditions, such as tumors that compress the cauda equina, tight filum terminale, diastematomyelia, or a massive herniated disc.[46]

Hamstring tightness is the cause of the peculiar gait that has become pathognomonic in the child with spondylolisthesis.[46] Indeed, the clinical picture can be so striking that Phalen and Dickson[46] were stimulated to describe it as a distinct syndrome. It may not be accompanied by pain and may be the sole reason the patient and family seek orthopaedic evaluation.[20] The excessively tight muscles keep the pelvis tilted backwards and do not permit hip flexion sufficient for a normal stride. Consequently, the patient has a stiff-legged and short stride gait with the pelvis being rotated forward with each step; New-

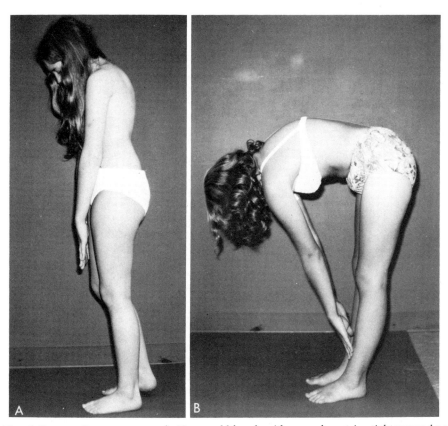

Figure 5–72.   A, Preoperative appearance of a 12-year-old female with severe hamstring tightness and a symptomatic Grade III spondylolisthesis. The patient is attempting to touch her toes, demonstrating marked restriction of forward bending. B, Eighteen months following surgery, she has complete resolution of hamstring tightness. The patient is now capable of full flexion of the hips with the knees in extension.

man[44] described this as a "pelvic waddle." The child may prefer to jog or run rather than walk or to walk up on the toes with the knees bent.

The physical examination may be normal in a child with spondylolysis or mild (Grade I or II) spondylolisthesis, or if the patient is symptomatic, restricted forward flexion of the hips (tight hamstrings) may be the only finding (Figs. 5–71 and 5–72). Distortion of the pelvis and trunk begin to be clinically apparent in the late stages of Grade II and are usually present when the slip reaches Grade III.[31, 60] The lumbar offset and lordosis can be severe and usually are accompanied by a backward tilt of the pelvis that may result from the tight hamstrings. When viewed from the front, the patient's lower abdomen appears to be thrust forward, forming a transverse abdominal crease at the umbilicus (Fig. 5–73). The ilia appear flared when viewed from the back, and the buttocks are heart-shaped and flattened

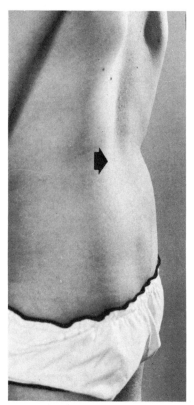

Figure 5–74. Flattening of the buttocks and the flaring of the ilia, typical clinical findings in the latter stages of spondylolisthesis. The palpable step-off (arrow) is the prominent fifth lumbar spinous process, due to the sliding forward of the fourth with the spondylolisthesis.

(Fig. 5–74). There may be a palpable step-off or depression over the fifth lumbar spinous process, which remains prominent while the fourth lumbar spinous process is carried forward with the anterior displacement of the vertebral bodies (Fig. 5–74). A lumbar "sag" or scoliosis is found in the majority of symptomatic patients and is due to reflex spasm and splinting from the lumbar irritation (Fig. 5–75). Generally this is not a structural curve and resolves with reclining or remission of symptoms.[48] Occasionally this curve can become structural and can form the basis of a thoracolumbar or double fixed deformity.[43]

Roentgenographic Findings

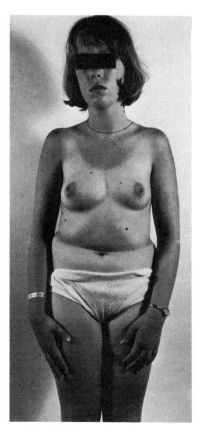

Figure 5–73. Grade III spondylolisthesis. Forward thrust of the lower abdomen forming a transverse abdominal crease at the umbilicus typically found in Grades III and IV.

POSTERIOR ELEMENTS. Spondylolysis refers to the radiolucent defect in the pars interarticularis. If the defect is large, it can be seen on nearly all roentgenographic views of

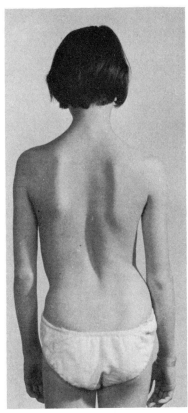

Figure 5–75. Typical "lumbar sag" associated with spondylolisthesis and usually found in the majority of symptomatic patients. It is probably caused by reflex spasm and splinting from lumbar irritation. This is generally not a structural curve, as it usually resolves with reclining or remission of symptoms.

the facets appear to sublux on the roentgenogram. If the slip continues, the pars interarticularis may become attenuated like pulled taffy — the "greyhound" of Hensinger[20] (Fig. 5–76B), and a defect may appear in the center (Fig. 5–78). The pedicles as well may appear elongated and may contribute further to the forward subluxation. In conditions that lead to structural bone weakness, such as osteogenesis imperfecta, lengthening of the pedicles is a more frequent occurrence. Wiltse[61] suggests that they are different manifestations of the same disease process, as he and, more recently, Wynne-Davies[65] have found both lesions present in family members, the spondylolytic being an acute stress fracture of the pars interarticularis and the dysplastic or elongated type representing a chronic stress reaction with gradual attenuation of the pars. Recognition of the dyplastic type is clinically important, since children with this type of spondylolisthesis are more prone to recurrent symptoms and clinical deformity if the condition is allowed to progress.[11, 20]

Roentgenographically, in the dysplastic type, the entire posterior neural arch, including the spine of the fifth lumbar vertebra, appears to slide forward with a marked offset (Fig. 5–69). If the lamina and posterior elements are present, progression will be limited to 25 per cent or there will be a cauda equina paralysis.[64] More often, further displacement of the vertebral body occurs owing to a break in the neural arch (Fig. 5–78). In contrast, in spondylolisthesis due to spondylolysis, the fifth lumbar spinous process and posterior elements maintain their position while forward displacement of the fourth lumbar spinous process occurs (Fig. 5–70). Deficiency of the posterior elements is a common occurrence in spondylolisthesis. Easily observable defects, such as dysraphic or malformed laminae, have been found in 32 to 94 per cent of these patients; if discovered on routine lumbosacral views, they should prompt more detailed roentgenographic investigation.[29, 65]

Sherman and associates[53] described the unusual occurrence of reactive sclerosis and hypertrophy of one pedicle and lamina and a contralateral spondylolysis in the same vertebral segment. They suggest that this represents a physiologic response to stress, the result of repeated trauma in the presence of an unstable neural arch, which will respond to conservative measures and symptomatic treatment. Roentgenographically, this may be confused with the reactive sclerosis associat-

the lumbar spine. If it is unilateral, as occurs in 20 per cent of patients[61] or if it is not accompanied by spondylolisthesis, it can be a very subtle finding requiring special techniques. Oblique views of the lumbar spine are often necessary to view this area in relief and apart from overlying bony elements. The "Scottie dog" of Lachapele with the defect appearing at the terrier's neck is a helpful visual aid to those inexperienced with the oblique roentgenogram (Fig. 5–76A). The edges of the defect are smooth and rounded, suggesting a pseudarthrosis rather than acute fracture; the width of the gap, of course, depends on the degree of spondylolisthesis (Fig. 5–77).

Confusion can occur when spondylolisthesis develops without spondylolysis — the dysplastic type (Fig. 5–69).[44, 64] This is a common finding in children who are symptomatic (26 to 35 per cent).[11, 20, 43] In this situation, rather than a gap or defect in the pars interarticularis,

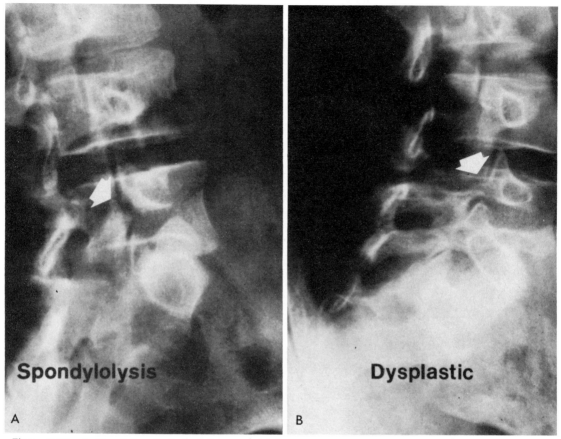

Figure 5–76. *A,* Pars interarticularis defect, spondylolysis (arrow) as seen on oblique roentgenographic view, typically found with the isthmic type of spondylolisthesis (type II). *B,* Similar oblique view of a patient with dysplastic (congenital) spondylolisthesis demonstrating elongation and attenuation of the pars interarticularis, perhaps a prespondylotic lesion.

ed with an osteoid osteoma. This becomes an important concern since excision of a sclerotic pedicle that is associated with a contralateral spondylolysis may increase instability. The presence of a nidus should confirm the diagnosis of an osteoid osteoma. A bone scan will not be helpful in differentiating between the two, since both will exhibit an increased isotope uptake owing to the presence of increased bone activity.

VERTEBRAL BODY. Forward subluxation of the vertebral body (spondylolisthesis) is best visualized on the lateral roentgenogram. Meyerding[37] devised a simple system for grading displacement. The top of the sacrum is divided into four equal sections. A slip in the first quarter of the sacrum is Grade I and one in the last quarter is Grade IV. A more exact method of measurement suggested by Taillard[56] measures the displacement of the olis-

thetic vertebra over the subjacent vertebral body and expresses the result in a percentage. This method is valuable in recording small changes in position, but clinically this is seldom necessary. Many patients have a significant change in position from standing to supine, average +15 degrees (ranging from +30 degrees to −10 degrees).[32, 39] Consequently, if a child is to be observed for progression of a spondylolisthesis, the roentgenographic technique must be the same at each visit. The standing lateral view is preferred.[7]

There are two kinds of slipping in spondylolisthesis: (1) tangential — the fifth lumbar vertebra slides forward on the first sacral vertebra, graded I through IV according to Meyerding classification; and (2) angular — the body of L5 tilts on the sacrum,[56] also referred to as angle of slipping,[7] roll,[11] kyphosis, or gibbus.[52] The angle of slip is measured

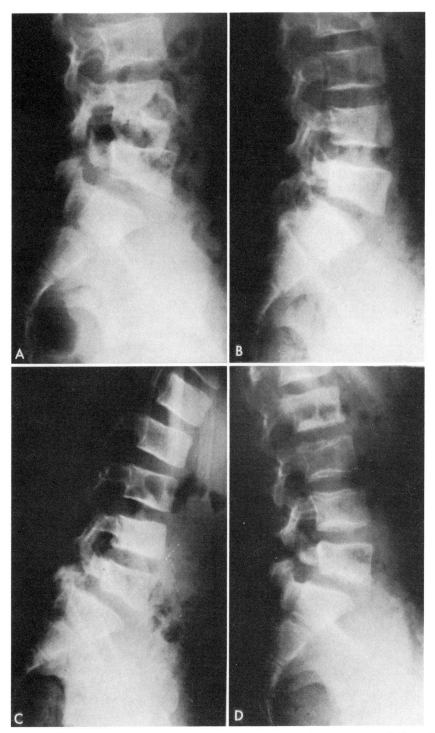

Figure 5–77.   Nine-year-old discovered to have spondylolisthesis. *A*, Lateral roentgenogram. *B*, Extension view at the same age demonstrating that the gap can be closed and the fifth lumbar body reduced by positioning. *C*, Flexion. *D*, Extension. Note the widening of the defect and progression of the spondylolisthesis. The patient is no longer able to reduce the gap or subluxation of the body with extension. (Roentgenograms provided courtesy of James A. Averett, Jr., M.D., Atlanta, Georgia.)

by the method described by Boxall and associates.[7] The angle is formed by a line drawn parallel to the inferior aspect of the fifth lumbar vertebral body and a line drawn perpendicular to the posterior aspect of the body of the first sacral vertebra (Fig. 5–80).

Children with spondylolisthesis appear to have more flexibility or looseness at the L5-S1 junction than their adult counterparts (Fig. 5–77A and B). This increased mobility is reflected in the roentgenographic and anatomic appearance of their vertebral bodies. There is gradual erosion of the anterior as well as the posterior aspect of the sacrum (Fig. 5–79),[7, 11, 29, 58] the sacrum becoming domed or peaked in the middle (Figs. 5–79 and 5–80).[20, 48] This inhibition of growth or erosion is mirrored in the trapezoid shape of the body of L5[29, 58, 62, 63] (the dorsal height of the vertebra being less than the ventral height) (Fig. 5–70), and the amount of wedging seems to be direct-ly related to the degree of slip.[6] This wear pattern suggests a teeter-totter type of instability of the lumbar vertebrae on the sacrum. As the slip advances to the higher grades, the sacrum and posterior aspect of the pelvis become more vertical (anterior inclination),[7, 20] again reflecting instability in combination with tight hamstrings and backward pulling of the pelvis (Figs. 5–81 and 5–82),[2] and the lumbar spine moves forward, increasing the lordosis,[6, 62, 63] giving rise to the typical clinical findings. In severe displacement, the lumbar body may appear to be precariously balanced on the sacrum and ready to cascade into the pelvis, but fortunately this is rare.

Although the foregoing discussion was limited to the typical spondylolisthesis of the fifth lumbar vertebra, vertebral forward displacement may occur at all levels of the spine. The next most common is the fourth lumbar vertebra and in most series represents 5 per cent of the total.

RISK FACTORS. Progression of the spondylolisthesis occurs between the ages of 10 and 15 and is quite uncommon in the adult (Fig. 5–77).[7, 11, 16, 29, 62] With time the anterior lip of the sacrum may develop a sclerotic buttress as a defensive measure to resist the slip (Fig. 5–82). Taillard[56] suggested that these changes portend a good prognosis in that further displacement is unlikely. Subsequent authors support his contention, finding this appearance more common in spondylolisthesis Grade I and II,[6, 29, 43] in adults,[6, 44] and uncommon in children.[20, 46] Boxall and associates[7] have called attention to the "angle of slip" (Fig. 5–80) of the fifth lumbar vertebral body on the first sacral body. They found that this angle accurately reflected the risk factors for continued progression, deformity, and symptoms.[7]

Frequently, it is impossible to accurately assess the potential for further displacement on the roentgenographic appearance alone. Comparison views, standing versus supine, in some instances will demonstrate instability and provide valuable information for prognosis and treatment. Similarly, flexion-extension views of the lumbosacral junction may be obtained to evaluate the presence of excessive motion (Fig. 5–77).

Myelographic Evaluation. Children with spondylolisthesis seldom require myelographic evaluation. In this age group, herniation of the nucleus pulposus rarely accompanies spondylolisthesis. Reviews of children with spondylolisthesis have consistently reported that

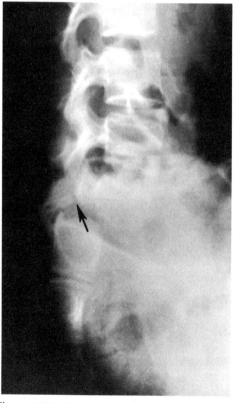

Figure 5–78. Spondylolisthesis due to subluxation of the facets. The pars interarticularis has become attenuated like pulled taffy, and a defect has appeared in the center (arrow). The break in the neural arch may permit further subluxation.

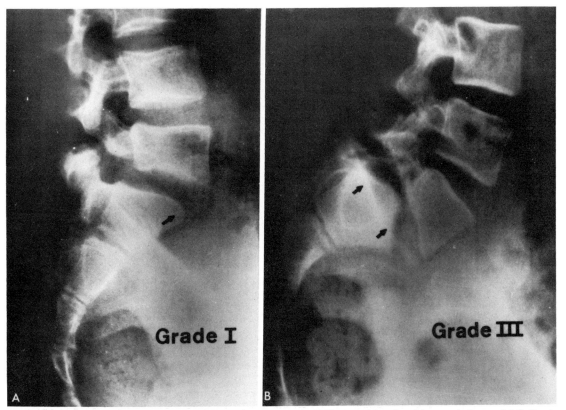

Figure 5–79. Instability of the body of L5 on the sacrum. *A,* A 10-year-old male with a grade I spondylolisthesis, demonstrating mild anterior erosion of the sacrum (arrow). *B,* A 13-year-old male with a grade III spondylolisthesis, demonstrating mild anterior erosion of the sacrum (arrow).

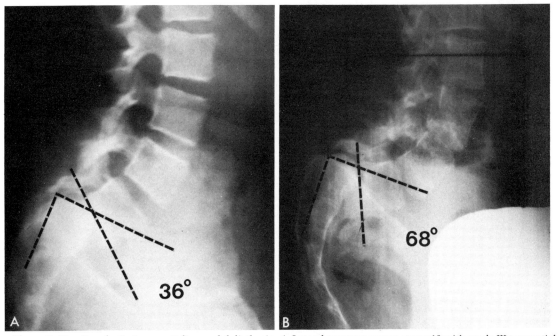

Figure 5–80. Dysplastic (congenital) spondylolisthesis. *A,* Lateral roentgenogram at age 10 with grade III tangential slip and significant angle of tilt (36°) of L5 on the sacrum. *B,* Same patient at age 13 untreated. Note moderate progression of the tangential slip and marked increase in the angle of tilt (68°), with increase in the lumbar lordosis and anterior inclination of the sacrum. The patient now has perineal anesthesia and a neurogenic bladder.

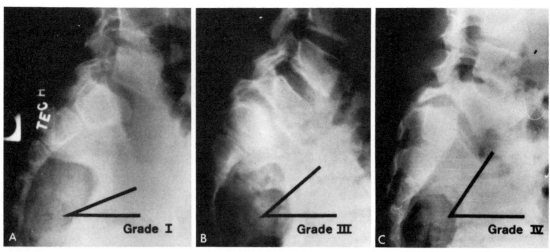

Figure 5–81. Three patients with different degrees of spondylolisthesis, *A, B,* and *C* (grades I, III, and IV). As the slip advances, the sacrum and pelvis become more vertical, in part owing to the backward pull of the tight hamstrings. The lumbar spine moves forward with increasing lordosis, giving rise to the typical clinical appearance. Often it is easier to understand the clinical problem if one considers the lumbar spine to be stable and observes the degree of motion of the pelvis.

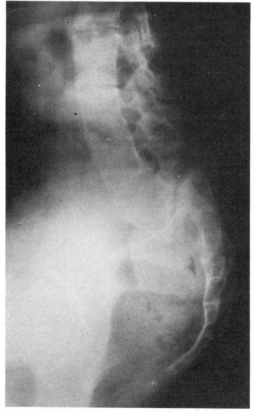

Figure 5–82. In this situation, the forward slide of the fifth lumbar body has been slowed by the sclerotic reaction between L5 and the sacrum. The sclerotic buttress forming on the anterior lip of the sacrum is a defensive measure to resist progression of the spondylolisthesis.

none of the patients have myelographic evidence of disc protrusion, and in those explored for herniation, none was found.[1, 7, 20, 55, 58] Although hamstring spasm or tightness is a frequent occurrence, objective signs of specific nerve root compression are generally absent. A myelogram should be considered if the patient's symptoms or neurologic signs do not resolve with bedrest. In this situation, it is incumbent to rule out the possibility of a coexistent lesion such as a neoplasm. Similarly, bladder and bowel dysfunction or perineal hypesthesia would justify further investigation.

If a myelogram is performed in the patient with spondylolisthesis due to a pars defect (isthmic, type II), on the lateral view the spinal canal is typically found to be indented anteriorly by the posterior aspect of the body of the first sacral vertebra.[7] In contrast, if the neural arch is intact and pulled forward with the fifth lumbar body (dysplastic, type I), a posterior partial block of the contrast material is likely.[44]

Treatment

SPONDYLOLYSIS

Although spondylolysis originates in children between five and ten years of age, relatively few are symptomatic or seek medical attention. It is not surprising, therefore, that children and teenagers usually respond to simple conservative measures.[20] Restriction of vigorous activities and back and abdominal strengthening exercises are usually successful in controlling those with mild backache and hamstring tightness. Patients with more severe or persistent complaints may require bedrest, immobilization in a cast or brace, and non-narcotic analgesics. Hamstring tightness is an excellent clinical guide to the success or failure of the treatment program. The majority of affected children can be expected to have excellent relief of symptoms or only minimal discomfort on long-term follow-up examination.[58, 61]

We would agree with Wiltse[61, 63] that any child or adolescent discovered to have spondylolysis, especially those under 10 years of age, should be followed closely. We do not advise those with asymptomatic spondylolysis or those with minimal symptoms to restrict their activities; 7.2 per cent of asymptomatic young men age 18 to 30 years have the pars defect,[38] and relatively few have persistent symptoms. Thus, limitation of activity in a growing child would not seem justified.

It must be emphasized that it is quite uncommon for spondylolysis to be symptomatic in adolescence, and the physician should resist the temptation to credit it exclusively as the cause of symptoms. Rather, one should vigorously explore for other causes of back pain. The differential diagnosis includes disc space infection, osteoid osteoma, spinal cord tumor, herniated disc, rheumatoid spondylitis, and muscle and neurologic disorders. As uncommon as these conditions are in childhood, when viewed from the total causes of back pain, they are equally as common as symptomatic spondylolysis in the teenager. One should be particularly wary of the child whose symptoms do not respond to bedrest or who has objective neurologic findings. In this situation, myelographic and electromyographic evaluation should be considered.

A small percentage of young people with spondylolysis do not respond to conservative measures or are unwilling to curtail their activities and may require surgical stabilization. If surgery is found necessary, lateral column fusion from the fifth lumbar vertebra to the sacrum employing iliac bone is usually sufficient (p. 277). Nachemson[41] reported solid healing of the defect using a bone graft coupled with an intertransverse fusion. Buck[9] proposed a technique for direct repair of the defect, employing screw fixation and iliac

bone graft. He emphasized that this procedure is indicated only for gaps of less than 3 or 4 mm., but in this situation it avoids the need for spinal fusion. We have no experience with this procedure, but it would appear useful in this group. The Gill procedure or laminectomy (or both) is never indicated without an associated fusion in children.[54] Removal of the posterior elements may in fact be harmful, leading to increased instability and spondylolisthesis in the postoperative period.

ASYMPTOMATIC SPONDYLOLISTHESIS

Children or adolescents with asymptomatic spondylolisthesis discovered on routine roentgenograms pose a perplexing problem. Unfortunately, precise guidelines are not available concerning the likelihood of further progression, back pain, degenerative arthritis, or the indications for prophylactic surgical stabilization. The physician should share these uncertainties with the patient and parents at the initial visit and should follow the child closely for signs of progression.

The potential for further progression during the growing years is well documented and is directly related to the age of the patient. Children who have had an episode of back pain due to spondylolisthesis of any grade have a higher incidence of recurrent episodes ending in permanent restriction of activities or the need for surgical stabilization.[58] Females seem to be at greater risk of further slipping and progression to more severe grades.[7, 11, 54] The roentgenographic appearance may provide a clue to the prognosis. Those who develop a sclerotic buttress on the anterior lip of the sacrum are less likely to progress than those with a dome-shaped, vertical sacrum and trapezoid fifth lumbar vertebral body.[4, 7, 20] The angle of slipping[7] of kyphosis of L5-S1 appears to be an excellent indicator of the risk factors.[7] Those with 50 per cent or greater spondylolisthesis (grades III and IV) are at high risk and should be considered for surgical stabilization.[2, 7, 20] In the higher grades, the risk of further deformity of pelvis and trunk may provide the sole stimulus to surgical stabilization.

Should activities be restricted? Wiltse[60] has suggested that activities need not be limited with slips of less than 25 per cent but that the patient should prepare for a vocation that does not require heavy lifting or strenuous activity. With slips greater than 25 per cent, he recommends that contact sports and activities that carry a high probability of back injury be avoided and that the same vocational goals be set. These guidelines must be tempered by the realization that many teenagers are resistant to leading such a restricted lifestyle or changing vocational plans.

SYMPTOMATIC SPONDYLOLISTHESIS

A great deal of information has been accumulated pertaining to the child with symptomatic spondylolisthesis, and thus results of treatment and prognosis are more predictable. Conservative measures are unsuccessful in controlling symptoms or postural deformity in more than half of these children. In grades III and IV, many children will require surgical intervention.[7, 20, 58, 61]

Indications for surgery are as follows: (1) pain unrelieved by conservative measures, (2) progression of subluxation, (3) symptomatic spondylolisthesis greater than 50 per cent (grades III and IV) in an immature patient, and (4) postural deformity or significant gait abnormalities due to tight hamstrings unrelieved by physical therapy.

All should have a period of hospitalization and enforced bedrest prior to surgery.[7, 20, 54] Symptoms should improve with this program, and if not, further investigation (myelography or electromyography) should be considered to rule out a coexistent lesion.

Immobilization in a lightweight plaster or plastic jacket has been a helpful contribution to the preoperative evaluation.[20] The response to immobilization can provide useful information concerning the efficacy of surgical stabilization to the physician, family, and patient.

OPERATIVE MANAGEMENT. Previously, posterior spinal fusion was performed to control spondylolisthesis, but this yielded a high percentage of pseudarthrosis[31, 58, 60] and further slip following surgery.[29] Owing in part to the abnormal and loose posterior element, there is not a sufficient bed of stable bone. At present, the bilateral-lateral column or transverse process fusion[57] is preferred since it provides a wide lumbosacral bed[43, 58, 60, 61] and improved rate of fusion.[7, 20] The bilateral-lateral column fusion technique requires more dissection with an increase in operating time. However, we feel these controlled problems are outweighed by the greatly improved chances of a successful arthrodesis.[20] Interestingly, adults have not shared this same degree of success, with a fusion rate of 67 per cent.[55] In patients with Grade I or II spondylolisthesis

(Fig. 5–79A), the body of L5 is not tilted, and fusion of the transverse process of the fifth lumbar vertebra to the ala of the sacrum is sufficient. With tilt of the vertebral body (L5-S1 gibbus), usually occurring in Grades III and IV (Fig. 5–69B), the transverse process of the fourth lumbar vertebra should be included in the fusion (Figs. 5–83 and 5–84).

The Gill procedure is never indicated by itself in children and adolescents with spondylolisthesis. Complete removal of the posterior elements may potentiate instability and is associated with a high incidence of further progression of the slip in the postoperative period[3, 6, 30, 31, 34, 58, 60, 61] and a significantly increased incidence of pseudarthrosis.[54] Although removal of the neural arch does not preclude a good clinical result, there is a higher incidence of poor results (pseudarthrosis, progression of slip, recurrence of symptoms) and of patients who require reexploration.[31, 54] Gill[16] himself did not recommend the procedure for children since presumably they have not developed the reactive (degenerative) changes that provide the postoperative stability found in adults.

Laminectomy is seldom indicated owing to the low incidence of associated herniated nucleus pulposus or nerve root impingement.[1, 7, 20, 55, 58] In general, if the patient's symptoms are related to activity and are improved or resolved with bedrest or immobilization in a cast or brace, stabilization of the spine alone will achieve excellent long-term remission of symptoms, including the disappearance of the hamstring tightness.[7, 20] We would therefore disagree with the recommendation of Barash and associates[3] that laminectomy and sacral osteoplasty be considered in all patients with severe hamstring spasm. If symptoms or clinical findings persist despite bedrest or immobilization or if the patient has difficulty with neurologic control of the bowel or bladder, then one should obtain a myelographic examination and, if positive, should recommend exploration of the spinal canal and decompression. Furthermore, lateral mass fusion does not interfere with the posterior elements and will not hinder decompression later if it becomes necessary.

Surgical Procedure (Fig. 5–83). The patient is positioned in a manner that avoids pressure on the abdomen, thus minimizing venous pressure and resultant increased blood loss. Hamstring tightness can prevent proper positioning and can be circumvented by flexing the hips and knees. We have employed a

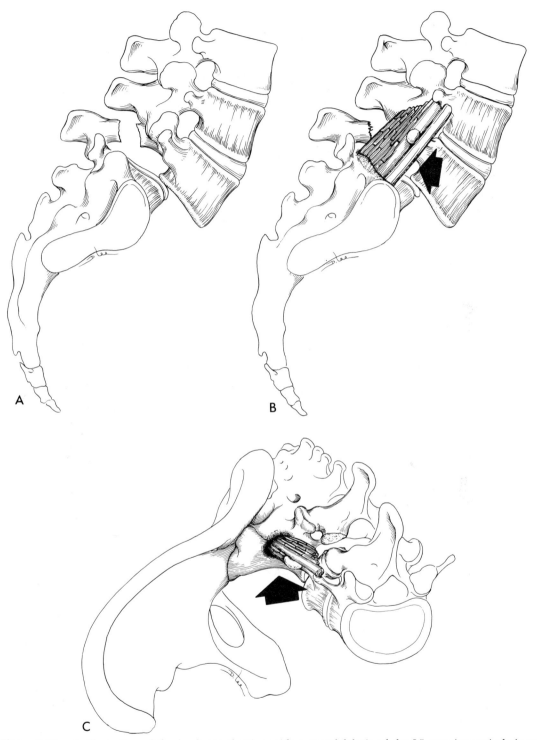

Figure 5–83. *A,* Illustration of the lumbosacral spine with a spondylolysis of the L5 pars interarticularis and spondylolisthesis. *B,* The surgical procedure preferred by the authors. A large window has been made in the ala of the sacrum (arrow) in which a large piece of cortical bone has been placed and which extends to the transverse process of the most proximal vertebra to be fused. This forms the floor of the bone graft on which the cancellous portion of the graft is placed. It is important that the graft nearly parallel the forces through the L5-S1 joint. *C,* View of the graft in place.

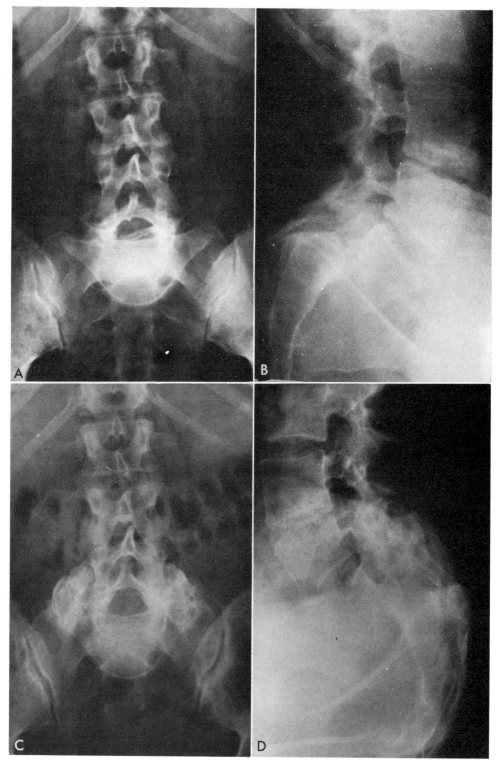

Figure 5–84. Nineteen-year-old with a grade III spondylolisthesis. *A* and *B*, Preoperative roentgenographic appearance. *C* and *D*, Appearance three years following bilateral-lateral column fusion. There has been no further progression of the spondylolisthesis, and the patient enjoys complete remission of symptoms. This result is to be anticipated by this method.

slightly curvilinear transverse incision between the iliac spines that centers over the lumbosacral junction. It is cosmetically acceptable and facilitates lateral dissection of the lumbar spine and exposure of an iliac crest to obtain the bone graft. Subperiosteal dissection involves only the vertebrae involved in the arthrodesis. It must be remembered that many patients will have spina bifida and loose posterior elements.[6, 11, 44, 62, 65] Thus, appropriate care must be taken as the deeper structures are dissected to avoid entering the spinal canal. The transverse processes are dorsally cleared of soft tissue, and the tips are circumferentially exposed as well as the ala of the sacrum bilaterally. For Grades I and II, exposure of the fifth lumbar vertebra to the sacrum will be sufficient; for Grades III and IV, exposure of the fourth lumbar vertebra will be required. The lateral columns of the vertebrae and the transverse processes are carefully decorticated. The facets remain intact, and the laminae are not disturbed. A hole is gouged in the superior ala of the sacrum, and a large cortical strip is placed in it and under the tip of the most proximal transverse process, forming the floor of the graft bed. The remaining space is filled with cancellous strips. It is important to position the graft as anteriorly as possible in order to parallel the compressive forces through the L5-S1 articulation (Fig. 5–84). If postoperative cast reduction is planned, the inferior cortical strip should be omitted, as it may impinge on the L5 root.[8] Similarly, the presence of an elongated pars or malformed facets may impede a satisfactory reduction and should be adequately freed or resected.[8]

POSTOPERATIVE MANAGEMENT. The patient is nursed in the supine position with the knees and hips flexed to decrease hamstring spasm. The patient is usually comfortable in a few days, and a cast is applied. To prevent further displacement, we routinely immobilize the child postoperatively in a bilateral pantaloon spica for three to four months.[20] Release of the posterior soft tissue attachments consequent to the surgical procedure can temporarily increase instability and may be further aggravated by early weight-bearing; thus, the cast insures against progression of spondylolisthesis and pseudarthrosis and provides a reliable means of controlling an active teenager. In this age group, this period of immobilization does not represent an economic disadvantage and with few exceptions[54] is physiologically well tolerated.[7, 20] This degree of restriction is probably not necessary in the skeletally mature adolescent or those with a mild slip who have a low potential for displacement. It has been reported by Stauffer and Coventry[55] that in the adult a solid arthrodesis can be obtained even though the patient's legs are not immobilized. The patient is not permitted to return to vigorous activities or contact sports during the first postoperative year, and then only if there is roentgenographic evidence of solid bony fusion.

Results of surgery are generally very good for this patient group. The mild neurologic changes usually disappear in the majority of patients.[7, 20] Hamstring tightness can be expected to resolve completely in the majority and to a large extent in the remainder, usually within the first 12 to 18 months.[7, 20] Patients are able to resume full and unrestricted activity, including track, cheerleading, horseback riding, swimming, and diving.[7, 20] Very few complain of limitation of spine motion. A high percentage can be expected to have a solid roentgenographic appearance of the fusion within the first year (Fig. 5–85) with no detectable motion on flexion-extension views.[20] An increased incidence of pseudarthrosis is associated with spina bifida[7] and a poor quality transverse process fusion. Some young people's vertebrae will remodel and further improve with growth.[7] A few inexplicably may have progression of the slip, despite an apparently solid arthrodesis.[7, 20] This is more likely to occur in those with a high angle of slipping (tilt), high percentage of slipping (tangential), midline fusion, and poor quality transverse process fusion.[7]

REDUCTION OF SPONDYLOLISTHESIS. The degree of angular slipping (L5-S1 gibbus) is the primary determining factor in the clinical deformity, the vertical sacrum and flat buttock, transverse abdominal groove, and increased lumbar lordosis. Thus, reducing the kyphosis at L5-S1 may achieve an excellent clinical result with only a slight change in the degree of tangential slip. A number of closed reduction techniques have been employed. Pelvic suspension and traction (halofemoral and halopelvic) have not generally been successful in changing the L5-S1 relationship nor in maintaining the reduction in the postoperative period. In addition, they may lead to significant complications.[7, 11, 17, 20, 29, 46, 60] Newman reported three patients who developed bladder dysfunction during postoperative traction, one in whom the dysfunction was permanent despite immediate release of traction.[44]

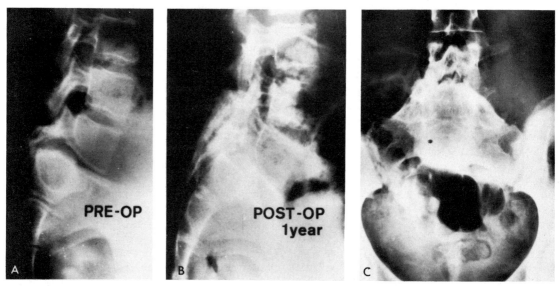

Figure 5–85. *A,* Roentgenographic appearance prior to bilateral-lateral column fusion, L4 to the sacrum, of an 11-year-old female with type I dysplastic spondylolisthesis and grade III spondylolisthesis. *B* and *C,* Postoperative appearance at age 12, demonstrating a solid fusion and no further progression of the spondylolisthesis. The patient was immobilized in a bilateral pantaloon spica for three months following the surgery to prevent further slippage.

Surgical reduction with instrumentation as described by Harrington can result in significant improvement but is technically difficult and has been associated with significant risk of neurologic complications.[8, 17, 44] Similarly, the reduction is not always maintained and can lead to an increase in thoracic lordosis.[7] Instrumentation that uses the sacral ala as a buttress precludes the use of a bilateral-lateral fusion technique, increasing the risk of pseudarthrosis.[52] Combined posterior and anterior surgical reduction as described by Bradford[8] can result in an excellent correction but is only indicated in the most severe cases.

It has been noted that recumbency alone improves reduction,[7, 11, 20] and recently, excellent results have been reported using cast reduction.[7, 38, 52] Previous attempts at closed reduction have focused on repositioning L5 on the body of S1, whereas this technique is the reverse in that the body of S1 is repositioned beneath L5. The cast is applied on a frame, which permits distraction of the trunk and hyperextension of the pelvis. With the patient supine, an elongation force is applied to the trunk, and the lower extremities hang free or with slight support, hyperextending the hips, allowing the pelvis to pivot on the crossbar (Fig. 5–86). The hip capsule and musculature

pulls the pelvis forward, rotating the sacrum beneath L5 to approximate the normal lumbosacral angle, reducing the L5-S1 kyphosis. Reduction may be further encouraged by positioning a localizer against the sacrum. Excessive pressure on the sacrum must be avoided, however. After the trunk portion of the cast is completed, the lower extremities are returned to a more comfortable position, and the bilateral pantaloon portion is completed. A major drawback is that this position may be uncomfortable and poorly tolerated by the patient. One can demonstrate that reduction is possible preoperatively, and serial casts may be applied to encourage further improvement.[52] The tangential slipping of L5 on the sacrum may not change; however, the technique can achieve a significant improvement in the L5-S1 kyphosis or angle of slip of the lumbosacral junction (Fig. 5–87). Appearance is improved by decreasing the vertical sacrum, apparent flatness of the buttocks, and restoring a more natural lumbar lordosis. Importantly, the reduction may decrease the chance of pseudarthrosis and late slip by decreasing the angle of slip.[7] Patients who undergo reduction of the spondylolisthesis with fusion should remain at bedrest for three to four months.[7, 20]

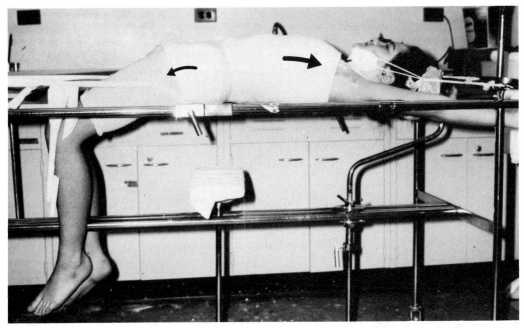

Figure 5–86. Cast reduction of spondylolisthesis. The patient is placed on the cast frame in the supine position. An elongation force is applied to the trunk (arrow). The lower extremities hang free or with slight support, hyperextending the hips and allowing the pelvis to pivot (arrow) on a crossbar. The hip capsule and musculature pulls the pelvis forward, rotating the sacrum beneath L5 to approximate the normal sacral angle. Reduction may be further increased by positioning a localizer against the sacrum. The trunk portion of the cast is completed and molded carefully to maintain the reduction. The lower extremities are returned to a more comfortable position, and the bilateral pantaloon portion is completed.

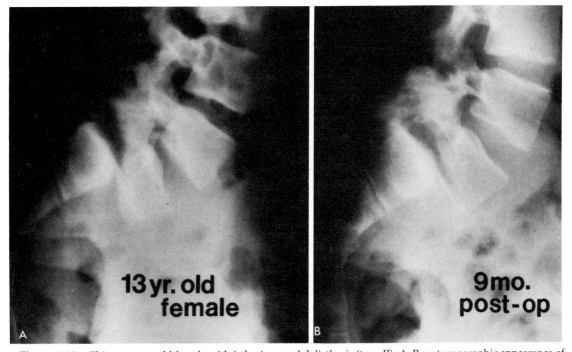

Figure 5–87. Thirteen-year-old female with isthmic spondylolisthesis (type II). *A,* Roentgenographic appearance of the spine prior to surgical stabilization. Note the degree of tangential subluxation and angle of tilt. *B,* Roentgenographic appearance at nine months after bilateral-lateral column fusion and cast reduction. Slight improvement in "tangential" slip; significant improvement in "angle of tilt," and clinically an excellent improvement in appearance.

Scoliosis and Spondylolisthesis

The lumbar scoliosis "list," "spasm," "antalgic," or "sag" (Fig. 5–75) commonly associated with symptomatic spondylolisthesis (23 to 36 per cent of cases) is secondary to lumbar muscle spasm.[6, 7, 13, 20, 29] It usually remits with recumbency or relief of symptoms. This curve can be expected to resolve following surgical stabilization of the spondylolisthesis and, in general, can be ignored.[7, 13, 20, 48] In rare instances of delayed treatment, the curve may become structural with permanent wedging of the vertebrae and discs.[13] Less commonly, a structural curve develops directly related to the pars defect, referred to by Tojner[57] as "olisthetic scoliosis" to indicate a low torsional-type curve. Patients with this curve pattern usually have more rotation, and the maximal torsion is at the spondylolytic vertebra, not the apical vertebra of the scoliosis as would be expected in an idiopathic curve of similar magnitude.[13] Spondylolysis or spondylolisthesis and spina bifida occulta occur with the same frequency in patients with idiopathic scoliosis as the general population.[10, 13] For details regarding management of structural scoliosis when it occurs with spondylolysis and spondylolisthesis, the reader is referred to Chapter 6.

Summary

Spondylolysis is a common problem found in 5 per cent of the general population. The etiology is a combination of two factors: (1) hereditary predisposition to the lesion due to a congenital deficiency of the sacrum and posterior structures and (2) developmental factors, such as trauma, posture, or certain repetitive activities, which may precipitate a stress fracture of the pars interarticularis of susceptible individuals. Although the lesion occurs in the growth years, very few develop symptoms during childhood and adolescence. For the child who develops symptoms, the onset usually coincides with the adolescent growth spurt,[7, 11, 20] and similarly progression of spondylolisthesis occurs between the ages of 10 and 15.[6, 11, 16, 29] When symptoms develop, the child may complain of low back pain and, to a lesser extent, posterior buttock and thigh pain, usually without a neurologic deficit. A few seek medical attention because of the postural deformity or abnormal gait secondary to hamstring tightness. Symptoms are usually initiated by strenuous activity and are relieved by limitation of activity or rest.

Children with spondylolisthesis appear to have more flexibility or looseness at the L5-S1 junction than their adult counterparts (Fig. 5–77). This increased mobility is reflected in the radiologic appearance of the vertebrae. There is gradual erosion of the anterior as well as the posterior aspect of the sacrum,[29, 44] and the sacrum becomes domed or peaked in the middle.[48] This inhibition of growth is mirrored in the trapezoid shape of the body of L5[23, 58, 62, 63] and is directly related to the degree of slip.[6] The wear pattern suggests a teeter-totter type of instability of the fifth lumbar vertebra on the sacrum (Fig. 5–79). The sclerotic buttress appearance or reactive changes common in adults[6, 43] are very uncommon in children.[20, 25] As the slip advances to the higher grades, the sacrum and posterior aspect of the pelvis become more vertical (anterior inclination), again reflecting instability in combination with tight hamstrings and backward pulling of the pelvis (angle of tilt),[3, 6, 20] giving rise to the marked physical changes and localized kyphosis of the lumbosacral spine. There is considerable evidence to suggest that when the spondylolisthesis exceeds 50 per cent, there are many dynamic and anatomic factors at work to potentiate continued deformity and symptoms in the growing adolescent. This is reflected clinically by the frequent failure of conservative measures in controlling symptoms and the need for surgical intervention in a significant percentage of patients once the slip exceeds Grade II.[7, 11, 20, 29, 58]

In the adult patient with spondylolisthesis, degenerative changes and nerve root irritation would seem to be the prime source of the symptoms. In children, however, symptoms are related to chronic instability of the L5-S1 joint. Stabilization of the spine, therefore, would appear to be the treatment of choice for the majority of symptomatic children. This may be accomplished by nonoperative means, such as cast or brace application, or in the refractory patient by surgical stabilization using a method that reliably results in arthrodesis, such as the bilateral-lateral column fusion. Procedures intended to relieve nerve root irritation unaccompanied by fusion, such as the Gill procedure or laminectomy, are contraindicated. By the same token, those conditions that led to instability preoperatively are still present in the postoperative period. Thus, immobilization and bedrest must be an integral part of the postoperative regimen.

References

1. Adkins, E. W. O.: Spondylolisthesis. J. Bone Joint Surg. *37B*:48–62, 1955.
2. Baker, D. R., and McHollick, W.: Spondyloschisis and spondylolisthesis in children. J. Bone Joint Surg. *38A*:933, 1956.
3. Barash, H. L., Galante, J. O., Lambert, C. N., and Ray, R. D.: Spondylolisthesis and tight hamstrings. J. Bone Joint Surg. *52A*:1319–1328, 1970.
4. Blackburn, H. S., and Belikas, E. P.: Spondylolisthesis in children and adolescents. J. Bone Joint Surg. *59B*:490–494, 1977.
5. Borkow, S. E., and Kleiger, B.: Spondylolisthesis in the newborn. Clin. Orthop. *81*:73–76, 1971.
6. Bosworth, D. M., Fielding, J. W., Demarest, L., and Bonaquist, M.: Spondylolisthesis: A critical review of a consecutive series of cases treated by arthrodesis. J. Bone Joint Surg. *37A*:767–786, 1955.
7. Boxall, D., Bradford, D. S., Winter, R. B., and Moe, J. H.: Management of severe spondylolisthesis in children and adolescents. J. Bone Joint Surg. *61A*:479–495, 1979.
8. Bradford, D. S.: Treatment of severe spondylolisthesis. A combined approach for reduction and stabilization. Spine *4*:423–429, 1979.
9. Buck, J. E.: Direct repair of the defect in spondylolisthesis. J. Bone Joint Surg. *52B*:432–437, 1970.
10. Cowell, M. J., and Cowell, H. R.: The incidence of spina bifida occulta in idiopathic scoliosis. Clin. Orthop. *118*:16–18, 1976.
11. Dandy, D. J., and Shannon, M. J.: Lumbosacral subluxation (Group I spondylolisthesis). J. Bone Joint Surg. *53B*:578–595, 1971.
12. Deyerle, W. M.: Lumbar nerve-root irritation in children. Clin. Orthop. *21*:125–136, 1970.
13. Fisk, J. R., Moe, J. H., and Winter, R. B.: Scoliosis, spondylolisthesis and spondylolysis. Their relationship as reviewed in 539 patients. Spine *3*:234–245, 1978.
14. Frieberg, S.: Studies on spondylolisthesis. Acta Chir. Scand. (Suppl.) 55, 1939.
15. Garceau, G. J.: The filum terminale syndrome (the cord-traction syndrome). J. Bone Joint Surg. *35A*:711–716, 1953.
16. Gill, G. G., Manning, J. G., and White, H. L.: Surgical treatment of spondylolisthesis without spine fusion. J. Bone Joint Surg. *37A*:493–520, 1955.
17. Harrington, P. R., and Tullos, H. S.: Spondylolisthesis in children: Observations and surgical treatment. Clin. Orthop. *79*:75–84, 1971.
18. Harris, R. I.: Spondylolisthesis (Hunterian lecture). Ann. R. Coll. Surg. Engl. *8*:259–297, 1951.
19. Harris, R. I.: *In* Nassim, R., and Burrows, H. J.: Modern Trends in Diseases of the Vertebral Column. London, Butterworth and Co. Ltd., 1959.
20. Hensinger, R. N., Lang, J. R., and MacEwen, G. D.: Surgical management of spondylolisthesis in children and adolescents. Spine *1*:207–216, 1976.
21. Herbiniaux, G.: Traite sur divers accouchemens laborieux, et sur les polypes de la matrice. Bruxelles, J. L. DeBoubers, 1782.
22. Hitchcock, H. H.: Spondylolisthesis: Observations on its development, progression, and genesis. J. Bone Joint Surg. *22*:1–16, 1940.
23. Jackson, D. W., Wiltse, L. L., and Cirincione, R. J.: Spondylolysis in female gymnasts. Clin. Orthop. *118*:68–73, 1976.
24. Kettlekamp, D. B., and Wright, G. D.: Spondylolysis in the Alaskan Eskimo. J. Bone Joint Surg. *53A*:563–566, 1971.
25. Kilian, H. F.: Schilderungen neuer Beckenformen and ihres Verhaltens in Leben. Mannheim, Verlag von Bassermann und Mathey, 1854.
26. LaFond, G.: Surgical treatment of spondylolisthesis. Clin. Orthop. *22*:175–179, 1962.
27. Lance, E. M.: Treatment of severe spondylolisthesis with neural involvement. (A report of two cases.) J. Bone Joint Surg. *48A*:883–891, 1966.
28. Laurent, L. E.: Spondylolisthesis. Acta Orthop. (Suppl.) 35, 1958.
29. Laurent, L. E., and Einola, S.: Spondylolisthesis in children and adolescents. Acta Orthop. Scand. *31*:45–64, 1961.
30. Laurent, L. E., and Osterman, K.: Spondylolisthesis in children and adolescents: A study of 173 cases. Acta Orthop. Belgica, *35*:717–727, 1969.
31. Laurent, L. E., and Osterman, K.: Operative treatment of spondylolisthesis in young patients. Clin. Orthop. *117*:85–91, 1976.
32. Lowe, R. W., Hayes, D. T., Kaye, J., Bagg, R. J., and Luekens, C. A., Jr.: Standing roentgenograms in spondylolisthesis. Clin. Orthop. *117*:80–84, 1976.
33. Lusskin, R.: Pain patterns in spondylolisthesis. A correlation of symptoms, local pathology, and therapy. Clin. Orthop. *40*:123–136, 1965.
34. Marmor, L., and Bechtol, C. O.: Spondylolisthesis: Complete slip following the Gill procedure: A case report. J. Bone Joint Surg. *43A*:1068–1069, 1961.
35. McKee, B. W., Alexander, W. J., and Dunbar, J. S.: Spondylolysis and spondylolisthesis in children: A review. J. Can. Assoc. Radiol. *22*:100–109, 1971.
36. Meyerding, H. W.: Spondylolisthesis. Surg. Gynecol. Obstet. *54*:371–377, 1932.
37. Meyerding, H. W.: Low backache and sciatic pain associated with spondylolisthesis and protruded intervertebral disc. J. Bone Joint Surg. *23*:461–470, 1941.
38. Moreton, R. D.: So-called normal backs. Indust. Med. Surg. *38*:216, 1969.
39. Monticelli, G., and Ascani, E.: Spondylolysis and spondylolisthesis. Acta Orthop. Scand. *46*:498–506, 1975.
40. Munster, J. K., and Troup, J. D. G.: The structure of the pars interarticularis of the lower lumbar vertebrae and its relation to the etiology of spondylolysis. J. Bone Joint Surg. *55B*:735–741, 1973.
41. Nachemson, A.: Repair of the spondylolisthetic defect and inter-transverse fusion for young patients. Clin. Orthop. *117*:101–105, 1976.
42. Neugebauer, F. L.: A new contribution to the history and etiology of spondylolisthesis. New Syndenham Society Selected Monographs, *121*(3):1–64, 1888.
43. Newman, P. H.: The etiology of spondylolisthesis. J. Bone Joint Surg. *45B*:39–59, 1963.
44. Newman, P. H.: A clinical syndrome associated with severe lumbosacral subluxation. J. Bone Joint Surg. *47B*:472–481, 1965.
45. Pease, C. N., and Najat, H.: Spondylolisthesis in children. Clin. Orthop. *52*:187–198, 1967.
46. Phalen, G. S., and Dickson, J. A.: Spondylolisthesis and tight hamstrings. J. Bone Joint Surg. *43A*:505–512, 1961.
47. Renaud, M. P.: Personal communication.
48. Risser, J. C., and Norquist, D. M.: Sciatic scoliosis in growing children. Clin. Orthop. *21*:137–155, 1961.
49. Robert, Monatsschrift für Geburtskunde und Frauenkrankheiten. *5*:81, 1855.

50. Roche, M. B.: Healing of bilateral fracture of the pars interarticularis of a lumbar neural arch. J. Bone Joint Surg. *32A*:428–429, 1950.

51. Rowe, G. G., and Roche, M. B.: The etiology of separate neural arch. J. Bone Joint Surg. *35A*:102–109, 1953.

52. Scaglietti, O., Frontino, G., and Bartolozzi, P.: Technique of anatomical reduction of lumbar spondylolisthesis and its surgical stabilization. Clin. Orthop. *117*:164–175, 1976.

53. Sherman, F. C., Wilkinson, R. H., and Hall, J. E.: Reactive sclerosis of a pedicle and spondylolysis in the lumbar spine. J. Bone Joint Surg. *59A*:49–54, 1977.

54. Sherman, F. C., Rosenthal, R. K., and Hall, J. C.: Spine fusion for spondylolysis and spondylolisthesis in children. Spine *4*:59–67, 1979.

55. Stauffer, R. N., and Coventry, M. B.: Posterolateral lumbar spine fusion. J. Bone Joint Surg. *54A*:1195–1204, 1972.

56. Taillard, W.: Le spondylolisthesis chez l'enfant et l'adolescent. Acta Orthop. Scand. *24*:115–144, 1955.

57. Tojner, H.: Olisthetic scoliosis. Acta Orthop. Scand. *33*:291–300, 1963.

58. Turner, R. H., and Bianco, A. J., Jr.: Spondylolysis and spondylolisthesis in children and teenagers. J. Bone Joint Surg. *53A*:1298–1306, 1971.

59. Watkins, M. B.: Postero-lateral bone grafting for fusion of the lumbar and lumbosacral spine. J. Bone Joint Surg. *41A*:388–396, 1959.

60. Wiltse, L. L.: Etiology of spondylolisthesis. Clin. Orthop. *10*:48–60, 1957.

61. Wiltse, L. L.: Spondylolisthesis in children. Clin. Orthop. *21*:156–163, 1961.

62. Wiltse, L. L.: Spondylolisthesis: Classification and etiology. Symposium on the Spine. American Academy of Orthopaedic Surgeons, St. Louis, C. V. Mosby Co., 1969, pp. 143–168.

63. Wiltse, L. L., Widell, E. H., and Jackson, D. W.: Fatigue fracture: The basic lesion in isthmic spondylolisthesis. J. Bone Joint Surg. *57A*:17–22, 1975.

64. Wiltse, L. L., Newman, P. H., and MacNab, I.: Classification of spondylolysis and spondylolisthesis. Clin. Orthop. *117*:23–29, 1976.

65. Wynne-Davies, R., and Scott, J. H. S.: Inheritance and spondylolisthesis: A radiographic family survey. J. Bone Joint Surg. *61B*:301–305, 1979.

LUMBAR AND SACRAL AGENESIS

Sporadic case reports of congenital lumbar and sacrococcygeal agenesis have appeared in the literature since Hohl first described the condition in 1852.[2] In this century, complete or partial lumbar absence has proved quite uncommon with fewer than 25 patients recorded in the literature.[9] These children are severely handicapped and with few exceptions require extensive care.[10] In contrast, sacrococcygeal agenesis occurs with greater frequency with over 200 patients reported and has a wide variation in clinical appearance.[13] The patient with partial sacral agenesis may not have a detectable deficit, whereas those with complete sacral absence are significantly deformed. Consequently, there are sufficient clinical data to guide the orthopaedist in the treatment of the less involved and more familiar distal agenesis. The less common lumbar and complete sacral agenesis present complex problems in management to which satisfactory solutions are not yet available.

Etiology

The etiology of these malformations has not been completely delineated; however, current experimental work may soon provide clues to the causal agent.[14] Despite the relative rarity of occurrence in humans, rumplessness is not an unusual event in the lower vertebrates. The deformity may occur both by spontaneous mutation or genetic transmission and has been studied in chickens, pigs, mice, and the Manx cat.[13] Genetic transmission is uncommon in humans in comparison to other vertebrates. Pouzet (1938) reported an instance of father-son inheritance, and only two other families have since been found.[7, 13] Many patients with lumbosacral agenesis, however, are physiologically unable to reproduce. Andrish did not find evidence of sacral agenesis in a roentgenographic study of parents of affected children; however, he did find a high incidence of minor scoliosis.[1]

A variety of noxious agents have been used to induce the condition in the embryo, including lithium salts, vitamin A deficiency, and physical agents, such as radiation and high temperatures. However, the most intriguing research to date is that of Duraiswami,[4] who induced rumplessness in developing chicks by the injection of insulin into the egg. Introduction of insulin during the first two days of incubation was followed by vertebral changes, such as rumplessness, whereas later injections caused other skeletal aberrations. Clinically, it has been noted that a significant number of children afflicted with distal vertebral agenesis are offspring of diabetic mothers or have a strong family history of diabetes.[1, 3, 11, 14] Blumel and associates,[3] who conducted a nationwide survey of patients with sacral agenesis, discovered an 18 per cent incidence of maternal diabetes. Passarge and Lenz[11] in their review of the literature calculated a 14 per cent incidence.

After the initial insult in early embryonic life, the pelvis and lower extremities fail to develop normally. This has been characterized by Frantz and Aitken[6] as failure of induction. The nervous tissue does not develop normally, and as a consequence, the lower extremities are not stimulated (induced) to develop properly. This theory does not provide a complete explanation, as the child with myelodysplasia has a distinctly different clinical appearance yet similar incomplete nerve development, nor does it account for the peculiar partial sparing of sensation and retention of proprioception found even in the most severely involved children. This sparing suggests that some elements of the nervous system have continued to grow despite the lagging behind of the musculoskeletal system. Renshaw[14] suggests that the lesion is in the development of the caudal notochord sheath and ventral spinal cord; these structures normally induce the formation of the vertebrae and motor nerves. The sensation remains intact as the thoracic neural elements are derived from neural crest tissue, which is spared.

Clinical Findings

The clinical appearance of the child is dependent on the level of the vertebral lesion. Those with a partial sacral or coccygeal agenesis may be asymptomatic. In contrast, the patient with lumbar or complete sacral agenesis is severely deformed, characteristically having rigid flexion contractures of the hips, knees, and ankles, accompanied by paralysis and extreme atrophy of the pelvis and lower extremities. The posture of the lower extremities has been likened to the "sitting Buddha" flexion-abduction contractures of the hips, knees flexed to 60 degrees with popliteal webbing and the feet tucked under the buttocks in equinovarus (Fig. 5–88). Inspection of the back reveals a bony prominence, which is the last vertebral segment, and often gross motion between it and the pelvis.[1] The buttocks are narrowed and compressed with dimpling two to three inches lateral to the gluteal cleft. The anus is patulous and horizontal. When the patient sits unsupported, the pelvis rolls up under the thorax (Fig. 5–89A). Flexion-extension may occur at the junction of the spine and pelvis rather than the hips.[1] Ambulation must be performed by the hands (Fig. 5–89B).

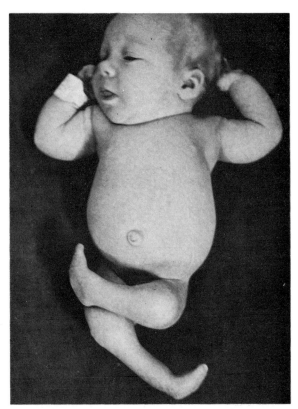

Figure 5–88. Newborn with agenesis of the lumbar spine and sacrum. Note the "sitting Buddha" posture of the lower extremities, flexion-abduction contractures of the hips, knees flexed with popliteal webbing, and feet tucked under the buttocks in equinovarus.

The neurologic deficit is one of the most unusual features of this condition. Motor paralysis is profound, with no voluntary, involuntary, or reflex activity, and anatomically corresponds within one level to what might be expected from the vertebral loss.[1, 14, 16] In contrast, the sensory disturbance does not parallel the motor or vertebral lesion.[16] Even the most severely involved patients have sensation to the knees and spotty hypesthesia distally. Trophic ulcerations of the feet are quite uncommon, suggesting at least protective sensation. Smith[16] found in cadavers with sacral agenesis that the nerves demonstrate extraordinary pertenacity, often crossing and recrossing the midline to reach the lower extremities. Unfortunately, bladder incontinence is a consistent feature in even the relatively minor hemisacral defect, but the mechanism is not the same in each patient.[8, 16, 17] Severe constipation with the absence of the normal sense of rectal distention is a common bowel problem.[18]

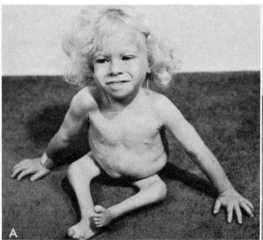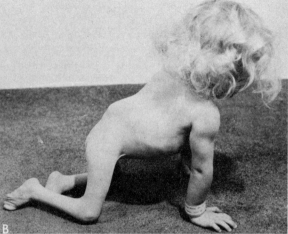

Figure 5-89.   Same patient, age four. (Roentgenograms, Fig. 5-96). *A,* Persistent flexion contractures of the hips and knees; when the patient sits unsupported, the pelvis rolls up under the thorax. *B,* Inspection of the back reveals the bony prominence which is the last vertebral segment. Buttocks are narrowed and compressed.

Recently, bladder dysfunction in these children has been studied extensively. There are no clinical or radiologic parameters that provide a reliable guide to identifying the variable patterns of urinary function.[8, 16, 17] Perineal sensation is preserved in almost all patients, and normal anal sphincteric activity does not exclude neurogenic bladder disease.[8] A few children with spastic sphincters are able

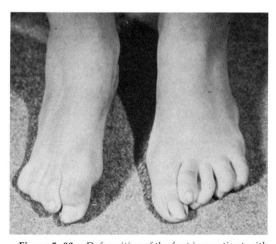

Figure 5-90.   Deformities of the foot in a patient with partial sacral agenesis (Fig. 5-93, roentgenograms) and a low-level neurologic lesion. These are often mistaken as resistant clubfeet or as secondary to arthrogryposis. It is not unusual for these children to be misdiagnosed for several years until the problems of toilet training call attention to the sacral anomalies.

to restrain dribbling for short periods, which Smith termed "pseudocontinence."[16] Each patient exhibits an individual mixture of either upper or lower motor neuronal deficits or both, and perineal electromyography must be used to obtain the correct diagnosis.[8]

With low-level lesions, the foot and leg deformities are similar to those found in the patient with a resistant clubfoot or arthrogryposis (Fig. 5-90). It is not unusual for these children to be misdiagnosed for several years or until the problems of toilet training call attention to the sacral anomalies. They are frequently confused with the arthrogrypotic, and indeed there are strong clinical similarities suggesting a common etiology. The arthrogrypotic, however, has full sensation in the lower extremities, control of bowel and bladder, and normal vertebral architecture. The severely afflicted child with arthrogryposis has involvement of the upper extremities as well.

Scoliosis (Fig. 5-91), hemivertebrae, spina bifida, and meningocele are commonly associated spinal anomalies.[1, 14] Visceral anomalies have been reported in approximately 35 per cent and are usually confined to the anogenital region, the most common being an imperforate anus, and the urinary tract, usually problems related to bladder dysfunction, such as hydronephrosis, vesicourethral reflux, and diverticula, but fused or absent kidney, exstrophy, and hypospadias also may be found (Fig. 5-92).[8, 16-18]

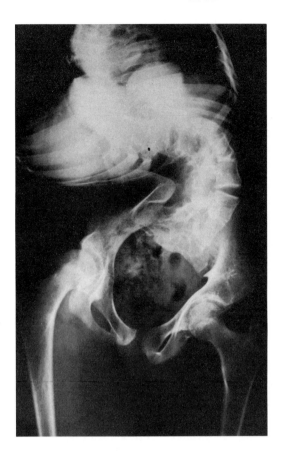

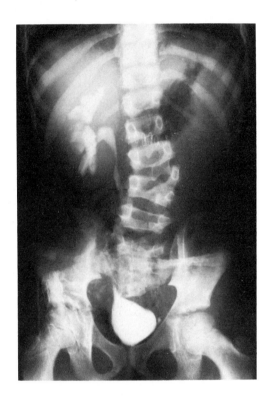

Figure 5–91 (at left). Partial absence of the sacrum and severe congenital scoliosis. Spinal anomalies such as hemivertebrae, spina bifida, and meningocele are commonly associated with lumbosacral defects. Visceral anomalies have been reported in approximately 35 per cent of these children and are usually confined to the anogenital area, particularly the urinary tract.

Figure 5–92 (at right). Intravenous pyelogram in a six-year-old female with a partial sacral agenesis and congenital scoliosis secondary to hemivertebrae. Note an absent left kidney and right hydronephrosis secondary to ureteropelvic obstruction. The patient's renal problems were not appreciated for several years, and she has chronic renal disease.

Roentgenographic Appearance

When the lesion involves the lumbar spine, in general there will be complete absence of all vertebral development, including the sacrum, below the affected area (Fig. 5–93). Lesions of the sacrum are less consistent, however, and approximately one third of the patients have the defect on only one side (Fig. 5–94).[16] Smith[16] has called this a hemisacrum and has described patients with total and subtotal unilateral absence of sacral segments. When the lesion is above the twelfth thoracic level, it is usually incompatible with life, but a few survivors have been reported,[15] the highest level of involvement being the ninth tho-

racic vertebrae.[9] Generally, there are some recognizable lumbar vertebrae present.

With lumbar or complete sacral agenesis, there is usually no bony connection of the spine to the pelvis, but a synarthrosis or sacralization of the terminal lumbar segments may occur and provide iliolumbar stabilization (Fig. 5–95).[14] The spinopelvic articulation should be carefully examined with flexion-extension roentgenograms, as the stability of this junction may have important implications in treatment and habilitation (Fig. 5–96).[7, 14] If the sacrum is absent, the pelvis is narrow, and the ilia usually articulate together posteriorly (amphiarthrosis) (Fig. 5–95A). Normally formed hip joints, dislocated hips (30 per

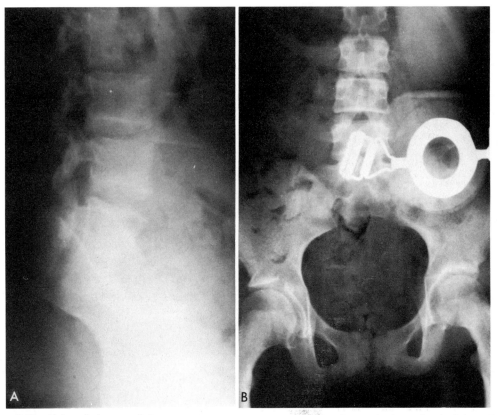

Figure 5–93. Subtotal absence of the sacrum, apparent transverse amputation at the lower level of the pelvis. *A,* Lateral roentgenographic view. *B,* Anterior-posterior. Note collecting device for urinary diversion.

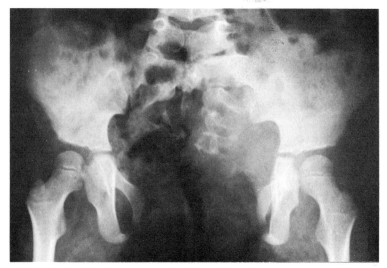

Figure 5–94. Partial agenesis of the sacrum demonstrating a left hemisacrum. Approximately one third of the sacral defects are unilateral. Note the severe diastasis pubis.

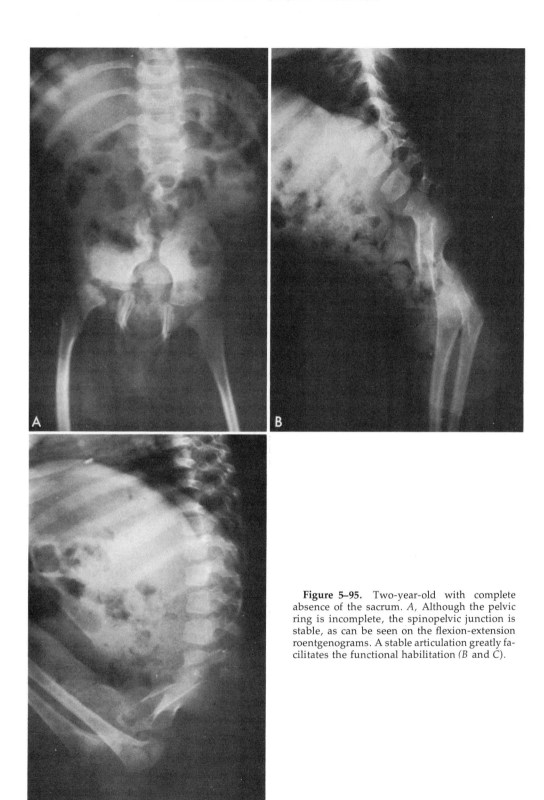

Figure 5–95. Two-year-old with complete absence of the sacrum. *A,* Although the pelvic ring is incomplete, the spinopelvic junction is stable, as can be seen on the flexion-extension roentgenograms. A stable articulation greatly facilitates the functional habilitation (*B* and *C*).

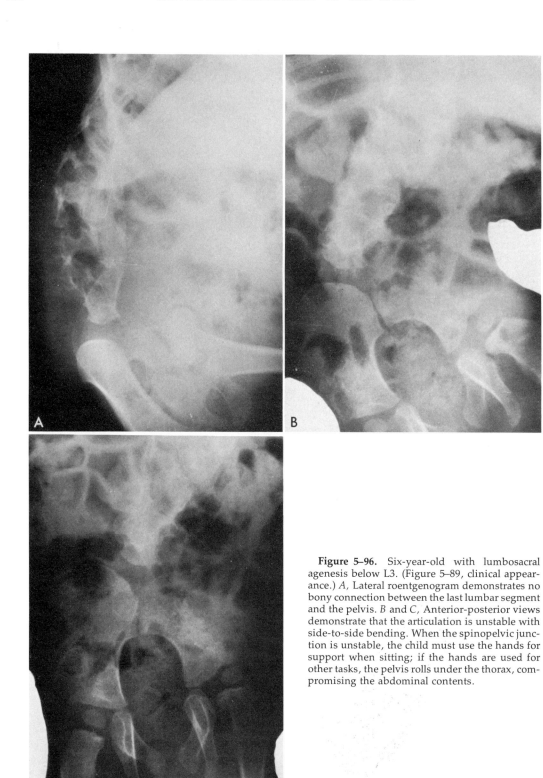

Figure 5–96. Six-year-old with lumbosacral agenesis below L3. (Figure 5–89, clinical appearance.) *A,* Lateral roentgenogram demonstrates no bony connection between the last lumbar segment and the pelvis. *B* and *C,* Anterior-posterior views demonstrate that the articulation is unstable with side-to-side bending. When the spinopelvic junction is unstable, the child must use the hands for support when sitting; if the hands are used for other tasks, the pelvis rolls under the thorax, compromising the abdominal contents.

cent), and coxa vara have all been reported with no consistent pattern.[1, 14] The femur and tibia are normally formed but atrophic. The bony architecture of the knee and ankle are normal and well defined.

Treatment

SUBTOTAL SACRAL AGENESIS

The treatment program varies with the level of involvement and as a consequence must be highly individualized. The following broad concepts may be helpful in the management of these children, however.

If the sacropelvic ring is intact (Fig. 5–93A), the patient generally will have a stable spinopelvic junction and potentially is a functional walker with minimal or no brace support.[1, 7] With the lower defects, the significant deformities are limited to the feet and legs and resemble those found in arthrogryposis or in the patient with a severe resistant clubfoot. So, too, the treatment is similar; early (at birth) aggressive correction of deformity should be the rule; much can be lost even in the slightest delay. Initially, this includes serial corrective plaster casts in conjunction with stretching and exercises to bring the feet plantigrade and the knees in extension. Later, braces and plaster night splints are needed to minimize the recurrence of deformity. As in arthrogryposis, soft tissue releases have limited application. Banta[2] noted that in his patients, massive release of flexion contractures about the knee only succeeded in gaining an average of 10 degrees of extension. He recommends osteotomy to obtain correction of the knee flexion deformity. Two-pin tibial traction supplemented with posterior knee release has been helpful in obtaining knee extension.[1] Correction should be obtained early and maintained with adequate bracing during the growing years to prevent the recurrence of deformity. Bony realignment of the foot with metatarsal osteotomy, triple arthrodesis, and often talectomy have been helpful in correcting foot deformities in the older child. Many of these children do not require bracing in adult life, as the relative stiffness of the joints provides enough intrinsic stability.

Reconstructive procedures such as muscle transfers are seldom indicated in these patients. Anatomic dissections of resected specimens reveal complete fatty replacement of skeletal muscle and thin, atrophic tendons.[6] Similarly, reduction of a congenitally dislocat-

ed hip may be successful in selected patients but must be tempered with a realistic appraisal of the potential functional capabilities of the child.[14] All efforts must be directed at maintaining adequate range of motion of the hips. Even those with complete lumbosacral agenesis who may be wheelchair bound will require 90 degrees of hip flexion.

An important part of the management of these children is recognition and treatment of the urinary abnormalities. It must be remembered that there is a high incidence of associated defects,[8, 16-18] which may lead to serious renal impairment. Urinary tract infection is common,[13] and advanced urinary tract disease may cause continued damage in an otherwise normal-appearing child. As a result, there may be a delay in diagnosis and nonremediable upper tract deterioration and severely limited therapeutic options (Fig. 5–92).[8, 17] The orthopedist must work in concert with the urologist and pediatrician, or the extensive orthopaedic habilitation program will be of limited benefit to the patient. If the urinary tract has not been evaluated, it is the responsibility of the orthopedist to see that this is accomplished.

LUMBAR AND TOTAL SACRAL AGENESIS

These children are severely handicapped and present several challenging and complex problems in management. As yet there is lack of agreement as to what constitutes the best method of treatment, owing in part to the small number of patients and paucity of long-term follow-up results.

Frantz and Aitken[6] have popularized an aggressive surgical approach to the lower extremities that is based on their extensive experience with patients who have lower limb amelia or phocomelia. These congenital amputees develop fast, skillful hand-walking patterns that are helpful within the confines of the home and use prostheses at school. It seemed to Frantz and Aitken that the grossly deformed, functionless limbs were inhibiting to the patient with lumbosacral agenesis and proposed subtrochanteric amputation. Handwalking was thus facilitated, and the patient could be fitted with a bucket-type prosthesis to stabilize the spinopelvic junction. The children are trained in a "swing-to" gait with crutches. Others have supported this procedure and are pleased with the long-term functional results and the appropriateness of surgery.[5, 6] The procedure is not recommended for the less severely involved children.

Banta[2] and, more recently, Andrish[1] have pursued a program directed at the conservation and straightening of the deformed lower extremities and a vigorous bracing program. They emphasize that the peculiar sensory sparing and preservation of proprioception found with this anomaly are of great value in standing and walking in braces and are quite different from the absence of sensation found in myelodysplasia. This neurosensory perception must be sacrificed when a thoracolumbar bucket prosthesis is used. Success of a bracing program, however, is dependent upon achieving adequate alignment of the extremities and requires vigorous early correction of the deformities by both surgery and closed means.[1, 2] The orthopaedist must be watchful to prevent recurrent deformities, which are detrimental to proper brace fit. Children who are free of hip and knee contractures remain functional walkers, particularly those who have some motor power below the knees.[1] Banta[2] reports that his patients have continued to demonstrate improvement in gait and balance over a five-year follow-up period. The true measure of success or failure of either program will have to await the assessment of how these children function in adult life. For the present, however, all need not be considered for high amputations.

SPINOPELVIC INSTABILITY

A serious problem is the spinopelvic instability that occurs when the pelvic ring is incomplete. This must be evaluated early with lateral flexion-extension roentgenograms, as a stable articulation greatly facilitates habilitation of function (Fig. 5–95). If the spinopelvic junction is unstable, the child may require the hands for trunk support when sitting (Fig. 5–96).[5, 12] When the hands are used for other tasks, the pelvis rolls up under the thorax, compromising the abdominal contents. Elting[5] has reported severe obstructive uropathy due to kinking of the ureters from spinopelvic instability. Perry[12] has noted that maintenance of satisfactory hip function and the prevention of flexion contractures is impossible with a grossly unstable spinopelvic junction. If, however, the spine is stabilized, then muscle stretching and surgical release will result in more satisfactory hip function and less chance for recurrence of contractures. Andrish, however, found that the degree of spinopelvic instability appeared to lessen with growth and that gradual formation of a ball and socket–

type articulation occurred.[1] He noted that motion between the spine and pelvis seem to aid in ambulation by compensating for the decrease in hip motion and flexion contractures.

Attempts at bracing to achieve stability of the spinopelvic articulation have not been generally successful. For those patients who require stabilization, Perry has described a technique for vertebropelvic fusion. Good results were obtained in four patients, permitting them to return to a satisfactory brace program and avoiding subtrochanteric amputation. The incidence of pseudoarthrosis from surgery in this area is high, however, and again long-term results will be necessary to evaluate its success or failure. This procedure should be performed only by surgeons who have a great deal of experience in spine surgery.

References

1. Andrish, J., Kalamchi, A., and MacEwen, G. D.: Sacral agenesis: A clinical evaluation of its management, heredity, and associated anomalies. Clin. Orthop. *139*:52–57, 1979.
2. Banta, J. V., and Nichols, O.: Sacral agenesis. J. Bone Joint Surg., *51A*:693–703, 1969.
3. Blumel, J., Evans, E. B., and Eggers, G. W. N.: Partial and complete agenesis or malformation of the sacrum with associated anomalies: Etiologic and clinical study with special reference to heredity; a preliminary report. J. Bone Joint Surg. *41A*:497–518, 1959.
4. Duraiswami, P. K.: Experimental causation of congenital skeletal defects and its significance in orthopaedic surgery. J. Bone Joint Surg. *34B*:646–698, 1952.
5. Elting, J. J., and Allen, J. C.: Management of the young child with bilateral anomalous and functionless lower extremities. J. Bone Joint Surg. *54A*:1523–1530, 1972.
6. Frantz, C. H., and Aitken, G. T.: Complete absence of the lumbar spine and sacrum. J. Bone Joint Surg. *49A*:1531–1540, 1967.
7. Freedman, B.: Congenital absence of the sacrum and coccyx; Report of a case and review of the literature. Brit. J. Surg. *37*:299–303, 1950.
8. Koff, S. A., and Deridder, P. A.: Patterns of neurogenic bladder dysfunction in sacral agenesis. J. Urol. *188*:87–89, 1977.
9. Mongeau, M., and Leclaire, R.: Complete agenesis of the lumbosacral spine: A case report. J. Bone Joint Surg. *54A*:161–164, 1972.
10. Nicol, W. J.: Lumbosacral agenesis in a 60 year old man. Br. J. Surg. *59*:577–579, 1972.
11. Passarge, E., and Lenz, W.: Syndrome of caudal regression in infants of diabetic mothers: Observations of further cases. Pediatrics *37*:672–675, 1966.
12. Perry, J., Bonnett, C. A., and Hoffer, M. M.: Vertebral pelvic fusions in the rehabilitation of patients

with sacral agenesis. J. Bone Joint Surg. *52A*:288–294, 1970.

13. Reeve, A. W., and Mortimer, J. G.: Lumbosacral agenesis or rumplessness. N. Z. Med. J. *73*:340–345, 1971.
14. Renshaw, T. S.: Sacral agenesis: A classification and review of twenty-three cases. J. Bone Joint Surg. *60A*:373–383, 1978.
15. Rosenthal, R. K.: Congenital absence of the coccyx, sacrum, lumbar vertebrae and the lower two thoracic vertebrae. Bull. Hosp. Joint Dis. *29*:287–292, 1968.
16. Smith, E. D.: Congenital sacral anomalies in children. Aust. N. Z. J. Surg. *29*:165–176, 1959.
17. White, R. I., and Klauber, G. T.: Sacral agenesis: Analysis of 22 cases. Urology *8*:521–525, 1976.
18. Williams, D. I., and Nixon, H. H.: Agenesis of the sacrum. Surg. Gynecol. Obstet. *105*:84–88, 1957.

SPINE DEFORMITY IN INDIVIDUALS WITH SKELETAL DYSPLASIA

There are a variety of skeletal and extraskeletal disorders that result in short stature, many of which are associated with spine deformities. This is not unexpected, as any disorder that interferes with the metabolism of bone or its architecture may lead to structural weakness and collapse. In the extremities this unpredictable structural quality results in bowing and shortening of the long bones, and in the spine, it results in kyphosis, lordosis, scoliosis, and, importantly, instability. It is important to understand the natural history of the spine problems associated with a specific dysplasia or syndrome, as these deformities may be the cause of early disability and even death. Many of these conditions can be identified at birth (Table 5–3), and preventable and occasionally fatal spine deformities may be avoided.

Short stature and thoracolumbar kyphoscoliosis are prominent features of many of these disorders and may occur in any of the skeletal dysplasias, as the normal ossification is disturbed and the vertebral bodies are weak and poorly formed. All vertebrae are dysplastic; however, the apex of the kyphosis is usually at the dorsolumbar junction, seemingly the weakest part. Hyperlordosis and spinal stenosis are also common accompaniments. In the past, kyphosis, scoliosis, or vertebral instability have been allowed to progress to such a degree that neurologic deficit has resulted. Any unexplained chronic motor weakness or retardation of motor milestones should raise the suspicion of occult myelopathy in these individuals, even in the absence of the classic signs of neurologic deficit.

Treatment may be difficult in these individuals because of the unpredictable nature of the bony structural weakness combined with ligamentous laxity. Lumbar lordosis is a generalized finding in most of these conditions and seldom requires treatment. In the young child one should be wary of the thoracolumbar kyphosis, which is a feature of nearly all the dysplasias. Significant kyphoscoliosis is a prominent feature, particularly of the dystrophic and metatrophic dysplasias, and may require early bracing or posterior spinal fusion to prevent or retard progression of deformity.

The odontoid hypoplasia characteristic of spondyloepiphyseal dysplasia congenita and mucopolysaccharidosis type IV (Morquio's) should alert one to obtain lateral flexion and extension views of the cervical spine. Early atlantoaxial fusion should be considered if instability is discovered. Sharply angulated cervical kyphosis associated with dystrophic dysplasia and Larson's syndrome should also be observed carefully, and if there is indication of progression or even minimal myelopathy, cervical fusion should be considered.

Achondroplasia

Achondroplasia is the most common and easily recognized of the bony dysplasias. The typical clinical features, apparent at birth, include a large skull, prominent forehead, kyphosis of the thoracolumbar spine, increased lumbar lordosis, nearly horizontal sacrum, large buttocks, and extremely short arms and legs. The condition is an autosomal dominant, but 80 per cent of patients are new mutations occurring at a relatively constant rate.[16] In general, the achondroplastic dwarf is intelligent, agile, deceptively strong, and can be expected to have a near normal life expectancy.[16]

It was thought that the typical deformities of achondroplasia were limited to the skull and extremities. In 1925, Donath and Vogl[8] first demonstrated the peculiar narrowing of the spinal canal that has now become a hallmark of this condition. The spinal cord and cauda equina are of normal size, but the lumen of the vertebral canal is severely reduced in both the sagittal and the transverse diameter, as the pedicles are unusually thick and short. This spinal stenosis (particularly in the lumbar region) (Fig. 5–97) is a consistent finding in all achondroplastic dwarfs, and as a consequence all have the potential for significant neurologic compromise with only minor encroachment of the spinal canal.[1, 4, 18] Although no accurate incidence data are available, most authors[1, 3, 9, 18] believe that these complications are relatively common in the adult achondroplast and are usually due to gradual worsening of a dorsolumbar gibbus, spurring from osteoarthritis, or herniation of a degenerative disc. Lumbar narrowing is not pathognomonic for achondroplasia, however, and can occur in other conditions, such as diastrophic dysplasia and hypochondroplastic dysplasia.

CLINICAL FINDINGS

CHILDREN. If the more lethal forms of chondrodystrophy are excluded (achondrogenesis, thanatophoric dwarfism, and asphyxiating thoracic dystrophy), we find that the true achondroplast is relatively free from neurologic problems during childhood.[16] One exception should be noted, and that is hydrocephalus. Head enlargement with mild dilatation of the ventricles is a consistent finding in achondroplasia.[6, 7] Head growth curves usually exceed the 97th percentile but parallel the normal slope for age.[6] When true hydrocephalus occurs, it is frequently due to mechanical obstruction of cerebrospinal fluid at the foramen magnum.[6, 7, 13] Basal synostosis of the skull (brachycephaly) is a characteristic finding in the young achondroplast[1] and can lead to narrowing and distortion of the foramen magnum.[6] High cervical cord compression has also been reported and is suggested as an unrecognized cause of the high perinatal mortality in achondroplasia.[4, 6, 7, 17] Signs and symptoms of progressive quadriparesis frequently are found in those infants with hydrocephalus, suggesting a common etiology. As a consequence, the achondroplastic neonate and infant must be carefully monitored with

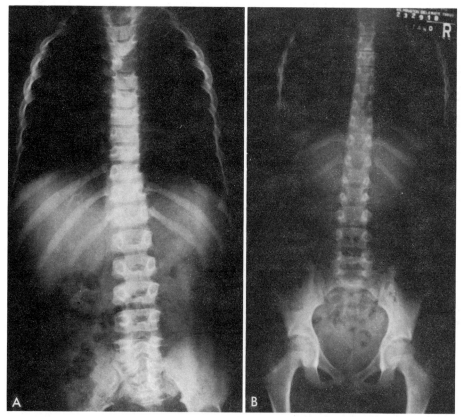

Figure 5–97. *A,* Twelve-year-old achondroplastic dwarf. Note marked narrowing of the interpedunculate distance, particularly in the lumbar and sacral portions of the spinal canal. *B,* Appearance of a normal spine at the same age.

frequent head circumference measurements and examination for signs and symptoms of quadriparesis.

Diagnosis of impending neurologic compromise is hampered by the fact that many normal achondroplastic children have delayed acquisition of motor skills and developmental milestones for reasons not yet understood.[6] Mental retardation, seizure disorders, and other neurologic abnormalities are not normally associated with achondroplasia, however, and when present should stimulate an intensive investigation.[6]

ADULTS. In the adult achondroplast, neurologic complications are more commonly due to compression of the neural elements in the dorsal and lumbar spine, rarely from constriction at the foramen magnum and basilar impression.[4, 10, 15] The spinal cord itself is of normal size and shape, but the spinal canal is stunted in both the transverse and sagittal dimensions. In the majority of patients, this snug fit is well tolerated, but any encroachment of the lumen can cause significant neurologic compromise. Children and young adults are usually spared this complication, but with aging a minor disc protrusion or slight spurring from osteoarthritis can have a devastating effect.

Onset of symptoms is usually in the third of fourth decade, but patients have been reported as young as 12 and as old as 60.[13, 18] The earliest symptoms are usually severe lumbosacral backache and radicular pain in the lower extremities. Low back pain, per se, is a nonspecific finding, as it is a common complaint in the adult achondroplast and is probably related to the hyperlordosis.[2] If the symptoms are progressive, objective neurologic findings should be sought for on physical examination. If the level of spinal cord impingement is above or at the conus medullaris (such as the dorsolumbar gibbus), the signs and symptoms will be those of an upper motor neuron lesion: hyperreflexia, spasticity, and disturbance of bowel and bladder function. If the lesion is in the region of the cauda equina (such as a herniated disc), lower motor neuron signs will be found: absent reflexes, muscle weakness, and paresthesia. Many achondroplasts have been reported who present with evidence of both upper and lower motor neuron involvement, and in this situation, there are multiple levels of impingement owing to a long kyphosis or degenerative osteoarthritis.

Initially, these complaints are intermittent, often with exacerbations and remissions over an extended period (two to three years), but if allowed to continue, the neurologic deficit will be irreversible.[13, 18] The slow progressive course of chronic cord compression is generally associated with multiple areas of narrowing due to osteoarthritis or gradual collapse of a dorsolumbar kyphosis due to disc degeneration.[1, 3, 4, 9, 18] Occasionally, the onset of the neurologic deficit is abrupt without any previous history of symptoms. In this situation, the clinician should suspect an acute disc herniation and a lesion localized to one vertebral level.[13]

Spinal curvature other than the typical hyperlordosis is common in the adult achondroplast (70 per cent).[2] Approximately one third have a mild to moderate scoliosis (less than 45 degrees). Onset is usually in late childhood, but few progress to severe degrees of curvature requiring treatment. One third can be expected to have kyphosis or kyphoscolisis. Here the prognosis is guarded, with a significant percentage (36 per cent) developing a severe deformity.[2] The majority of patients with neurologic impairment have kyphosis. With the exception of a sharply angulated gibbus, however, there is no correlation between the degree of kyphosis and the incidence or severity of neurologic involvement.[9] Kyphosis is only one factor that should be considered in those who have neurologic symptoms. More than half of the achondroplasts with spinal cord compression have a normal or mildly kyphoscoliotic spine.[2, 4, 13] Admittedly, these statistics are based on a small sample size but are consistent with the experience of several authors.[1, 3, 9, 12, 13]

The unique roentgenographic appearance of the spine and pelvis in the achondroplastic dwarf is a reliable diagnostic aid irrespective of the age of the patient.[5, 12] This is particularly helpful in the newborn period, when the classic clinical features are less apparent and errors in diagnosis are more common. The most consistent radiologic finding is narrowing of the interpedicular distance in the lumbar spine (Fig. 5–97). Normally the distance between the pedicles increases from the upper to lower lumbar vertebrae with L5 being the widest; however, in achondroplasia, the reverse is true. The pedicles throughout the spine are 30 to 40 per cent thicker than normal, reducing the transverse dimension of the achondroplast's spinal canal by approximately one third.[14] The pedicles are shorter but not to the same degree; thus, measured anterior-posterior distance is near normal except in the L4 and L5 area.[14] The nerve root foramina are narrowed owing to enlargement of the inferior facets.[14] The vertebral bodies are concave on their dorsal surface, and the end plates appear to mushroom outward. The intervertebral discs are increased in thickness so that at one year the ratio of vertebral body to disc is 1:1 instead of the normal 3:1.[5]

The lumbosacral angle is increased in the newborn, and the plane of the sacrum becomes nearly horizontal after the child begins to walk.[12] In infants, a mild kyphosis is a common finding in the region of the thoracolumbar junction (Fig. 5–98).[11-13] This deformity can be expected to return to normal as the child begins to walk and develops the

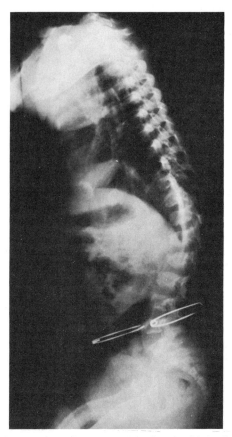

Figure 5–99. Three-year-old achondroplastic dwarf with kyphosis. The longer curve extending over several segments is more common. Treatment of this curvature in the early years may prevent complications due to deterioration of the kyphosis in adult life.

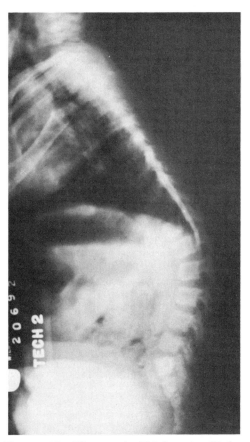

Figure 5–98. Nine-month-old infant. A mild thoracolumbar kyphosis is a common finding at this age. This curvature can be expected to reverse in 70 per cent of achondroplastic dwarfs as the child begins to ambulate and develop the typical hyperlordosis of the lumbar spine.

typical hyperlordosis of the lumbar spine. In approximately 30 per cent of patients, the kyphosis persists and may progress to a severe deformity.[2] Two patterns emerge: (1) a long kyphosis extending over several segments (Figs. 5–99 and 5–100)[2, 9, 11, 12] or, less commonly, (2) a sharply angulated gibbus over a single wedged vertebra (Fig. 5–101).

The pelvis is also distinctive in the newborn. The ilia are square with some rounding of the corners and narrowing of the lower part. The sciatic notch is short, and the overall configuration of the pelvis is short and squat. The acetabula are horizontal, and ossification of the proximal femoral epiphysis is delayed.[5] With continued growth, the pelvis remains broad and short, the femoral head is normal, and the acetabulum is concentric. The tibia and femur are obviously shorter and bowed.

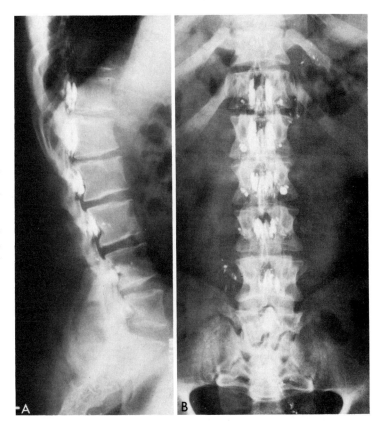

Figure 5–100. Sixteen-year-old achondroplastic with a long arcuate type of kyphosis. The patient had an insidious onset of pain and intermittent claudication with progressive neurologic symptoms and signs, ultimately requiring laminectomy. More than one half of the achondroplasts with spinal cord compression have a normal or mild kyphoscoliotic spine.

MYELOGRAPHIC EXAMINATION

When the achondroplast develops signs or symptoms of nerve root or cord compression, a myelogram is indicated. This procedure is best done by introducing the contrast material into the suboccipital area and allowing it to flow down the vertebral canal. Lumbar spinal puncture is notoriously unsuccessful and hazardous, as the narrow canal is crowded with the neural elements.[1, 4, 18] There is seldom free flow throughout the canal, and the contrast material tends to puddle in the concavities of the vertebral bodies between the prominent discs. Often the contrast material is blocked at T11-12, giving the initial impression that this is the area of maximal constriction. In the patient with long-standing symptoms, multiple areas of narrowing are the rule, and a myelogram indicating a single localized block should be critically reviewed.

TREATMENT

During the childhood and adolescent years, the achondroplastic dwarf is usually free from any spine-related problems and seldom requires orthopaedic attention. The adolescent achondroplast may develop scoliosis, but the curvature is of moderate degree and seldom requires bracing or surgery for control.[3] More than one third have persistent kyphosis at the dorsolumbar junction, however. A significant percentage may be expected to progress during the growing years to a severe deformity and significant disability in adult life.[2]

The progressive nature of the deformity and the potential for serious sequelae justify aggressive treatment of kyphosis in the immature individual with achondroplasia.[3, 9, 12] Early intervention with a Milwaukee brace is recommended, particularly in the young child with a sharply angled gibbus or wedge vertebrae (Fig. 5–101A), to decrease the deformity or at least halt progression of the kyphosis. Recently, bracing of the lumbar spine in conjunction with stretching of the hip flexion contractures has been used for the hyperlordosis with initial encouraging results.

In the adult achondroplast, the effects of aging, postural stress, and trauma may alter the previously stable relationship between spi-

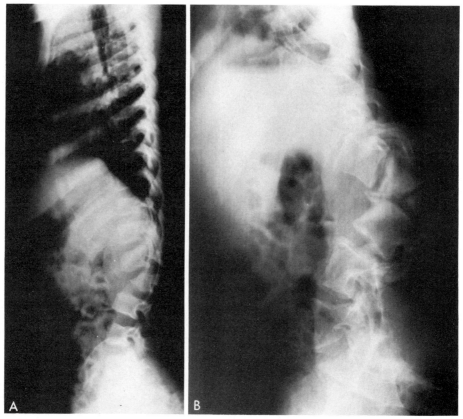

Figure 5–101. *A,* Five-year-old achondroplastic dwarf with a sharply angulated gibbus over a single wedged vertebra. *B,* Sharply angulated gibbus at the dorsolumbar (L1) junction in a 22-year-old female with achondroplastic dysplasia. She had back pain and radicular symptoms with standing and sitting for several years. In the past six months the pain has become persistent, extended to the lower extremities, and increased with sitting or standing. Neurologic examination revealed a decreased sensation to pinprick and light touch over the lateral aspects of both legs and increased muscular tone, positive Babinski's sign, and ankle clonus. Electromyogram confirmed spinal cord compression in the lower thoracic level.

nal cord and canal. This is especially true in the lumbar spine, where there is little tolerance for even minor encroachment. Low back pain is a common complaint of the older achondroplast, owing to the extreme hyperlordosis of the lumbar spine,[2] but relatively few develop objective signs of nerve root compression, and most respond satisfactorily to conservative measures.[2]

When nerve root or spinal cord impingement occurs and fails to respond to conservative measures, surgical intervention is required. In those patients who have an acute onset of symptoms, a herniated disc should be suspected. If this can be verified by clinical and myelographic examination, laminectomy and disc excision should be performed promptly. Encroachment of the nerve root by the inferior facets is common.[14] The nerve canal should be explored and foraminotomy should be performed if stenosis is demonstrated.[14]

More commonly, the patient has a long history of increasing symptoms and a diffuse neurologic deficit, increasing weakness, or intermittent claudication, sensory impairment, or bladder and bowel difficulty. This pattern is suggestive of multiple areas of compression from osteoarthritic spurring or a dorsolumbar kyphosis. A myelogram in this situation is less reliable, as the contrast material seldom flows freely and may falsely implicate one area when several are involved. It is important to ascertain the exact cause of the neurologic symptoms prior to planning a surgical procedure. If symptoms are due to narrowing of the canal from osteoarthritic spurs or multiple disc protrusions, then posterior decompression may be beneficial. If the cause is a progressive kyphosis or gibbus with anterior impingement, laminectomy alone will not be sufficient. In this situation, efforts should be directed to decreasing the curvature and posterior stabilization or, in the case of the sharply angulated gibbus, to anterior decompression and anterior stabilization.

If enlargement of the spinal canal is deemed necessary, the surgeon should avoid a limited posterior decompression, as this will not provide permanent or complete relief of symptoms. A complete decompression from the tenth thoracic to the first sacral vertebra with total unroofing of the spinal canal is preferred.[1, 9-11, 18] The laminectomy should extend above the area of mild kyphosis, as commonly this is the area of maximal compression.[1, 9, 18] Similarly, the laminectomy should be wide, including the medial portion of the inferior facets and foraminotomy should be performed if there is encroachment of the nerve canal.[14] Extensive removal of the posterior vertebral elements may seriously compromise structural stability and allow further increase of the kyphosis, and consideration should be given to anterior fusion.

There is a serious risk of injury to the spinal cord during the surgery itself; the short pedicles, acute angle of the lumbosacral junction, and virtual absence of an epidural space increases the technical difficulty of the procedure. Extensive removal of anterior osteophytes or bulging discs from a posterior approach is not recommended and frequently leads to serious deterioration of the patient's condition postoperatively.[18]

The postoperative results are dependent on the duration and severity of the patient's symptoms. If the spinal cord has been compressed for a long period, there is less potential for complete recovery. In general, extensive surgical decompression has been successful only in halting progression of the neurologic deficit, and only a few have shown reversal of the lesion.[1, 9, 10, 13, 18] This has prompted several authors[1, 3, 9, 18] to recommend strongly earlier operative intervention. In the past there has been a rather passive approach to the problem. We would like to make a strong plea for a more aggressive attitude with early brace intervention to halt the progression of the kyphosis and earlier surgical intervention to stabilize the spine and possibly prevent the neurologic sequelae. The problems are quite similar to those seen in congenital kyphosis, and the same management recommendations should apply.[11]

References

1. Alexander, E., Jr.: Significance of the small lumbar spinal canal: Cauda equina compression syndromes due to spondylosis. J. Neurosurg. *31*:513–519, 1969.

2. Bailey, J. A.: Orthopaedic aspects of achondroplasia. J. Bone Joint Surg. *52A*:1285–1301, 1970.

3. Bailey, J. A.: Disproportionate Short Stature: Diagnosis and Management. Philadelphia, W.B. Saunders Co., 1973.

4. Bergstrom, K., Laurent, U., and Lundberg, P. O.: Neurological symptoms in achondroplasia. Acta Neurol. Scand. *47*:59–70, 1971.

5. Caffey, J.: Achondroplasia of pelvis and lumbosacral spine: Some roentgenographic features. Am. J. Roentgenol. *80*:449–457, 1958.

6. Cohen, M. E., Rosenthal, A. D., and Matson, D. D.: Neurological abnormalities in achondroplastic children. J. Pediatr. *71*:367–376, 1967.

7. Dennis, J. P., Rosenberg, H. S., and Alvord, E. C., Jr.: Megalencephaly, internal hydrocephalus and other neurological aspects of achondroplasia. Brain *84*:427–444, 1961.

8. Donath, J., and Vogl, A.: Untersuchungen über den chondrodystrophischen Zwergwuchs. Arch. Intern. Med. *10*:1–44, 1925.

9. Duvoisin, R. C., and Yahr, M. D.: Compression spinal cord and root syndromes in achondroplastic dwarfs. Neurology (Minneap.) *12*:202–207, 1962.

10. Hancock, D. O., and Phillips, D. G.: Spinal compression in achondroplasia. Paraplegia *3*:23–33, 1965.

11. Kopits, S. E.: Orthopaedic complications of dwarfism. Clin. Orthop. *114*:153–197, 1976.

12. Langer, L. O., Jr., Baumann, P. A., and Gorlin, R. J.: Achondroplasia. Am. J. Roentgenol. *100*:12–26, 1967.

13. Lutler, L. D., and Langer, L. O.: Neurologic symptoms in achondroplastic dwarfs — surgical treatment. J. Bone Joint Surg. *59A*:87, 1977.

14. Lutler, L. D., Lonstein, J. E., Winter, R. B., and Langer, L. O.: Anatomy of the achondroplastic lumbar canal. Clin. Orthop. *126*:139–142, 1977.

15. Luyendijk, W., Matricali, B., and Thomeer, R. T. W. M.: Basilar impression in an achondroplastic dwarf: Causative role in tetraparesis. Acta Neurol. Chir. *41*:243–253, 1978.

16. McKusick, V. A.: Heritable Disorders of Connective Tissue, 4th ed. St. Louis, C.V. Mosby Co., 1972.

17. Potter, E. L., and Coverstone, V. A.: Chondrodystrophy fetalis. Am. J. Obstet. Gynecol. *56*:790–793, 1948.

18. Vogl, A.: The fate of the achondroplastic dwarf (neurologic complications of achondroplasia). Exp. Med. Surg. *20*:108–117, 1962.

Spondyloepiphyseal Dysplasia

Spondyloepiphyseal dysplasia is a congenital chondrodystrophy involving vertebrae and the epiphyses of the long bones that can lead to irregular epiphyseal ossification and eventually joint incongruities. Clinically, the patients are short-statured from shortening of the limbs and trunk and are prone to early degenerative osteoarthritis, particularly of the spine and hips.[8, 9, 11] The clinical and roentgenographic appearance (dysostosis multiplex) is similar to that found in the patient with Morquio's syndrome, but the spondyloepiphyseal dysplastic does not yet have a recognizable biochemical abnormality.[10, 11] Lamy and

Maroteaux[7] identified spondyloepiphyseal dysplasia as a separate entity in 1960; previously, these patients were included under the broader classification of multiple epiphyseal dysplasia described by Fairbank[3] in 1946.

There are nearly as many variations of spondyloepiphyseal dysplasia as families reported, and further classification is not practical. They can be roughly divided into two groups: (1) spondyloepiphyseal dysplasia congenita, an autosomal dominant trait that can be recognized at birth and represents the most severe form[9, 10] and (2) spondyloepiphyseal dysplasia tarda, an X-linked recessive trait found only in males with the onset of clinical findings in late childhood.[8, 11] Children with spondyloepiphyseal dysplasia regardless of type usually have normal intelligence.

CLINICAL FINDINGS

The most important feature of spondyloepiphyseal dysplasia is the delayed onset of the clinical and roentgenographic findings.[5] The degree of involvement influences the time of recognition, with the most severely involved (congenita form) suspected clinically at birth but requiring roentgenographic confirmation.[8] For the less severely involved (tarda form), growth retardation is the first clinical clue and usually is suspected between the ages of two and five (Fig. 5–102). Occasionally, the mildly involved child will have relatively normal appearance except for short stature, which may not be recognized until adolescence,[8] and that often is the only presenting complaint.

A short trunk due to decreased vertical height of the vertebral bodies is common to all forms of spondyloepiphyseal dysplasia.[11] The average adult height for persons with spondyloepiphyseal dysplasia congenita can be expected to be from 37 to 52 inches,[10] and for persons with spondyloepiphyseal dysplasia tarda, it will be from 52 to 62 inches.[9] Similarly, the configuration of the spinal deformity varies with the degree of involvement. Scoliosis is more commonly found in the patient with spondyloepiphyseal dysplasia tarda. Dorsal kyphosis and exaggerated lumbar lordosis are more typical of the congenita form.[9]

All have peripheral joint involvement. The hips are the most frequently involved,

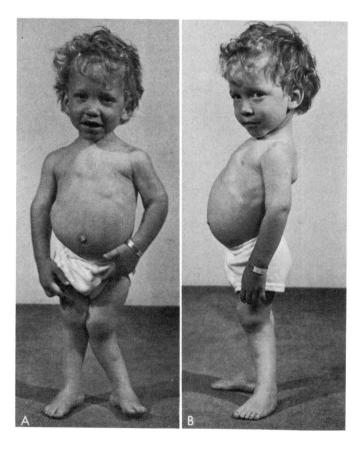

Figure 5–102. *A* and *B*, Clinical appearance of a five-year-old with spondyloepiphyseal dysplasia. Normal appearance of the head and face, short stature, short limbs, and genu valgum. Characteristically, these changes occur gradually with growth, and the child usually appears normal at birth.

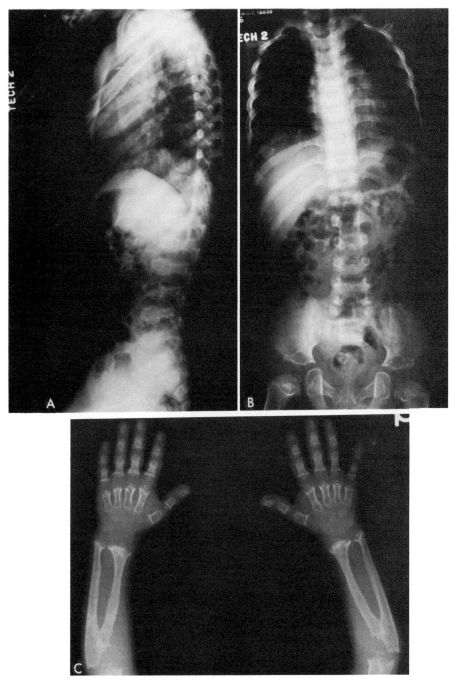

Figure 5–103. Six-year-old with spondyloepiphyseal dysplasia. *A,* Lateral view notes the pronounced vertebral changes, irregularity of the end plates, and disc protrusions resembling Schmorl's nodes. Adolescents commonly have delayed development of the ring apophysis causing the "central tongue" appearance of the lumbar vertebral bodies. Involvement of all vertebral bodies is a constant feature and may be complete flattening (platyspondylia) or limited only to anterior wedging. *B,* Anterior-posterior view. Progressive change in the bony architecture can be expected with further growth. Note changes in the proximal femoral epiphysis resembling Perthes disease. *C,* Similar involvement of the elbow and wrist. Twenty-six year old with spondyloepiphyseal dysplasia tarda. Height 4 feet, 11 inches with strong family history of short stature. Previously diagnosed as Morquio's syndrome. Also treated for bilateral Perthes disease.

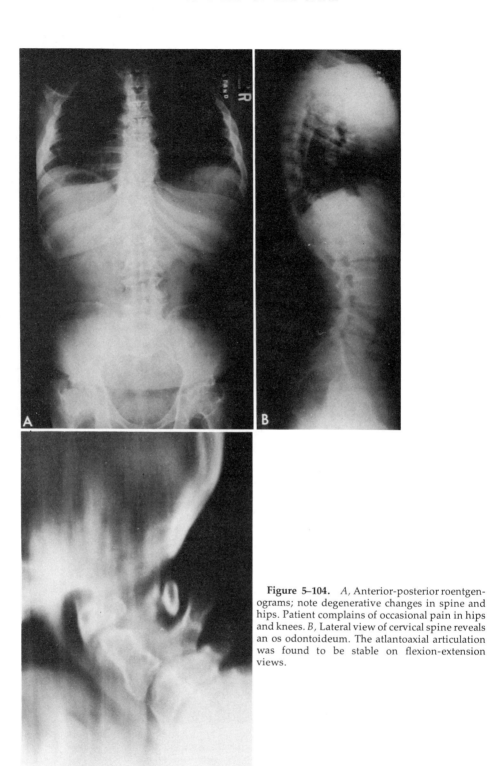

Figure 5–104. *A,* Anterior-posterior roentgen-ograms; note degenerative changes in spine and hips. Patient complains of occasional pain in hips and knees. *B,* Lateral view of cervical spine reveals an os odontoideum. The atlantoaxial articulation was found to be stable on flexion-extension views.

with a restricted range of motion. In addition to shortening of the extremities, the severely involved patient may demonstrate extreme joint laxity, waddling gait, genu varum or valgum, and pes planus. Myopia and retinal detachment are common in spondyloepiphyseal dysplasia congenita.[10]

Back pain and joint pain are common complaints during the growing years, particularly adolescence. The pain is usually intermittent and aching in nature, aggravated by activity and relieved by rest. Later as young adults, patients may develop the typical symptoms and signs of degenerative osteoarthritis of the spine and hips.

The clinical appearance of the child with spondyloepiphyseal dysplasia congenita closely resembles that of Morquio's syndrome but can be distinguished by the absence of keratinsulfaturia.

ROENTGENOGRAPHIC FINDINGS

In all forms of spondyloepiphyseal dysplasia, the vertebral changes are quite striking, often resembling those found in Morquio's syndrome, but may not be apparent until adolescence.[8, 10] All vertebral bodies are affected, but the degree of involvement reflects the severity of the disease, from severe flattening (platyspondylia) to mild anterior wedging (Fig. 5–103).[2, 8, 11] The adolescent

commonly has delayed development of the ring apophysis, causing the "central tongue" appearance, particularly in the lumbar region (Fig. 5–103A).[2, 5, 8] This is also the age when thoracic kyphoscoliosis may begin. This may progress slowly to moderate or severe kyphoscoliosis in the adult.[8] The vertebral end plates are commonly irregular, with disc intrusions resembling Schmorl's nodes, especially in the tarda form. The roentgenographic appearance is quite similar to Scheuermann's disease (Fig. 5–103). An unusual feature of the tarda form is the eburnation of the vertebral end plates in conjunction with a dysplastic appearance of the body. This roentgenographic appearance at first glance resembles intervertebral disc calcification and is occasionally confused with ochronosis.[8] Abnormalities of the odontoid are a frequent finding in the congenita form and are similar to those found in Morquio's syndrome.[8, 11] All patients should be evaluated with lateral flexion-extension views of the cervical spine to ascertain the stability of the atlantoaxial joint (Figs. 5–104B and 5–105). The late spine changes, as with the other affected joints, are those of degenerative osteoarthritis (Figs. 5–104 and 5–105).[8, 11]

The hips are the most commonly involved peripheral joints, followed by the knees and ankles, but any or all joints may be involved. Delay in epiphyseal ossification is common to all forms (Fig. 5–103). When ossification

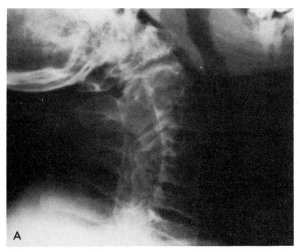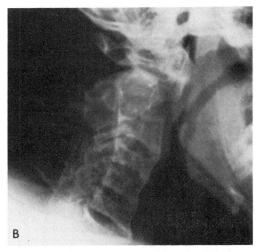

Figure 5–105. Nineteen-year-old male with spondyloepiphyseal dysplasia has intermittent neck and occipital pain. Extension *(A)* and flexion *(B)* lateral films of his cervical spine show an os odontoideum and subluxation of C1 on C2 similar to that seen in Morquio's syndrome. Note the degenerative changes in the remainder of the cervical spine and lack of motion.

occurs, it is from multiple centers within the epiphysis and has been characterized as "mulberry-shaped" or having a flocculent appearance. The roentgenographic appearance of the hips may be quite similar to that found in Perthes' disease. This mistake in diagnosis can be avoided by roentgenographic survey of the spine, knees, and ankles, particularly in the child who presents with bilateral Perthes' disease. With growth, irregularity of the femoral head may be apparent, but with wide variation from fairly round to severe degenerative osteoarthritis.[8] Wedging of the distal tibial epiphysis is common and may contribute to valgus collapse of the foot and severe pes planus.

TREATMENT

Many of these children have back pain during the growing years, particularly adolescence.[1, 2] Treatment is symptomatic, and the patient usually responds to conservative measures.[1, 2] Symptoms generally subside with maturity for the less severely involved patients. A few have persistent symptoms of degenerative osteoarthritis, particularly of the spine and hips.[2, 8, 11]

Spine complications are infrequent and generally are limited to the congenita form. Scoliosis and kyphosis usually are mild but may be progressive, and all patients must be carefully observed during adolescence. Successful management with the Milwaukee brace has been reported, and a few have required surgical stabilization.[3]

Aplasia of the odontoid with resultant instability is a frequent finding in the congenita form of spondyloepiphyseal dysplasia and is responsible for myelopathy and quadriparesis in up to one third of this group.[5, 6, 9] The cervical myelopathy may occur in infancy, causing respiratory problems or delayed motor development milestones. Those with C1-C2 instability (Fig. 5-105) should have posterior cervical fusion.

References

1. Bailey, J. A.: Disproportionate Short Stature: Diagnosis and Management. Philadelphia, W.B. Saunders Co., 1973.
2. Diamond, L. S.: A family study of spondyloepiphyseal dysplasia. J. Bone Joint Surg. 52A:1587–1594, 1970.
3. Fairbank, H. A. T.: Dysplasia epiphysealis multiplex. Proc. R. Soc. Med. 39:315–317, 1946.
4. Fisher, R. L.: Unusual spondyloepiphyseal and spondylometaphyseal dysplasias of childhood. Clin. Orthop. 100:78, 1974.
5. Ford, N., Silverman, F. N., and Kozlowski, K.: Spondyloepiphyseal dysplasia (pseudo-achondroplastic type). Am. J. Roentgenol. 86:462–472, 1961.
6. Kopits, S. E.: Orthopaedic complications of dwarfism. Clin. Orthop. 114:153, 1976.
7. Lamy, M., and Maroteaux, P.: Les Chondrodystrophies Geno-typiques. Paris, L'expansion Scientifique Française, 1960.
8. Langer, L. O., Jr.: Spondyloepiphyseal dysplasia tarda: Hereditary chondrodysplasia with characteristic vertebral configuration in the adult. Radiology 82:833–839, 1964.
9. McKusick, V. A.: Heritable Disorders of Connective Tissue, 4th ed. St. Louis, C.V. Mosby Co., 1972.
10. Spranger, J. W., and Langer, L. O., Jr.: Spondyloepiphyseal dysplasia congenita. Radiology 94:313–322, 1970.
11. Weinfeld, A., Ross, M. W., and Sarasohn, S. H.: Spondyloepiphyseal dysplasia tarda: A cause of premature osteoarthritis. Am. J. Roentgenol. 101:851–859, 1967.

Less Common Skeletal Dysplasias

Scoliosis, kyphosis, or both may occur in nearly every type of dwarfism, and our discussion will be limited to those conditions in which spinal deformity is a prominent feature (Table 5–4): diastrophic dysplasia, hypochondrodysplasia, the Kniest syndrome, metatropic dwarfism, Larsen's syndrome, and pseudoachondroplasic dysplasia. Spine deformities

TABLE 5–4. OSTEOCHONDRAL DYSPLASIAS* WITH SPINE DEFORMITIES

Identifiable at Birth
More Common
    Achondroplastic dysplasia
    Metatropic dysplasia
    Diastrophic dysplasia
    Spondyloepiphyseal dysplasia congenita
    Larsen's syndrome
Less Common
    Kniest's dysplasia
    Parastremmatic dysplasia
    Chondrodysplasia punctata
Manifested Later in Life
More Common
    Hypochondroplastic dysplasia
    Pseudochondroplastic dysplasia
    Spondyloepiphyseal dysplasia tarda
Less Common
    Metaphyseal chondrodysplasia
    Spondylometaphyseal dysplasia (Kozlowski)
    Dyggve-Melchior-Clauson dysplasia

*The Paris International Nomenclature of Constitutional Diseases of Bone (as revised in 1977).

occur in other less frequently encountered bone dysplasias: spondylometaphyseal dysplasia (Kozlowski type),[7] parastremmatic dwarfism,[15] the Stickler syndrome,[16] and the Conradi-Hünermann syndrome.[16] The orthopaedic management, however, is similar.

DIASTROPHIC DYSPLASIA

Diastrophic comes from the Greek word for bent or twisted and aptly describes the physical findings. The children typically have joint contractures and dislocations as well as resistant clubfeet and may be confused with arthrogryposis[8] or Larsen's syndrome. Distinguishing features manifest at birth are a crumpled or cauliflower deformity of the ears, cleft palate, and a hypermobile thumb, described as a hitchhiker's thumb.[8, 18] The condition is an autosomal recessive. Progressive rigid kyphoscoliosis is a common finding (Fig. 5–106); it may develop in the first year of life or by age five or six and may seriously compromise cardiopulmonary function.[6, 8, 18] Many have cervical spina bifida occulta, exaggerated lumbar lordosis, and lumbar spinal stenosis. Cervical kyphosis, which may be severe, is present in at least 25 per cent of those with diastrophic dysplasia (Fig. 5–107).[5, 8, 18]

As the scoliosis tends to be progressive, early posterior spinal fusion is recommended if bracing does not control the curve.[6] Posterior cervical fusion or posterior and anterior cervical fusion is frequently indicated in those with cervical kyphosis.[5] These individuals are extremely short-statured, but despite their contractures, dislocations, and rather resistant clubfeet, they are generally ambulatory. If they are not, this should alert the physician to the possibility of meylopathy secondary to the spinal deformities.

HYPOCHONDROPLASIA

Hypochondroplastic dysplasia resembles a mild form of achondroplasia with normal-sized trunk and disproportionate shortening of the extremities. There is a generalized ligamentous laxity with limitation of elbow extension and forearm supination.[14] The spine changes are those of mild achondroplasia with increased lumbar lordosis and narrowing of the lumbar interpedicular distance. Spine problems in these individuals are uncommon, but when present they are similar to those of achondroplasia. This is a dominantly inherited condition that is rather common and easily overlooked as a variant of normal development. The abnormality usually is not discovered in infancy but at about school age.

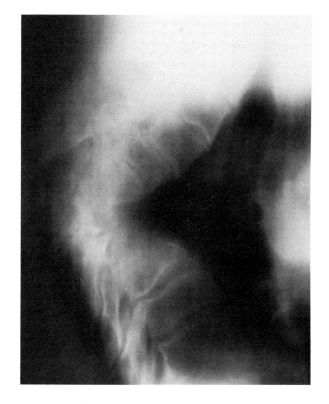

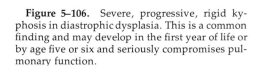

Figure 5–106. Severe, progressive, rigid kyphosis in diastrophic dysplasia. This is a common finding and may develop in the first year of life or by age five or six and seriously compromises pulmonary function.

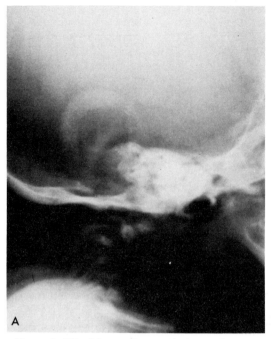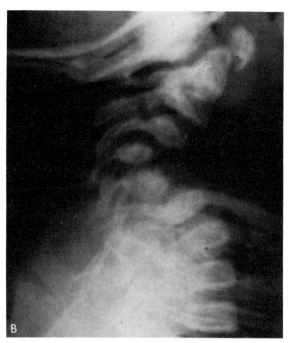

Figure 5–107. Many patients with diastrophic dysplasia have cervical kyphosis, which may be severe and is present in at least 25 per cent of those with diastrophic dysplasia. *A,* A newborn with severe cervical kyphosis who ultimately died within the first two weeks of life from pulmonary problems. *B,* An older patient with similar findings. This is quite similar to the cervical kyphosis seen in Larson's syndrome, which is usually secondary to hypoplastic anterior elements and unusual segmental anomalies.

KNIEST DYSPLASIA

Kniest dysplasia is a short trunk type of short stature that is probably inherited as an autosomal dominant. Patients with this condition resemble those individuals with metatropic dysplasia, but they have several distinguishing features.[12] The face is flat, especially in the midface, and the eyes are wide-set. Cleft palate is common, as are limited joint motion and myopia, which may be severe enough to lead to retinal detachment. The kyphoscoliosis develops in early childhood but is usually not as progressive as in metatropic dysplasia. There is a prominent lumbar lordosis and accompanying hip flexion contracture, which produce a characteristic stance. Epiphyseal and metaphyseal changes are evident at birth, which give the femurs the radiographic "dumbbell" shape. The vertebrae are elongated, flattened, and wedged, especially in the dorsal spine. The scoliosis or kyphosis is usually mild but may be progressive and should be carefully observed during growth.

LARSEN'S SYNDROME

This syndrome is characterized by multiple congenital dislocations, particularly of the hips and knees. The individuals have a prominent forehead with abnormal facies, short metacarpals, and segmentation anomalies of the cervical and thoracic spine.[10, 17] The mode of inheritance is unclear, but recent reports suggest that it may be dominantly inherited.[4, 11] The spine problems in this syndrome are potentially hazardous, with reports of death due to cervical instability.[11] The frequently hypoplastic anterior elements and wide cervical spina bifida may lead to unstable, sharply angulated cervical kyphosis with or without thoracic lordosis. There also may be decreased interpedicular distance in the thoracic region, mild to moderate thoracic or thoracolumbar scoliosis, and lumbar lordosis. Early posterior and/or anterior cervical fusion is indicated for those patients with progressive cervical kyphosis.[11] Delayed motor development in these individuals should make one suspicious of cord compression due to progressive deformity or impingement by the hypermobile vertebral segments.

METATROPIC DYSPLASIA

Metatropic dysplasia is a type of short spine dwarfism characterized by a progressive kyphoscoliosis and deformed chest.[9] The name denotes the principal deformity. The infant has short limbs and a long trunk as in achondroplasia, but the trunk rapidly shortens owing to progressive kyphoscoliosis or "metamorphosis."[9] In infancy, the vertebral bodies are small, flattened, or diamond-shaped; these anomalies are most marked at the dorsolumbar junction.[9] Later, platyspondylia and anterior wedging predominate, frequently with a humplike buildup of bone in the central and dorsal portions of the vertebral end plates, and resemble the changes seen in spondyloepiphyseal dysplasia. The rapidly progressive kyphoscoliosis can lead to severe shortening and respiratory failure.[1, 9] Infantile mortality is increased owing to respiratory failure secondary to a reduced thoracic volume and mobility from the narrowed thorax. Early and aggressive treatment of the scoliosis to prevent the respiratory compromise would seem to be indicated. The scoliosis in metatropic dysplasia is generally resistant to brace treatment.[13]

PSEUDOACHONDROPLASTIC DYSPLASIA

As indicated in the name, the body habitus of these patients resembles achondroplasia, except the skull and facial features are normal and the findings in the hand are not similar.[3] Roentgenographically, the spine and epiphyses are more typical of spondyloepiphyseal dysplasia tarda, and there is no decrease in the interpedicular distance of the lumbar spine. These manifestations are frequently not recognized at birth but are discovered between two and five years of age, when the growth retardation becomes apparent, Exaggerated dorsal kyphosis and lumbar lordosis are constant features.[3] Mild to moderate scoliosis occurs in some and may require bracing. Recently, Cooper and coworkers found the cartilage cells of pseudoachondroplasia to be storing an abnormal material. They feel this alteration in metabolism most likely produces a soft cartilage that can deform markedly under stress.[2] The resulting vertebral deformation, particularly in the anterior vertebral margin, may lead to severe kyphosis, and neurologic complications have been reported.[2, 3]

No laboratory tests are available to differentiate the pseudoachondroplastic type from the achondroplastic dwarf, and errors in diagnosis are common. To determine the correct diagnosis, three differential points should be considered: (1) the child with pseudoachondroplasia characteristically has late onset and gradual development of clinical features, whereas the achondroplastic dwarf can be recognized at birth; (2) all children and adults with pseudoachondroplasia have a clinically and radiologically normal head and face; and (3) the fingers may be short but never show the trident configuration of achondroplasia.[3]

References

1. Bailey, J. A.: Disproportionate Short Stature: Diagnosis and Management. Philadelphia, W.B. Saunders Co., 1973.
2. Cooper, R. R., Ponsetti, I. B., and Maynard, J. A.: Pseudoachondroplastic dwarfism. J. Bone Joint Surg. 55A:475, 1973.
3. Ford, N., Silverman, F. N., and Kozlowski, K.: Spondyloepiphyseal dysplasia (pseudoachondroplastic type). Am. J. Roentgenol. 86:462, 1961.
4. Habermann, E. T., Sterling, A., and Dennis, R. I.: Larsen's syndrome: An heritable disorder. J. Bone Joint Surg. 58A:558, 1976.
5. Herring, J. A.: The spinal disorders in diastrophic dwarfism. J. Bone Joint Surg. 60A:177, 1978.
6. Kopits, S. E., and Parovic, M. N.: Orthopaedic complications of dwarfism. Clin. Orthop. 114:153, 1976.
7. Kozlowski, K.: Metaphyseal and spondylometaphyseal chondrodysplasia. Clin. Orthop. 114:83, 1976.
8. Langer, L. O.: Diastrophic dwarfism in early infancy. Am. J. Roentgenol. 98:399, 1965.
9. LaRose, J. H., and Gay, B. D.: Metatropic dwarfism. Am. J. Roentgenol. 106:156, 1969.
10. Larsen, L. J., Schottstead, E. R., and Bost, F. C.: Multiple congenital dislocations associated with characteristic facial abnormality. J. Pediatr. 37:574, 1958.
11. Micheli, L. J., Hall, J. E., and Watts, H. G.: Spinal instability in Larsen's syndrome. J. Bone Joint Surg. 58A:562, 1976.
12. Rimoin, D. L., Siggers, D. C., Lachman, R. S., and Silberberg, R.: Metatrophic dwarfism and Kniest syndrome and pseudoachondroplastic dysplasia. Clin. Orthop. 114:70, 1976.
13. Rimoin, D. L., and Horton, W. A.: Short statures. Parts I and II. J. Pediatr. 92:523–528, 697–704, 1978.
14. Scott, C. I.: Achondroplastic and hypochondroplastic dwarfism. Clin. Orthop. 114:18–30, 1976.
15. Spranger, J. W., Langer, L. O., and Wienedeman, H. R.: Bone Dysplasias. An Atlas of Constitutional Disorders of Skeletal Development. Philadelphia, W.B. Saunders Co., 1974.
16. Spranger, J. W.: Epiphyseal dysplasias. Clin. Orthop. 114:46, 1976.

17. Steele, H. H., and Kohl, E. J.: Multiple congenital dislocations associated with other skeletal abnormalities (Larsen's syndrome/three siblings). J. Bone Joint Surg. *54A*:75, 1972.

18. Stover, C. N., Hayes, J. T., and Holt, J. H.: Diastrophic dwarfism. Am. J. Roentgenol. *89*:914, 1963.

Storage Diseases

MUCOPOLYSACCHARIDOSES (MPS)

The mucopolysaccharidoses are inherited metabolic disorders of connective tissue in which afflicted individuals are unable to produce or, in some instances, degrade a specific complex carbohydrate. As a consequence, an excess of the metabolite is retained within the cells as well as excreted in the urine. Improved techniques in biochemical analysis have greatly facilitated early diagnosis, particularly in the patient whose findings are suggestive but who does not yet exhibit the classic clinical and roentgenographic appearance. Successful tissue culture of fibroblasts from MPS patients has provided information regarding pathogenesis and possibly will lead to improved methods of treatment.[4] Classification of these disorders is presently changing owing to the rapidly expanding pool of information.[4, 14] The original six groups (Hunter, Sanfilippo, Scheie, Morquio's, Hurler's, and Maroteaux-Lamy) have been subdivided to include several variations.[14]

Only three develop significant changes in the spine — Morquio's, Hurler's, and Maroteaux-Lamy — and thus form the basis of this discussion. All three have an autosomal recessive inheritance pattern and exhibit dwarfism due to shortening of the spine and limbs from epiphyseal involvement. These children appear normal at birth, and as more of the abnormal metabolite is accumulated, they gradually develop the typical clinical features. Depending on the degree of involvement and index of suspicion of the examiner, the diagnosis is usually suspected by the age of two or three. The conditions are progressive, but the expressivity is variable even among affected family members; thus, prognosis and management must be individualized.

HURLER'S SYNDROME (MPS I). This condition is rapidly progressive, and afflicted children usually die before 10 years of age.[14] Prominent features include dwarfing, mental retardation, corneal clouding, and hepatosplenomegaly. The basic defect is failure to degrade dermatan sulfate and heparin sulfate with excessive urinary excretion and storage in the cells.

The children have flexion contractures and limited motion of all peripheral joints. The neck is short so that the head appears to rest on the shoulders. One of the early features of Hurler's syndrome is usually a prominent gibbus at the dorsolumbar junction.[3] Roentgenographically, the vertebral body at the apex of the kyphosis is wedged with anterior beaking (Fig. 5–116) possibly owing to anterior herniation of the disc.[1, 16] This is not accompanied by similar changes in the adjacent vertebrae and may be due to pressure from hyperflexion when these hypotonic children first sit.[16]

Orthopaedic treatment of the joint contractures or spinal deformities is of limited benefit. The severe mental retardation, blindness, and cardiopulmonary complications usually serve to limit functional activity and any need for operative intervention.

MORQUIO'S SYNDROME (MPS IV). Morquio's syndrome is the most common of the mucopolysaccharidoses and, in contrast to achondroplasia, is the prototype of dwarfism that becomes apparent later in infancy and childhood. These patients have normal mentation, are physically active, and many survive to adult life. The deformities, particularly of the lower extremities and spine, often require treatment, and consequently the condition is familiar to the orthopaedist. Keratin sulfate excretion in the urine is excessive, and the condition is often referred to as keratosulfauria. The clinical and roentgenographic findings in Morquio's syndrome are similar to those found in spondyloepiphyseal dysplasia. Previously, the two conditions were often confused, but now they can be differentiated by laboratory tests.

Usually at the age of three or four, the children have developed the characteristic clinical appearance (Fig. 5–108). The neck is short and hyperextended with the head appearing to rest on the shoulders. The facies are characteristic; broad mouth, prominent maxilla, short nose, and widely spaced teeth. Corneal clouding and hearing defects are quite common. There is a prominent sternal kyphos, flaring of the rib cage, and occasionally a dorsal kyphosis. The peripheral joints appear to be enlarged and prominent owing to poor surrounding musculature. Unlike Hurler's syndrome, a good range of joint motion is usually maintained, and hypermobility of joints is a common finding.[14]

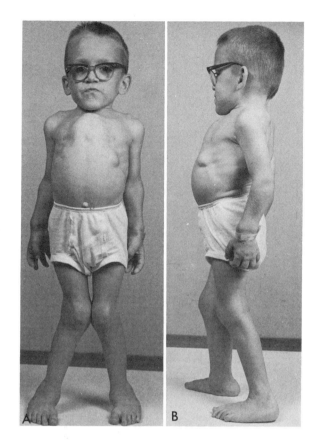

Figure 5–108. *A* and *B,* Clinical appearance of a nine-year-old with Morquio's syndrome. The neck is short and hyperextended, with the head appearing to rest on the shoulders. The facies is characteristic: broad mouth, prominent maxilla, shortened and widely spaced teeth. There is a prominent sternal kyphosis, flaring of the rib cage, genu valgum, and flat feet. The peripheral joints appear to be enlarged and prominent owing to the poor surrounding musculature.

Many have abnormalities of the odontoid[2, 14] with either hypoplasia or frank absence, which can lead to atlantoaxial instability and neurologic disturbances (Fig. 5–112).[2, 9, 12, 14] Universal platyspondylia is the most characteristic roentgenographic feature in this condition. Anterior beaking and wedging of the vertebral bodies can be seen at all levels (Fig. 5–109A and B), particularly at the dorsolumbar junction (Figs. 5–110 and 5–111). In the older patient, ligamentous laxity, a decreased anteroposterior diameter of the canal, and increased wedging of the vertebral bodies or gibbus at the dorsolumbar junction combine to increase the chance of spinal cord compression similar to the achondroplast.[2, 13, 14] Clinical evidence is scanty but suggests that neurologic problems in the first two decades are related to odontoid abnormalities. In later life, symptoms due to the kyphosis or gibbus tend to predominate.[2]

The ilia are flared superiorly but are dramatically narrowed inferiorly by the enlarged acetabulum. The femoral epiphysis is initially present, but fragmentation and flattening quickly ensue with disappearance of the femoral head, usually in adult life (Fig. 5–109C and D).[14] Genu valgum can be severe with adaptive changes in the knee joint and ligamentous laxity (Fig. 5–108A).

Treatment. Recent reports indicate that atlantoaxial instability is more common in Morquio's syndrome than previously recognized.[2, 5, 8, 9, 11, 12, 14] McKusick[13] suggests that all will eventually develop significant spinal cord compression at the atlantoaxial articulation. This may result from either anomalous development of the odontoid or laxity of the transverse atlantal ligament.[2, 9, 14] In one study,[2] five of eight patients developed neurologic signs and symptoms from cervical spinal cord compression, and in another study,[12] six of 11 patients developed these manifestations. The earliest indication of impending quadriparesis may be quite subtle and overlooked. Kopits[9] reports that the majority of patients present only with generalized progressive weakness, manifested as lack of physical endurance, history of frequent falling, or asking to be carried. Later, these patients exhibit the typical findings of spinal cord compression with hyperreflexia, spasticity, and loss of bladder and bowel control. If the condition is allowed to continue, the child eventually be-

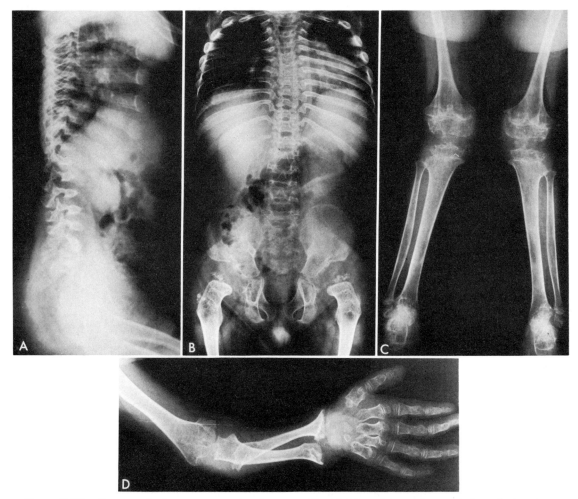

Figure 5–109. Roentgenologic appearance of a nine-year-old with Morquio's syndrome. *A,* Lateral view demonstrates universal platyspondyly with anterior beaking and wedging of the vertebral bodies at all levels. *B,* Anteriorposterior view. The femoral epiphysis is initially present, but fragmentation and flattening quickly ensue. *C,* Typical appearance of the knees and ankles, with marked genu valgum. *D,* Appearance of the elbow, wrist, and hand.

comes bedridden, quadriparetic, and dies from neurologic impairment of respiration.[9, 12] It must be emphasized that weakness is a nonspecific complaint. Keratin sulfate is stored in the neural cells, and this may be, at times, the cause of the patient's progressive deterioration rather than spinal cord compression. Atlantoaxial instability must be documented prior to any surgical considerations. In this regard, lateral flexion-extension laminagraphic techniques are necessary (Fig. 5–112). Gas myelography has been used by Kopits[10] to visualize the spinal cord and surrounding structures with excellent results (Fig. 5–116).

If significant spinal cord compression is found, reduction and surgical stabilization are indicated. Reduction should be accomplished prior to surgery. Kopits[8] has recommended the halo-cast or halo-brace, but this may compromise an existing marginal pulmonary function which is common in patients with atlantoaxial instability.[8, 12] As the skull is dysplastic, the likelihood of complications from the halo, such as protrusion of the pins, is increased.[12] Occiput to C2 fusion is usually required, and, despite the dysplastic appearance of the bone, a solid arthrodesis usually can be achieved.[16] Dramatic neurologic improvement should not be expected, as the existing damage may be irreversible.[12] The surgery should be viewed as a means of stabilizing the condition and preventing further irritation to the spinal cord.[10, 12] Spinal cord compression at the level of the thoracolumbar gibbus (Fig. 5–113) is an infrequent complication usually limited to the older patient[2, 13] and similar to that found in achondroplasia. Similarly, treatment of the developing gibbus during childhood with an appropriate spinal orthosis may arrest its progress and may prevent late complications (Fig. 5–114).[2]

MAROTEAUX-LAMY SYNDROME (MPS VI). This condition is more recently recognized and uncommon; consequently, the clinical features, treatment, and prognosis have not been well delineated. The metabolic error results in abnormal excretion of urinary dermatan sulfate. These children have joint contractures and stiffness similar to those found in Hurler's syndrome. Cardiac involvement is common and can result in early death.[2] Odontoid dysplasia and atlantoaxial instability with resultant spinal cord compression similar to those found in Morquio's syndrome have been described,[14] but not as frequently. The

roentgenographic appearance of the spine is vertebral flattening, not as severe as that seen in Morquio's syndrome. These findings are variable even among family members and as yet do not reliably distinguish this condition from the other mucopolysaccharidoses (Fig. 5–115). Kyphosis at the dorsolumbar junction can occur, but as yet has not been reported to be progressive.

GANGLIOSIDOSIS, MUCOLIPIDOSIS

Mucopolysaccharidoses are the most common and best studied of the storage diseases. In addition, many unusual and uncommon storage diseases that affect the vertebrae can lead to kyphosis, especially dorsolumbar gibbus, such as the gangliosidoses and mucolipidoses and their subgroups.[15]

In infancy there is usually a hook-shaped deformity of the vertebral body at the thoracolumbar junction (Fig. 5–116). Later, as the

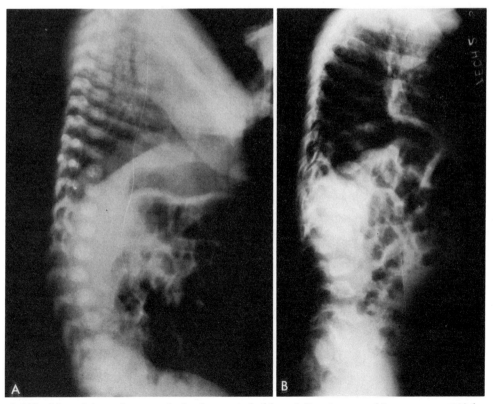

Figure 5–110. Morquio's syndrome: early development of gibbus. *A*, Roentgenographic appearance at 10 days of age demonstrates slight wedging of the second lumbar vertebra. Patient was suspected of having the disease, as he has affected older sibs. *B*, Roentgenographic appearance at age five showing further beaking of the vertebrae and changes typical of Morquio's syndrome. Note subluxation of the first lumbar on the second lumbar vertebral body.

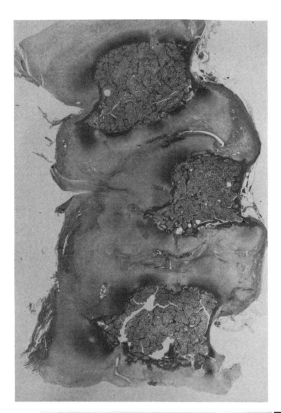

Figure 5–111. Photomicrograph; cross section of the typical beaked vertebra found in Morquio's syndrome. Patient expired secondary to respiratory failure. Note the herniation of the intervertebral material into the bony substance.

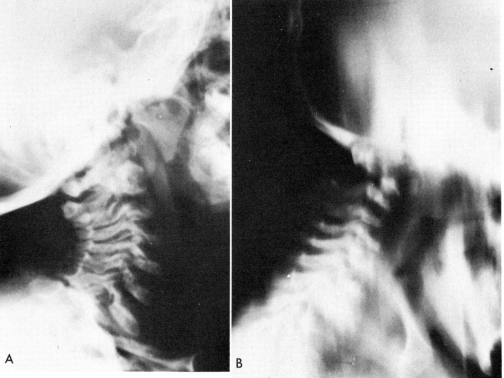

A

B

Figure 5–112. Five-year-old with Morquio's syndrome discovered to have progressive weakness and long tract signs in the upper and lower extremities. *A,* Routine lateral examination demonstrates the dysplastic appearance of the bone but otherwise normal configuration of the cervical spine. *B,* With flexion of the neck and employing lateral laminagraphic techniques, forward displacement of the atlas on the axis can be demonstrated. The patient was placed in a halo-pelvic apparatus to accomplish reduction, and posterior fusion (occiput to C2) was performed.

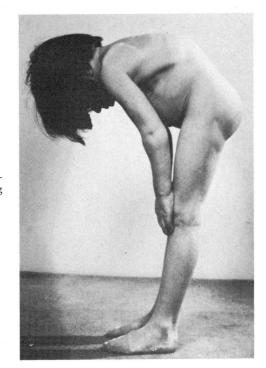

Figure 5–113. Eight-year-old with Maroteaux-Lamy syndrome. Note accentuation of the thoracolumbar gibbus during forward flexion.

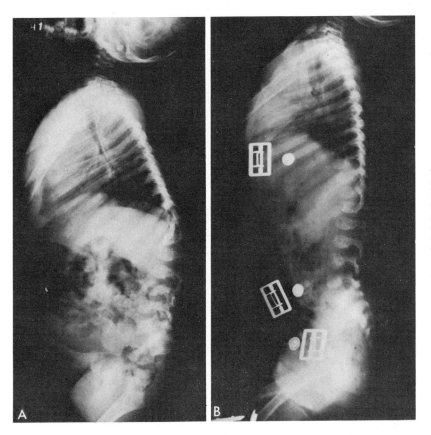

Figure 5–114. Two-year-old with Maroteaux-Lamy syndrome and a thoracolumbar gibbus. *A,* Sitting lateral roentgenogram with kyphosis centered at the wedged twelfth thoracic vertebral body. *B,* Treatment with a lightweight spinal orthosis demonstrates partial correction.

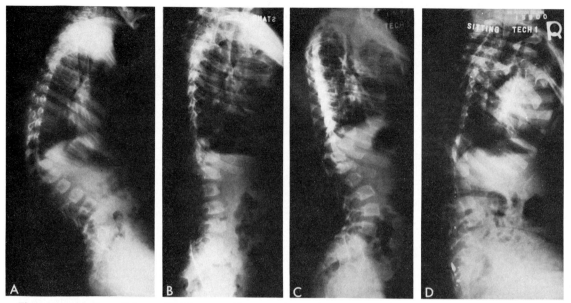

Figure 5–115. Four siblings with Maroteaux-Lamy syndrome. Lateral views of the spine demonstrate four distinct variations in spine configuration. *A*, Long arcuate kyphosis. *B*, Vertebral changes, but normal alignment. *C*, Gibbus at a single vertebral level. *D*, Mild long kyphosis.

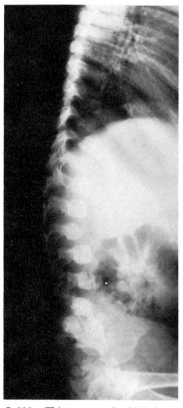

Figure 5–116. Thirteen-month-old infant evaluated for delay in motor development and subluxation of the hips. Lateral roentgenogram of the spine demonstrates a beaking of the L2 vertebral body. This is a definite pathologic finding and is compatible with storage disease such as mucopolysaccharidosis, mucolipidosis, or hypothyroidism. Further clinical and laboratory investigations are indicated. For this child, laboratory studies have confirmed the diagnosis of Hurler's syndrome.

child grows older, there is marked flattening of all the vertebral bodies, particularly in the anterior portion.[16] For the majority the prognosis is very poor,[13] and the spine changes are usually accompanied by joint abnormalities and mental retardation.[7] A clinical and roentgenographic picture would be quite similar to mucopolysaccharidosis (dysostosis multiplex) and can be differentiated by histochemical or chemical analysis.[7, 15]

In general, patients with gangliosidosis or mucolipidosis have a severe psychomotor retardation and such limited life expectancy that orthopaedic intervention is seldom indicated.

References

1. Begg, A. C.: Nuclear herniations of the intervertebral disc: Their radiological manifestations and significance. J. Bone Joint Surg. *36B*:180–193, 1954.
2. Blaw, M. E., and Langer, L. O.: Spinal cord compression in Morquio-Brailsford's disease. J. Pediatr. *74*:593–600, 1969.
3. Caffey, J.: Gargoylism (Hunter-Hurler disease, dysostosis multiplex, lipochondrodystrophy): Prenatal and neonatal bone lesions and their early postnatal evolution. Am. J. Roentgenol. *67*:715–731, 1952.
4. Danes, B. S., and Grossman, H.: Bone dysplasias, including Morquio's syndrome, studied in skin fibroblast cultures. Am. J. Med. *47*:708–720, 1969.
5. Einhorn, N. H., Moore, J. R., and Rowntree, L. G.: Osteochondrodystrophia deformans (Morquio's disease). Observations at autopsy in one case. Am. J. Dis. Child. *72*:536–544, 1946.
6. Gilles, F. H., and Deuel, R. K.: Neuronal cytoplasmic globules in the brain in Morquio's syndrome. Arch. Neurol. *25*:393–403, 1971.

7. Kelly, T. E.: The mucopolysaccharidoses and mucolipidoses. Clin. Orthop. *114*:116, 1976.
8. Kopits, S. E., and Steingass, M. H.: Experience with
   the "halo-cast" in small children. Surg. Clin. North
   Am. *50*:935, 1970.
9. Kopits, S. E., et al.: Congenital atlanto-axial dislocations in various forms of dwarfism. J. Bone Joint
   Surg. *54A*:1349–1350, 1972.
10. Kopits, S. E.: Orthopaedic complications of dwarfism. Clin. Orthop. *114*:153, 1976.
11. Langer, L. O., Jr., and Carey, L. S.: The roentgenographic features of the KS mucopolysaccharidoses
   of Morquio (Morquio-Brailsford's disease). Am. J.
   Roentgenol. *97*:1–20, 1966.
12. Lipson, S. J.: Dysplasia of the odontoid process in
   Morquio's syndrome causing quadriparesis. J.
   Bone Joint Surg. *59A*:340–344, 1977.
13. McKusick, V. A.: Heritable Disorders of Connective
   Tissue, 4th ed. St. Louis, C.V. Mosby Co., 1972.
14. Melzak, J.: Spinal deformities with paraplegia in two
   sisters with Morquio-Brailsford syndrome. Paraplegia *6*:246–258, 1969.
15. Spranger, J. W., Langer, L. O., and Wiedemann, H.
   R.: Bone Dysplasias. An Atlas of Constitutional
   Disorders of Skeletal Development. Philadelphia,
   W.B. Saunders Co., 1974.
16. Swischuk, L. E.: The beaked, notched, or hooked
   vertebrae: Its significance in infants and young
   children. Radiology *95*:661–664, 1970.

CHAPTER 6

Scoliosis and Kyphosis

DAVID S. BRADFORD, M.D.
Twin Cities Scoliosis Center

JOHN H. MOE, M.D.
Fairview Hospital, Univeristy of Minnesota

ROBERT B. WINTER, M.D.
Gillette Children's Hospital

INTRODUCTION

Lateral and posterior curvatures of the spine have been recorded in literature since the earliest medical writings and have been noted as well in skeletal remnants of prehistoric man. Hippocrates, one of the first to write on the subject, applied the name scoliosis to any curvature of the spine.[124] He described spinal deformity primarily from injury, but he did note that "curvature of the spine occurs even in healthy persons in many ways for such a condition is connected with its nature and use and besides there is a giving away in old age and on account of pain. But the outward curvature due to falls usually occurs when the patient comes down on his buttocks or falls on his shoulders and in this curvature, one of the vertebrae necessarily appears to stand out more prominently. . . ." Hippocrates also described an apparatus for forcibly reducing the deformity, but it did not appear to be very effective.[18] Over the ensuing centuries, attempts to treat the spinal deformity became more evident.

Paul of Aegina, one thousand years after Hippocrates' efforts, attempted to reduce the spinal deformity by bandaging the body to splints.[18] Ambroise Paré, in 1579,[196] was the first to attempt trunk support by anterior and posterior metal plates, made by armorers (Fig.

6–1).[196] By the eighteenth and nineteenth centuries, scoliosis became more recognized as a pathologic entity, and braces of various ingenious design were made for the torso in an attempt to prevent progression. Sitting habits were sometimes given as the cause of the adolescent scoliosis that we now term "idiopathic." A large number of school desks and chairs were subsequently designed to overcome the deformity (Fig. 6–2).[111] Exercises and vertical halter stretching (Fig. 6–3) were prescribed, along with the use of various types of body braces. Some of these braces included head caps and halters.

Hare, in 1849, described the use of traction to the head and pelvis in the horizontal position.[111] Plaster molds of his patients who had completed such treatment revealed re-

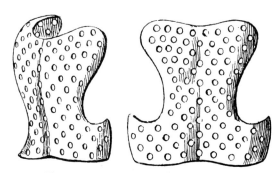

Figure 6–1. The Corset of Paré — (1579).

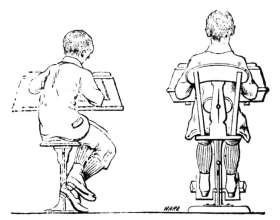

Figure 6–2. A typical text illustration indicating poor posture as a primary cause of scoliosis – 1830.

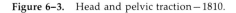

markable cosmetic improvement. He ascribed the deformity to poor sitting habits, to constitutional disorders, and to rickets. His treatment was to place the patient on an inclined plane of firm material, so designed that while a padded head halter was used padded side pressures were also applied. He also added padded straps pulling upward on the axillae and padded straps attached to the ankle. His spectacular results are open to question (Fig. 6–4). He felt that, while exercise treatment and constrictive body corsets and braces were of no value, proper dieting, respiratory exercises, and gymnastic exercises in bed were important. His work is of particular interest because he noted the difference between infectious disease of the spine and scoliosis.

Edward Lonsdale of London, in the same year, wrote a treatise on treatment of lateral curvatures of the spine.[154] He stated that the prevalence of the deformity in girls was directly related to a more sedentary life pattern. He stated that "it is most difficult to trace the cause," but felt that the postural habits of girls while sitting and sewing, constriction of the lungs by stays, carrying of young children on one arm principally, and excessively rapid growth in adolescence were causes of the deformity. General debility and weakness of certain muscles and the mechanical weight of the head and upper extremities were given as additional causes. For treatment, he advocated a special spinal support, which consisted of a pelvic hoop combined with an axillary crutch and a spring-supported pad against the rib prominence, a device almost identical to the Barr-Bushenfeldt brace of this century.[7, 18] In addition, he proposed a sling suspension against the rib deformity in the horizontal position. Unfortunately, he showed no end results of his treatment.

The first carefully fitted supports were made about 1895 by Friedrich Hessing of Ausgburg.[120] Albert Hoffa used this brace but emphasized the need of concomitant exercises to furnish active correction.[127] By the end of the nineteenth century, plaster of Paris applied as a circular jacket became an accepted method of holding correction of a curvature. Wullstein included the head and neck and combined multiple metal lateral pressure pads against bony prominences (Fig. 6–5).[274] Lewis Sayre[219] used vertical head suspension and a body cast (Fig. 6–6).[219] Frames for applying casts were designed for both vertical and horizontal distraction by Bradford and Brackett (Fig. 6–7). The horizontal frame had a lateral pad attached to a half-hoop, which was remarkably similar to the localizer frame that Joseph Risser first used in 1952.[207, 210, 211]

At the turn of the century two types of braces were developed. Most relied on passive support with axillary crutches, elastic bands for rib pressure, and even weights and pulleys. The active brace first proposed by Spitzy required that the patient either maintain elongation of the spine or suffer pain.[240] This brace, however, did not have holding pads. Earlier attempts at correction included the passive correction brace of Steindler and the ingenious lever system of Barr-Buschenfeldt.[18]

Figure 6–3. Head and pelvic traction – 1810.

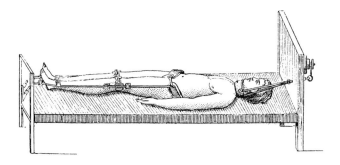

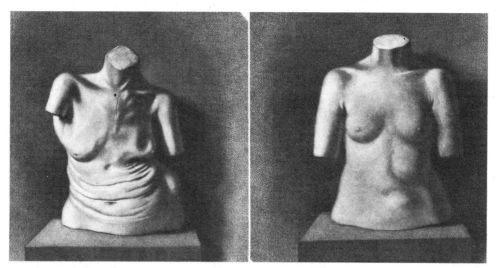

Figure 6–4. From Hare (1849), illustrating the effect of his treatment by traction. The validity of this dramatic result is subject to question.

A landmark of progress in the control and correction of progressive idiopathic curvature in the growing child was the development of the Milwaukee brace. This was originally designed by Blount and Schmidt as a substitute for the distraction plaster jacket.[20, 21] They substituted a circular neck ring with occipital and chin pads for the plaster collar and a molded leather pelvic girdle for a plaster girdle. They joined the two sections with turnbuckles incorporated into four uprights connecting the two and made it a removable distraction jacket. They placed an adjustable screw pressure pad against the rib prominence. The patient was kept supine, and the brace was removed for surgical fusion. It proved to be a success, and modifications were made.

The leather girdle was made more closely form-fitting. A single bar was placed anteriorly. The pressure pad against the thoracic rib prominence was attached by straps and an

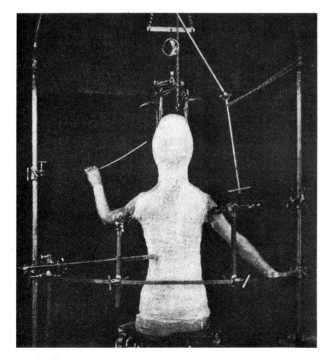

Figure 6–5. Plaster application technique, Wullstein — 1902.

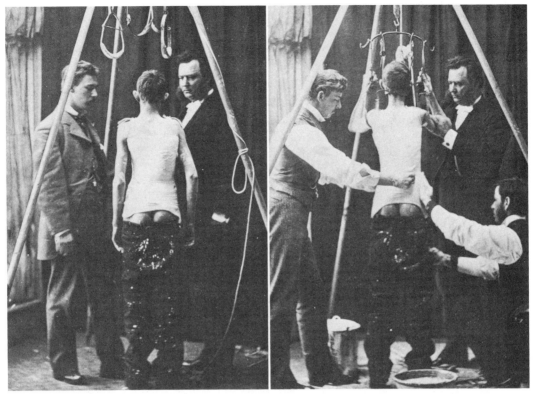

Figure 6–6. Plaster application by Sayre for scoliosis correction. (From Sayre Textbook on Scoliosis — 1870.)

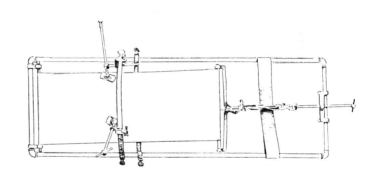

Figure 6–7. From Brackett and Bradford — 1890.

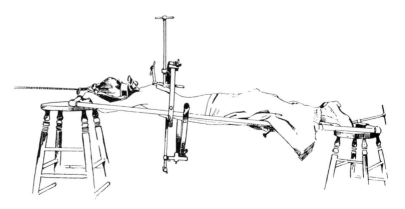

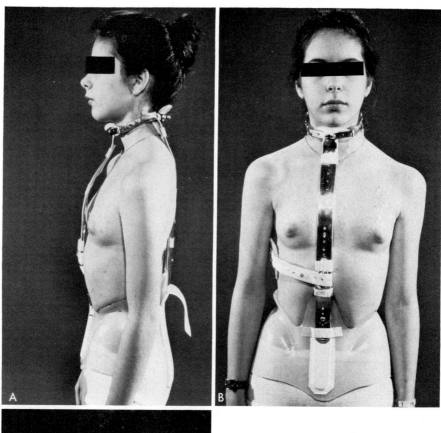

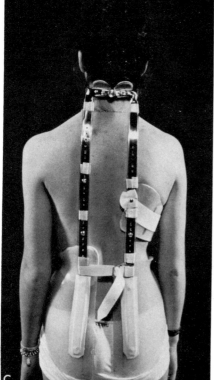

Figure 6–8. The current Milwaukee brace with plastic pelvic girdle.

anterior outrigger. The lumbar pad was modified. Soon the brace became more cosmetically acceptable. Both in Milwaukee and in Minneapolis-St. Paul, the modified brace was worn for long periods without surgery. It was discovered that the brace worn during growth could produce correction of the curve.

It has become increasingly apparent, however, from close review of patients under long-term follow-up observation that permanent correction by the use of the brace is not usual. Rather, the greatest success from brace wear lies in prevention of small curves from becoming larger curves. In the last several years, rather extensive modifications of the basic brace design have developed. These have included a change in the neck ring to a smaller throat mold, the use of newer thermaplastic materials, and a wider acceptance of thoracolumbar and thoracolumbosacral orthoses for flexible thoracolumbar or lumbar curvatures (Fig. 6–8).

The operative treatment of scoliosis began in 1914 when Russell Hibbs did his first scoliosis fusion.[121-123] He had previously performed a similar operation for tuberculosis of the spine in 1911. Albee in 1914 devised a fusion technique that consisted of tibial bone struts inserted into the split spinous processes.[4] Albee's operation did not appear as successful as that of Hibbs, who inserted bone graft into the intervertebral joints. Because of a rather high incidence of pseudarthrosis published by Hibbs and others, surgical correction of the deformity was not widely accepted in the 1930s and 1940s. In fact, Steindler gave up fusion completely and resorted to exercise and bracing in an attempt to establish better compensation and balance.[246] In the past two decades, improved fusion techniques and the successful development of spinal instrumentation have significantly advanced the operative management of the scoliosis patient. Harrington's instrumentation, first successfully used in 1960, truly revolutionized the operative management of spinal deformities.[112] In fact, now it has become the mainstay in surgical treatment in scoliosis. In 1956, Hodgson described the anterior approach to the spine for treatment of tuberculosis and later in 1965 described anterior opening wedge osteotomy for the treatment of congenital kyphosis.[125, 126] The anterior approach now has become the mainstay of treatment of structural kyphosis. New advances in the past decade, such as the halo hoop,[88] Dwyer instrumentation,[73,74] and Zielke instrumentation have revolutionized the treatment of structural spinal deformity.

CLASSIFICATION AND TERMINOLOGY[62, 67, 196, 208]

Curvatures may be classified by the area of the spine in which the apex of the curve is located: (1) cervical curve, apex between C1 and C6; (2) cervical thoracic curve, apex between C7 and T1; (3) thoracic curve, apex between T2 and T11; (4) thoracolumbar curve, apex between T12 and L1; (5) lumbar curve, apex between L2 and L4; (6) lumbosacral curve, apex between L5 and S1.

It should be noted that there are essentially two major types of curvatures, the nonstructural and the structural.[99, 128] Nonstructural scoliosis is nonprogressive. On examination with the patient bending toward the side of the apex of the curvature, the spine appears to completely correct clinically as well as radiographically. The cause of nonstructural lumbar scoliosis would be a shortened extremity on the side of the apex of the curvature. Vertebral rotation is not characteristic of nonstructural curvatures. However, these curves should be watched during growth since occasionally they may develop into a structural deformity.

A structural curvature, on the other hand, may not be voluntarily corrected, and seldom can it be passively or even forcibly fully corrected. Vertebral rotation into the convexity of the curvature is usual, and this may be manifested by a fixed thoracic prominence on the convex side of the curvature in the case of thoracic deformity. This may best be seen when the patient assumes a forward bend position. Most structural curvatures are of the congenital type. In idiopathic scoliosis, the development of structural changes is often dependent upon the rapidity and the severity of curve progression.

A classification of spinal deformity has now been accepted by the Scoliosis Research Society.[57, 58, 90] These deformities may occur simply or in combination. Deformities may be classified according to magnitude, location, direction, and etiology. The direction of the curvature is designated by the side of the convexity of the deformity.

Idiopathic Scoliosis[130-133]

This group forms by far the largest number of patients. The diagnosis is unknown. It has been suggested that environmental factors may play a role in the infantile group, while hereditary and familial factors are operative in the adolescent group.[47, 275, 276] Three groups are identified according to the age of recognition.

INFANTILE. This type of idiopathic scoliosis is rare in America but is common in England and Northern Europe. It is present at birth or appears shortly thereafter. Curvatures noted in children under the age of three are classified in this group. Eighty to 90 per cent of these curves resolve spontaneously; no therapy is needed. Of the remainder, most progress during childhood and become extremely severe problems. The rib angle difference measurement of Mehta[167] may sometimes distinguish the progressive from the nonprogressive infantile idiopathic curves. Infantile idiopathic curves are predominantly left thoracic and are more frequent in males.

JUVENILE. In this category, the onset of the curve begins after age three but before puberty. The separation of the early juvenile from the late infantile types is impossible unless adequate early standing radiographs are available. These curvatures are mainly right thoracic and are commonly first recognized at about age six. Males and females are equally involved. In contrast to the infantile idiopathic group, these usually progress throughout infancy. If untreated, severe deformity is to be expected.

ADOLESCENT. By definition, a curve starting after the onset of puberty is included in this category. A right thoracic curve predominates. In small curvatures, less than 10 degrees, the occurrence in males versus females is the same.[44, 45] However, in curvatures greater than 20 degrees or in progressive curvatures, females are far more frequently involved than males (6.4 females to 1.0 male, and 19.3 per cent females to 1.2 per cent males, respectively.)[71] A large number of these curves are structural when first seen. The flexibility and progression of these curves, however, are quite variable. The structural curvatures tend to progress during adolescence if untreated, while the nonstructural curves may remain flexible and rarely produce problems.

The etiology of idiopathic scoliosis is unknown. It is suggested from the studies of Wynne-Davies and Cowell, Hall, and MacEwen that a definite familial tendency exists.[64, 275, 276]

Structural Scoliosis

    I. Idiopathic
        A. Infantile (0–3 years)
            1. Resolving
            2. Progressive
        B. Juvenile (3–10 years)
        C. Adolescent (> 10 years)
   II. Neuromuscular
        A. Neuropathic
            1. Upper motor neuron
                a. Cerebral palsy
                b. Spinocerebellar degeneration
                    i. Friedreich's disease
                    ii. Charcot-Marie-Tooth disease
                    iii. Roussy-Lévy disease
                c. Syringomyelia
                d. Spinal cord tumor
                e. Spinal cord trauma
                f. Other
            2. Lower motor neuron
                a. Poliomyelitis
                b. Other viral myelitides
                c. Traumatic
                d. Spinal muscular atrophy
                    i. Werdnig-Hoffmann
                    ii. Kugelberg-Welander
                e. Myelomeningocoele (paralytic)
            3. Dysautonomia (Riley-Day)
            4. Other
        B. Myopathic
            1. Arthrogryposis
            2. Muscular dystrophy
                a. Duchenne (pseudohypertrophic)
                b. Limb-girdle
                c. Facioscapulohumeral
            3. Fiber type disproportion
            4. Congenital hypotonia
            5. Myotonia dystrophica
            6. Other
  III. Congenital
        A. Failure of formation
            1. Wedge vertebra
            2. Hemivertebra
        B. Failure of segmentation
            1. Unilateral (unsegmented bar)
            2. Bilateral
        C. Mixed
   IV. Neurofibromatosis
    V. Mesenchymal disorders
        A. Marfan's
        B. Ehlers-Danlos
        C. Others
   VI. Rheumatoid disease
  VII. Trauma
        A. Fracture
        B. Surgical
            1. Post-laminectomy
            2. Post-thoracoplasty
        C. Irradiation

VIII. Extraspinal contractures
  A. Postempyema
  B. Post-burns
IX. Osteochondrodystrophies
  A. Diastrophic dwarfism
  B. Mucopolysaccharidoses (e.g., Morquio's syndrome)
  C. Spondyloepiphyseal dysplasia
  D. Multiple epiphyseal dysplasia
  E. Other
X. Infection of bone
  A. Acute
  B. Chronic
XI. Metabolic disorders
  A. Rickets
  B. Osteogenesis imperfecta
  C. Homocystinuria
  D. Others
XII. Related to lumbosacral joint
  A. Spondylolysis and spondylolisthesis
  B. Congenital anomalies of lumbosacral region
XIII. Tumors
  A. Vertebral column
    1. Osteoid osteoma
    2. Histiocytosis X
    3. Other
  B. Spinal cord (see neuromuscular)

Nonstructural Scoliosis

I. Postural scoliosis
II. Hysterical scoliosis
III. Nerve root irritation
  A. Herniation of nucleus pulposus
  B. Tumors
IV. Inflammatory (e.g., appendicitis)
V. Related to leg length discrepancy
VI. Related to contractures about the hip

Kyphosis

I. Postural
II. Scheuermann's disease
III. Congenital
  A. Defect of formation
  B. Defect of segmentation
  C. Mixed
IV. Neuromuscular
V. Myelomeningocele
  A. Developmental (late paralytic)
  B. Congenital (present at birth)
VI. Traumatic
  A. Due to bone and/or ligament damage without cord injury
  B. Due to bone and/or ligament damage with cord injury
VII. Postsurgical
  A. Post-laminectomy
  B. Following excision of vertebral body
VIII. Post-irradiation
IX. Metabolic
  A. Osteoporosis
    1. Senile
    2. Juvenile
  B. Osteomalacia
  C. Osteogenesis imperfecta
  D. Other

X. Skeletal dysplasia
  A. Achondroplasia
  B. Mucopolysaccharidoses
  C. Neurofibromatosis
  D. Other
XI. Collagen disease
  A. Marie-Strümpell
  B. Other
XII. Tumor
  A. Benign
  B. Malignant
    1. Primary
    2. Metastatic
XIII. Inflammatory

Lordosis

I. Postural
II. Congenital
III. Neuromuscular
IV. Post-laminectomy
V. Secondary to hip flexion contracture
VI. Other

Patient Evaluation[1]

EARLY EVALUATION OF SCOLIOSIS — SCHOOL SCREENING. Evaluation of a patient for scoliosis may be done quickly by a trained school nurse or a physical education teacher (Fig. 6–9). School children may be checked annually with this test, preferably from ages 10 to 16; girls may wear a halter, and boys may be checked without a shirt. The examiner should view the patient from the back, side, and front and should note particularly any evidence of rib hump prominence on a forward bending test. Very minor differences between two sides can be appreciated. If a deformity is detected, the child should be referred to the family physician, and standing radiographs of the spine should be taken where indicated. If scoliosis is diagnosed, the child is referred to the orthopaedic surgeon or crippled children's clinic for further evaluation and treatment.

ORTHOPAEDIC EXAMINATION. The orthopaedic examination of a patient with scoliosis should be detailed. A careful history must be taken and should include specifically inquiries as to pain, neurologic symptoms, family history, and growth spurt and menarche. All diseases known to be associated with a high incidence of scoliosis, that is, connective tissue diseases, should be ruled out. Once the history is completed, an examination of the patient is undertaken. The patient should remain undraped except for a small pair of

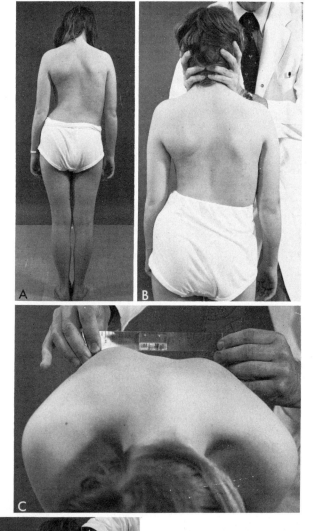

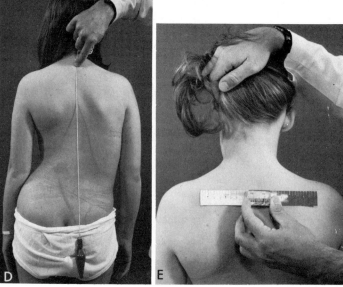

Figure 6–9. *A,* The patient must be viewed from a short distance to fully evaluate the deformity. From the rear view *all* clothing should be removed, when permissible. Here is shown a typical right thoracic idiopathic curve. Note the lowering of the right shoulder, the fullness and scapular prominence over the right thorax, the decreased distance between the arm and the right thorax, and the increased distance between the left arm and thorax. The left pelvis seems higher than the right, but this is due to flank fullness on the right and flank depression on the left. The pelvis is level and the "high hip" commonly referred to by parents is apparent, not real. The thorax is depressed on the left. *B,* Mobility of the spine can be quickly checked by hand suspension. *C,* The difference in the height of the thoracic cage should be recorded with a spirit level at the same distance from the spine. This is best determined in the thorax with the patient bent toward the examiner. The lumbar prominence is best checked from behind. One must be certain that the arms are dropped vertically and that the fingertips are together. *D,* A plumb line dropped from the mid-occiput or from the seventh (prominence) cervical vertebra demonstrates a list of the body toward the right. The distance from the gluteal crease to the line of deviation should be recorded. *E,* Shoulder level and low neck asymmetry should be checked and recorded.

Legend continued on opposite page.

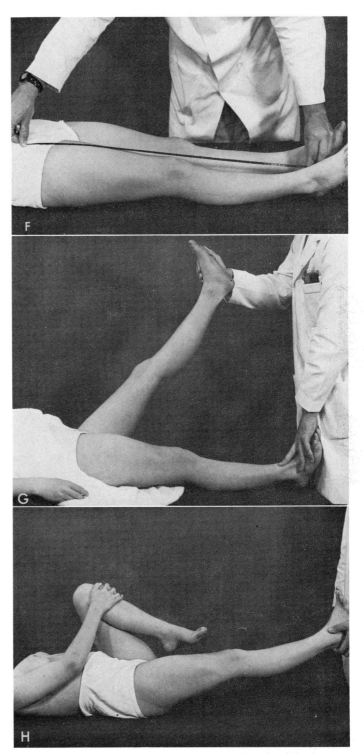

Figure 6–9 *Continued.* *F,* The length of the lower extremities should be measured as accurately as possible. *G,* Tightness of the hamstrings, pectoral muscles, and heel cords should be recorded. *H,* Always check for hip flexion contractures.

Illustration continued on following page.

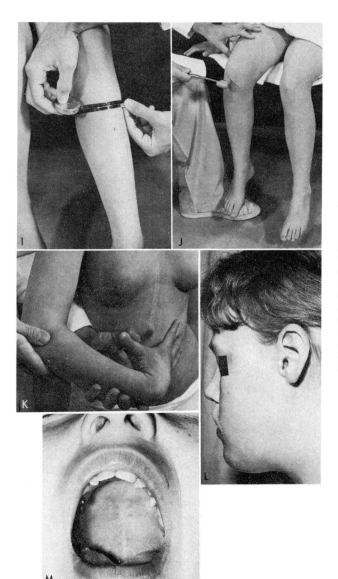

Figure 6–9 *Continued.* *I,* Evidence of atrophy or hypertrophy should be determined by measurement. *J,* A complete neurological evaluation should be done on every patient. *K,* All skin discolorations (cafe-au-lait) and scars (cardiac or other surgery) should be noted and recorded. Hypermobility of fingers and thumb should be tested. *L,* Abnormalities of the ears, nose, eyes and extremities should be carefully noted. *M,* Abnormalities of bite, teeth and palate should be recorded. Likewise, the wearing of corrective orthodontic appliances should be recorded.

underpants and a loose gown that is open in the back. The examiner should view the entire body from the front, side, and rear, noting (1) scapular asymmetry and unilateral prominence; (2) waist asymmetry or fullness; (3) shoulder level; and (4) asymmetry in the distance between the arms and the torso. The patient is then asked to bend forward at the hips toward the examiner, dropping both arms vertically, holding the fingertips together. The examiner then notices any asymmetry of the rib cage. A high rib cage on one side is indicative almost invariably of a thoracic curvature (Fig. 6–10). The patient is then viewed in the same manner from the rear, noting asymmetry in the height of the lumbar area,

which likewise denotes a rotational prominence of the lumbar spine and, hence, spinal deformity. The height of the rib or lumbar prominence should be recorded. A plumbline should be dropped from the lower cervical spinous process at the C7 cervical vertebra, and the distance from the vertical string to the gluteal cleft is a measurement of spinal imbalance. The patient is then requested to bend to each side. Extreme spinal spasm with inability to bend normally from side to side may be indicative of intraspinal irritative lesions, such as a spinal cord tumor, osteoid osteoma, or herniated disc. The skin is examined for pigmented lesions, subcutaneous tumors, hairy patches, angiomas, and scars. Café au lait

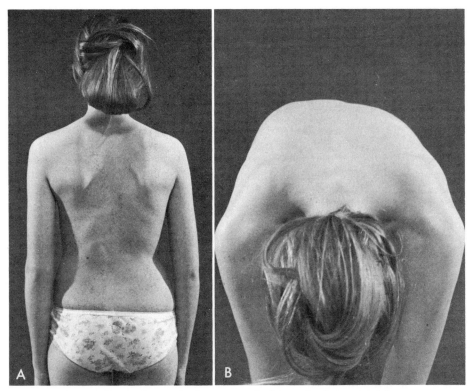

Figure 6–10. Careful examination by a school nurse resulted in early diagnosis of this curvature (10 degrees). Note spine asymmetry in the flexed position (*B*).

spots may be a manifestation of generalized neurofibromatosis. A hairy patch over the sacrum or lower lumbar spine is indicative of diastematomyelia until proved otherwise, and abnormal scarring with extreme elasticity may be a manifestation of Ehlers-Danlos syndrome. Abnormalities of the extremities, appendages, mouth, and palate should be noted, and joint motions and contractures, especially in the hips should be recorded. Measurements of leg lengths and circumferences and straight leg raising tests should be carried out. Tight hamstrings with low back pain and spasm may be a manifestation of spondylolisthesis. Finally, a complete and careful neurologic examination, especially of the lower extremities, should be carried out and recorded. The patient's intelligence and mental status should be noted during the examination. Sitting and standing heights should be taken and recorded along with the arm span.

ROENTGENOGRAPHIC EVALUATION. Roentgenographic evaluation of a child with spinal deformity is essential. In a young child, the entire spine and pelvis may be visualized on a 14 × 17″ film. Older children and adolescents should have longer films (14

× 36″). The whole spine is seen on the roentgenograph, and the relationship between the head, shoulders, upper trunk, and pelvis may be appreciated. Unnecessary exposure to x-rays should be avoided. For patients referred to the orthopaedist with a clinical diagnosis of scoliosis or kyphosis and a demonstrated clinical deformity, we prefer to take only an AP and lateral roentgenogram at a six foot distance (14 × 36″ film) and to review these roentgenograms before ordering additional ones. In the presence of a significant curvature (greater than 25 degrees), a routine scoliosis or kyphosis series may be taken.[265] This includes a supine view of the entire curve in the anteroposterior view taken with the patient bending maximally to the right and to the left. A calculation of curvature flexibility is of great assistance, for instance, in determining the length of the spinal fusion should surgery be deemed necessary. Additional roentgenograms would include the left hand and wrist to determine bone age.[100] Any abnormalities noted in the lumbosacral area might be better delineated with a Ferguson view. This view gives a true anteroposterior view of the lumbosacral joint. Any evidence of spondylolysis and spondylolisthesis would require oblique views in the lumbosacral area. A standing lateral roentgenogram of the lumbosacral area in cases of spondylolisthesis is essential in order to accurately calculate the magnitude of the deformity and the true slip angle.

Lateral roentgenograms of the spine are best taken with both of the patient's arms resting at the shoulder level on an adjustable bar. This insures a constant standard view from which future comparisons may be made. The lateral roentgenogram likewise should include the entire spine and must be of excellent quality in order to visualize the upper thoracic vertebra as well as the lumbosacral area. A hyperextension lateral view of the thoracic or lumbar spine is taken with the patient in a supine position with a Styrofoam block centered at the apex of the kyphosis. This allows one to calculate the flexibility of the deformity. Traction roentgenograms may prove helpful in the supine position should the patient have a very severe curvature (greater than 100 degrees). In these cases, side bending views may not give a true indication of flexibility of the deformity.

Leg length inequality can produce a lum-

bar curve while the patient is standing. In a similar manner, a roentgenogram taken when the child is standing with poor posture and unequal weight distribution may demonstrate a functional curve. Such curves are of no significance unless they are structural. A short leg or unequal weight bearing will not produce a structural cruve but may give the examiner a false indication of the magnitude of the structural component.

Further diagnostic roentgenograms will depend upon the etiology of the problem. Tomograms are particularly helpful in evaluating congenital deformity or the extent of a bone tumor. A myelogram is indicated in the presence of interpediculate widening in order to rule out the diagnosis of spinal dysraphism, syringomyelia, diastematomyelia, or cord tumor. In the presence of neurologic abnormality associated with scoliosis, myelography likewise is indicated. Intravenous pyelography is particularly useful in the presence of congenital spine deformity.[160, 268, 270] A high association of urologic abnormalities with congenital deformity makes this test a necessity for routine evaluation.

CURVATURE MEASUREMENTS (Fig. 6–

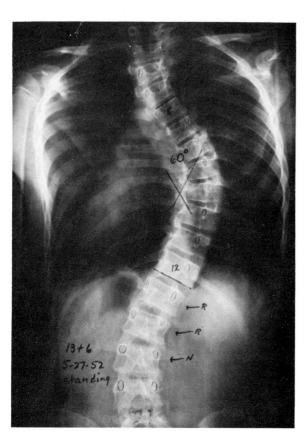

Figure 6–11. The Cobb method for measuring scoliotic curvatures. The end vertebrae are those maximally tilted into the concavity of the curvature (T5 and T12). Rotation continues into L1 and L2, and the first neutral vertebra is L3. Fusion must extend to the neutral vertebra (L3) in order to prevent progression (see text).

11).   Once the roentgenograms have been obtained and a spinal curvature has been noted, curve measurements are made according to the Cobb method. The end vertebrae are determined. These vertebrae are the last ones that are tilted into the concavity of the curvature being measured. When they are parallel, the one farthest from the apex of the curve is the end vertebra. Once the caudal and cranial end vertebrae of each curve are identified, the curvature is measured by drawing a line along the end plate of the upper vertebra and along the end plate of the lower vertebra. If these end plates are indistinct, the pedicle may be used instead. The angle formed by these two lines is measured and consists of the curve measurement. All curvatures should be measured. Vertebral rotation may be determined by the method of Nash and Moe and may be graded I, II, III, or IV depending upon the severity of rotation.[187]

SKELETAL MATURITY.   Skeletal maturity may be measured not only by the patient's physiologic appearance but also radiographically by the bone age, iliac epiphysis, and vertebral ring apophysis. The bone age is determined by comparison of the wrist and hand roentgenogram with the standards found in the Greulich and Pyle atlas.[100] The iliac epiphysis ossification originally described by Risser may be calculated. The iliac crest is divided into four quarters, and the epiphyseal excursion grade is determined — grade I for 25 per cent, grade II for 50 per cent, grade III for 75 per cent, and grade IV for complete excursion; grade V occurs when the excursion is complete and the fusion of the epiphysis to the ilium is likewise complete. The vertebral ring epiphysis may be noted on the lateral roentgenogram of the vertebra. This consists of a separate ossification area that fuses to the vertebral body once vertebral maturation is complete. This appears to coincide well with complete cessation of vertebral growth.

PULMONARY FUNCTION IN SCOLIOSIS

A deformed and rigid thoracic cage that is present in moderate to severe thoracic scoliosis results in a restrictive type of lung disease characterized by a reduction in lung volume, vital capacity, and maximum voluntary ventilation.

Hippocrates, in the last half of the fifth century, was one of the first to recognize that patients with scoliosis commonly have respiratory illness and frequently die prematurely.[124] Schneevogt, in 1854, found that patients with spinal deformities had reduced vital capacities.[54] Flagstad and Kallman, in 1928, noted that the vital capacity was most reduced when the curvature was in the thoracic spine.[54] Chapman subsequently demonstrated that lung volumes were decreased, but cardiac function remained normal until late in the course of the disease or until preterminal changes occurred in lung function.[54]

It is well established that the individual with scoliosis dies not from anatomic deformity but from cardiopulmonary failure. Nilsonne and Lundgren, in evaluating a group of patients with severe scoliosis who had been observed over a period of 50 years, found the mortality to be twice as high as in a corresponding group of controls.[190] Pulmonary or cardiac failure was the cause of death in 60 per cent of the scoliotic group. Of the surviving group, 50 per cent had disabling symptoms that prevented them from working.

Considering increased morbidity as well as mortality associated with untreated scoliosis, it is mandatory that the physician managing scoliosis problems have a workable understanding of the pathophysiology of pulmoanry disease in these patients.[9, 12, 84, 92, 185, 190] Pulmonary function evaluation can be an invaluable aid in determining the pretreatment risk of the scoliosis patient as well as in preventing post-therapy complications.[259]

Pulmonary function may be evaluated in several ways. One may classify pulmonary function studies as those that deal with static values, dynamic values, functional efficiency values, and radioactive xenon values.[205] Static values of importance are the total lung capacity, the vital capacity, and the residual volume. The total lung capacity is that amount of air that a person can voluntarily trap into his lungs. It is made up of two parts; the portion that, regardless of how hard we exhale, we cannot get out of our lungs (residual volume) and the portion that we can exhale after a maximum inspiratory effort (vital capacity) Fig. 6–12).

The vital capacity can be measured quite simply with the aid of a spirometer. In the healthy subject without spine deformity the standing height and age are considered satis-

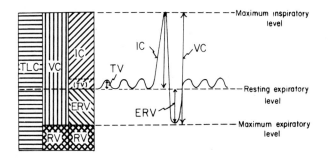

Figure 6–12. Pulmonary function. Relationship between the vital capacity (VC), residual volume (RV), tidal volume (TV), expiratory and inspiratory reserve volumes (ERV, IRV), and total lung capacity (TLC). (Adapted with permission from The Lung. Clinical Physiology and Pulmonary Function Tests, Comroe, J. H., Jr., Forster, R. E., II, DerBois, A. B., and Carlsen, E. (eds.), Chicago, Year Book Medical Publishers, p. 8.)

factory standards on which to predict normal lung volumes. However, in the patient with scoliosis the lateral curvature has decreased the patient's standing height. If the standing height is used to predict normal vital capacity under these circumstances, the result will be far less than that in the undeformed individual. Measured lung volumes in the scoliotic patient (which are normally reduced) might, therefore, appear to be normal. Traction or surgery might add to this inaccuracy, since lengthening the spine would raise the predicted vital capacity. Because the observed vital capacity is expressed as a percentage of the predicted vital capacity, surgery or traction may falsely appear to have caused pulmonary function deterioration. Therefore, it became obvious

that a reliable method must be devised to predict nondeformed height. Several methods have been described.[12, 252, 278] The most satisfactory, we feel, is that of Hepper.[21] Hepper analyzed the arm span and height in 288 normal subjects, aged 16 to 63. He found that the arm span/height ratio was 1.03:1 for men and 1.1:1 for women, with a standard deviation of ±0.02. Johnson and Westgate (Fig. 6–13) extended these studies and felt that the difference in mean ratios between sex and age groupings was not significant.[135] They arrived at a ratio of 1.03:1 (standard deviation ±0.02), which could be applied to all subjects when calculating height from arm span. Furthermore, because of the large error of estimate inherent in predicting vital capacity (±12 per

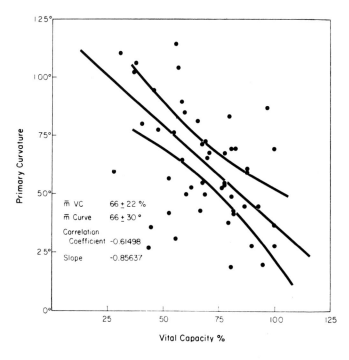

Figure 6–13. Reduction in vital capacity with increasing curvature. A ratio of 1.03 (standard deviation of ±0.02) can be applied to all subjects when calculating height from arm span. Non-deformed height must be used when calculating predicted vital capacity. Observed vital capacity is then expressed as a percentage of predicated. (From Johnson, B. E., and Westgate, H. D.: Methods of predicting vital capacity in patients with thoracic scoliosis. J. Bone Joint Surg. *52A*:1433, 1970.)

cent), they classified patients with up to 20 per cent reduction in vital capacity as normal. A vital capacity between 60 and 80 per cent was classified as a mild restriction, a value between 40 and 60 per cent, moderate restriction, and below 40 per cent, severe restriction.

Dynamic values refer to those studies relating to a patient's pulmonary function in a limited period of time. One of the most important values is the one second, timed vital capacity. The normal value is 80 per cent. With obstructive pulmonary disease, the value is decreased accordingly. Maximum inspiratory and expiratory flow rates and maximum breathing capacity also provide data on the patient's functional ability and may prove abnormal, particularly in obstructive pulmonary disease.

The functional efficiency of the lung may be tested by the volume of the dead space in relation to the total lung volume (this is normally 35 per cent) and by the alveolar-arterial oxygen gradient. There is normally about a 10 mm. gradient between alevolar oxygen pressure (Pao_2) and arterial oxygen pressure (Pao_2) in the normal adult. If the gradient (PaO_2/Pao_2) is increased, it means that blood is being shunted through the lung without being oxygenated.

Radioactive xenon[133] is an insoluble gas with a very short half-life. It may be forced into solution, then injected into the superior vena cava, and as it passes out of the blood into the alveoli, it can be measured by radioactive counters placed over the chest. The patient may also breathe xenon[133] and, by the same method, the aeration of the lung can thus be calculated. In essence, xenon[133] can furnish data on aeration/perfusion ratios of the lung, lung volumes, and ventilation and perfusion of the lobes. In the supine position there is a relatively even distribution of aeration and perfusion from the base of the lung to the apex. In the erect position there is a decrease in perfusion from the base to the apex, while with increased activity perfusion increases throughout until the apices themselves are perfused.

Effect of Scoliosis on Pulmonary Function

In the scoliotic patient, it has been well established that the total lung capacity and vital capacity are reduced.[9, 52, 70, 81, 89, 163, 251, 258] Until late in the pathologic process, the residual volumes are normal. Westgate and Mankin found that in idiopathic scoliosis the reduction in vital capacity was significantly correlated with the severity of the curvature.[164, 258, 260] Shannon and others found a reduced total lung capacity in all patients with curvatures exceeding 65 degrees.[230] Patients with curvatures exceeding 90 degrees had a vital capacity reduced by a much greater amount than the total lung capacity. Reduction in lung volumes appears to be related to several factors. Patients with poor muscle function (poliomyelitis) are known to have a greater reduction in their vital capacity than patients with similar curvatures and normal muscle function.[83] The chest deformity per se may also be a factor in compression of normal lung tissue, thereby limiting lung volume. It has been noted that only a few patients with curvatures less than 65 degrees have reduced vital capacities.[163, 266] Reduction in vital capacity has also been shown to be related to the severity of lordosis associated with scoliosis.[266] Finally, a third factor might involve the elastance of distensibility of the thoracic cage.[52] Caro has noted that strapping of the chest in normal individuals results in diminution of the maximum expiratory flow rate, maximum breathing capacity, and the vital capacity. Bergofsky has found that in adults with scoliosis the work of breathing was five times that of normal patients.[9] He felt that the compliance of the respiratory system in older patients was reduced. Ting and Lyons have since published work to support this contention.[251]

Whereas the vital capacity provides essential information on pulmonary function in the scoliotic patient, the timed vital capacity is usually of little help. The patient's vital capacity may be reduced, but since there is little obstructive component, he will exhale the reduced volume at a normal rate. Maximum breathing capacity also has been found to be reduced in scoliotic patients, the degree of reduction being directly proportional to the degree of curvature.[251, 260] Maximum expiratory flow rates are also reduced, yet evidence of obstructive pulmonary disease is lacking. Dayman and Fry and Hyatt have shown that in normal subjects, gas flow changes proportionately with the degree of inflation of the lung.[68, 85] Since the inflation capacity may be reduced in thoracic scoliosis, a decrease in flow rates may also be expected.[89]

Arterial hypoxemia is noted with more severe curvatures (greater than 65 degrees). This develops secondary to venoarterial shunting and altered regional perfusion. The shunting may be due to two causes. The lung tissue adjacent to the convex portion of the curvature is small and infantile and frequently contains atelectatic areas that are consequently poorly ventilated. On the other hand, perfusion in the scoliotic lung is also altered.[70] Bjure has noted that in 42 per cent of scoliotic patients studied, the airways started to close at lung volumes greater than the functional residual capacity, the usual resting expiratory level.[12] Those alveoli that were therefore closed would not be ventilated, and blood perfusing them would not be oxygenated. As the curvature increased above 55 to 65 degrees, Riseborough and Shannon have reported an increase in shunting as well as dead space, the greater changes occurring in the smaller, convex lung.[205] Westgate also has found the lung on the convex side to be the worse affected, while Dollery and colleagues and Littler and associates found no significant difference in perfusion and ventilation between the lung on the convex or concave side of the curvature.[70, 152, 257]

Surgical Correction: Pulmonary Considerations

Immediately following surgery, lung volumes and flow rates may be reduced by 10 to 30 per cent from pain, drugs, and metabolic alterations brought about by blood transfusions and surgery.[259] Makley and coworkers have demonstrated a striking reduction in pulmonary function, particularly in vital capacity and maximum breathing capacity, after the application of a preoperative Risser localizer cast.[163] They found a mean decrease in vital capacity of 500 cc. and a decrease in maximal breathing capacity of 10 to 20 liters. It was of interest to note that the halo apparatus did not decrease vital capacity. Patients with borderline pulmonary function, therefore, require preoperative therapy consisting of intermittent positive pressure breathing, use of blow bottles, coughing, respiratory physiotherapy, and, occasionally, postoperative ventilatory support.[237] A 40 per cent reduction in vital capacity and maximum breathing capacity greatly increases the risk of postoperative

complications and respiratory failure.[258] This group of patients may likewise have documented laboratory evidence of respiratory failure consisting of Pao_2 of less than 50 mm. Hg on 100 per cent oxygen, a $Paco_2$ greater than 65 mm. Hg, and a pH of less than 7.250. Patients demonstrating signs of respiratory failure as well as right heart failure are not necessarily unacceptable surgical candidates.

Surgical correction may in some cases improve the cardiopulmonary status.[13] Halofemoral traction is an excellent means of assessing the operability of these patients. Following halofemoral traction, improvement in pulmonary function studies may prove striking, and surgery then may be successfully undertaken (Table 6–1, Fig. 6–14). Inoperability is established when right heart failure or respiratory failure are precipitated or unrelieved by traction.

Results of Surgical Correction on Pulmonary Function

Numerous investigations have been undertaken to evaluate the effects of scoliosis correction on pulmonary function. Westgate and Moe,[260] as well as Henche and colleagues[117] have shown a decrease in vital capacity following surgical correction of the scoliosis deformity. No significant change in lung function following surgical correction has been noted by Makley,[163] Cook,[61] Meister,[168] and Vallbona.[252] On the other hand, studies by Boyer,[26] Winter,[266] and Lindh and Bjure[150] have noted improvement in vital capacity following surgical correction of the deformity (Fig. 6–15).

Case report

D.J. was first seen at Gillette Hospital in May, 1970, at the age of fifteen plus five. He had worn a Milwaukee brace for approximately two years. On initial examination he showed a right thoracic scoliosis with a marked thoracic lordosis. His original curve at the time he was first seen was 30 degrees and had increased to 40 degrees before he began the Milwaukee brace. In the brace the curve reduced to 37 degrees, but steadily increased even while wearing the brace, to the point where on his arrival at Gillette the curve measured 70 degrees. Because of the marked thoracic lordosis, pulmonary function measurements were obtained. He demonstrated

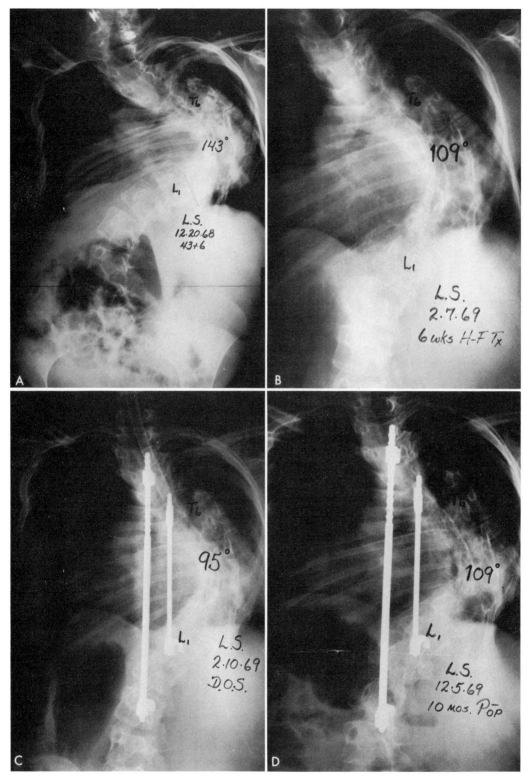

Figure 6–14. Scoliosis curvature measurements in patient (L.S.) with poliomyelitis and pulmonary failure. *A,* Initially; *B,* post traction; *C,* post surgery; and *D,* post cast removal.

Illustration continued on following page.

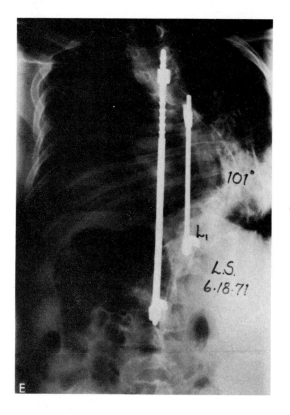

Figure 6–14 *Continued. E,* Patient at follow-up (see Table 6–1).

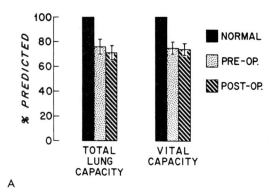

A

DEAD SPACE IN KYPHOSCOLIOSIS

Pa_{CO_2} (mmHg) 34±1 33±1

V_D / V_T 0.33 0.23

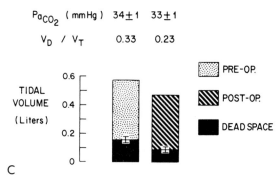

C

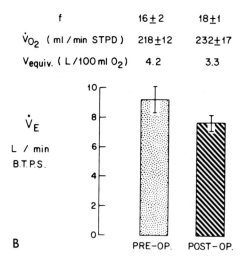

	f	16±2	18±1
$\dot{V}_{O_2}$ (ml / min STPD)		218±12	232±17
$V_{equiv.}$ (L /100 ml O_2)		4.2	3.3

B

Figure 6–15. Pulmonary function studies in thirteen kyphoscoliosis patients before and one year after surgery which consists of spine fusion and Harrington rod instrumentation. *A,* Little change is apparent in lung volumes. *B,* Minute ventilation decreased by 26 per cent. *C,* Dead space fell by 40 per cent. (From Riseborough, E. J., and Shannon, D. C.: The effects of scoliosis on pulmonary function and the changes occurring in the lungs following surgical correction of idiopathic scoliosis. *In* Post-graduate Course on the Management and Care of the Scoliosis Patient. Hugo A. Keim, M.D. [ed.], New York Orthopedic Hospital, 1970.)

TABLE 6–1. EFFECT OF HALOFEMORAL TRACTION ON PULMONARY FUNCTION
(L.S. 43 yr. Post Polio ♀)*

	Room Air 12/12/68	14 Days Traction 1/14/69	14 Days Postoperative 2/24/69	5½ Months Postoperative 7/22/69
VC (cc.)	850 (33%)	1250 (49%)	1150 (45%)	1575 (61%)
FEV$_1$ sec. (cc.)	600			
MBC (L/min.)	24 (36%)	35 (51%)	33 (50%)	38 (59%)
Pao$_2$ mm. Hg	40	58	55	60
Paco$_2$ mm. Hg	54	50	41	38
pH mm. Hg	7.44	7.49	7.43	7.41

Curve – Scoliosis 123°
      Kyphosis 90°

*This table demonstrates cardiorespiratory failure and, consequently, inoperability in a 43-year-old post-polio patient. At home she was confined to a bed or chair with oxygen continuously. Following traction, operability was indicated by improved vital capacity (VC), maximum breathing capacity (MBC), Pao$_2$, and Paco$_2$.

moderately severe restrictive lung disease with a respiratory capacity (vital capacity) of 51 per cent of normal. The preoperative testing showed a vital capacity of 2200 cc., and following surgery this had increased to 4320 cc. or 74 per cent of vital capacity, a gain of 2120 cc. The maximal breathing capacity preoperatively was 32 liters per minute and postoperatively 62 liters per minute. The Pao$_2$ preoperatively was 79 mm. Hg and postoperatively 85 mm. Hg, a slight increase. Orthopedic treatment consisted of preliminary stretching in Cotrel traction. This gave a correction to 50 degrees. He was operated on, and one week postoperative a supine roentgenogram showed a curve of 34 degrees. He was placed in a postoperative Risser cast with extremely large anterior and posterior windows for breathing, and in this cast his curve measured 35 degrees. He was then ambulated in the postoperative Risser cast. The standing roentgenogram in the cast measured 34 degrees. Two years following surgery, his AP standing roentgenogram showed the curve measuring 37 degrees, representing only a 3 degree loss since the time of surgery, comparing supine with final standing roentgenogram. Measurements of the lateral roentgenograms presurgery showed a lordosis of −40 degrees, and postoperatively this has been reduced to −19 degrees, or a gain of 21 degrees correction. It is tempting to speculate that correction of his lordosis improved his pulmonary function (Fig. 6–16).

Shannon, Riseborough, and Kazemi[229] have noted from their studies that minute ventilation following surgery was 26 per cent less to achieve the same degree of alveolar ventilation at the same metabolic rate, and this was accompanied by an increase in arterial Po$_2$. Dead space fell by approximately 40 per cent (Fig. 6–15). They felt this improvement was primarily in the alveolar dead space and not in the anatomic dead space.[205] Finally, regional distribution of ventilation and blood flow, studied by xenon bolus technique, remained normal in patients with curvatures of less than 65 degrees. This distribution failed to show improvement postoperatively in those patients with an initial curvature greater than 70 degrees (increased blood flow in upper lung and decreased flow in the dependent areas).

The fact that a regional change in aeration had not occurred (in spite of a calculated 40 per cent improvement in dead space) was interpreted as indicating that the dead space alteration had occurred throughout the lung. Gas exchange, therefore, was substantially improved, but the persistence of abnormal blood flow in those patients with the more severe curvatures suggests that permanent vascular changes had occurred prior to surgery. This also implies that surgical correction of the scoliotic spine should be undertaken prior to alterations in pulmonary vascular perfusion or before the curvature exceeds 65 degrees.

Summary

An understanding of pulmonary function in patients with thoracic scoliosis is essential for those who treat this deformity. Adequate evaluation of pulmonary function preopera-

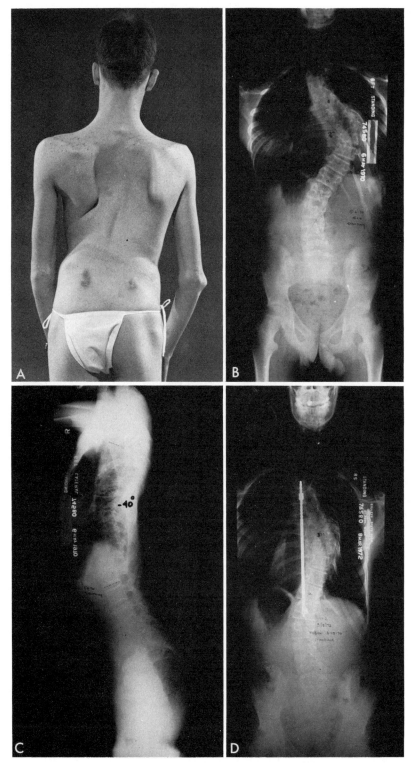

Figure 6–16. *A* and *B,* Severe thoracic lordoscoliosis in a fifteen-year-old male. *C,* Thoracic lordosis is evident, measuring minus 40 degrees. *D,* Following correction of his curvature, marked improvement in pulmonary function is evident. (See text.)

Legend continued on opposite page.

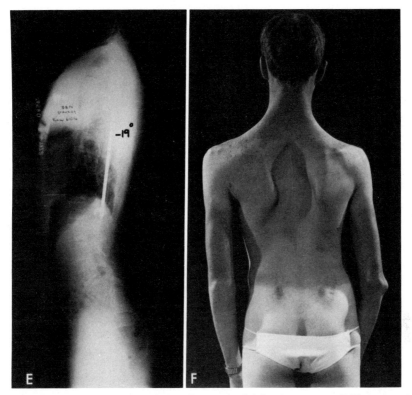

Figure 6–16 *Continued.* *E,* Thoracic lordosis is greatly improved following surgery. *F,* The cosmetic result is satisfactory.

tively may prevent life-threatening complications in the postoperative period. Respiratory failure may be gradual in onset, and careful postoperative monitoring of arterial blood gases may be needed in the borderline patient. Patients who at first seem inoperable may demonstrate satisfactory improvement in halo-femoral traction so that surgery may be safely carried out.

TREATMENT OF IDIOPATHIC SCOLIOSIS

The treatment of idiopathic scoliosis has undergone marked changes in the past decade. Through a better understanding of the natural hisory of spine deformity and a better understanding of the long-term results of operative and nonoperative treatment, indications for treatment as well as the specific types of treatment have changed. This is particularly true in the adolescent idiopathic curvatures in which school screening efforts have demonstrated that the vast majority of small curvatures (less than 20°) are not progressive and therefore do not require treatment.

Treatment of idiopathic scoliosis may be divided into three modalities: observation, bracing, and surgery. The indications for the type of treatment to a large extent depend on the age of the patient and the magnitude of the curvature and whether or not progression has been demonstrated or is expected. Treatment should be undertaken in order to prevent progression, improve deformity, prevent or lessen pain, and prevent or improve pulmonary dysfunction.

Infantile Idiopathic Scoliosis

Infantile idiopathic scoliosis is uncommon in this country but is relatively common in Great Britain. It appears sometime between birth and three years of age and may be either progressive or nonprogressive, and it ultimately resolves. The vast majority of cases (85 per cent) spontaneously disappear without treatment.[134, 153, 228]

Treatment is unnecessary for the nonprogressive type, but progressive infantile idiopathic scoliosis and all curvatures greater than 30 to 35 degrees must be vigorously treated. Those patients with a rib vertebral angle difference of 20 degrees or greater have a likelihood of showing progressive deformity, and they likewise should be treated. The treatment of choice is a Milwaukee brace, and this may be fitted to the child as young as six months of age. The brace mold may be taken in a child under ketamine anesthesia. A satisfactory alternative to bracing is a Risser cast applied under anesthesia. The pelvic section must be changed frequently in order to accommodate growth. Rather than using the conventional throat mold and occipital pads, a padded neck ring is useful. The Milwaukee brace must be worn until the curve is maximally corrected and appears stable. A few patients will respond well throughout growth and will never require arthrodesis. However, this occurs infrequently, for the vast majority of the patients will eventually require spinal fusion. The curve should never be allowed to increase beyond 60 degrees. Arthrodesis should be reserved for those curvatures of more than 40 degrees at approximately ten years of age or younger patients in whom the curve continues to progress despite all nonoperative measures. It has been our contention that it is preferable to have a slightly shortened straight spine than a very short crooked one. It should be remembered that even after arthrodesis the Milwaukee brace must often be continued to prevent lengthening of the curvature and bending of the fused area. More recently when faced with progressive curvatures in this age group unresponsive to nonoperative management, we have used internal instrumentation with a subcutaneous Harrington device without spinal fusion. The patient is kept in a brace, and every six to twelve months the subcutaneous rod is lengthened in order to maintain correction of the curvature. The fusion has thus been delayed until the preadolescent period, allowing further spinal growth while maintaining correction of the deformity.

Juvenile Idiopathic Scoliosis

By definition, scoliosis with an onset after age three but before the onset of puberty is referred to as juvenile idiopathic scoliosis. Although some juvenile curvatures of minor degrees show spontaneous improvement, the vast majority in our experience do not. Some curvatures may remain static, whereas others may progress relentlessly throughout growth. Since it is impossible to tell which curves will be progressive and which ones will not, we have been more inclined in the past several years to observe those curvatures less than 25 degrees. Any curvature greater than 30 degrees should be braced immediately, whereas those curvatures less than 20 degrees may be watched and followed with serial roentgenograms. Most curvatures in the range of 20 to 30 degrees would be braced if 5 degrees or more of progression has been demonstrated. The best treatment for curvatures less than 60 degrees is the Milwaukee brace. The results of Milwaukee brace treatment in this age group are excellent; quite often one may achieve stable correction after one to two years in a brace, permitting part-time brace wear thereafter. The brace should not be completely discontinued while the child is still growing. During the period of the adolescent growth spurt, curvatures have a tendency to increase, and return to full-time brace wear may be necessary at this time.

Juvenile idiopathic scoliosis that progresses despite brace or cast treatment will require surgical arthrodesis. Curvatures should not be allowed to progress beyond 60 degrees, and fusion should be carried out if this occurs regardless of the age of the patient. As in infantile idiopathic scoliosis, Milwaukee brace treatment may be necessary following fusion in order to prevent lengthening of the curve and bending of the fusion area. Likewise, in this age group we have used a subcutaneous rodding technique in order to allow continued spinal growth with maintenance of correction until the preadolescent or adolescent growth period. At this time, surgical arthrodesis with internal instrumentation is carried out.

Adolescent Idiopathic Scoliosis

Adolescent idiopathic scoliosis is the most common cause of spine deformity seen in the United States. By definition the onset occurs approximately at puberty. The most common curve pattern is a right thoracic curve extending from T4, T5, or T6 to T11, T12, or L1. The most common end vertebrae are T5 and T12. The second most common curvature pattern is a right thoracic and left lumbar curve, the third most common being a thoracolumbar curve, and the fourth most common being a double thoracic curve, that is, a high left thoracic associated with a right thoracic curvature.

The natural history of adolescent idiopathic scoliosis is again quite varied. The vast majority of these curvatures under 30 degrees progress little if at all. According to a recent study, it was noted that of 36 patients seen after menses began, only one curve progressed.[55] Of 59 patients seen before the onset of menses, the progression was as follows: 92 per cent of double major curves, 70 per cent of thoracolumbar curves, 58 per cent of thoracic curves, and 29 per cent of lumbar curves.

The treatment of adolescent idiopathic scoliosis is either observation, bracing, or surgery. Exercises alone do not appear to influence the curvature, nor do they influence the curvature associated with infantile idiopathic or juvenile idiopathic scoliosis. For curvatures less than 20 degrees we prefer to simply observe them since the vast majority of these curvatures do not progress. Curvatures from 20 to 30 degrees demonstrating at least 5 degrees of progression would be managed with a Milwaukee brace. Curvatures greater than 30 degrees would be braced when first seen. Curvatures greater than 40 degrees tend to respond poorly to the brace; therefore, for curvatures from 40 to 50 degrees and greater we would lean more towards surgical correction of the deformity.

Adult Idiopathic Scoliosis

Patients seen in the adult period (greater than 21 years of age) with evidence of spine deformity may require treatment. Again, the indications for treatment would be progression of the deformity, severe back pain, and progression or impairment of pulmonary function. Cosmetic deformity alone occasionally may be an indication for treatment. Treatment for the most part is surgical. If the patient presents with pain associated with the deformity, however, nonoperative treatment with analgesics and anti-inflammatory medications should be used as a first step. Facet blocks under local anesthesia with steroid injection are also helpful. Occasionally a trial of immobilization with a body cast or a plaster jacket may be beneficial in relieving the discomfort. Physical therapy may likewise be helpful. Surgical arthrodesis, however, may be necessary, especially in the presence of con-

tinued pain and progressive deformity. It must be remembered that surgery in the adult is technically more difficult than in children and adolescents; the bone is softer, complications are greater, and pseudarthrosis is more frequent.

The Milwaukee Brace in Scoliosis[15-22, 170, 172, 176, 178, 179]

The standard orthosis for the treatment of idiopathic scoliosis is the Milwaukee brace. Initially designed by Drs. W. P. Blount and A. C. Schmidt in 1945, the Milwaukee brace has become the mainstay of nonoperative treatment. The Milwaukee brace design must have a well-formed pelvic girdle, two posterior uprights, and a single anterior upright. These are joined together with a neck ring at the upper end with a throat mold anteriorly and two occipital pads posteriorly. The neck ring should be closely fitted and the throat mold should come within 1 cm. of the front of the throat with the occipital rest fitting snugly under the occiput. In the infant the throat mold and occipital rest may be substituted by a well-fitted and well-padded neck ring. One should be careful that this does not produce pressure against the mandible. Pads are added appropriately to correct the curvatures that are present. For the typical right thoracic curve, an L-shaped thoracic pad is positioned on those ribs leading to the apex of the curvature. For a lumbar curve, a lumbar pad is applied to the transverse process area above the iliac crest just over the apex of the lumbar curve. It is best to fit this pad inside the pelvic girdle. For high thoracic curves involving the T1 to T5 area, a shoulder ring may be used. Sometimes a trapezius pad associated with an axillary sling may be preferable. If the patient has an associated kyphosis with the scoliosis, a posterior margin of the pad should be placed underneath the posterior upright, thus adding correction to the kyphosis. If the patient has a scoliosis with a slightly lordotic thoracic spine, the pads should be positioned pure laterally in order to prevent aggravation of the thoracic lordosis.

When beginning brace treatment, it is sometimes necessary to apply a left axillary sling to counteract the lateral forces of the right thoracic pad. The axillary sling facilitates the patient's maintaining the neck in the center of the neck ring. With time, however, as the patient learns to compensate and to center the neck over the neck ring, the axillary sling may be discontinued.

Prefabricated pelvic sections are now being utilized in many centers and have proved helpful if the patient's shape fits the standard model. Some orthotists even still prefer to use leather for the pelvic section with metal bands over the iliac crest area. It is not important what the pelvic section is actually made from provided it is well fitted and comfortable.

Certain conditions must be avoided in Milwaukee brace fabrication: (1) A poorly fitted pelvic girdle that is too loose and too short, particularly posteriorly, is a frequent source of failure. A well-made Milwaukee brace cannot be made to stand upright. The posterior portion must be low over the buttocks in order to produce a pelvic tilt, and the anterior portion of the pelvic girdle must be above the pubis so that the pelvic tilt can be easily produced by the patient. (2) A poorly contoured upright producing a bird cage effect is a source of great irritation to the patient. It is not necessary to have much room between the upright and the chest wall either anteriorly or posteriorly, but there must be enough room to allow full chest expansion. The fit of the uprights must be attached to the pelvic girdle in such a way that the patient does not stoop forward. If this does occur, the patient may stand in a round-shouldered or forward thrusting position, aggravating the tendency for thoracic roundback deformity. (3) A high-riding occipital pad should be avoided. (4) Excessive pressure over bony prominences must be avoided as well. Particular care should be taken to avoid the thoracic pad being positioned under the posterior upright in cases where true thoracic lordosis is present. If this does occur, aggravation of lordosis will result. In cases of thoracic lordosis with scoliosis, the pad must be positioned laterally and not purely posteriorly.

INDICATIONS

In general the Milwaukee brace is effective for mild to moderate curvatures in the range of 20 to 40 degrees (Fig. 6–17). Occasionally curvatures from 40 to 60 degrees in the infantile or early period may be managed in a Milwaukee brace, but in the adolescent, curvatures grater than 40 degrees respond poorly to brace treatment. It must be appreciated that the brace is primarily a device to prevent small curves from becoming larger curves and not a device to permanently cor-

rect larger curves into small curves. In fact, earlier results showed that the brace was a corrective device.[179] However, long-term follow-up results have shown that although bracing would initially improve a curvature, at long-term follow-up the curve average was the same as that at the start of treatment.[53] Curvatures above 40 degrees occasionally may be treated in a Milwaukee brace provided the child still has growth remaining, but the results in our experience have been poor. Other factors besides curve magnitude should be taken into consideration when deciding on whether a patient is a brace candidate. One should consider growth, type of curvature, cosmesis, socioeconomic factors, patient, family, and the capabilities of the prosthetist.

The physiologic age is of great importance in determinig the success or failure of Milwaukee bracing. Chronological age is obviously of no value. A young girl at age 14 may be skeletally mature with a bone age of 16 and, therefore, would not be a brace candidate. Another girl of 14 chronological age may have a bone age of 12 and not be menstruating and, therefore, would be an ideal candidate. All factors relative to growth and development should be evaluated. These include bone growth as determined by the Greulich and Pyle atlas, menstrual history, breast development, pubic hair development, Risser sign, and evaluation of the ring apophysis in the vertebral bodies.[100] In girls the onset of breast development and pubic hair development are usually simultaneous and mark the start of a growth spurt. Menstruation usually occurs about two years later and generally occurs about 70 per cent of the way through the growth spurt. The Greulich and Pyle atlas is not helpful in determining the end of spinal growth. The Risser sign (completion of excursion of the iliac epiphysis) also correlates poorly with the end of spinal growth. The most important indicator of spinal maturity is closure of the ring apophysis of the vertebral bodies. It can be said with great certainty that there is no indication for Milwaukee brace use in anyone with closure of the ring apophysis. Curvatures may be treated when the iliac epiphysis has completed excursion but is not fused to the ilium. More likely than not, however, this treatment will not be beneficial.

The curvature itself is important. Single curves, that is, right thoracic or left lumbar curves, are more deforming than double curves. Fusion of single curves is easier, and

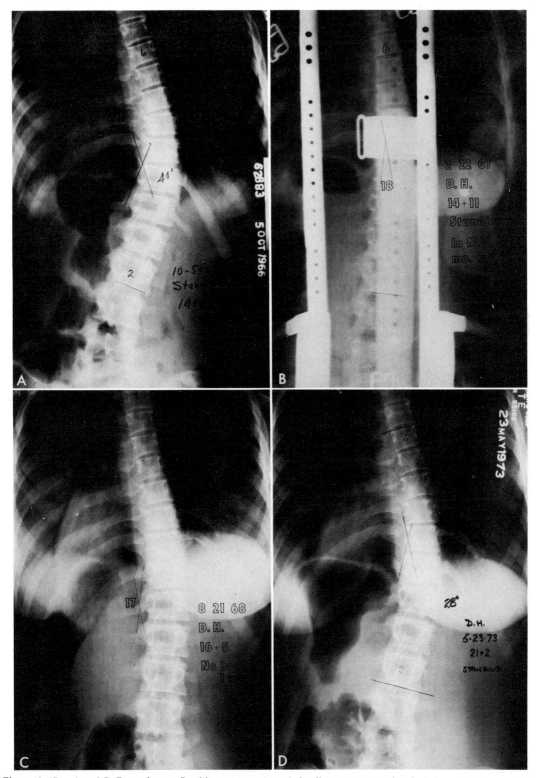

Figure 6–17. *A* and *B*, Forty degree flexible curvature in a skeletally immature individual demonstrating a satisfactory result with Milwaukee brace treatment. The brace was worn for two years. *C* and *D*, Five year follow-up demonstrates an excellent result with only a 9 degree loss of correction.

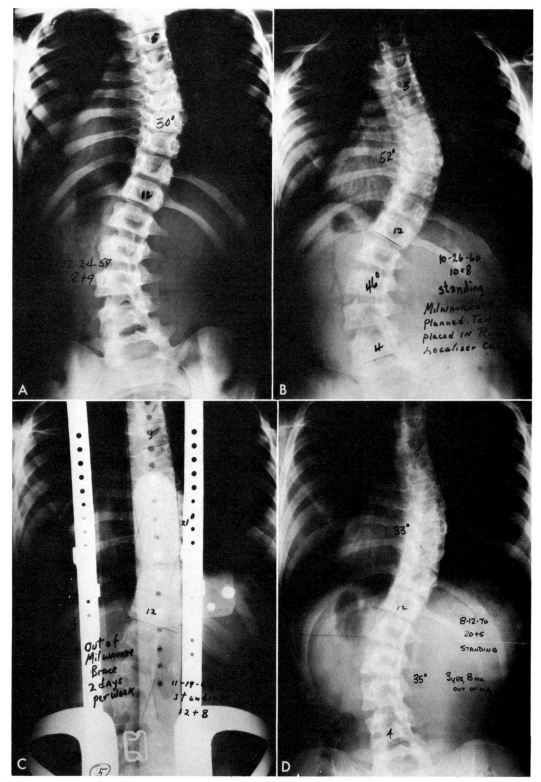

Figure 6–18. *A* and *B,* Thirty degree curvature in an eight-year-old female had, in two years, progressed to 52 degrees when first seen by the orthopedist. Since this was a mobile curvature in a skeletally immature patient, Milwaukee brace treatment was carried out. *C,* Two years later the patient had progressed to part-time brace wear. *D,* At age 20 years and 3 months, over three years out of the brace, the correction remains quite satisfactory.

Legend continued on opposite page.

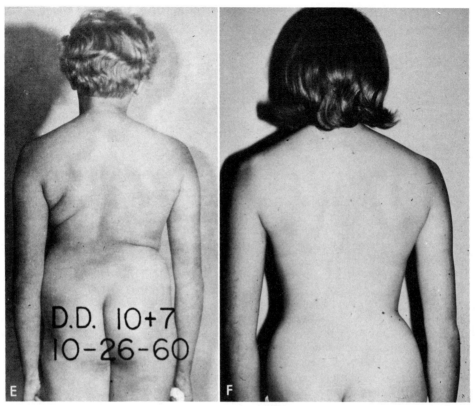

Figure 6–18 *Continued.*   The final result at age 18 years and 3 months (*F*), compared with the original photograph at age 10 years and 7 months (*E*), is excellent.

especially for thoracic curves, less disabling than fusion of a right thoracic, left lumbar curvature. Generally speaking, we will accept double structural curvatures (right thoracic and left lumbar) up to 50 degrees, whereas single curvatures of more than 45 or 50 degrees are more likely surgical candidates. The double thoracic curve pattern (left thoracic T1 to T5, right thoracic T5 to T12) described by Moe responds poorly to brace treatment. Often correction of the right thoracic curve will aggravate the high left thoracic curve. Therefore, double thoracic curves of more than 45 degrees respond best to surgical arthrodesis. Thoracic lordosis associated with scoliosis is often best managed with spinal fusion. The Milwaukee brace may aggravate the lordotic component, leading to progressive deformity with marked decrease in the anteroposterior chest width (Fig. 6–16).

Cosmesis may well be a factor in helping one decide whether surgery or bracing is advisable. If the patient has a 45 degree curvature with a 3 cm. rib hump deformity or greater, bracing will not produce as satisfacto-

ry a result as surgery. Very short curvatures do not respond as well to bracing as long curvatures, such as a 50 degree curve of five segments versus a 50 degree curve of eight segments (Fig. 6–18).

Finally, one should consider the patient's acceptance of the brace, the socioeconomic conditions of the family, and the availability of a knowledgeable and competent prosthetist. It has been our experience that children from poor areas usually will not wear a brace, and in such situations, especially if the curvature rests in a gray zone (40 to 50 degrees), surgical arthrodesis is preferable.

MANAGING THE PATIENT IN A MILWAUKEE BRACE

Once the patient is fitted for the brace, we instruct the patient to begin full-time brace wear immediately, that is, 23 hours of every 24, allowing this short time for bathing and personal hygiene. Brace wear should be started on a full-time rather than a part-time basis because the adjustment is much quicker and patient acceptance is much greater when a full-time program is begun immediately. Slow weaning only prolongs the period of adjustment and makes brace wear sometimes less acceptable to the patient. The patient is seen every three to four months for a follow-up visit and repeat roentgenograms to be certain that loss of correction is not occurring and the brace is still fitting satisfactorily. A physical therapy program associated with brace wearing has in our hands proved very helpful.[19] It is not known whether brace wear associated with exercises is indeed superior in terms of correction to that of brace wear alone. However, patient acceptance appears greater with the therapist as part of the team. Furthermore, the therapist is of great assistance in helping the patient adjust to the brace and learn brace care. The exercises carried out consist of conditioning exercises in and out of the brace with specific movements in the brace that will reduce the major curve, decrease the lumbar and thoracic lordosis, reduce the rib hump, and force out the opposite chest wall, which we usually term the thoracic valley. The physical therapist instructs the patient on how to do a pelvic tilt, flattening the lumbar spine while increasing the abdominal muscle power by sit-up exercises. The patient must also learn push-ups while maintaining the pelvic tilt and must learn how to shift away from the right thoracic pad to correct a right thoracic curve and at the same time expand the thoracic valley on the concave side. A lumbar curve can likewise be improved through a lateral shift. In addition, a patient must learn how to expand the chest fully, pressing the thoracic rib hump against the thoracic pad and exerting maximal pressure while expanding the thoracic valley. This sometimes appears effective in helping to decrease the rib hump, and it should be done many times daily.

A minimum of one year of full-time brace treatment should be carried out before any consideration should be given to weaning the patient from the brace. At the end of one year of brace treatment, if the curvature has been improved by at least 50 per cent, a careful weaning program may begin. We first allow the child approximately three to four hours a day out of the brace and demonstrate at that time by roentgenogram that no more than a 3 to 4 degree loss of correction has occurred. In a similar manner, gradual weaning is continued, never more than three hour increments each three months. Maximal weaning could progress to 12 hours out of the brace at the end

of the second year of treatment. Provided correction has not been lost, night-time wear is then continued until growth is complete. Such early weaning may not be possible, and most patients require the brace full-time for two to three years. It must be emphasized that the brace program must be adapted to each patient individually; and there is no cookbook rule that may be applied to all patients (Fig. 6–19). As a general rule, we have found that optimal results are usually obtained if a full-time brace schedule continues until (1) vertical height has been achieved as determined by serial height measurements and (2) the Risser sign shows full capping.[59] In girls these two factors coincide, but in boys another 2 cm. of vertical growth develops after full capping of the iliac epiphysis.[5]

Occasionally the patient may totally object to any sort of brace wear in spite of demonstrated progression of the curvature. The curvature may not be severe enough to require surgery (less than 40 to 50 degrees), although it may be expected that no treatment would result in a more severe deformity ultimately requiring surgery. In these rare situations, part-time brace wear — after school and at night-time only — may be an acceptable alternative to the patient and family. Although this would not be a recommendation as the optimal form of therapy, this treatment is probably better than no treatment at all. Continued progression of the curvature in these circumstances in spite of part-time brace wear would again be an indication for surgical arthrodesis.

In summary, adolescent idiopathic curvatures less than 40 degrees may respond well to brace treatment provided the patient is physiologically immature, the patient and family are cooperative, and an excellent brace has been constructed. Early juvenile and infantile curvatures up to 60 degrees may be managed successfully with a brace. Curvatures less than 20 degrees as a general rule should not be treated unless progression has been demonstrated.

LUMBAR AND THORACOLUMBAR BRACES IN IDIOPATHIC SCOLIOSIS

Recently a surge of interest has developed in using underarm braces for treating idiopathic scoliosis. This is not a new concept. However, with the advent of newer thermoplastic materials, the underarm braces appear to be better designed and more effective

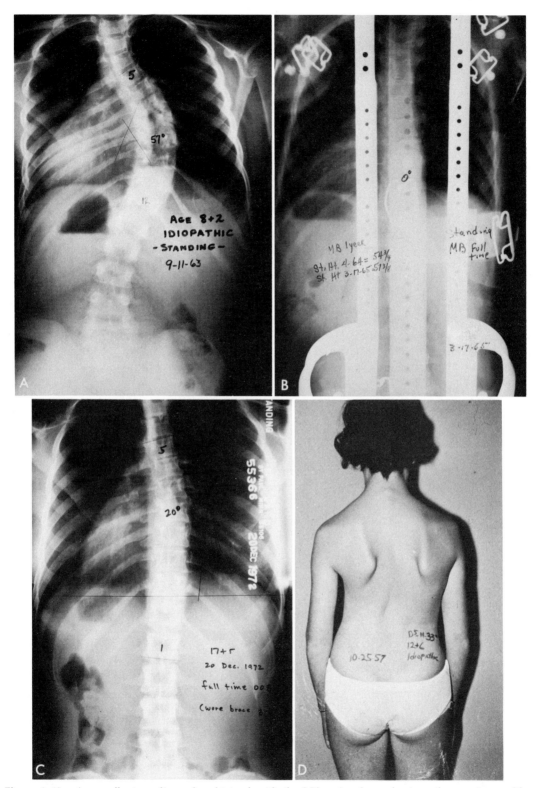

Figure 6–19. An excellent result can be obtained with the Milwaukee brace for juvenile curvatures, although prolonged brace wear may be necessary. This patient wore the brace for eight years and her correction has been satisfactorily maintained. *A,* Initial x-ray. *B,* Milwaukee brace worn full time for one year. *C,* At age 17 years and 5 months, one year out of brace, the result is satisfactory. *D,* The original photograph.

Illustration continued on following page.

in controlling idiopathic curvatures. Although several authors have reported good results from the use of these body jackets for thoracic as well as lumbar curvatures, we have found these braces to be most effective for flexible lumbar and thoracolumbar curvatures less than 40 degrees.[49, 59] However, if used in thoracic curvatures, these orthoses may decrease pulmonary function and lead to significant chest wall deformity. These braces should be worn just as a Milwaukee brace, and the treatment schedule should be precisely the same (Fig. 6–20).

CAST CORRECTION

Since the advent of plaster of Paris in the mid-nineteenth century, cast correction has been extensively used in the nonoperative and operative treatment of scoliosis. Perhaps the greatest contributions to successful cast correction were made by Risser, first with the turnbuckle cast and later with the localizer cast.[211] We have modified the localizer cast to incorporate the heavy muslin sling of Cotrel of Berck-Plage, and our present cast technique

should properly be called the Risser-Cotrel cast.[62, 63] This technique may be used in the nonoperative management of scoliosis, although if possible bracing is preferable. We rarely, if ever, use a preoperative cast for correction but find the greatest use of a cast in the postoperative period (Fig. 6–21). Occasionally the halo may need to be incorporated into the cast. A low profile halo has proved very helpful in our experience.[6]

Operative Management of Idiopathic Scoliosis

The surgical management of idiopathic scoliosis has undergone remarkable changes in the past 10 to 15 years. Indications have become more precisely defined, techniques have been greatly advanced, and as a consequence results have been vastly improved. The following section will present the indications for surgery, the use of preliminary traction, selection of fusion area, the technique of arthrodesis, and the postoperative management.

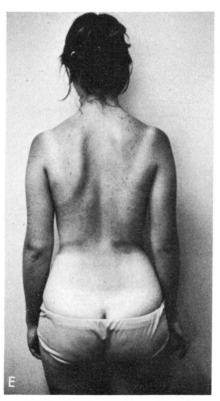

Figure 6–19 *Continued.* *E,* Patient at age 17 years and five months.

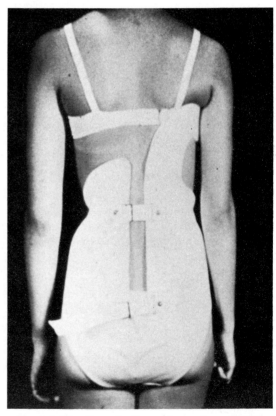

Figure 6–20. Example of an underarm brace (TLSO—thoracolumbar sacral orthosis).

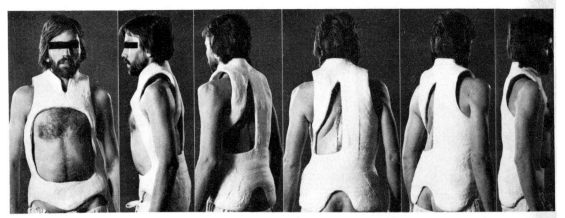

Figure 6–21. A postoperative cast.

INDICATIONS

The indications for surgery, as defined earlier, are progressive deformity uncontrolled by brace wear or too far advanced for brace treatment, back pain uncontrolled by conservative management, pulmonary dysfunction, and cosmesis. In the younger individual, pain is not a prominent symptom, and as a consequence the indication for surgery is based primarily on the magnitude of the curvature and the possibility of further difficulties in the future. It has been our contention that adolescent curvatures greater than 45 or 50 degrees are best managed by surgery. As noted in the section on natural history, patients with curvatures greater than 50 degrees at the end of growth often may show progression of their curvature during adult life. With progression of the curvature, respiratory insufficiency may develop. Thoracic curves greater than 60 degrees are usually associated with a progressive decline in pulmonary function as noted earlier. Furthermore, correction of these curvatures in the adult cannot be expected to always improve pulmonary function. It is better, therefore, to prevent pulmonary function deterioration than it is to try to correct it. Looking at all these factors together, we feel that curves of 45 to 50 degrees in the adolescent are best managed with spinal fusion and Harrington instrumentation. It should be remembered that this concept is not absolute; there are some curvatures of 50 degrees, for instance, the double right thoracic, left lumbar curve, that appear to be well balanced and unassociated with significant deformity or decrease in pulmonary function. These curves are best left alone. However, some patients with 40 degree curvatures presenting with severe thoracic lordosis and marked rib hump deformity and a slight decrease in vital capacity are best managed, we feel, with surgery. Treatment should be individualized to the patient.

TRACTION — INDICATIONS AND METHODS

Since the first description of the halo skull traction method by Perry and Nichol in 1959, its use in scoliosis treatment has been widespread.[198] Although originally designed as a means of gaining and maintaining head and neck position when attached to a body cast in the paralytic patient, it rapidly found use in the treatment of cervical fractures and deformity for rheumatoid arthritis.[87] Its advantages lie in the rigid fixation of the head and neck. Subsequently, Moe incorporated bilateral femoral traction with the halo to gain preoperative correction of spinal deformity.[268] We have found at this time that halofemoral distraction is most useful as a means of gaining further correction in two-stage procedures, such as spinal osteotomies followed by traction and second-stage spinal fusion with Harrington instrumentation, and in determining the operability of poor risk scoliotic patients with cardiopulmonary failure. Following a period of distraction, reassessment of operability may demonstrate such improvement in cardiopulmonary function that the patient may safely undergo correction and spinal fusion (Fig. 6–14). Finally, in the very severe spine deformity (greater than 100 degrees) preoperative halofemoral distraction may be of some benefit in gaining correction prior to surgery.

If it is thought that skeletal traction is indicated, one may often omit the femoral pins

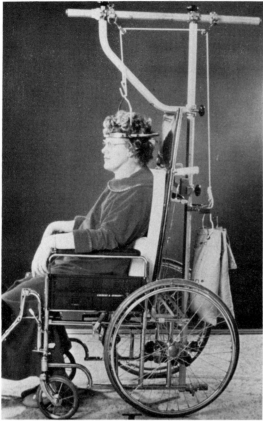

Figure 6–22. Halo wheelchair distraction described by Stagnara is a useful traction technique, especially in the adult patient. The patient may be ambulatory during the day, facilitating personal care and even showering. Thromboembolic complications appear lessened.

tion of plaster cast without restriction of chest expansion. However, the major disadvantages, such as limited access to the iliac area and a high frequency of complications, limit its usefulness. Pin track infections are common; bowel perforation and nerve palsy (brachial plexus, abducens, glossopharyngeal, and hypoglossal) have been reported. A rare but catastrophic complication is the delayed onset of paraplegia. The etiology is unknown but appears to be on a vascular basis and is associated with excessive distraction forces.[165] Degenerative arthritis of the cervical spine is a frequent complication.

FUSION AREA

Proper selection of the fusion area is one of the most important aspects of the surgical procedure. Too short a fusion will result in lengthening the curvature and bending of the graft. Too long a fusion will result in needless restriction of spinal mobility. In general, one should fuse the structural major curvature and should avoid fusing compensatory curvatures. The fusion should be limited to the end vertebra of the structural curvature provided the end vertebra demonstrates neutral rotation. Side bending roentgenograms are of great help in determining the structural curve from the nonstructural or compensatory curvature, particularly the structural right thoracic from the compensatory left lumbar curve pattern. If a right thoracic curve proves to be the structural one, then fusion should extend as stated from end vertebra to end vertebra. If the rotation continues for several segments distal to the end vertebra, all vertebrae that are rotated in the same direction as the spinal vetebra should be included in the fusion. The rule for selection of the fusion area, therefore, is to fuse from end vertebra to end vertebra but also from neutral vertebra to neutral vertebra in regards to rotation (Fig. 6–23). There are some exceptions to this rule. Rotation that extends beyond the measured curvature may correct somewhat with cast correction or side bending as noted on roentgenograms. When this is noted, the fusion area may be safely shortened by one segment, especially if the patient is skeletally mature. On the other hand, if the patient is a child and still has significant growth remaining, it is better to select the more distal vertebra rather than the more proximal one.

This rule does not apply to low lumbar curvatures, and we have found that the closer the curvature approaches the sacrum, the less

and place the patient in a halo wheelchair with the body weight providing countertraction as described by Stagnara (Fig. 6–22).[241] When the patient is not in the halo wheelchair, a Cotrel strap may provide appropriate countertraction in bed, preventing the necessity for femoral pins. As a rule we prefer distraction beginning at approximately 6 kilos, adding increments of 1 kilo per day until 10 to 12 kilos of traction are being used. Forces in children should be decreased accordingly. The halo may be used without difficulty in children two and a half to three years of age.

We no longer use the Cotrel head halter and pelvic harness as a unit. We have not found it helpful in preoperative traction or as a traction device between two-stage surgical procedures. Likewise, the use of the halo hoop apparatus as described by Dewald and Ray[69, 192, 192a] has proved rarely helpful in our experience. The technique does provide control, correction of the deformity, and elimina-

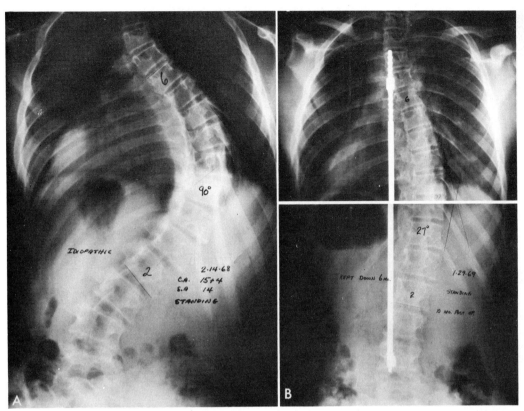

Figure 6–23. *A,* Although the end vertebra in the curvature is L2, the neutral vertebra is L4. Fusion must, therefore, extend to the neutral vertebra in order to prevent progression and assure an excellent result. *B,* The correction in this case has been superb (68 per cent of the original curve).

important is the extended rotation. We would favor stopping the fusion in most cases at L4 and rarely, if ever, fusing to L5. Fusion to the sacrum for idiopathic scoliosis is not indicated. It may occasionally be required if there is a symptomatic spondylolysis or spondylolisthesis at the lumbosacral junction associated with a lumbar curvature that requires arthrodesis. However, if there is an asymptomatic spondylolysis at L5, the fusion may stop at L4 and one may disregard the spondylolysis. It is important that the solution to each problem be individualized and each treated separately dependent on symptoms.[82]

The two most difficult problems are the double thoracic curve pattern and the right thoracic, left lumbar curve pattern. In the double thoracic curve pattern, distraction and fusion of the right thoracic T5 to T12 curve may aggravate the high left thoracic T1 to T5 curvature (Fig. 6–24). Decision on whether to fuse the upper thoracic curve may be determined on the erect preoperative roentgenogram. If the upper thoracic curve shows that the T1 vertebra is tilted toward the convexity of the right thoracic curve or that the first rib

on the left side is higher than the first rib on the right, then the upper curve should be included in the fusion area. In the case of a right thoracic, left lumbar curve, the question of whether to fuse the left lumbar curve with the right thoracic is a difficult one. If both curves are of approximately equal magnitude on standing roengenograms and are equal on the supine bending roentgenograms, then both curvatures must be fused (Fig. 6–25). If the lumbar curve demonstrates greater flexibility than the thoracic curve, that is, if it corrects to a greater degree on side bending than the thoracic curvature, the fusion of the thoracic curve alone should be sufficient.

Surgical Technique[97, 98, 111-113, 115, 116, 171, 173, 177]

The primary aim of surgical arthrodesis of the spine is to promote a physiologic state in the skeletal tissue that will ultimately result in bone formation, maturation, and union. To achieve this aim, it is necessary to meticulously clean the bony elements of all soft

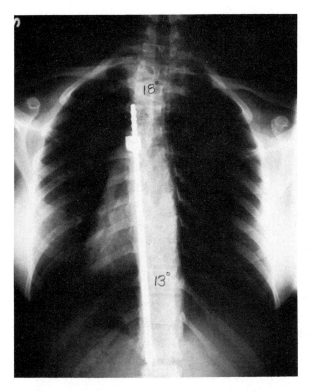

Figure 6–24. In patients with a double thoracic curvature, failure to fuse the high thoracic curvature may lead to increased neck deformity. This case should have been fused to T1, inserting the hook into the right T1-T2 facet area.

tissue debris, to completely decorticate and destroy the facet joints, and finally, to add copious amounts of autogenous iliac bone grafting throughout the fusion area.

For adequate exposure of the spine with minimal blood loss, the patient must be well positioned. We prefer positioning the patient on a four-poster or Hall frame, which allows the abdomen to hang free. This position is extremely valuable, for it decreases interabdominal pressure, minimizing blood loss, We no longer find the preoperative cast very useful (Fig. 6–26). Following skin preparation and draping, a straight incision is made through the superficial skin layer. The intradermal and subcutaneous area is injected with epinephrine 1:500,000. This reduces capillary bleeding and helps to reveal the fascial planes. The incision is carried down to the fascia, exposure being facilitated by self-retaining Adson cerebellar retractors. The small vessels are cauterized, and the incision is then amply made over the spinous processes, taking great care to remain within the cartilage gap and not to deviate into the paraspinal musculature. A Cobb elevator is then used to facilitate subperiosteal stripping of the spinous processes and the lamina (Fig. 6–27). Tendinous attachments of the short rotator muscles along the inferior lamina may be cut with a small knife.

Resection must be meticulous, and if one stays subperiosteally, bleeding should be negligible. Sponge packing is useful. We find it most helpful to begin distally and work proximally since the oblique attachments of the short rotator muscles and ligaments are most easily detached from the lamina in this direction. It is preferable to separate subperiosteally only to the facet joints on the first dissection with a Cobb elevator, to continue the dissection to the end of the transverse processes on the second dissection. Stripping far laterally on the initial step often tears muscle as well as segmental vessels just lateral to the facet joint, resulting in excessive blood loss. A metallic marker is placed in the spinous process in the lower-most vertebra, and roentgenogram is taken to confirm the correct level.

The facet joints should be cleared of all ligamentous and capsular attachments by using sharp curets. In the thoracic spine the facet is uncovered by cutting and stripping the most inferior portion of the inferior facet with a clockwise and caudally directed force. With removal of this small piece of bone, that is, the inferior facet, the exposed cartilage of the superior facet is readily visualized. One may then sweep the curet medially, removing remaining ligamentous attachments. In the ver-

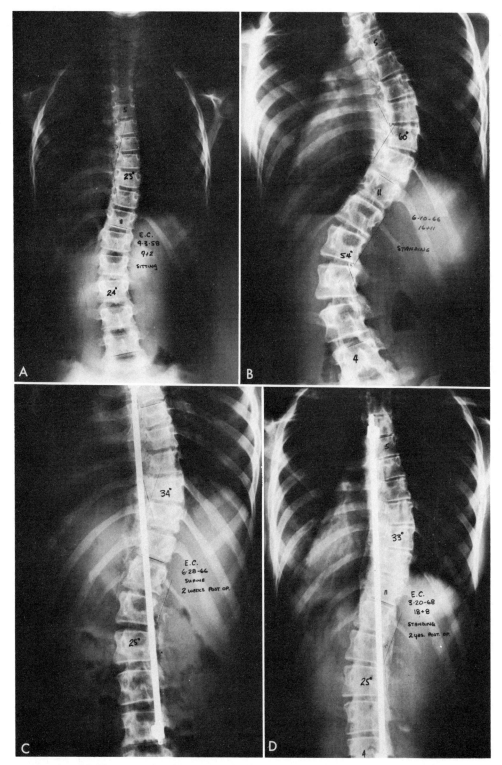

Figure 6–25.   *A* and *B,* This series demonstrates a relentless progression of spinal curvatures from the age of nine. At age 16 years and 11 months, both curvatures had become structural, and fusion of each curve was necessary. *C,* A single rod was adequate for instrumentation. We generally prefer the dollar sign rod when instrumenting two curvatures. Two overlapping rods, one for each curvature, may lead to kyphosis at the junction of the two curvatures. *D,* The final result two years postoperatively shows no loss of correction.

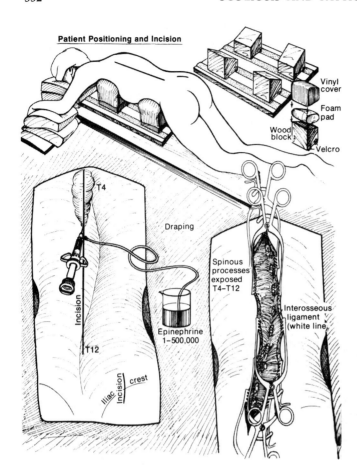

Patient Positioning and Incision

Figure 6–26. Patient positioning and incision. (From Moe, J. H., Winter, R. B., Bradford, D. S., and Lonstein, J. E.: Scoliosis and Other Spinal Deformities. Philadelphia, W. B. Saunders Co., 1978.)

Figure 6–27. Exposure. (From Moe, J. H., Winter, R. B., Bradford, D. S., and Lonstein, J. E.: Scoliosis and Other Spinal Deformities. Philadelphia, W. B. Saunders Co., 1978.)

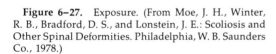

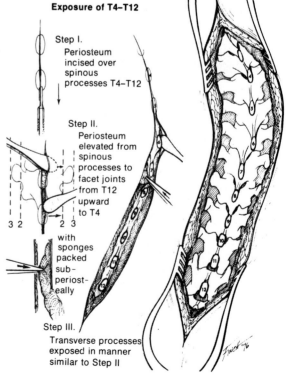

tebra selected for upper hook insertion, a small portion of the inferior articular process is removed with a small osteotome. The portion should be slanted cephalad and should encompass nearly all the width of the articular surface. A Harrington hook #1254 is then gently inserted with a hook driver, making sure that it passes between the joint surfaces. As it engages the center of the pedicle just cephalad, it is gently tapped to indent the pedicle. One must be certain that the width of the hook occupies the width of the articular surface. This hook is now removed, and a dual hook with a central flange (#1262) is similarly inserted. This hook is firmly impacted into the pedicle.

The lower hook is inserted under the lamina of the vertebra selected. The ligamentum flavum is first removed, and using a short Kerrison rongeur, the superior margin of the lamina edge is then cut, allowing insertion of a #1254 hook. Great care should be taken not to damage the pars interarticularis or to remove too much bone from the lamina.

After both hooks are inserted, the iliac crest is exposed through the same incision or an additional incision overlying the iliac crest. Cortical and cancellous bone is then obtained from the outer table of the ilium. The iliac area is then packed off for later closure.

Attention is next directed to the fusion area, and the joints on the concavity are completely destroyed by one of a variety of techniques (Figs. 6–28 and 6–29).[93-95, 181] We

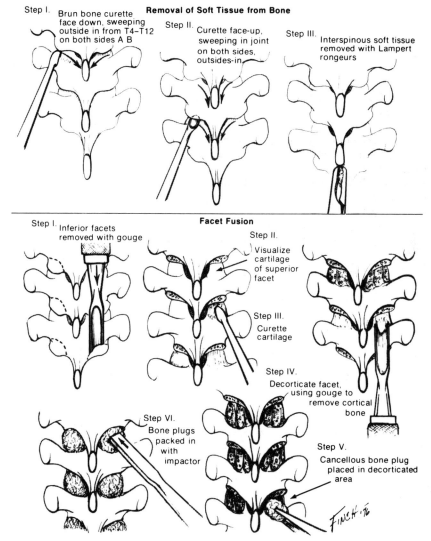

Figure 6–28. Removal of soft tissue from bone. (From Moe, J. H., Winter, R. B., Bradford, D. S., and Lonstein, J. E.: Scoliosis and Other Spinal Deformities. Philadelphia, W. B. Saunders Co., 1978.)

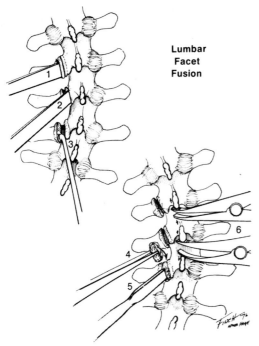

**Lumbar
Facet
Fusion**

Figure 6–29. Lumbar facet fusion. (From Moe, J. H., Winter, R. B., Bradford, D. S., and Lonstein, J. E.: Scoliosis and Other Spinal Deformities. Philadelphia, W. B. Saunders Co., 1978.)

Bony Decortication

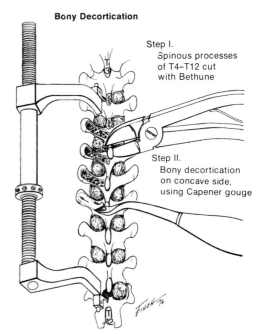

Step I.
Spinous processes
of T4–T12 cut
with Bethune

Step II.
Bony decortication
on concave side,
using Capener gouge

Figure 6–30. Bony decortication. (From Moe, J. H., Winter, R. B., Bradford, D. S., and Lonstein, J. E.: Scoliosis and Other Spinal Deformities. Philadelphia, W. B. Saunders Co., 1978.)

prefer to pack large amounts of cancellous bone into the facet joints after they are destroyed and then proceed with careful decortication of the concave side of the curvature. If the curvature is much greater than 80 degrees and fairly rigid, a Harrington outrigger may be useful to facilitate facet resection, bone grafting, and decortication (Figs. 6–30 and 6–31). As a general rule, however, it is not necessary. A distraction bar of appropriate length is placed between the two hooks, and distraction is carried out. Only experience can indicate to the operating surgeon the point at which the safe, maximal distraction has been obtained. Suffice it to say that distraction should not be carried out to the point of bony disruption or to the point of rod bending. An 18 gauge wire or a C-ring may then be placed around the Harrington rod to prevent it from telescoping within the hook. Joint fusion and decortication of the convex side of the curvature is then carried out.

If there is a significant rib hump deformity (greater than 3 to 4 cm.), a Cotrel transverse process osteotomy may be carried out. This technique is sometimes found useful in facilitating correction of the rib hump deformity. The transverse processes are osteotomized on

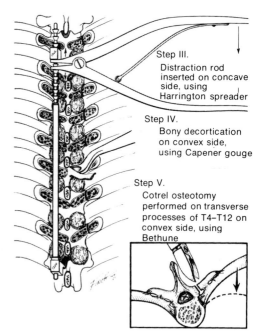

Step III.
Distraction rod
inserted on concave
side, using
Harrington spreader

Step IV.
Bony decortication
on convex side,
using Capener gouge

Step V.
Cotrel osteotomy
performed on transverse
processes of T4–T12 on
convex side, using
Bethune

Figure 6–31. Bony decortication. (From Moe, J. H., Winter, R. B., Bradford, D. S., and Lonstein, J. E.: Scoliosis and Other Spinal Deformities. Philadelphia, W. B. Saunders Co., 1978.)

the convex side of the curvature as vertically as possible at their base with a sharp rib cutter. The process is then hinged superiorly and laterally, allowing the rib to swing forward at the costovertebral articulation.

Prior to wound closure, a Stagnara wake-up test is performed by the anesthesiologist. We have found this simple test the most effective spinal cord monitor currently available. It allows instantaneous knowledge as to the competency of motor pathways to the lower extremities. Once the patient does move the feet on request, anesthesia is then deepened, and the wound is closed in a routine fashion.

ADJUNCTS TO THE HARRINGTON SYSTEM

Adjuncts to the Harrington system include compression rod assembly, segmental wiring (Luque), and a transverse loading device (DTT) first designed by Dr. Gordon Armstrong of Ottawa, Canada.

A contracting hook assembly is not routinely used at our scoliosis center for the treatment of idiopathic curvatures. It is somewhat cumbersome to put in place, but increased stability of correction is greater with the addition of the contracting assembly to the distraction device. It is detrimental when one is dealing with a true thoracic lordosis associated with scoliosis, since the compression effect may aggravate lordosis. It is routinely used in patients who have a kyphotic component to their scoliosis since this device effectively decreases kyphosis (Fig. 6–32).

The transverse loading device is indeed a helpful addition to the Harrington system. It improves fixation, stability, and the fusion rate and has in our experience improved on occasion the amount of correction that may be obtained (Fig. 6–33). However, certain problems associated with the use of the DTT must be appreciated. Overcorrection with increased deformity of the neckline is possible if one is dealing with a double thoracic curve and one fuses only the right thoracic curvature. Hook

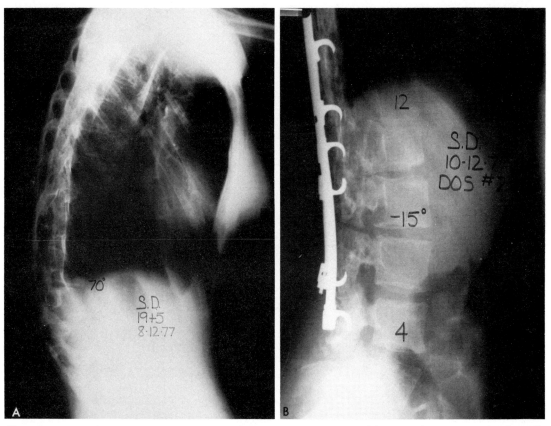

Figure 6–32. *A,* This patient had previously undergone unsuccessful spinal fusion and instrumentation for scoliosis. Her rods were removed, and progressive thoracolumbar kyphosis developed two degrees to a pseudarthrosis. *B,* Multiple osteotomies along with a Harrington compression and distraction rod effectively corrected with kyphosis. Healing was satisfactory.

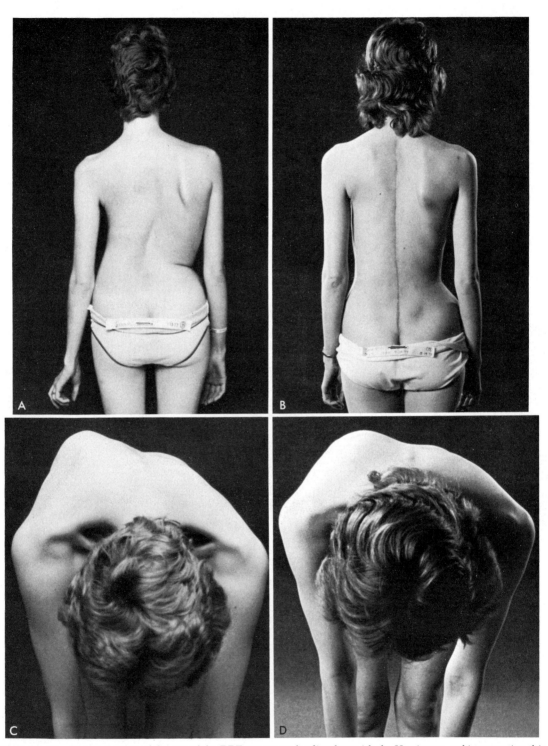

Figure 6–33.   Demonstration of the use of the DDT transverse loading bar with the Harrington rod in correcting this severe structural scoliosis. *A, C,* and *E* are pretreatment views; *B, D,* and *F* are post-treatment views. The arthrodesis appeared quite solid with no loss of correction nineteen months postoperatively.

Illustration continued on following page.

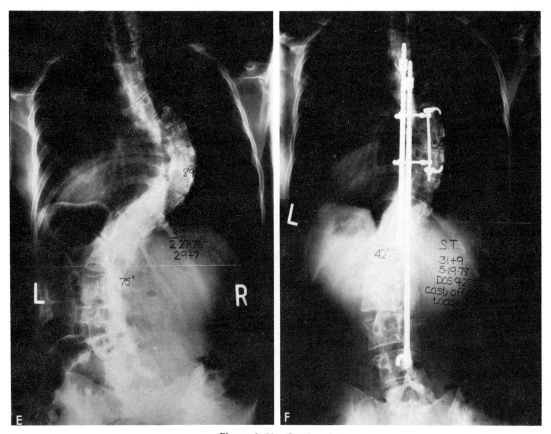

Figure 6–33 *Continued.*

dislodgment may occur more frequently because of a transverse compression effect. Also, increased vertebral rotation may be possible as well as loss of lumbar lordosis if this device is used in the lumbar spine. If one is attempting to maintain lumbar lordosis with fusions extending into the lumbar spine, one is advised to use the compression assembly on the concave side in order to maintain lordosis and facilitate curve correction along with the distracting assembly rather than just the distracting assembly alone.

ANTERIOR SPINAL FUSION[39, 109, 125, 145, 192, 262]

Anterior spinal fusion has over the past ten years come to play a very valuable role in the treatment of severe pain deformities. Prior to the pioneering work of Hodgson from 1955 to 1965, orthopaedic surgeons had a great reluctance to operate on the anterior part of the spine. Hodgson demonstrated from tuberculosis surgery that this approach was feasible and in fact was the most appropriate one.[270]

THE ANTERIOR APPROACH FOR THE MANAGEMENT OF SCOLIOSIS

The indications for the anterior approach for the management of scoliotic spinal deformities are relative and by no means absolute. It is apparent that this approach offers greater improvement in correction and greater stability (especially if combined with the posterior approach) than is possible by posterior techniques alone. The question one must ask, therefore, is whether the improvement in correction and stability provided by this procedure justifies the greater risk of complications. We have found that anterior surgery, along with instrumentation if possible, is most appropriate when applied to the following situations: paralytic deformity with pelvic obliquity, deformity with deficient posterior elements (such as myelomeningocele), cerebral palsy with spasticity, severe lumbar and thoracolumbar deformity in the adult, and congenital deformity with hemivertebra.

PARALYTIC DEFORMITY. Paralytic spinal deformity usually can be managed successfully by posterior procedures alone. For more severe deformities involving the lumbar or thoracolumbar area (generally curvatures greater than 75 degrees) with pelvic obliquity, the anterior approach with Dwyer fixation is preferable. Not only may greater correction be possible, but pelvic obliquity also is managed much better, and the pseudarthrosis rate appreciably decreases. Anterior fusion with instrumentation is rarely, if ever, sufficient as a single procedure. A second-stage posterior spinal fusion and Harrington rod instrumentation to the sacrum are essential (Fig. 6–34). Pulmonary function must be carefully assessed preoperatively, since a thoracotomy in the presence of severe pulmonary failure may be ill-advised.[25, 192]

DEFICIENT POSTERIOR ELEMENTS. In patients with myelomeningocele and postlaminectomy scoliotic deformity, the anterior approach with arthrodesis and internal fixation is most desirable. Because customary posterior techniques are associated with a high incidence of pseudarthrosis, the necessity for the anterior approach is readily apparent.[181]

CEREBRAL PALSY. Scoliosis secondary to cerebral palsy with spasticity has proved difficult to control with stabilization by customary posterior procedures alone. The combined approach, consisting of anterior spinal fusion of the lumbar or thoracolumbar curves followed by a second-stage posterior fusion from the upper thoracic spine to the sacrum, has in our experience resulted in a lower incidence of pseudarthrosis with better correction and control of pelvic obliquity.[2, 23]

IDIOPATHIC SCOLIOSIS IN THE ADULT. Lumbar and thoracolumbar curvatures in the adult may be managed successfully by the anterior approach with spinal fusion and internal fixation followed by a second-stage posterior spinal fusion with Harrington rod instrumentation. This method should be reserved primarily for the severe structural lumbar or thoracolumbar curvature greater than 75 to 80 degrees that is associated with a flexible or insignificant thoracic curvature (less than 30 degrees). Adult patients have a higher incidence of pseudarthrosis, and the anterior approach coupled with a posterior spinal fusion and Harrington rod instrumentation as a second stage can improve correction, increase stability, and insure a greater likelihood of successful arthrodesis. Whether to do this in the adolescent patient (less than 20 years of age) with a deformity less than 60 degrees remains a question in our opinion. With the anterior approach and Dwyer fixa-

tion, the degree of correction is better, and the length of fusion may be shortened. Yet, unless one is versed in these techniques, the complications may well prove greater than those of the posterior approach alone. The surgical scar and wound appearance are certainly less cosmetically desirable. Furthermore, the anterior approach does not guarantee a successful arthrodesis, and if used alone without supplemental posterior spinal fusion and instrumentation or without well-executed surgery, the pseudarthrosis rate appears to be higher.[181]

CONGENITAL HEMIVERTEBRA AND UNSEGMENTED BAR. The presence of a hemivertebra is not an indication for its removal. Most spinal deformities with a congenital hemivertebra can, in fact, be managed successfully with localized fusion rather than excision. However, in a patient with a lumbar hemivertebra and a fixed pelvic obliquity with a lateral translation of the thorax, hemivertebral excision is recommended. Severe structural deformity in the thoracic spine from a hemivertebra or a congenital segmented bar may also be difficult to manage by the posterior approach. Anterior wedge osteotomy with second-stage posterior wedge resection and spinal fusion may prove the only feasible method of management. We generally prefer to accept a greater measure of deformity in the thoracic spine and treat with early fusion by the posterior approach alone, since vertebral excision in the thoracic spine is associated in our experience with a much greater risk of paraplegia.[147, 181, 235]

ANTERIOR APPROACH FOR THE MANAGEMENT OF KYPHOSIS

The anterior approach is indicated for treating kyphosis of any etiology and for decompressing the spinal cord when the compression is anterior.

In our experience the most common cause of severe kyphosis is congenital. These kyphoses usually present with a fairly sharp angular deformity that is associated with a very high incidence of pseudarthrosis when treated by conventional posterior arthrodesis. The pseudarthrosis rate in congenital kyphosis greater than 60 degrees treated by posterior fusion alone has been reported as high as 60 to 80 per cent.[270] On theoretical grounds this might be expected since the tensile forces in a posterior fusion for kyphosis would prove too great to allow bony fusion and maturation. Only by anterior fusion would the fusion mass

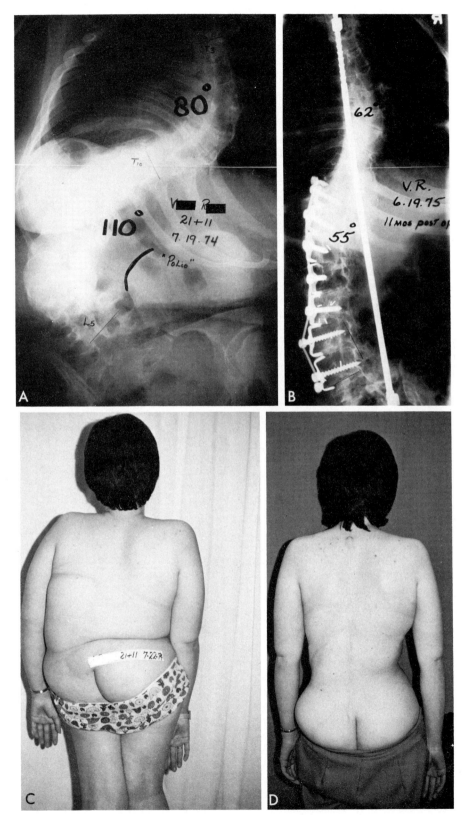

Figure 6–34. Dwyer anterior approach with a second-stage posterior spinal fusion and Harrington rod instrumentation is particularly useful in patients with paralytic spinal deformity. The correction of pelvic obliquity is superior to that obtained with other methods. *A* and *C* are preoperative views; *B* and *D* are postoperative views.

be under compression and, therefore, would be more likely to heal and solidify.

When posterior elements are lacking, such as in postlaminectomy kyphosis or kyphoscoliosis secondary to myelomeningocele, the anterior approach is necessary. Anterior surgery also may be utilized to remove tumors or infectious disease as well as to decompress the spinal cord. Exposure by the posterior approach is difficult and hazardous, if not impossible, since the cord simply cannot be retracted out of the way as can other tissues. The most common causes of cord compression relating to spine deformity are congenital kyphosis and kyphoscoliosis secondary to neurofibromatosis. These two diseases account for approximately 80 per cent of cord compression problems. In both, posterior laminectomy techniques usually fail, resulting in increased paralysis secondary to an increased kyphosis. This is caused by the laminectomy procedure per se, which (1) removes valuable stabilizing bone, resulting in increased deformity, and (2) is inadequate to furnish the exposure necessary to eliminate the anterior bony prominence. Anterior transthoracic spinal cord decompression with simultaneously performed anterior spinal fusion has proved to be the procedure of choice for these difficult problems.

Anterior fusions alone are no guarantee to a solid arthrodesis. Pseudarthroses can and have occurred in our experience. Most of the pseudarthroses were technical problems caused either by insertion of an ineffective graft too short to encompass the full length of the kyphosis or by failure to augment the graft by additional rib or fibular grafts associated with autogenous iliac bone for the more severe kyphotic deformities.[41]

The need to perform an osteotomy to correct the fixed deformity of the spine may necessitate an anterior approach. This is relevant in those cases in which posterior corrective technique would be of little use, that is, hemivertebra excision of a fixed kyphotic deformity. In the rigid congenital scoliosis secondary to hemivertebra, it is sometimes possible and necessary to remove the hemivertebra in order to correct the deformity. This may be done in two stages or as a combined procedure. In the presence of a fixed kyphotic deformity, such as Scheuermann's disease, it may be necessary to remove the intervertebral disc completely as the initial procedure, packing the intervertebral disc space with cancellous bone and then proceeding with a second-stage posterior fusion with Harrington instrumentation some two weeks later. This combined approach allows for a greater degree of correction, improved stability, and a greater likelihood of successful arthrodesis. Finally, when performing anterior surgery, it is usually in our experience necessary to augment the anterior fusion with a posterior fusion as well and preferably with posterior instrumentation. In those situations in which there is good correctability over the kyphotic curvature as demonstrated on hyperextension roentgenograms, one may do the posterior fusion first with instrumentation and then an anterior fusion as a second procedure, filling in the anterior defects with bone grafts or with an anterior strut graft. For the fixed, rigid deformity, however, it is best to do the anterior approach first and then the posterior arthrodesis.

In summary, anterior fusion is indicated in scoliosis for severe deformity associated with paralysis, deficient posterior elements, cerebral palsy, idiopathic scoliosis in the adult, and removal of congenital hemivertebra. Anterior fusion is also indicated in kyphosis of an etiology and for decompression of the spinal cord or nerve tissues when the compression lies anterior. The techniques of anterior spine surgery have been well described and, therefore, will not be discussed here. The reader is referred to standard textbooks and references on this material.[29, 30, 39, 181]

ANTERIOR INSTRUMENTATION.[29, 30, 39, 73, 74, 108, 109] The use of anterior instrumentation and fusion for correction of spinal deformity has proved an innovative and powerful method in the management of scoliosis. Although the technique is demanding, advantages are readily apparent. These procedures offer improved correction over more customary posterior approaches, greater degree of stability, more certain arthrodesis, especially if posterior elements are missing, and, in the case of the Zielke device, improved derotation of the spine.

These devices are best reserved for the thoracolumbar and lumbar curvatures and have particular use in paralytic curvatures in which the posterior bony mass is deficient or absent, such as in myelomeningocele (Fig. 6–34). Anterior instrumentation occasionally may be helpful in lumbar and thoracolumbar curves in adolescence, but as a general rule it is more helpful in idiopathic curvatures in adults, for the correction achieved is superior, the immobilization is shortened, and the incidence of pseudarthrosis is less, especially if it is combined with a posterior spinal fusion with Harrington instrumentation as a second-stage procedure.

It should be stressed that the anterior instrumentation techniques are primarily a method of correction. They will not guarantee a solid anterior arthrodesis. We have found that in most cases a Dwyer procedure must be supplemented with a posterior spinal fusion with Harrington rod instrumentation. Careful attention to the details of anterior fusion is essential. The cartilage end plates must be completely removed, and the intervertebral disc space should be carefully packed with autogenous bone in order to prevent pseudarthrosis. A Dwyer procedure is totally contraindicated in the presence of kyphosis, and, in fact, without kyphosis some degree of loss of lumbar lordosis will be produced by this device. The Zielke device appears particularly advantageous, for derotation of the spine is superior to that achieved with the Dwyer procedure, and lordosis may be better maintained with the device. Anterior instrumentation has a particular advantage in idiopathic curvatures in that the length of the fusion may be shortened somewhat, maintaining greater spine mobility. However, the surgical scar is inferior in terms of cosmesis to that of the posterior approach, and this should be taken into consideration. Finally, we have found that in the case of adults with osteoporotic bone, improved fixation with these devices may be achieved by the use of methylmethacrylate.

It is sufficient to say that these procedures may prove the most formidable and demanding that the orthopaedist has encountered. We have generally recommended a team approach with a thoracic or general surgeon assisting in the exposure. Complications with these procedures include infection, paraplegia, hemorrhage, metal failure, and pseudarthrosis. In reserving this procedure for the indications previously described, paraplegia should not be a problem provided the metal and screw placement is proper and the segmental vessels are ligated and divided on the midlateral surface of the vertebral bodies well away from the intervertebral foramen. In paralytic scoliosis associated with thoracolumbar curvatures and pelvic obliquity, fusion to the sacrum is necessary. Using anterior instrumentation devices, one is unable to fuse to the sacrum, and, therefore, posterior spinal fusion with Harrington instrumentation to the sacrum as a second-stage procedure is essential.

CONGENITAL SPINE DEFORMITY

Congenital spine deformities are those due to congenitally anomalous vertebrae. Patients with congenital deformities differ greatly from those with idiopathic scoliosis. There are greater varieties of deformity, the curvatures are more rigid, there are frequently more associated anomalies, and the hazards of treatment can be greater.

Classification

"Open" spinal defects, such as myelomeningocoele, are such a distinct problem that these will be discussed separately later in this chapter. The "closed" defects of development, that is, those with intact neural arches and no paralytic component, will be discussed here.

The main distinctions are defects of vertebral formation and defects of vertebral segmentation. Deformities are also classified according to the presence of scoliosis, kyphosis, or lordosis.

If a defect of segmentation involves all of an articulation between two vertebrae, no deformity is produced, and there is no growth at that level. These are commonly called "bloc" vertebrae. Multiple bloc vertebrae will produce torso shortening but usually no curvature.

Asymmetric defects of segmentation produce varying deformities depending on their location. An anterior defect of segmentation ("anterior unsegmented bar") will produce a kyphosis. A posterior defect of segmentation will produce a lordosis, and a lateral defect of segmentation will produce a scoliosis. The most common of these is a lateral defect with scoliosis. A kyphosis is less common, and a lordosis is quite rare.

Defects of vertebral body formation can be purely anterior, resulting in kyphosis, purely lateral, resulting in scoliosis, or anterolateral, resulting in kyphoscoliosis. The most common is a lateral defect of formation, or hemivertebra. These may be single or multiple.

Mixed defects are frequent, with the patient demonstrating both defects of segmentation and defects in formation. These can occur in different areas of the spine or in the same area (Fig. 6–35).

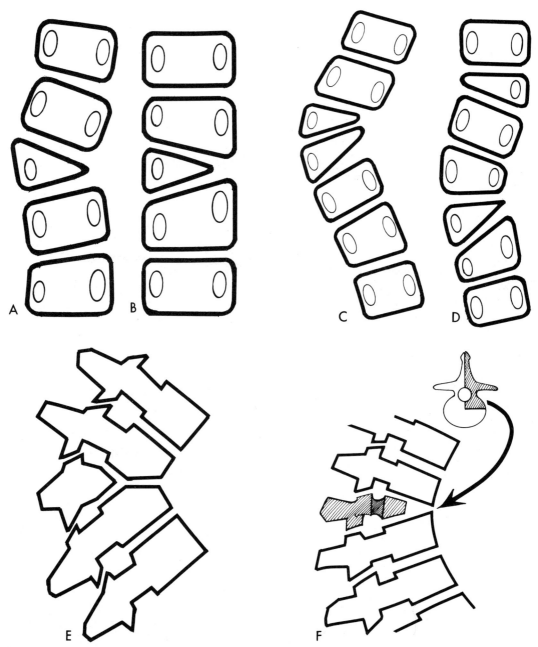

Figure 6–35. *A,* A nonincarcerated single hemivertebra. *B,* An incarcerated hemivertebra. There is no curvature. Progression is less likely than with the type seen in *A. C,* Two hemivertebrae on the same side and adjacent to one another. A significant curve is present. Progression is very likely. *D,* Double, balanced hemivertebrae. Progression of each curve may or may not take place. *E,* An anterior failure of formation with resulting kyphosis. Progression is inevitable. *F,* An anterolateral failure of vertebral formation resulting in kyphoscoliosis. Progression is inevitable.

Legend continued on opposite page.

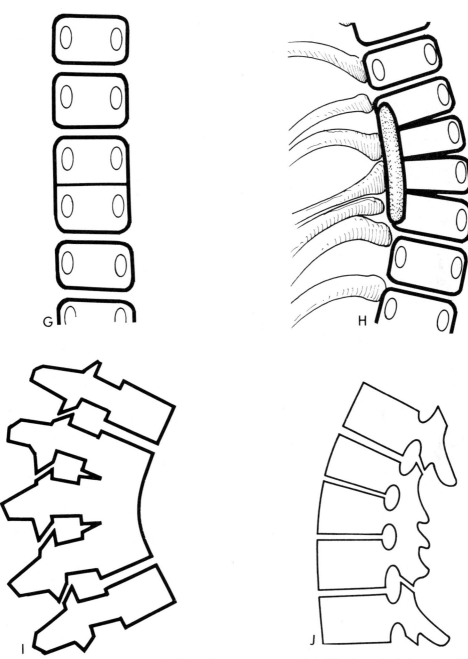

Figure 6–35 *Continued.*   *G,* Symmetrical defect of segmentation with a "bloc" vertebral formation. *H,* A lateral failure of segmentation (unilateral unsegmented bar). *I,* An anterior defect in segmentation (anterior unsegmented bar). *J,* Congenital lordosis due to a failure of posterior element segmentation.

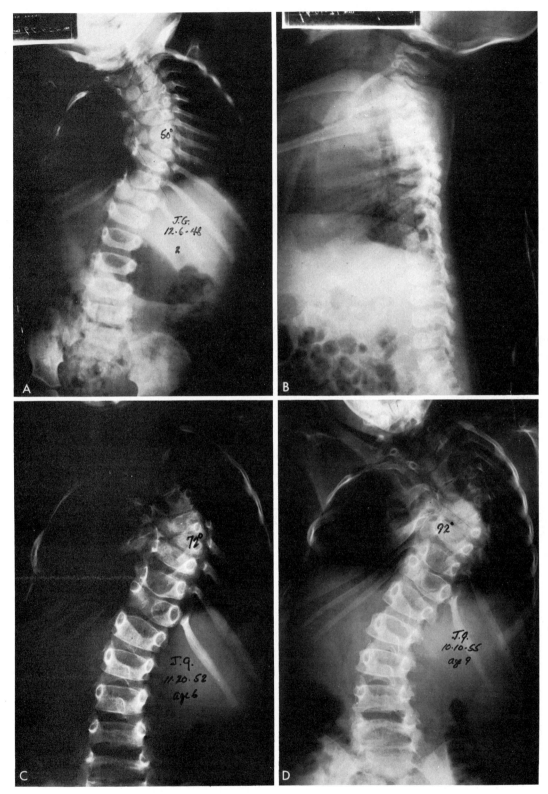

Figure 6–36 *See legend on opposite page.*

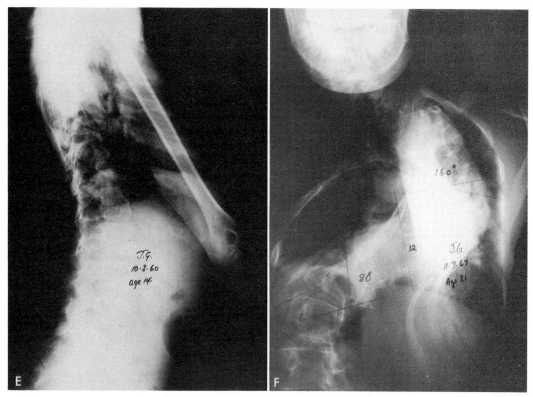

Figure 6–36. *A,* Two-year-old male with a 50 degree congenital scoliosis due to a combination of failure of formation plus failure of segmentation. Growth potential on the convex side greatly exceeds that on the concave side.

B, A lateral roentgenogram at age two demonstrates thoracic lordosis. This is a bad prognostic omen for pulmonary function.

C, AP view at age six years reveals increase of the curve to 72 degrees. No treatment had been given. The failure of segmentation is now more evident.

D, By age nine years, the curve has reached 92 degrees. The ribs on the left are "fused" together, a further indication of a failure of segmentation of the spine. The patient still received no treatment.

E, Lateral view at age 14 shows severe lordosis of the entire spine. This has progressed compared to the original roentgenogram.

F, AP standing roentgenogram at age 21. The curve is now 160 degrees, with a marked and rapid increase during the adolescent growth spurt. The patient presented to the authors at this time because of severe cor pulmonale. He died at age 22, a victim of his untreated scoliosis.

Natural History

CONGENITAL SCOLIOSIS

Much of the confusion that previously existed about the natural history of congenital scoliosis has been eliminated. Several studies have indicated that most congenital scolioses are progressive. Approximately 25 per cent do not progress and customarily do not need treatment. Twenty-five per cent progress mildly. The majority, however, do progress and require treatment of some type.

Certain types of anomalies are more predictable than others. The unilateral unsegmented bar is the most obvious of all the anomalies in terms of predictable progression. The existence of multiple hemivertebrae on the same side is also a very predictably progressive anomaly. Although at first glance it appears to be different from the unilateral unsegmented bar, it is actually similar in that there is a relatively normal growth potential on the convexity and a virtually absent growth potential on the concavity. This leads to a steadily progressive curvature. These two lesions are so predictably progressive that early fusion can be carried out on a prophylactic basis (Fig. 6–36).

Other anomalies are less predictable and usually must be permitted to "declare themselves." This means that a careful period of observation is necessary in which the patient is seen at regular intervals, usually every six months, with radiologic examination in the

upright position at each visit. The roentgenograms are very carefully measured by the
Cobb technique, and each roentgenogram is
then compared with both the last film and the
original film. If progression is taking place,
then treatment is definitely indicated. If, however, progression is not occurring, then treatment usually would not be indicated, provided
that the curve is originally mild. Progression
takes place at the rate of approximately five
degrees per year and, therefore, when seeing
the child at six month intervals, the physician
expects to see a change of only 2.5 degrees at
each visit. This is customarily attributed to
"measurement error" but usually can be appreciated when the current film is compared to
the original film and not just to the roentgenogram at the last visit.

Most of the errors seen in the treatment of
congenital scoliosis are errors of observation.
By this we mean that the physician fails to
realize that the curvature is progressing. The
second most common error is failure to act
when progression is seen to be taking place.
This is an error of judgment. Errors in the
treatment process are less common than
errors of observation or judgment.

We have a very simple rule concerning
congenital spine deformities: *Do not permit
progression*. Once a curve begins to progress,
it will not cease to do so until the end of
growth. Therefore, we must do all within our
power, either nonoperatively or operatively,
to stop that progression.

Many physicians mistakenly believe that
a curve can be allowed to progress and then,
at a certain point in time or a certain number
of degrees of curvature, treatment can be
instituted with the expectation that significant
improvement will take place. This is an unrealistic philosophy in the treatment of congenital
spine deformities. Congenital deformities tend
to be very rigid, and once a deformity develops, it is extremely difficult to recorrect the
spine to the original position. The average
surgical correction in idiopathic or paralytic
curves is 50 to 60 per cent, but in congenital
curves it is only 15 to 20 per cent.

Although some anomalies are highly predictable, the majority are not, and careful
follow-up examination with serial anteroposterior and lateral roentgenograms at six month
intervals remains the most important technique for following these patients (Fig. 6–
37).

CONGENITAL KYPHOSIS

The natural history of congenital kyphosis tends to be more malignant than that of
congenital scoliosis.[270] Kyphosis due to an
anterior defect of segmentation (anterior unsegmented bar) is most commonly seen at the
thoracolumbar junction. Mild to moderate deformities are produced, but paraplegia has not
been reported (Fig. 6–38).

Kyphosis due to failures of vertebral
body formation is more common and usually
much more severe. These are frequently associated with some scoliosis but may be purely
kyphotic.

When located in the upper thoracic spine,
particularly around the T4 to T9 level, paraplegia is frequently noted with progressive
deformity. Except for tuberculous kyphosis,
congenital kyphosis is the most common
cause of spinal cord compression due to spine
deformity. Kyphotic deformities at the thoracolumbar junction are less frequently associated with paraplegia.

Paralysis most frequently occurs at the
time of the growth spurt (ages eleven or
twelve) and is usually associated with a rapid
increase in the deformity. Early diagnosis and
appreciation of the severity of the problem is
crucial in the proper management of these
patients (Figs. 6–39 and 6–40).

CONGENITAL LORDOSIS

Congenital lordosis is fortunately a very
rare problem. When present in the thoracic
spine, the posterior defect of segmentation
coupled with anterior growth results in progressive loss of pulmonary function and often
early death (Fig. 6–41).

ASSOCIATED ANOMALIES

A patient with a congenital deformity,
regardless of type, often has other congenital
anomalies in other organ systems. In our
experience, the most common associated anomalies are found in the genitourinary tract.
These are so common that we have found
routine intravenous pyelography to be necessary on all patients with congenital spine deformity regardless of the type, severity, or
location of the curve. Many of the lesions are
unilateral kidneys or duplications, which are
not life-threatening, but a significant percentage have life-threatening obstructive urop-

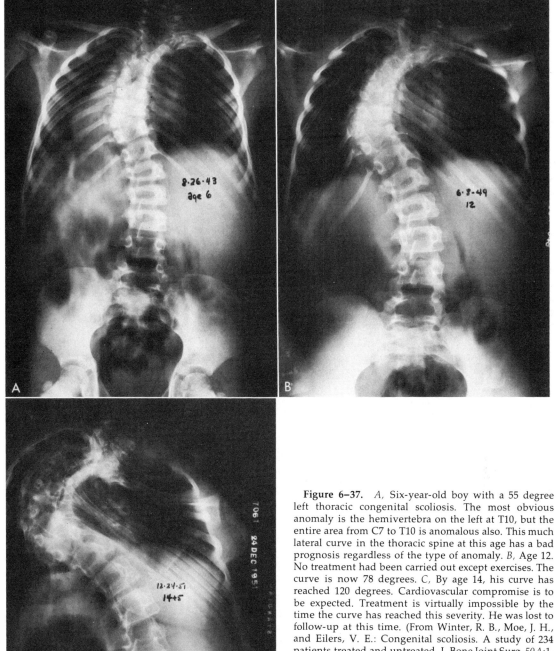

Figure 6–37. *A,* Six-year-old boy with a 55 degree left thoracic congenital scoliosis. The most obvious anomaly is the hemivertebra on the left at T10, but the entire area from C7 to T10 is anomalous also. This much lateral curve in the thoracic spine at this age has a bad prognosis regardless of the type of anomaly. *B,* Age 12. No treatment had been carried out except exercises. The curve is now 78 degrees. *C,* By age 14, his curve has reached 120 degrees. Cardiovascular compromise is to be expected. Treatment is virtually impossible by the time the curve has reached this severity. He was lost to follow-up at this time. (From Winter, R. B., Moe, J. H., and Eilers, V. E.: Congenital scoliosis. A study of 234 patients treated and untreated. J. Bone Joint Surg. *50A*:1, 1968.)

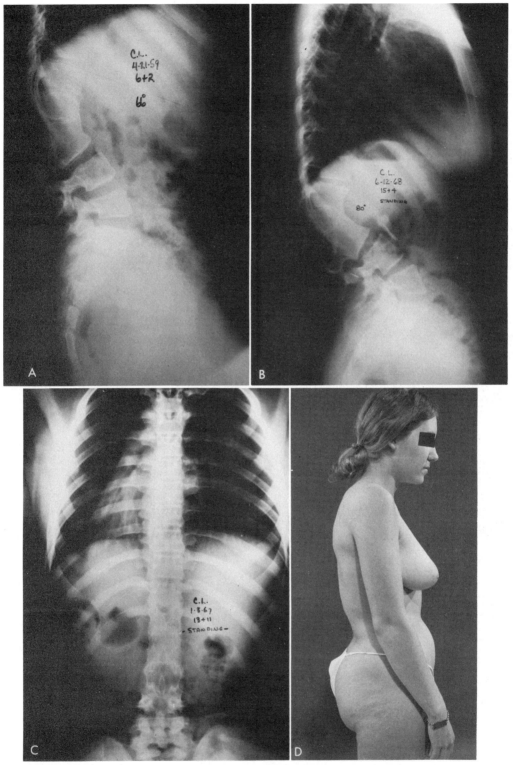

Figure 6–38. *A,* Congenital kyphosis due primarily to anterior failure of segmentation 66 degrees at age six. *B,* The same patient at age 15. The curve has slowly increased to 80 degrees. *C,* At age 13, the AP view shows no scoliosis, typical of the patient with congenital kyphosis due to anterior failure of segmentation. *D,* at age fifteen, she shows only a minimal kyphosis. No treatment was felt necessary at this time. (From Winter, R. B., Moe, J. H., and Wang, J. F.: Congenital kyphosis, its natural history and treatment as observed in a study of 130 patients. J. Bone Joint Surg. *55A:* 223–256, 1973.)

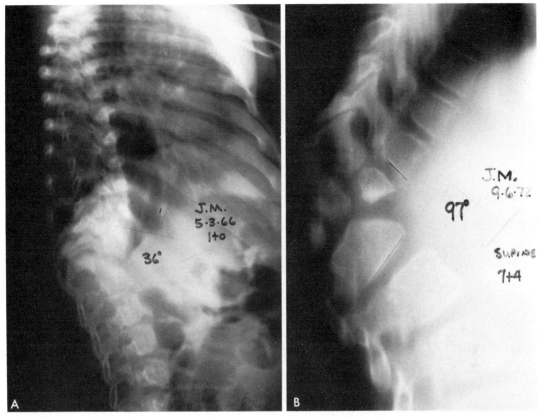

Figure 6–39. *A,* A one-year-old male with congenital kyphosis due to the absence of a vertebral body at the thoracolumbar junction. There is a 36 degree kyphosis. *B,* The same patient at age seven with a 97 degree kyphosis and early signs of cord compression.

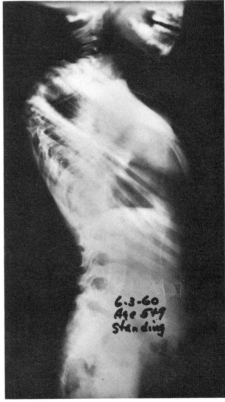

Figure 6–40. Severe congenital kyphosis in the thoracic spine. This girl developed paraparesis at age nine. (From Winter, R. B., Moe, J. H., and Wang, J. F.: Congenital kyphosis, its natural history and treatment as observed in a study of 130 patients. J. Bone Joint Surg. *55A:*223–256, 1973.)

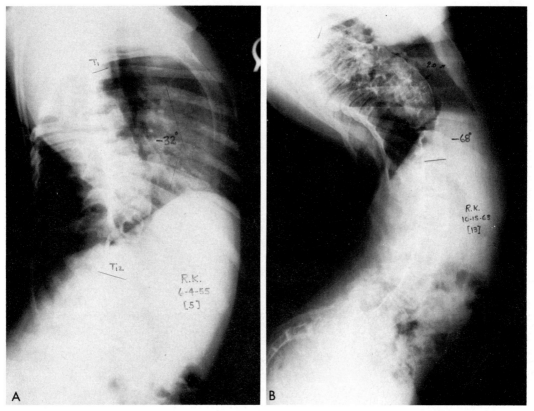

Figure 6–41. *A,* R.K., a five-year-old female with a congenital thoracic lordosis of minus 32 degrees. No treatment was given. *B,* R.K. at age 13. Her lordosis was now minus 68 degrees. Dyspnea was marked. She died at age 19 of respiratory failure.

athy, quite often silent until detected by routine intravenous pyelography.

A diligent search should be made for other anomalies. These may be previously unappreciated and may materially affect the risk of surgery for the spinal problem. Anomalies of the heart, chest wall, abdominal wall, and extremities are frequent. The Klippel-Feil syndrome and Sprengel's deformity are also very frequent.

Diastematomyelia, or some other form of spinal dysraphism, was observed in about 5 per cent of the congenital scoliosis patients at our hospitals. Very careful neurologic evaluation is mandatory in all patients with congenital spine deformities. A liberal use of myelography (especially the water-soluble type) has revealed many previously unsuspected lesions. We feel that myelography is indicated in (1) any patient with a hair patch on the back and *any* type of neurologic deficit or lower extremity abnormality; (2) any patient with bowel or bladder malfunction; (3) any patient

with widening of the spinal canal; (4) any patient with lower extremity abnormalities, such as clubfoot, flat foot, or vertical talus; (5) any patient with the suggestion of a midline bony spur in the canal; or (6) any patient with a gait abnormality or uneven feet.

Recent advances in water-soluble myelography and computerized tomography have revolutionized the radiologic evaluation of the spine, but the indications and results of these techniques have not yet been fully delineated.

The detection of a diastematomyelia, tight filum terminale, or other type of tethering lesion is of great importance in planning the surgical treatment of a patient with congenital spine deformity. Usually any tethering structure must be divided or removed by a competent neurosurgeon prior to the spinal corrective measures. The highest risk group for paralysis in the surgical treatment of spine deformity are those with congenital anomalies. Congenital kyphosis carries the highest risk of all. Distraction instrumentation must

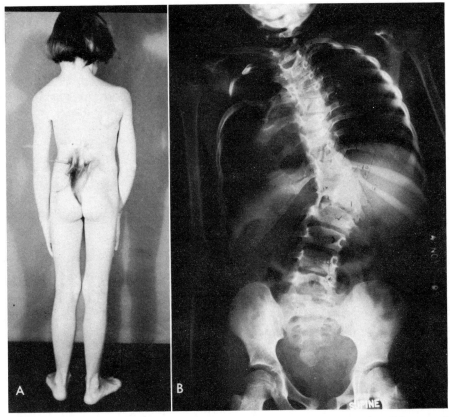

Figure 6–42. *A,* Nine-year-old girl with congenital scoliosis and a diastematomyelia. This type of hairy patch strongly indicates a congenital maldevelopment of the neural axis. *B,* AP roentgenogram demonstrating congenital scoliosis with unilateral failure of segmentation at T3, 4, 5, the same at T8, 9, 10, 11, 12, multiple hemivertebrae on the same side between T10 and L2, widening of the spinal canal at T12, L1, and a midline bony mass at L1. Myelography confirmed a diastematomyelia at L1.

be done with great care, including intraoperative neurologic evaluation (Fig. 6–42).

Treatment

There are only three methods of treatment available to the physician: (1) controlled observation, (2) orthotic treatment, and (3) surgical treatment. Controlled observation — periodic clinical and radiologic evaluation at six month intervals without actual treatment — already has been described. No patient should be discharged from observation until growth is complete.

NONOPERATIVE TREATMENT

Nonoperative treatment is orthotic treatment. Exercises, electrical stimulation, and any other form of nonoperative treatment are of no value. Braces are effective in some patients but not in others. In general, braces are effective for the treatment of flexible curves, a flexible curve being defined as one in which bending or stretching roentgenograms demonstrate definite improvement of the curve. Braces are totally ineffective for rigid curves — those curves having no improvement on bending or traction roentgenograms. Braces have been totally ineffective for congenital kyphotic or lordotic problems.

Braces are often used for treatment of the secondary curves in congenital scoliosis. Quite often, the primary congenital curve is rigid, but the secondary curve not only is flexible but also tends to become progressive in and of itself. We have seen many patients in whom the secondary curve has become more severe than the primary curve.

Braces are seldom the only form of treatment the patient will require. Usually the brace is used only to control the curve until the onset of the adolescent growth spurt when fusion is done.

The type of brace used depends upon the location of the curve. For curvatures with the apex in the lumbar or thoracolumbar area, some type of underarm brace is satisfactory. For curvatures with the apex in the midthoracic spine or higher, only the Milwaukee brace is sufficient.

The proof of the effectiveness of a brace is the control of the curve. If a progressive curve has its progression halted by the brace, then brace treatment should continue. If, however, the curve gets worse despite brace treatment, then fusion should be done.

Generally speaking, brace treatment for congenital scoliosis is less effective than for idiopathic scoliosis. It is unreasonable to think that a brace can control a curvature due to an unsegmented bar or multiple hemivertebrae on the same side of the spine. A brace cannot "create" growth where none exists (Fig. 6–43).

SURGICAL TREATMENT

CONGENITAL SCOLIOSIS. The most frequently required method of treatment of congenital scoliosis is spinal fusion. The questions confronting the treating surgeon are therefore ones primarily of timing and technique. What is the best time to fuse the congenitally scoliotic spine? Unfortunately, there is no simple answer to this question. It depends upon the types of anomalies present, the severity of the deformity, the nature of the progression, and the nature of the patient and his or her individual situation.

For example, a patient with a clearly defined unilateral unsegmented bar involving four vertebrae at age three years should undergo spinal fusion immediately. Nothing will be gained by waiting except an irreversible increase in deformity. Since the orthopaedic surgeon has not been granted the ability to create growth where none was provided by nature, then we are left with the only available alternative, which is to slow down or stop growth on the opposite side of the curve. This can be done only by fusion.

Another example would be a patient with a hemivertebra at the thoracolumbar junction that has been carefully observed for many years and noted to be nonprogressive. Under careful observation, the patient is noted to

have a curve increase at age twelve during the growth spurt. Fusion is now indicated in this patient at age twelve, whereas in the patient discussed before, fusion was indicated at age three.

The critical key to success is the performance of a good surgical arthrodesis. The entire curve must be fused, including all vertebrae rotated in the same direction as the apical vertebra. The sacrum is included in the fusion only when the sacrum acts as a segment of the primary curve. If the curve extends to a long area with continued growth, then further vertebrae should be added to the fusion.

Increase of curvature is prevented by a thick, broad fusion mass. Breadth of the fusion mass is achieved by a wide exposure from the tip of one transverse process to the tip of another transverse process. Thickness of the fusion mass is achieved by facet joint eradication, deep decortication, and the addition of abundant bone graft material. The facet joints must always be eradicated, especially in the convexity of congenital curves, since the posterior growth plates lie just beneath the facet articular cartilage. In particularly difficult curves, anterior convex fusion will aid in achieving a solid arthrodesis and can prevent the fusion from bending due to active anterior growth plates.

Autogenous iliac bone graft is the best, but if it is not available, then we use homogenous bank cancellous bone (from a rib or femoral head). Bank bone heals less rapidly but otherwise appears to be quite satisfactory. Parental bone is no better than bank bone.

Correction of the curve is best achieved by cast correction utilizing the Risser-Cotrel cast. This can be done prior to surgery, and the surgeon can operate through a window in the cast, or the cast can be applied at the time of surgery (if an anesthetic is necessary owing to the age of the child) or a week later with the patient awake.

Excellent results (Figs. 6–44 and 6–45) can also be obtained by using a Milwaukee brace as the correcting device. The authors prefer this technique for cervicothoracic congenital scoliosis. For curves in the cervical spine, a halo-cast is preferable (age three or older). For lumbar curves, an underarm cast is sufficient.

For more severe curves, correction is best obtained by skeletal traction utilizing a halo-wheelchair or halofemoral traction. Halopelvic traction is not recommended for con-

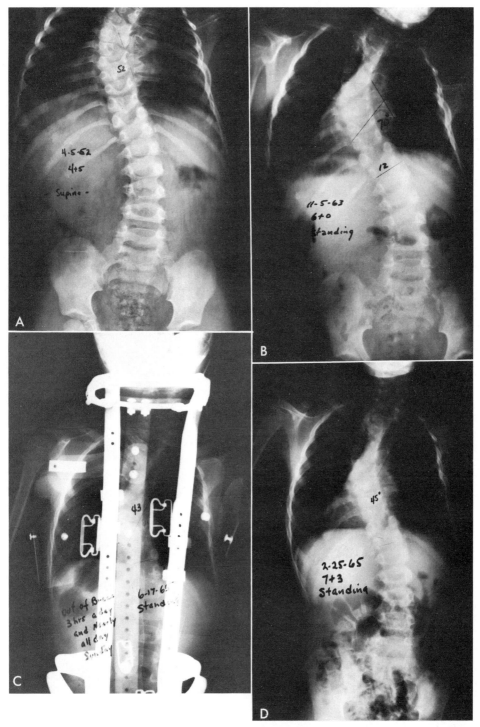

Figure 6–43. *A,* Four-year-old boy with a 52 degree congenital thoracic scoliosis (mixed unilateral failure of formation and segmentation). No treatment was given. *B,* Age six years. The curve now measures 70 degrees. A Milwaukee brace was prescribed. *C,* Age eight years. The curve now measures 43 degrees in the brace, an adequate correction. *D,* Age seven years. The curve measures 45 degrees standing out of the brace. This type of curve can be expected to increase during the adolescent growth spurt despite Milwaukee brace use, so he was fused prior to the growth spurt (at age 10).

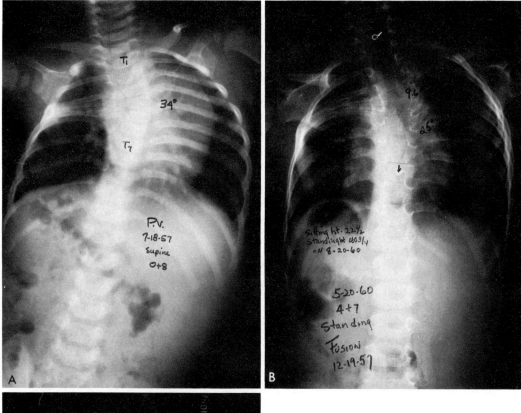

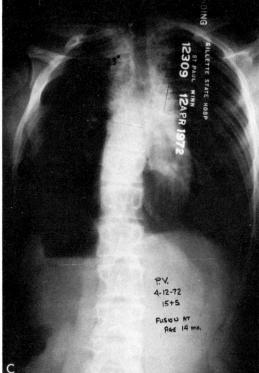

Figure 6–44.   *A,* Eight-and-one-half-month-old boy with a classic unilateral unsegmented bar (T3-T6). Progression is inevitable. Early fusion is mandatory. *B,* Age four years, seven months. Fusion from C7-T9 had been performed at age 14 months. The curve has been corrected from 34 degrees to 25 degrees. *C,* At age 15, 14 years post fusion, the curve measures 23 degrees.

Legend continued on opposite page.

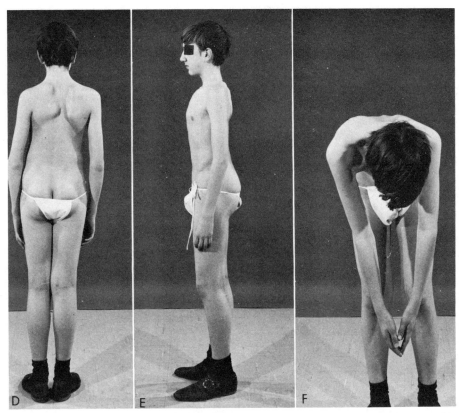

Figure 6–44 *Continued* *D,* Posterior photograph at age 13. Trunk shortening is present, but acceptable, and much preferable to a severe scoliosis. *E,* Lateral photograph at age 13. Note the absence of lordosis. *F,* Forward-bending photograph at age 13. Note the absence of any rib-hump deformity.

genital curves owing to the high risk of paraplegia or curve traction injury. The advantage of preliminary skeletal traction is the slow and gradual correction of the curve with the patient awake and able to indicate any neurologic problem. Traction for longer than two or three weeks has not proved beneficial in our experience. Harrington instruments can then be inserted as stabilizers to maintain the correction obtained by the awake traction. As stated previously, the result of Harrington distraction rods is dangerous in congenital scoliosis because of the high frequency of tethered cords and should be avoided if possible (Fig. 6–46 and 6–47).

One of the major problems confronting the surgeon today is whether or not to remove a hemivertebra. *The presence of a hemivertebra is not an indication for its removal.*

Most hemivertebra problems can be managed by localized fusion of the curvature rather than by excision. It is only those patients with severe deformity not improvable by any other means in whom hemivertebra excision should be considered. The primary indications are fixed pelvic obliquity and fixed lateral translation of the thorax. It is most safely performed in the lower lumbar spine, where one is dealing with the cauda equina and not the cord.

If hemivertebra excision is to be performed, the two-stage technique of Leatherman is recommended.[146, 147] In this, the anterior portion is removed at one operation, and the posterior portion is removed and the curve arthrodesis is done one to two weeks later. If possible, a small Harrington compression rod should be used to close the wedge posteriorly. Cast immobilization must continue until the fusion is absolutely solid, usually nine to twelve months after surgery. Hemivertebra excision should never be performed without at the same time doing a fusion of adequate length.

CONGENITAL KYPHOSIS. Kyphotic deformities cannot be managed by braces, and

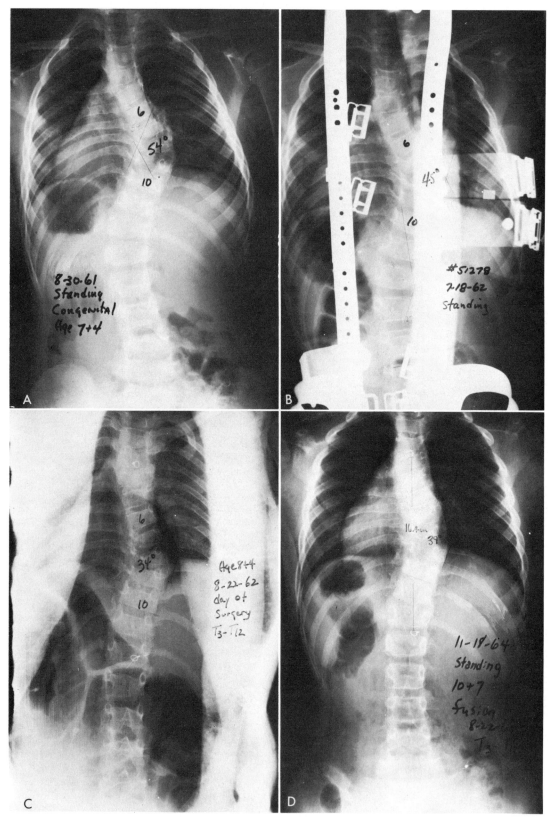

Figure 6–45. *See legend on opposite page.*

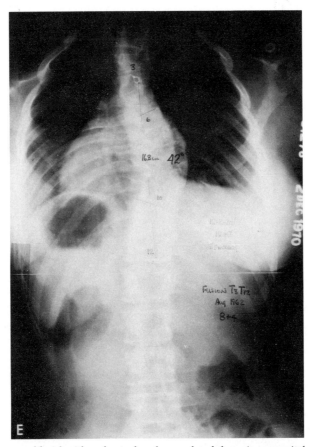

Figure 6–45. *A,* Seven-year-old girl with a short, sharply angulated thoracic congenital scoliosis. Such short, sharp curves tend to do poorly in a Milwaukee brace; cast correction and fusion is the procedure of choice and should be done at this age. A Milwaukee brace was attempted on this girl to see what result could be obtained. *B,* After one year in a well-fitted Milwaukee brace, the correction was inadequate, and fusion was scheduled. *C,* AP spine roentgenogram showing the correction obtained in a Risser localizer cast. *D,* Age 10 years and seven months. AP standing roentgenogram two years and three months following fusion. The curve is 39 degrees. The length of the fusion mass is 16.4 cm. on a standardized roentgenogram. *E,* Age 16 years and eight months, eight years following fusion. The curve measures 42 degrees, a slight loss due to "bending" of the fusion. The fusion mass measures 16.8 cm., an increase in length of only 4 mm. since age 10. Fusions do not grow. (From Winter, R. B., Moe, J. H., and Eilers, V. E.: Congenital scoliosis. A study of 234 patients treated and untreated. J. Bone Joint Surg. *50A*:26, 1968.)

early posterior fusion is the procedure of choice. Our best results have been those patients who underwent posterior fusion before the age of three years. Pseudarthrosis is so common that we frequently explore the fusion and add more bone six months after the initial operation (Fig. 6–48).

Those patients over age three and with angular kyphosis greater than 50 degrees usually cannot be stabilized by posterior fusion alone. Both anterior and posterior fusion are necessary. Anteriorly, the discs and anterior longitudinal ligament should be removed, and strut grafts must be inserted in the area of the angular kyphosis. The most com-

mon error is the failure to use enough bone graft material (Fig. 6–49).

In contrast to its use in patients with congenital scoliosis, halofemoral traction has proved quite dangerous in the treatment of congenital kyphosis. The traction pulls as much on the cord as it does on the bone and tends to pull the cord against the apex of the kyphosis, producing paralysis. Therefore, we have found it preferable to directly attach the kyphotic area. Internal correction of the kyphos by disc excision, ligament excision, and the use of a bone spreader has proved far safer than skeletal traction.

Patients presenting with paraplegia or

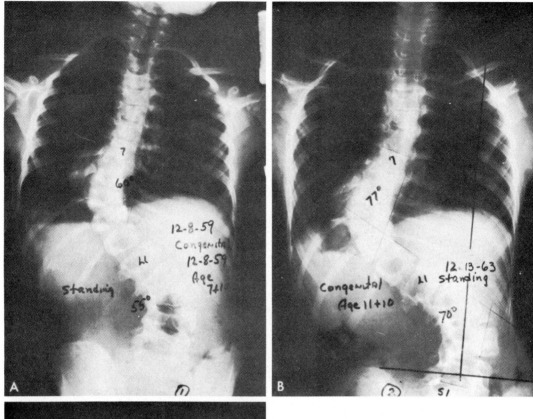

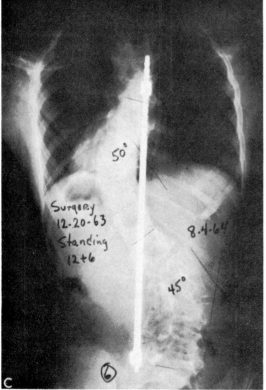

Figure 6–46. *A,* Seven-year-old girl with a left thoracic, right lumbar congenital scoliosis with decompensation to the left. Active treatment should have been carried out at this time, either operatively or nonoperatively, but unfortunately no treatment was given. *B,* Age 11 years, 10 months, at the time she was presented to the authors. This type of progression should not be permitted. Surgical correction and fusion are mandatory now. *C,* AP roentgenogram at time of cast removal following surgery. She had preoperative correction in a Risser cast, and was operated on through a window in the cast. The rod was inserted to maintain correction, not to obtain additional correction. Fusion to the sacrum was needed because of the fixed decompensation.

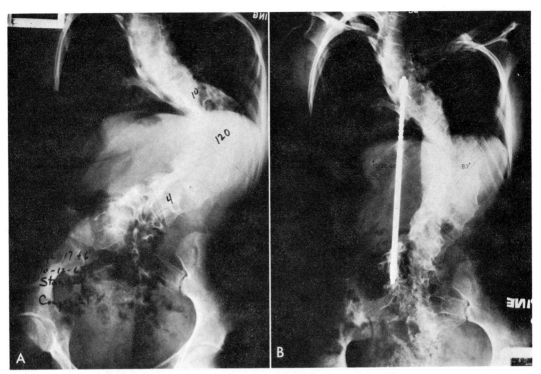

Figure 6–47. *A,* Seventeen-year-old girl with severe 120 degree scoliosis. It is a disgrace to ever permit a curve to become this severe. Halofemoral tract is the ideal way to correct such a curve. *B,* Two years after correction and fusion, and 18 months after a pseudarthrosis repair. She was corrected from 120 degrees to 80 degrees in the halofemoral traction. The Harrington rod was inserted only to maintain this correction, not to obtain more. (From Winter, R. B., Moe, J. H., and Eilers, V. E.: Congenital scoliosis. A study of 234 patients treated and untreated. J. Bone Joint Surg. *50A*:32, 35, 1968.)

paraparesis due to congenital kyphosis are difficult to manage. *Laminectomy is the worst thing that can be done, since it removes the only stabilizing structures present and does not decompress the cord.* The treatment of choice is anterior removal of the offending bone prominence that projects into the spinal cord. This can be done either through the Capener lateral rachiotomy approach or, preferably, through an anterior transthoracic exposure, which allows not only anterior decompression but anterior arthrodesis as well. Posterior fusion should also be done two to four weeks later. The stabilization by anterior and posterior fusion is as important as the decompression. Patients with early and mild evidence of cord compression can be managed by anterior and posterior fusion without direct cord decompression.

The most important method of treatment of paraplegia is to prevent it by early adequate fusion, never permitting the spine to develop an amount of kyphosis that will embarrass the spinal cord. Therefore, it is an orthopaedic responsibility to fuse and stabilize these serious kyphotic deformities (Fig. 6–50).

CONGENITAL LORDOSIS. Congenital lordosis is produced by anterior growth in the presence of a posterior defect in segmentation. The best treatment is early recognition and early anterior arthrodesis of the involved area. Nonoperative treatment is of no value.

Text continued on page 384

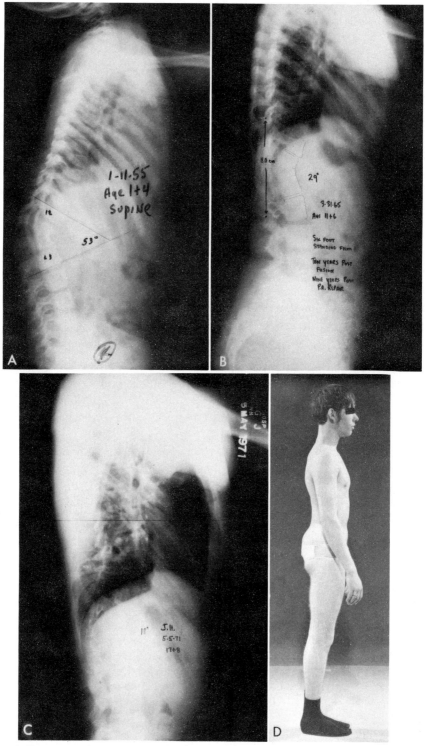

Figure 6–48. *A,* Sixteen-month-old boy with congenital kyphosis. Posterior fusion was done two months later. *B,* At age 11 years and 6 months, 10 years after fusion, and nine and one half years after pseudarthrosis repair, the kyphosis is 29 degrees. *C,* At age 17 years and 8 months, 16 years after fusion the kyphosis measures 18 degrees. *D,* Lateral photograph at age 17. Note the normal spine contours. There is no significant loss of trunk height. The fusion was from T8 to L2. (From Winter, R. B., Moe, J. H., and Wang, J. F.: Congenital kyphosis, its natural history and treatment as observed in a study of 130 patients. J. Bone Joint Surg. *55A*:253, 1973.)

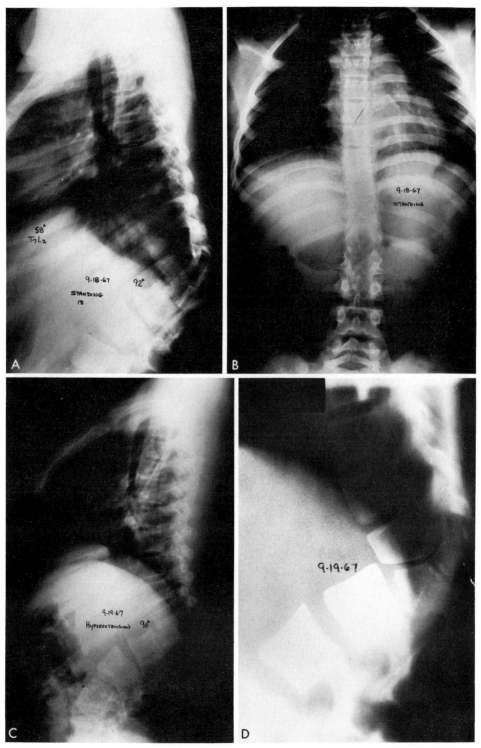

Figure 6–49. *A,* Thirteen-year-old girl with rapidly progressive congenital kyphosis. There were no neurologic symptoms yet. *B,* AP roentgenogram to show absence of scoliosis. *C,* Supine hyperextension roentgenogram shows minimal correctability. *D,* Lateral laminogram demonstrating total absence of body of T10, 60 per cent absence of body of T11, and contact of the anterior corners of bodies of T9 and T12. The small triangle of bone posteriorly at the apex is T10, of which there are only the pedicles and posterior elements.

Illustration continued on following page.

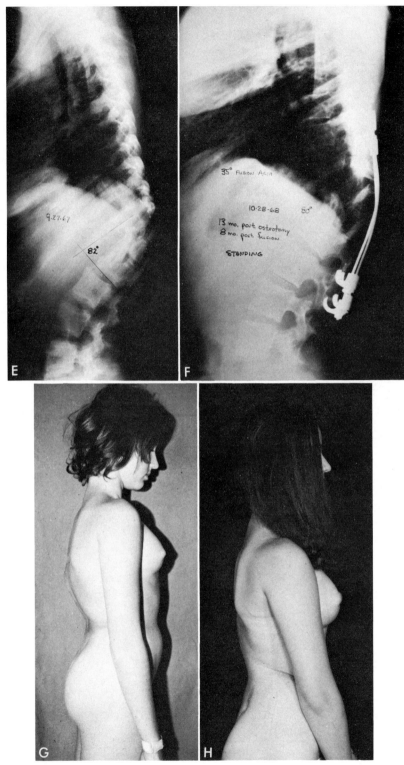

Figure 6–49 *Continued.* *E,* Following anterior discectomy and insertion of strut graft plus cancellous bone. *F,* Thirteen months following anterior fusion and eight months following posterior fusion. The delay between operations was due to a pressure sore from a cast. The two procedures are customarily done two weeks apart. *G,* Preoperative photograph. *H.* Photograph two years postoperative. (From Winter, R. B., Moe, J. H., and Wang, J. F.: Congenital kyphosis, its natural history and treatment as observed in a study of 130 patients. J. Bone Joint Surg.: *55A*:242, 1973.)

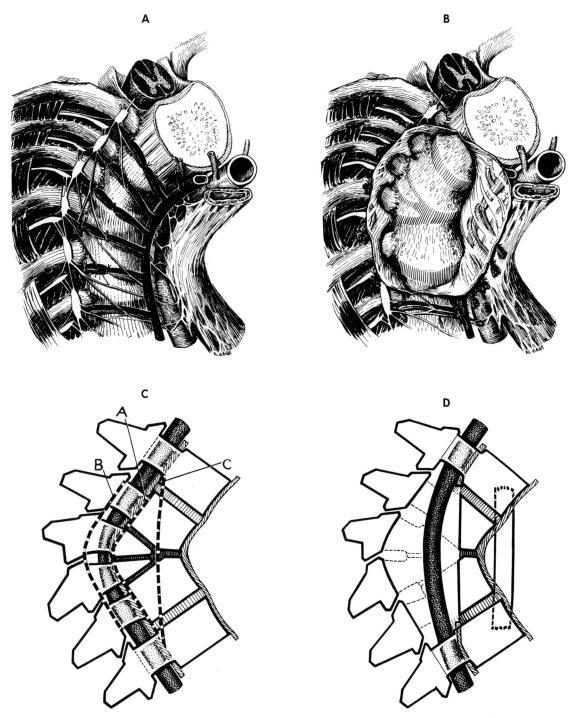

Figure 6–50. *A,* Anterior transthoracic approach to a congenital kyphosis. The segmental vessels are ligated opposite the midlateral aspect of the vertebral bodies. *B,* A flap of tissue composed of periosteum of the vertebral bodies and anulus fibrosus is elevated, protecting the great vessels. The lateral aspect of the vertebral bodies is exposed from the foramina to past the anterior longitudinal ligament, which is divided. *C,* A triangle of bone (here marked by "A" and "C") is removed, leaving only the cortex on the far side. If there is a significant scoliosis also, then the pedicles are also removed (line "B") from the *concave* side. *D,* The cord moves forward to a new position, free of the compressing bone. Anterior strut grafts plus cancellous bone are added to create a strong anterior fusion mass anterior to the anterior longitudinal ligament (which has been resected). A posterior fusion is done one month later (From Winter, R. B., Moe, J. H., and Wang, J. F.: Congenital kyphosis, its natural history and treatment as observed in a study of 130 patients. J. Bone Joint Surg. *55A*:250, 254, 1973.)

SCOLIOSIS AND KYPHOSIS: OTHER CAUSES

Neuromuscular Scoliosis

Neuromuscular scoliosis can be divided into the neuropathic and myopathic types, the neuropathic being far more common. The neuropathic types include those diseases of the upper and lower motor neurons. In the upper motor neuron lesions, one usually encounters spastic paraparesis or paraplegia, for example, with cerebral palsy or the child with traumatic paraplegia. Lower motor neuron diseases are associated with flaccid paralysis, poliomyelitis, and spinal muscle atrophy. The myopathic disorders include those abnormalities within the muscle itself.

Accurate diagnosis and general patient evaluation are most important in determining the proper approach to the spinal deformity. Is the neuromuscular condition static or progressive? Is apparent progression truly evident, or is the problem one of "pseudoprogression" due to increased body weight without concomitant increase in useful muscle mass? Has the proper diagnosis been made? Is the child's tight heel cord due to cerebral palsy, or is it really due to a spinal cord tumor?

Cerebral palsy is associated with spine deformity in 10 to 50 per cent of patients, the frequency rising in proportion to the severity of involvement. Spastic hemiparesis is almost never associated with scoliosis. Early curvatures in ambulatory individuals can be successfully treated in braces. Flexible, collapsing curvatures can be well-treated in sitting support orthoses, designed to passively support the child in an upright position until spinal "tone" is achieved. Highly structural curves will not respond to bracing and require surgical stabilization.

For purely thoracic curves (a relative rarity in cerebral palsy), standard techniques of posterior fusion with Harrington instrumentation are adequate. For severe thoracolumbar and lumbar curves, the best results are obtained by combined anterior instrumentation and fusion followed by a long posterior fusion with instrumentation to the sacrum (Fig. 6–34).

The commonest lower motor neuron diseases with scoliosis are poliomyelitis, myelomeningocoele, and spinal muscle atrophy. Myelomeningocoele deformities will be discussed later in this chapter. Poliomyelitis has virtually been eliminated from much of the world but is still a very significant problem in less developed countries. Because of its continued frequency and because of its many well-recognized sequelae, some pertinent points are worth reviewing.

One of the characteristics of poliomyelitis (and spinal muscle atrophy) is the production of muscular and fascial contractures. The iliotibial band is frequently contracted, leading to pelvic obliquity, hip flexion, knee flexion, and external tibial rotation. Release of this band at both the hip and distal thigh level is a prerequisite to scoliosis treatment (Fig. 6–51). If bilateral involvement is present, simultaneous bilateral release is recommended. Pelvic obliquity may thus be due to iliotibial band contracture only, to scoliosis only, or a combination of both.

Brace treatment of the paralytic scoliosis can be very helpful in delaying the need for fusion but virtually never is a total substitute for fusion. Brace treatment must begin early and must be pursued intensively to be effective. If the curvature is progressive despite bracing, surgical treatment is indicated regardless of age (Fig. 6–52).

Surgical treatment of the usual curve of poliomyelitis is best accomplished by posterior Harrington instrumentation and spinal fusion. The fusion area is usually much longer than in idiopathic scoliosis and must include the sacrum if there is pelvic obliquity due to the scoliosis. High thoracic curvatures may extend into the cervical spine, and fusion may extend into the cervical spine. Harrington instruments, however, must never be inserted proximal to T1. Halo-casts should be used when fusion extends into the cervical spine.

Severe thoracolumbar or lumbar curves associated with fixed pelvic obliquity are best treated by both anterior and posterior surgical procedures. The achievement of a level pelvis with a well-balanced spine above it is the ideal goal in the treatment of paralytic scoliosis (Figs. 6–53 and 6–54).

Curves due to spinal muscle atrophy are quite peculiar to the curves of poliomyelitis. Bracing is valuable in order to delay fusion, but the curve never should be allowed to progress beyond 50 degrees in the brace. Long fusions to the sacrum are mandatory. Rapid resumption of upright activity is imperative to prevent general deterioration. The chief error

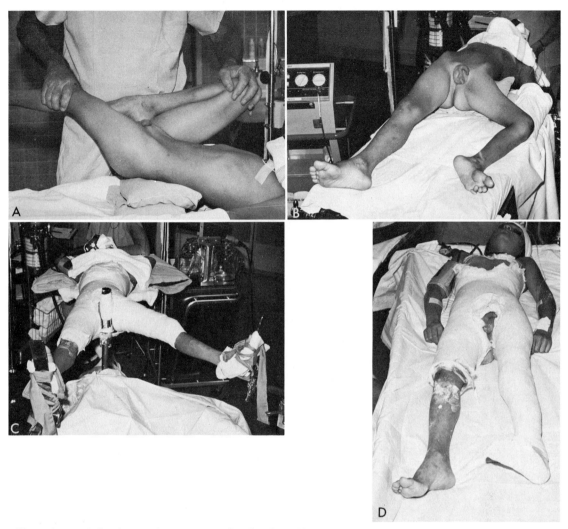

Figure 6–51. *A,* Paralytic scoliosis associated with pelvic obliquity requires careful analysis. Release of contractures if present must precede the treatment of the scoliosis. Testing for a tight iliotibial band. Note hip flexion contracture. The tight band and hip flexion contracture is demonstrable only with the leg held in adduction and slight internal rotation. *B,* The typical position assumed by patient with tight iliotibial band is one of abduction and external rotation. *C,* After cutting both upper and lower aspects of iliotibial band a Steinmann pin is incorporated into the plaster in the lower femur. This pin holds the pelvis down while the affected leg is held in abduction. Strong traction pulls down the high pelvis on the normal leg while a spica cast is incorporated. *D,* The affected leg is then brought into internal rotation and adduction as well as some hyperextension. In this patient it is incorporated in the cast; often it is only held in position as a long leg cast.

in treatment of curves due to spinal muscle atrophy is the mistaken belief that the neurologic disease is progressive.

Curves due to less common neurologic disorders, such as syringomyelia, Friedreich's ataxia, Charcot-Marie-Tooth disease, and spinal cord tumors must be evaluated on their own merits, but in general, progressive curves must be controlled by whatever means possible, either bracing or surgical. Any scoliosis progressing beyond 60 degrees must be fused, the only exceptions being terminal Duchenne muscular dystrophy and severely retarded, bedridden children.

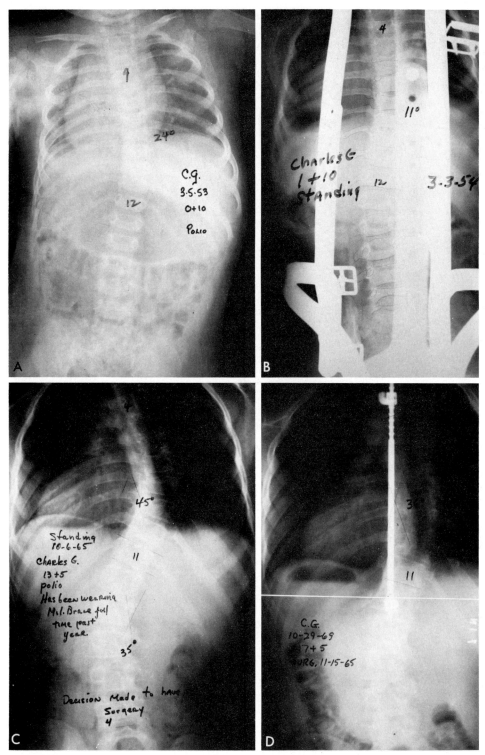

Figure 6–52. *A,* At 10 months of age, this boy already had a 24 degree scoliosis due to poliomyelitis at age two months. *B,* In a Milwaukee brace at age one year, 10 months, his curve is well-controlled at 11 degrees. *C,* At age 13, his growth spurt occurred, and his curve began to worsen despite the brace, which had successfully controlled the curve for 12 years. *D,* At age 17, four years after fusion, his scoliosis is stabilized, there is no fusion to the sacrum, and his torso length is normal.

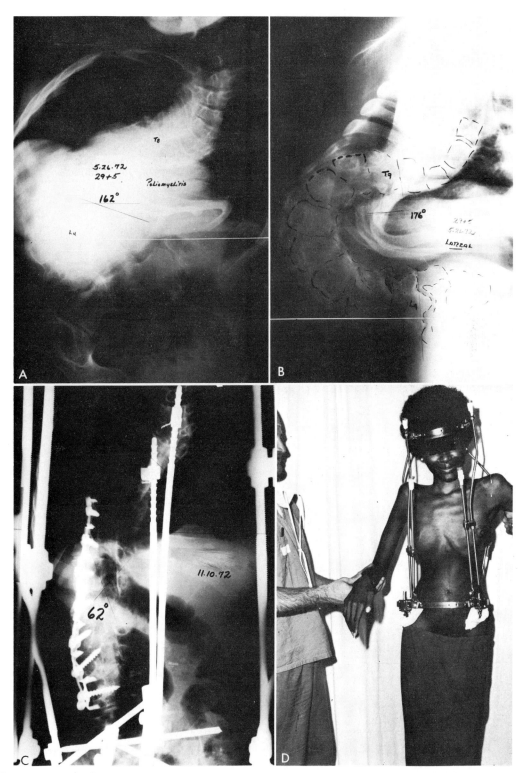

Figure 6–53. *A* and *B,* AP and lateral roentgenograms of the spine in a 29-year-old female with severe paralytic scoliosis. *C,* Surgery consisted of four procedures: (1) halofemoral distraction; (2) posterior osteotomies; (3) Dwyer anterior interbody fusion and instrumentation; and (4) posterior spine fusion and instrumentation from T4 to the sacrum. *D,* Postoperatively, she was put in a halo-hoop for six months to provide for better immobilization, and to correct residual pelvic obliquity.

Illustration continued on following page.

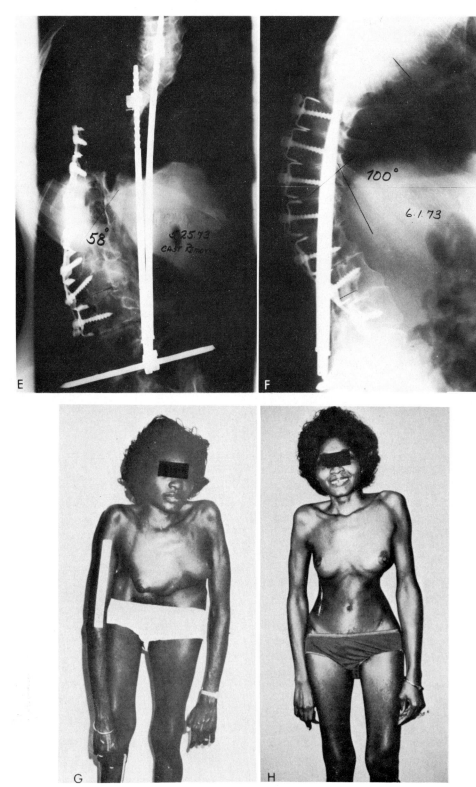

Figure 6–53 *Continued.*   *E* and *F,* Roentgenograms after cast removal (11 months after the original surgery) demonstrate solid fusion and maintenance of correction. *G* and *H,* Photographs before and after surgery demonstrating an excellent final result.

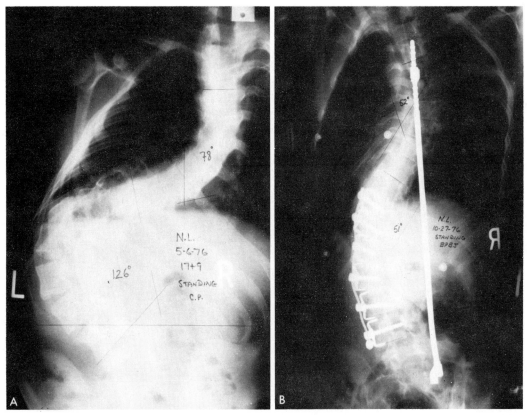

Figure 6–54. *A,* This 17-year-old male with spastic quadriplegia had an increasing scoliosis with pain at the apex of the lumbar curve. His torso was markedly displaced to the right. He was fully ambulatory, lived at home with his parents, and attended a special school. *B,* After a two-stage correction and fusion, he has achieved excellent torso balance. The fusion extends from T4 to the sacrum. An L4-L5 pseudarthrosis required subsequent repair.

Myelomeningocoele Spine Deformity

NATURAL HISTORY

Children with myelomeningocoele have a very high percentage of spine deformity, the incidence rising with higher levels of paralysis. With a T10-level paraplegia, the incidence of serious spinal deformity by adolescence is nearly 100 per cent. Children with L5-level paralysis have a 20 per cent incidence of scoliosis.

There are two main types of deformity seen, the congenital and the paralytic. Congenital deformities are those in which there are congenital vertebral anomalies in addition to the spina bifida. Hemivertebrae and unsegmented bars are typically seen. A very special and difficult problem is a congenital kyphosis at the level of the spina bifida. The congenital deformities are present at birth and may progress with growth. These follow the same course as congenital anomalies without myelomeningocoele.

The paralytic spine deformities are not present at birth but develop later in growth. They have a tremendous tendency to accelerate rapidly at the time of the pubertal growth spurt. This may occur relatively early in children with myelomeningocoele owing to their abnormal endocrine patterns (Fig. 6–55).

NONOPERATIVE TREATMENT

Nonoperative treatment of these children is difficult. Their multiple medical problems, and especially the skin insensitivity, have made bracing a great challenge. Nonoperative treatment by exercises, electrical stimulation, or stretching has never succeeded and should not be attempted.

Lindseth has recently reported improvement of paralytic curves by cerebral shunting to alleviate central canal enlargement.[151]

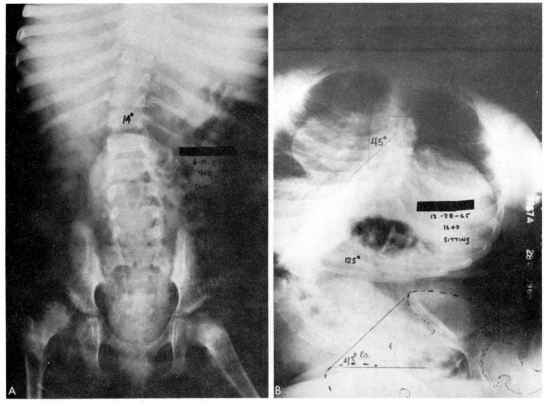

Figure 6–55. *A,* A nine-year-old female with myelomeningocele and a 14 degree left lumbar curve. *B,* The same patient at age 16 showing a 125 degree curve and severe pelvic obliquity.

The keys to successful brace treatment are (1) early brace application, (2) "total contact" fit, (3) very gradual adjustment to the brace, and (4) very careful monitoring of the patient. Successful brace treatment cannot be accomplished without conscientious and devoted parents.

Nonoperative treatment is only a temporizing measure in order to obtain adequate spine growth. Fusion is done whenever the brace fails to control the curve, in our experience usually at the growth spurt.

Nonoperative treatment has no benefit for congenitally anomalous vertebrae. These areas usually require early fusion, just as though there were no paralytic components.

Surgical treatment of the myelomeningocoele spine is probably the most difficult area of all spine deformities. It should never be attempted by the inexperienced surgeon. A total mastery of idiopathic and neuromuscular deformity techniques is an absolute prerequisite.

Traction has not proved beneficial in our hands. The skull is often thin, and defects can be present owing to cerebral shunts. The spinal cord is always tethered, and traction may produce or aggravate an Arnold-Chiari malformation. The bones of the lower extremities are osteoporotic and do not hold pins well. Bedrest is detrimental to the patient's general status, osteoporotic legs, and renal function.

Posterior instrumentation and fusion to the sacrum are mandatory. The fusions are long and must extend three or four levels above the uppermost vertebra of the primary curve. Structural secondary thoracic curves are common and, if present, must be included in the fusion area (Fig. 6–56).

Previous attempts to achieve satisfactory correction and fusion by the posterior approach alone have met with such a high failure rate that many surgeons are recommending that both anterior and posterior fusion should always be done. Although some excellent re-

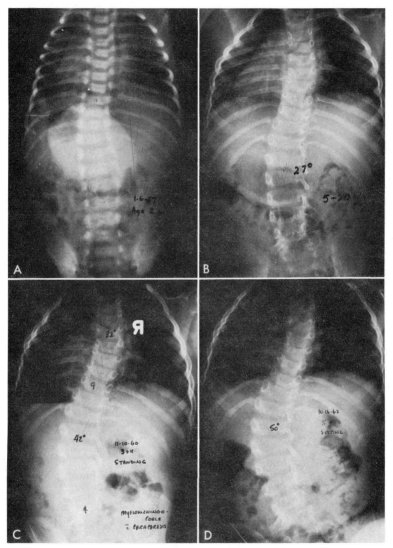

Figure 6–56. *A,* An AP roentgenogram at age two weeks showing the myelomeningocele sac and a 14 degree scoliosis, but no congenital anomalies. *B,* Age three years and four months. Curve now measures 27 degrees. No treatment was given. *C,* Age three years and eleven months. Patient is ambulatory with short leg braces and crutches. He has an incomplete L4 lesion, and normal intelligence. The curve now measures 42 degrees. *D,* Age five years and ten months. His curve has increased to 50 degrees. Still no spine treatment was given.

Illustration continued on following page.

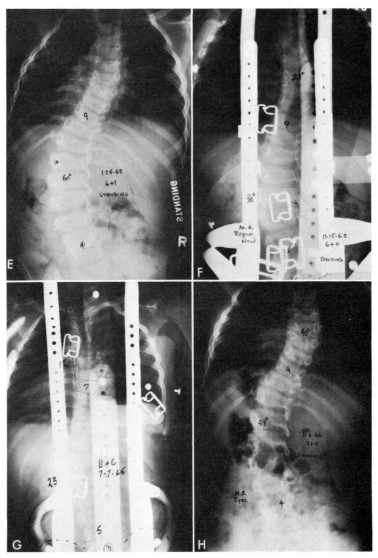

Figure 6–56 *Continued.*   *E,* Age six years and one month. The curve was now 60 degrees and a Milwaukee brace was prescribed. Although not of normal quality there was sensation in the area of brace contact. This type of progression is typical of the patient with myelomeningocele scoliosis. *F,* Age six years and eleven months. His curve responded well to the brace, now measuring 30 degrees. *G,* Two years later, the curve measures 23 degrees in the brace. *H,* An AP stand-ing roentgenogram out of the brace at age nine years, eleven months shows the primary lumbar curve at 43 degrees, and a thoracic curve of 40 degrees. Bracing was continued.

Illustration continued on opposite page.

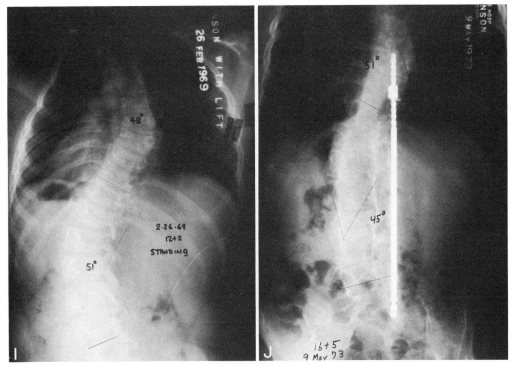

Figure 6–56 *Continued.   I,* Standing roentgenogram at age 12 years shows the two curves at 51 degrees (lumbar) and 48 degrees (thoracic). The curves are obviously deteriorating, and a long fusion is better for his age. *J,* At age 16 years and five months, four years after fusion from T4 to S1 with instrumentation of the T9-S1 area. The fusion is solid. (A transverse process fusion was done to avoid the spina bifida.) This represents a good blending of brace and surgical treatment for the optimal end result. Anterior fusion was not necessary in this patient.

sults have been achieved by posterior fusion alone, additional anterior fusion improves the success rate significantly.

The typical patient has a long, sweeping, paralytic thoracolumbar curve with pelvic obliquity. The achieving of a level pelvis is of paramount importance, and every effort must be directed toward this goal. Our best results have been from anterior fusion with Dwyer or Zielke instrumentation from about T10 to L4 or L5 and posterior instrumentation and fusion from a higher level down to the sacrum.

Postoperative management has been difficult, especially because of the anesthetic skin about the pelvis. Prolonged bedrest is detrimental owing to mental stagnation, renal stones, urinary tract infection, and extremity osteoporosis. We, therefore, do not use bedrest, casts, or immobilization of the hips.

Postoperative management with removable two-piece body jackets of polypropylene has given the best results (Fig. 6–57).

Myelomeningocoele congenital kyphosis is the most difficult of all deformities to treat. Braces have proved ineffective. Early apical resection and realignment with reconstitution of posterior muscle balance as advocated by Lindseth[151] have provided the best early treatment.

More major deformities in older children have been best treated by resection of the vertebrae proximal to the apex of the kyphosis, plus realignment, posterior instrumentation and fusion, and then anterior fusion. Early total fusion of the lumbar spine may lead to respiratory insufficiency due to continued growth of the internal organs at the expense of the thoracic cavity (Fig. 6–58).

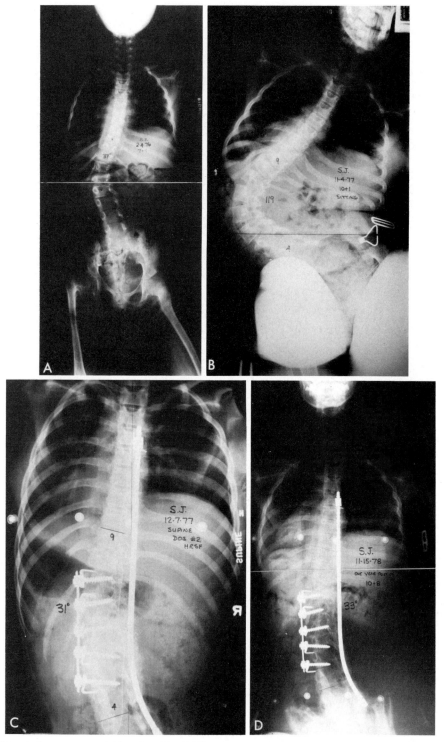

Figure 6–57. *A,* A seven-year-old female with a 37 degree curve on a supine film. *B,* The same patient at age 10 with a 119 degree curve on a sitting film. *C,* The patient after anterior fusion and Zielke instrumentation plus posterior fusion and Harrington instrumentation. Correction of the curve to 31 degrees and complete leveling of the pelvic obliquity has been achieved. *D,* The patient one year later demonstrating a 33 degree curve and slight relapse of the pelvic obliquity.

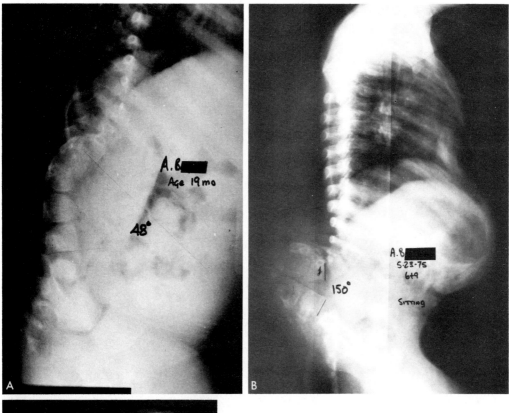

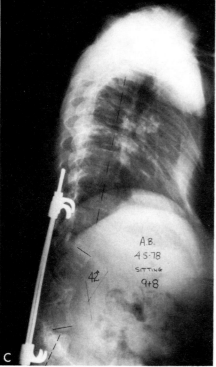

Figure 6–58. *A,* A 48 degree lumbar kyphosis in a child with myelomeningocele at age 19 months. *B,* The same patient at age six shows a severe, 150 degree kyphosis. She had a chronic pressure sore over the apex of the kyphosis. *C,* The same patient after surgical correction and stabilization. There is no external deformity. Sitting stability is much improved.

Neurofibromatosis Scoliosis

Scoliosis is a well-recognized component of von Recklinghausen's neurofibromatosis, occurring in about 20 to 25 per cent of the patients. It is also well known that the spine deformity in neurofibromatosis is particularly troublesome, often leading to paraplegia if left untreated or to pseudarthrosis when arthrodesis is attempted.

Although the patient with neurofibromatosis can have any of the other common types of spine deformity, it is the dystrophic curve that causes all the problems and deserves special mention. The dystrophic curve is short, sharply angulated, has severe rotation of the apical vertebrae, has scalloping of the vertebral margins, often has "penciling" of the adjacent ribs, and frequently is associated with a soft tissue neurofibroma lying adjacent to the vertebrae (Fig. 6–59).

These curves are usually progressive, often at a young age, and may progress after cessation of growth. If kyphotic, paraplegia may result. Neurofibromatosis kyphoscoliosis is second only to congenital kyphosis in the production of paraplegia (Fig. 6–60).

Brace treatment is of absolutely no benefit for dystrophic curves. The procedure of choice is fusion, regardless of age. Posterior fusion is sufficient for scoliotic deformities, but both anterior and posterior fusion are necessary for kyphoscoliotic problems.

Patients with severe deformities respond well to halofemoral traction owing to the flexibility of the curves. This is then followed by posterior instrumentation and fusion for scoliosis, and if kyphosis is present, anterior fusion as well. The best results in neurofibromatosis kyphoscoliosis have been achieved by doing the posterior procedure first and the anterior one second. This is contrary to congenital kyphosis, in which the front should be done first.

Pseudarthrosis is common. Exploration and augmentation of the fusion are recom-

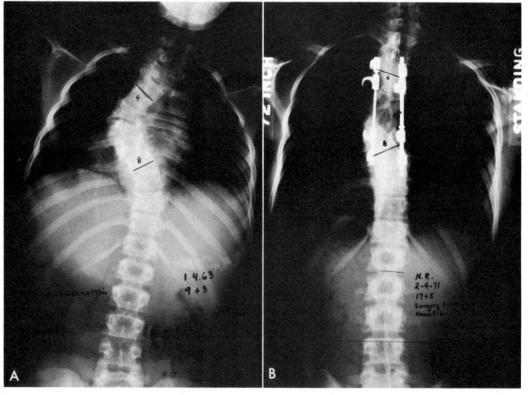

Figure 6–59. *A,* This patient with neurofibromatosis and an acutely angulated curve had only a moderate kyphosis. She was therefore fused posteriorly, using only a distraction and compression Harrington instrumentation. *B,* At age 17½, nine years after surgery, her spine remains well controlled by posterior spinal fusion. There is no increase in kyphosis.

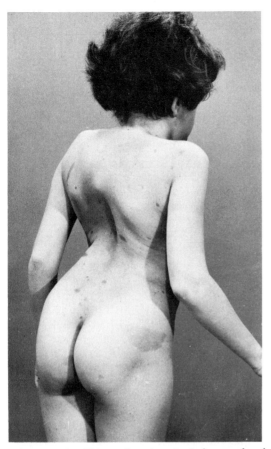

Figure 6–60. This patient is a typical example of kyphoscoliosis with multiple cafe-au-lait spots. She also demonstrated minimal spasticity. Treatment consisted of anterior and posterior spine fusion, with an excellent result and relief of her spasticity.

mended if there is loss of correction or any defect in the fusion mass on good oblique views.

If the patient has no kyphosis and is developing paraplegia, an intraspinal tumor is most likely. This should be removed by laminectomy, and a fusion should be done simultaneously (or a week later if necessary). Laminectomy alone should never be done in an area of dystrophic curve.

If paraplegia is associated with a kyphosis, the cord compression is more likely due to the kyphosis and not a tumor. If the paraparesis is mild and early, good results can be obtained by anterior and posterior fusion with cast correction and prolonged bedrest until the fusion is solid. Cord exposure is not necessary.

For more extensive degrees of paralysis, anterior cord decompression, anterior fusion, and then posterior fusion are necessary.

Spine Deformity Following Laminectomy

The occurrence of postlaminectomy spine deformity is rare except in children treated for spinal cord tumors. Several such series have been reported with an average of at least 50 per cent of the survivors having significant deformity.

Several types of deformity can occur, depending on the type of tumor, extent of paralysis, level of laminectomy, and extent of laminectomy. A short, angular kyphosis will result after a thoracic laminectomy in which the facets were removed bilaterally. A long, sweeping kyphosis will develop after a thoracic laminectomy in which the facets were preserved. Scoliosis is more related to paralysis than the laminectomy per se.

Prevention of severe deformity is critically important. Neurosurgeons must, whenever possible, not disturb the facet joints. Following surgery, the patient must be followed by an orthopaedic surgeon knowledgeable about spinal deformities. Developing deformities must be promptly braced. Deformities refractory to bracing must be fused.

One of the major problems in this area seems to be the reluctance of physicians to recognize that a progressive kyphosis is taking place. This is coupled with a reluctance to treat it aggressively. All too often the child is denied appropriate orthopaedic care on the mistaken premise that the lesion is fatal.

The main clinical problem is thoracic or thoracolumbar kyphosis. The optimal treatment is both anterior and posterior fusion. The anterior fusion should utilize one or more strut grafts, depending on the severity of the kyphosis. The posterior fusion must be lateral to the laminectomy. If possible, compression rods should be added for stability, but they must not press upon the cord area.

Postoperative support can be a Milwaukee brace, Risser cast, or halo-cast, depending upon the level and severity of the deformity. Halo-casts are essential for cervical and high thoracic deformities.

Scoliosis in Marfan's Syndrome

Scoliosis occurs in approximately 50 per cent of patients with Marfan's syndrome and may be quite severe, is often painful, and may result in pulmonary dysfunction. The patterns of deformity are quite similar to idiopathic scoliosis, usually tending to be either a single right thoracic major curve or a double major, right thoracic, left lumbar curve.

Brace treatment is appropriate for progressive curves of 20 to 40 degrees in growing children, but the end results have been less rewarding than for similar idiopathic curves. There is a smaller percentage of success, apparently due to the inability of the soft tissues to "stabilize," with nonoperative treatment.

Surgical treatment is preferable for patients with progressive curves over 40 degrees. Standard posterior fusion with Harrington instruments has given excellent results. Preoperative casting or traction usually has not been necessary. Anterior fusion has been needed only rarely, usually only in patients with a marked kyphosis at the thoracolumbar junction.

A detailed medical evaluation is mandatory before operating on a patient with Marfan's syndrome. Aortic aneurysms, aortic and mitral valve insufficiency, and lens dislocation must be carefully looked for. The only real contraindications to surgery are aortic aneurysm and untreatable aortic or mitral insufficiency. The patient with Marfan's syndrome should not be denied modern scoliosis surgery just because of the diagnosis.

Spine Deformity Following Irradiation

Irradiation for pediatric malignancies has long been known to be potentially productive of spine deformity. Recent studies of larger numbers of patients have more precisely delineated the nature of the problem. The vastly improved survival rate of the children has led to a larger number of children presenting to scoliosis centers with spine deformities. Usual tumors resulting in irradiation deformity are neuroblastoma and Wilms' tumor. Irradiation has also been used for spinal cord tumors, such as astrocytomas and ependymomas, but the late effects here are confused by the laminectomy and the paralytic components of the deformity.

The incidence of bony changes following irradiation have varied in different series. Studies from Boston Children's Hospital of 69 survivors of neuroblastoma reveal 56 per cent to have some type of structural spine deformity at review. If greater than 2000 rads of radiation were given, there was a 73 per cent deformity rate, and if less than 2000 rads were given, the deformity rate was 53 per cent. Kyphosis was noted in 13 per cent, and an increase in kyphosis to 50 per cent was observed in patients who also had undergone laminectomy. Many of these patients were not followed to maturity, and of those patients who were followed to maturity, 18 per cent were noted to have a scoliosis.[166]

Deformity may be either a scoliosis or a kyphoscoliosis. Many of the deformities are not severe and do not require treatment, but occasionally treatment is indicated because of progressive deformity, usually not manifest until the adolescent growth spurt.

Similar studies following irradiation for Wilms' tumor also have been reported from Boston by Riseborough and associates.[206] Of 81 patients who had follow-up examination, 59 had spinal deformity, 38 had scoliosis only, two had kyphosis only, and 19 had kyphoscoliosis. In all these patients the deformity remained slight until the growth spurt and then progressed; seven required fusion. Milwaukee brace wear was attempted in three, and all three trials failed. The incidence of deformity was related to the dose given.

It is important, therefore, to monitor patients having irradiation for tumors since statistically it would appear that the spine deformity is the most common late manifestation of irradiation for the tumors during childhood. Brace treatment should be attempted for progressing deformities, but it should not be expected to have a high degree of success. A curve of greater than 40 degrees is probably best treated by surgical fusion.

In our experience, those demonstrating both kyphosis and scoliosis have had a lower rate of success with a posterior fusion alone and are best treated by both anterior and posterior fusion.

The fusions may heal slowly owing to the poor circulation in the irradiated area, and a longer healing time must be anticipated.

Scheuermann's Juvenile Kyphosis and Postural Roundback Deformity

Kyphosis remains one of the most frequently neglected deformities that develop during childhood and adolescence. Parents and even physicians may recognize the presence of a roundback deformity of the spine but may ascribe it to a problem of poor posture. This is unfortunate in that the poor posture is usually a manifestation of severe structural alterations in the vertebral column. Early recognition and proper treatment of these patients can be expected to produce a superior result, not only in correcting the deformity but also in alleviating back complaints.

Juvenile kyphosis was a poorly understood concept until 1920, when Holger Scheuermann first demonstrated radiographically that the deformity was caused by wedge-shaped vertebrae.[220] In 1964, K. H. Sørensen further categorized the disease process and suggested that Scheuermann's definition apply to a kyphosis that includes three adjacent vertebrae with wedging of five or more degrees.[239] The etiology of Scheuermann's kyphosis, however, has remained unknown, and the speculations outlined in the literature are as diverse as the authors who have written about them. Scheuermann, in 1920, first proposed that this was a disease process caused by avascular necrosis of the cartilage ring apophysis of the vertebral body. With the onset of avascular necrosis of the vertebral body, growth inhibition occurred and, subsequently, kyphosis developed. However, this theory has never been widely accepted. Bick and Copel, in 1951, noted that the limbus, or ring apophysis, was not connected to the growth plate and, therefore, contributed nothing to the longitudinal growth of the vertebra.[10] Therefore, any changes or alterations that occurred in the limbus would not necessarily alter the growth potential of the vertebral body. Schmorl, in 1930, suggested that herniation of the intervertebral disc material through the growth plate produced the kyphosis.[224] The changes, he felt, first started as bulging of the disc material in the area of the nucleus pulposus, presumably because of developmental disturbances. Through preformed or traumatic tears in the end plates, part of the disc material was forced into the bony spongiosum, resulting in diminished height of the intervertebral disc. Disturbances in enchondral growth ultimately produced the kyphosis. This theory likewise has not been universally accepted. It is known that disc protusions may occur outside the area of the kyphosis in patients with Scheuermann's disease. Also, patients who have no evidence of Scheuermann's disease may have Schmorl's nodules. Mechanical factors have been impli-

cated in the development of the kyphosis. Scheuermann noted that the disease, in his experience, most often occurred in young agricultural workers who were involved in heavy labor.[220, 221] Scheuermann's kyphosis is known to occur in normal, healthy school children uninvolved in excessive physical labor. On the other hand, muscle contractures occasionally are noted in patients with Scheuermann's disease. Lambrinudi, in 1934, noted hamstring tightness in many patients and felt this was of significance in the development of the deformity.[143] Michelle felt that contractures of the iliopsoas muscle were instrumental in producing the deformity.[169] Although these findings are of interest, they may not be present in all patients with Scheuermann's disease, and their significance consequently remains unknown. A familial occurrence of Scheuermann's disease has been described (Fig. 6–61, A to E). It has not been established whether this observation is of genetic or environmental importance.

Of interest are the questions raised in the past concerning the relationship of Scheuermann's kyphosis to endocrine and nutritional abnormalities.[77, 158] In 1969 Muller and Gschwend[184] noted that in 22 patients with Turner's syndrome, 11 demonstrated radiographic changes in Scheuermann's kyphosis. Patients with Turner's syndrome are known to have severe osteoporosis not unlike that developing in the postmenopausal female.[46] Other workers have suggested that vitamin insufficiency is instrumental in the onset of Scheuermann's disease,[236] and other researchers have published work to suggest that patients with Scheuermann's disease may show alterations in bone metabolism.[86, 183] Recent work in our center has suggested that patients with Scheuermann's disease may indeed have a mild form of juvenile osteoporosis.[40] A dietary analysis suggested that deficiency of calcium may be a common finding in these patients.

PATHOLOGY

Surprisingly enough, there are remarkably little published data on the pathology of Scheuermann's disease either in the adolescent or adult. Gross and microscopic findings, however, have been noted and are of some interest.[31] When one examines a spine from a patient with Scheuermann's disease, one is immediately struck by the finding of a very

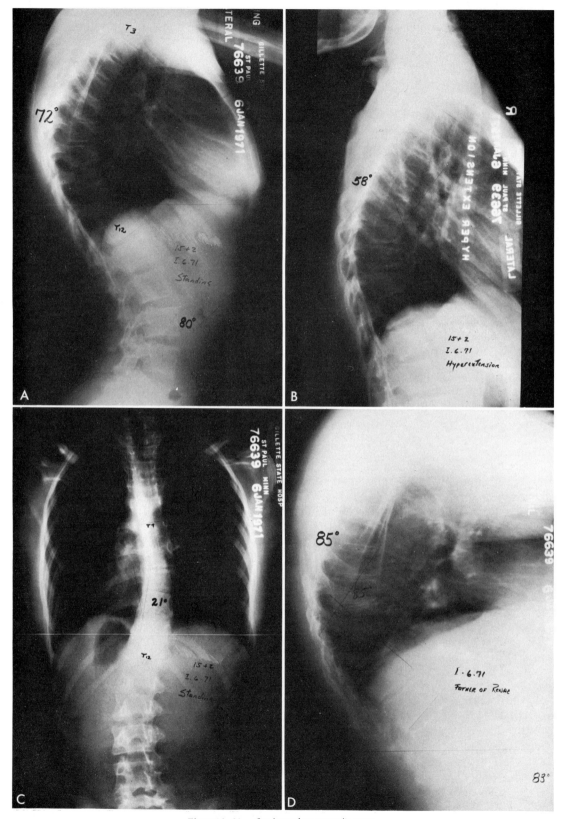

Figure 6–61. *See legend on opposite page.*

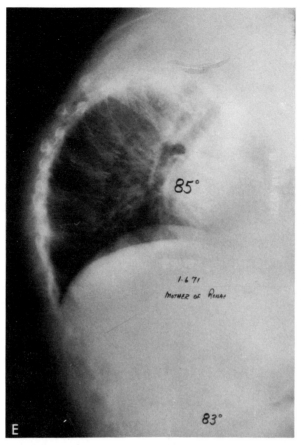

Figure 6-61. *A* and *B,* Fifteen-year-and-two-month-old female with Scheuermann's disease. Rigidity of kyphosis is noted by the poor correction on the hyperextension roentgenogram. *C,* Scoliosis, although mild, is present in one third of the patients. *D* and *E* demonstrate the occurrence of Scheuermann's disease in families, in this case the mother and father.

thickened and tightened anterior longitudinal ligament that appears almost to act as a bowstring across the anterior aspects of the vertebral bodies. This is not only characteristic of Scheuermann's kyphosis but also occurs in congenital, traumatic, or postirradiation kyphosis. The vertebral bodies, on the other hand, do appear markedly wedged as the roentgenograms would show, and the vertebral disc space is actually narrowed. The width of the disc itself appears to far exceed that of the vertebra at the anterior margin, yet once the disc material has been dissected, that portion between the vertebral bodies is truly narrowed. This discrepancy may best be compared to the effect created by a marshmallow that is compressed between two smooth plates. When the disc material and bony centrum are analyzed histologically, no evidence of avascular necrosis may be identified. On the other hand, a cartilage spongiosa demarca-

tion is very irregular and may be completely disrupted in areas where Schmorl's nodules have actually fractured the bony trabecula, allowing cartilage and disc material to extravasate into the bony centrum. The growth plate itself may be quite disordered as a result of this disruption.

CLINICAL DESCRIPTION

These are few definitive studies concerning the early pathogenesis of Scheuermann's disease. In fact, histologic material from patients during the active stage of the disease process is meager (Fig. 6-62). We have noted, from biopsy material obtained from a 16 year old patient with active Scheuermann's disease, evidence of Schmorl's nodules with protrusion of disc material through the end plate.[12] On the other hand, the disc material appears to be histologically normal.

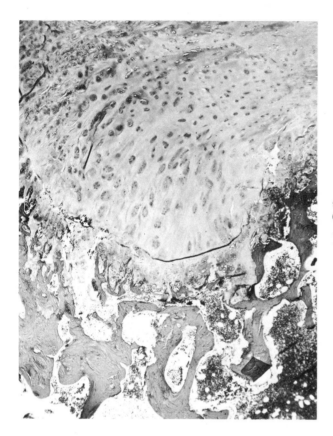

Figure 6–62. Herniation of nuclear material through the end plate into the bony spongiosa (Schmorl's nodule). (From Bradford, D. S., and Moe, J. H.: Scheuermann's juvenile kyphosis: A histologic study. Clin. Orthop. *160*:45, 1975.)

The reported incidence of Scheuermann's disease has varied between 0.4 per cent and 8.3 per cent of the general population, depending upon whether the diagnosis was based on radiographic or clinical criteria. From a review of 1338 cases reported in the literature, the male to female ratio appears to be equally divided. In recent studies, however, Bradford and others[34] have noted a female to male ratio of two to one. The age of onset of the disease is difficult to establish because radiographic changes typical of Scheuermann's disease are rarely demonstrable prior to age 11.

Initial complaints consist of deformity and pain at the apex of the kyphosis. The incidence of these complaints again has varied according to the series reported. Albanese and Guntz noted pain in only 20 per cent of their patients while Scheuermann and Nathan and Kuhns reported an incidence greater than 60 per cent.[3, 188, 220, 221] It is important to realize that many patients, when first seen, are totally unaware that they have a deformity and, in fact, have been urged to see a physician by family or close friends.

On examination a thoracic kyphosis with lumbar lordosis will be apparent (Fig. 6–63). We have found the prone hyperextension test to be of great value in judging the mobility and degree of fixation of the thoracic kyphosis. Direct tenderness or muscle spasm may be elicited over the apex of the curvature, and an associated scoliosis may be visualized in approximately 30 to 40 per cent of the cases. The pectoral and hamstring muscle groups often prove tight. Rarely, a neurologic examination may demonstrate spastic paraparesis secondary to cord compression.

ROENTGENOGRAPHIC FINDINGS

Roentgenographic evaluation of the patient with Scheuermann's disease must be thorough. A lateral roentgenogram of the spine with the arms held parallel to the floor and the hands resting on a support is most helpful in evaluating the curvature. A standing 14 × 36-inch anteroposterior roentgenogram is taken in order to rule out an associated scoliotic curvature. A supine hyperextension lateral roentgenogram of the thoracic spine, using a polyurethane plastic wedge placed at the apex

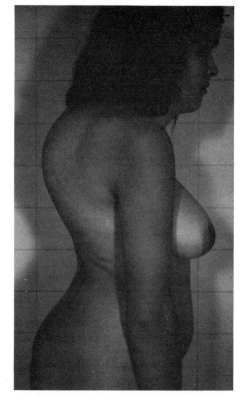

Figure 6–63. The clinical appearance of a patient with classical Scheuermann's disease. A severe thoracic kyphosis with a marked increase in normal lumbar lordosis is readily apparent.

of the curvature, facilitates this exposure and provides important information concerning the mobility of the curvature. A left hand roentgenogram should also be taken in order to assess the extent of skeletal maturation. The degree of kyphosis and lordosis and the amount of vertebral wedging is then calculated (Fig. 6–64). The angles are outlined by marking the end vertebra or that vertebra which is maximally tilted into the curve and drawn in a perpendicular line to the end plate. The angle thus formed is considered to be the kyphotic angle. The sacrum is considered to be the end vertebra for measurement of lordosis. Vertebral wedging is outlined in a similar fashion. The early characteristic findings of Scheuermann's disease include wedging, Schmorl's nodules, irregular end plates, and a mild scoliosis of 10 to 20 degrees, with or without vertebral rotation. Persistent vascular grooves may be present but appear to be related to immaturity of the vertebral body rather than to the characteristic finding of Scheuermann's disease. Late radiographic changes of Scheuermann's include a concave anterior border of the vertebral body, a flat-

tening of the vertebra, giving a relative increase in the anteroposterior dimension, and synostosis and exostosis forming between the vertebral bodies (Fig. 6–65). It is important to assess the skeletal age not only by the hand roentgenogram but also by noting the maturation of the iliac crest apophysis and the vertebral ring apophysis. The best radiographic criteria for the diagnosis of Scheuermann's disease have proved to be irregular end plates and vertebral wedging, along with an increase in the normal thoracic kyphosis. Accurate control studies demonstrating the normal range for kyphosis are, unfortunately, not available. From limited unpublished studies in our department we feel that a kyphosis between 35 and 40 degrees in a growing child is the upper limit of normal.[33]

DIFFERENTIAL DIAGNOSIS

Many authors have emphasized the problems occasionally encountered in differentiating Scheuermann's kyphosis from infectious spondylitis. However, with a thorough clinical and laboratory evaluation, as well as tomogra-

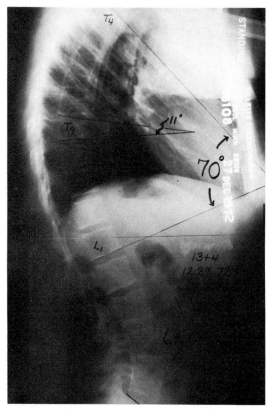

Figure 6–64. The method of measuring kyphosis, lordosis, and vertebral wedging according to the Cobb principle is outlined. The end vertebrae for the measurement of kyphosis are considered those vertebrae which are maximally tilted into the concavity of the curvature. Lordosis is measured from the lower kyphotic vertebra to the sacrum. Vertebral wedging is measured by drawing a line parallel to the bony end plates and calculating the angle thus formed. The early characteristic changes of Scheuermann's disease, Schmorl's nodules and irregular end plates, are noted.

phy of the spine, the true diagnosis should readily be established. Traumatic injuries to the spine occasionally present a confusing picture, but in these injuries usually only one vertebra is involved, while in Scheuermann's disease many vertebrae are involved (Fig. 6–66A). Osteochondrodystrophies, such as Morquio's and Hurler's disease, as well as postlaminectomy kyphosis, tumors, and congenital deformities of the spine, may be considered in the differential diagnosis (Fig. 6–66). Lumbosacral anomalies should always be ruled out. Spondylolisthesis at L5 and S1 can produce a severe lumbar lordosis and, consequently, a compensatory thoracic kyphosis. These patients may be completely asymptomatic except for a roundback deformity.

They will usually, however, not show radiographic changes of the vertebra found in Scheuermann's disease.

Finally, Scheuermann's disease should be distinguished from postural roundback deformity. Differentiation of these conditions in the preadolescent child prior to vertebral wedging may be difficult.[195] For a pure postural roundback we would include patients with a supple kyphosis without fixation who have no evidence of vertebral wedging, end plate irregularity, or disc protrusions (Fig. 6–67 A–C).

COMPLICATIONS OF SCHEUERMANN'S DISEASE

A kyphosis of less than 40 degrees is infrequently of cosmetic significance. However, if the curvature becomes greater the clinical deformity will be more pronounced, even in the obese individual. Deformities above 70 degrees are quite noticeable and, because of an increased compensatory lordosis (forward

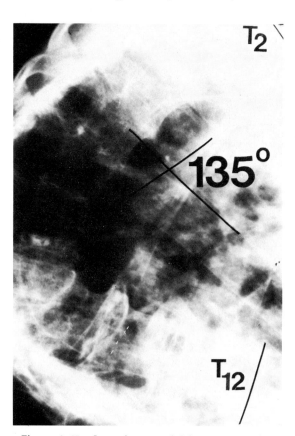

Figure 6–65. Late changes of Scheuermann's disease are well outlined. They include concave anterior borders of the vertebral body, synostosis and exostosis, between the vertebrae.

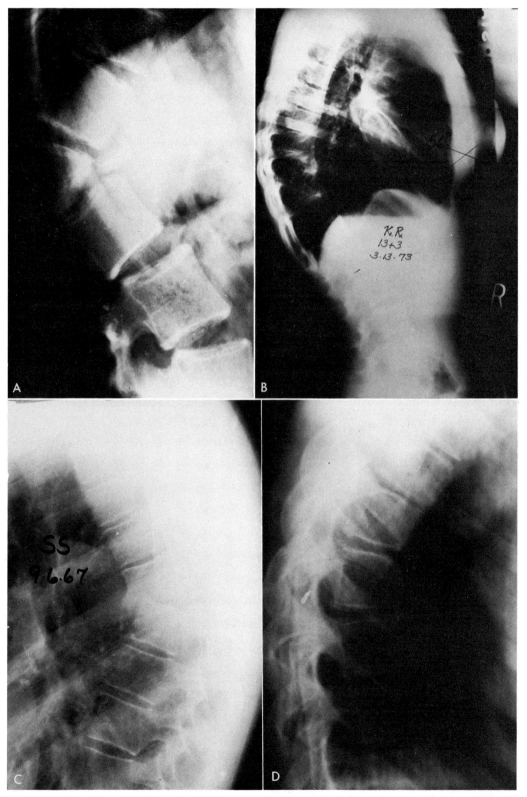

Figure 6–66. The differential diagnosis of Scheuermann's disease would include *A,* traumatic kyphosis; *B,* congenital kyphosis; *C,* tumors involving the vertebral bodies; and *D,* kyphosis secondary to infection with laminectomy.

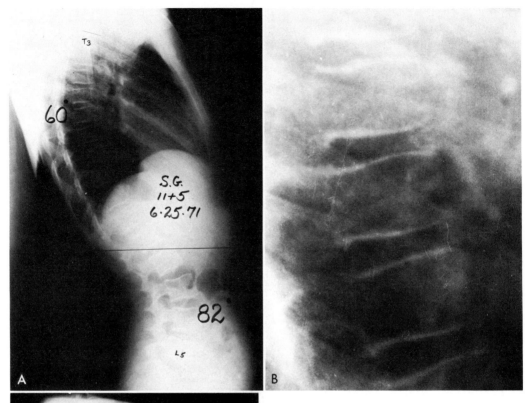

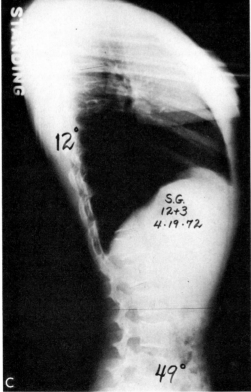

Figure 6–67. *A* and *B,* A pure postural round-back deformity may be confused with Scheuermann's kyphosis. However, in these patients the kyphosis is not fixed and the vertebrae do not show wedging or end-plate irregularity. *C,* These patients often may be managed quite satisfactorily by a program of exercises alone. (From Bradford, D. S., Moe, J. H., and Winter, R. B.: Kyphosis and postural roundback deformity in children and adolescents. Minn. Med. *56:*114–120, 1973, with permission of Minn. Med.)

protrusion of the cervical spine), they present a cosmetically objectionable appearance. Curves of this magnitude may even increase after skeletal maturation is complete. Pain at the apex of the kyphosis is present at one time or another in approximately one half of the patients before they reach age 20. This is mild and usually not disabling. However, after maturity the incidence of thoracic pain, although less, may be disabling in some patients. The incidence of low back pain, on the other hand, does not seem to be any higher than that found in the normal population. Neurologic complications in Scheuermann's disease, although rare, have been well outlined in the past.[27] A spastic paraparesis may develop secondary to cord compression or a herniated thoracic intervertebral disc at the apex of the curvature. Finally, one should always carefully examine the anteroposterior roentgenogram of the thoracolumbar spine in patients with Scheuermann's disease to be sure that widening of the interpedicular space is not present. Spinal epidural cyst may be associated with classical radiographic changes of Scheuermann's disease and may present with widening of the interpedicular space.[1, 56, 76] (Fig. 6–68 *A–C*).

TREATMENT

In considering whether treatment should be undertaken or not for Scheuermann's kyphosis, one should know the end result from adults who have not been treated. Complications relating to Scheuermann's disease are (1) cosmetic deformity, (2) back pain, and (3) neurologic deficit. One should also remember that any degree of kyphosis at the thoracolumbar or lumbar spine is abnormal since normally the spine in these areas is either neutral or lordotic.

It has been our experience that thoracic back pain in adults secondary to Scheuermann's disease may prove disabling and difficult to manage except by spinal fusion. It is known that the deformity, if not treated during adolescence, will often progress (Fig. 6–69). Therefore, we feel that treatment in the growing child is indicated in order to correct the deformity as well as to alleviate present symptoms and prevent future ones.

Various methods of treatment have been outlined in the past. Exercises alone have been suggested, but definite evidence of improvement in the deformity has not been es-

tablished.[188, 236] Exercises as a supplement to other forms of treatment, however, have been beneficial and may furnish a means of loosening muscle contractures.[42, 43, 248] Bedrest alone has been recommended, along with plaster shells or jackets, as has hyperextension treatment on a Bradford frame.[79, 80, 136, 188, 236, 248, 255] Combined methods of treatment have been advocated by many authors.[102, 188, 222, 248] These methods consist of a period of bedrest or traction to loosen the contractures, followed by the application of a plaster shell to straighten the kyphosis. The plaster jacket might be used to maintain the correction until growth is complete. On the other hand, a two-stage application of a plaster cast has proved to be an effective method.[8, 79, 105, 211, 247] The lordosis is straightened first with the patient bending forward while the lower part of the plaster is applied. Then, as a second stage, the plaster is extended to the upper part of the trunk, correcting the kyphosis. The cast is changed every three months for approximately one year. Stagnara and Perdriolle have noted a marked improvement in the degree of kyphosis in patients treated by this method.[242] Other authors have likewise found bracing and casting techniques to be extremely effective in the correction of the kyphosis.[103, 189, 202, 217, 218, 243]

The use of a Milwaukee brace in the nonoperative treatment of scoliosis was first reported by Blount in 1958.[20] Moe, in 1965, reported successful results in correcting the deformity of juvenile kyphosis with the use of a Milwaukee brace.[174] Recently, Bradford and colleagues have reviewed the results in 75 patients who have completed Milwaukee brace treatment for Scheuermann's kyphosis.[34, 37] The kyphosis improved by 42 per cent and the lordosis by 36 per cent of the pretreatment values (Fig. 6–70 *A–D*).

All except two patients who wore the Milwaukee brace as directed showed significant correction of their deformity. Factors that served to limit the degree of correction with the Milwaukee brace were an initial kyphosis greater than 65 degrees, vertebral wedging averaging greater than 10 degrees, and skeletal maturation as noted by closure of the iliac apophysis at the time treatment was instituted.

PLAN OF PATIENT MANAGEMENT. Following a complete history and physical examination, roentgenograms are obtained. The roentgenograms are taken with the patient standing in the lateral plane with the arms

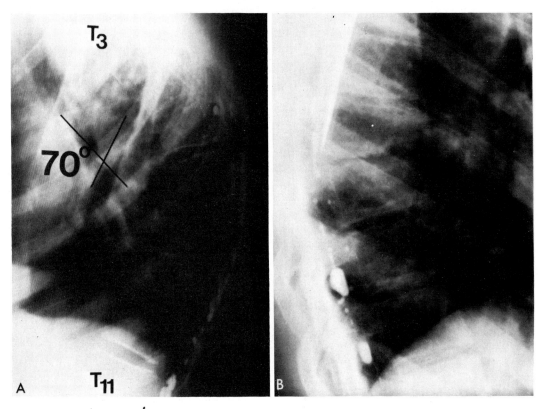

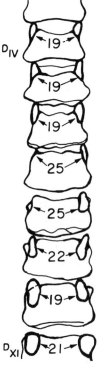

Figure 6–68. Neurologic complications in Scheuermann's disease are outlined. They include *A,* cord angulation at the apex of the curvature; *B,* herniation of a thoracic disc at the apex of the curvature; and *C,* a kyphosis in association with a spinal epidural cyst. In this instance a diagnosis can be suspected by the presence of a widened interpedicular space. (From Cloward, R. B., and Bucy, P. C.: Spinal extradural cyst and kyphosis dorsalis juvenilis. Am. J. Roentgenol., *38*:681–706, 1937).

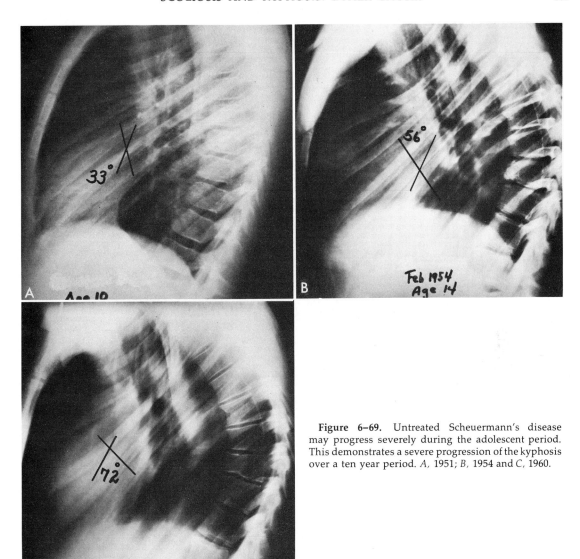

Figure 6–69. Untreated Scheuermann's disease may progress severely during the adolescent period. This demonstrates a severe progression of the kyphosis over a ten year period. *A,* 1951; *B,* 1954 and *C,* 1960.

outstretched parallel to the floor. A hyperextension roentgenogram is taken in the supine position, and the kyphotic angles are measured and compared. If an increased kyphosis is demonstrated to be rigid (less than 15 or 20 degrees of mobility on hyperextension), a Risser antigravity cast including the neck is applied. The cast is changed two or three times over the next two to three months in order to obtain more correction. A brace mold is made in between cast changes and is fabricated while the patient is in the plaster cast. Once the brace is completed, the cast is removed, and the brace is applied to the patient. An exercise program in the brace is initiated consisting of pelvic tilting exercises to decrease lumbar lordosis, muscle stretching exercises designed to overcome contractures, and thoracic extension exercises to build up the thoracic extensor muscle groups. The patient is allowed out of the brace two to three hours a day for personal hygiene and bathing (Figs. 6–71 to 6–73).

Repeat lateral standing roentgenograms in the brace are obtained at four-month intervals. If a scoliosis is present initially, repeat follow-up anteroposterior roentgenograms of the spine should be obtained as well at each follow-up visit. As a general rule, the kyphosis along with vertebral wedging are usually cor-

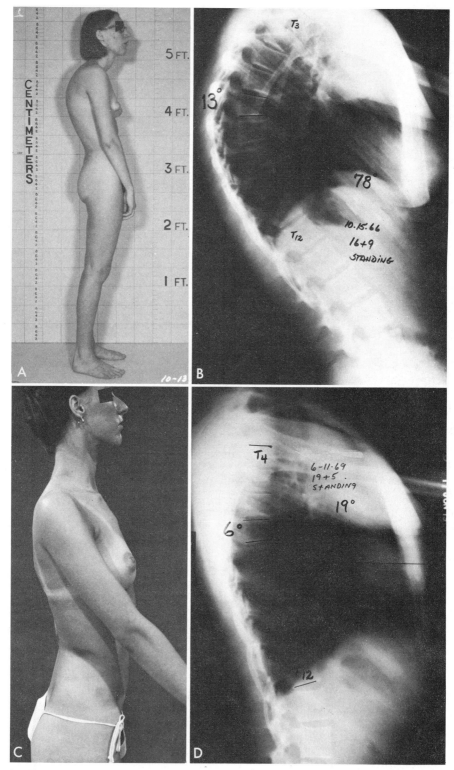

Figure 6–70.   The results of treatment of juvenile kyphosis with the Milwaukee brace are well outlined in this series of roentgenograms and photographs. *A* and *B*, Before treatment. *C* and *D*, Following 18 months in the Milwaukee brace the patient showed a marked improvement in her kyphosis and vertebral wedging, and her clinical appearance was excellent.

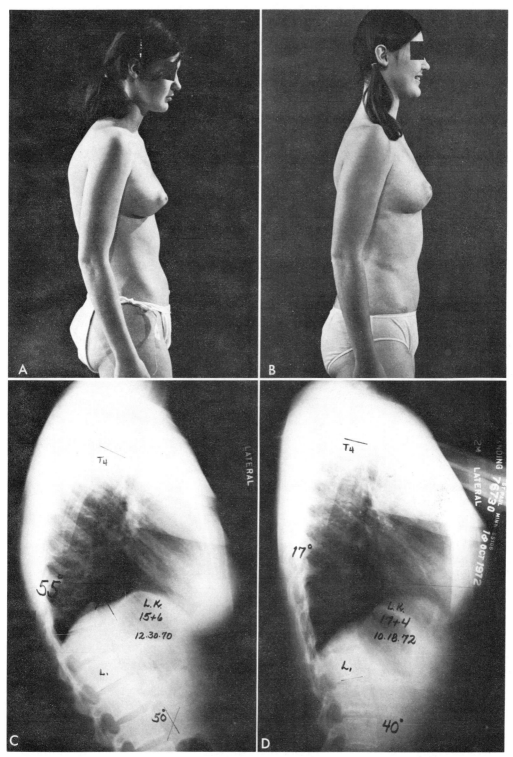

Figure 6–71. This sequence of figures demonstrates the clinical appearance of a patient before (*A* and *C*) and after (*B* and *D*) 20 months' treatment with the Milwaukee brace. The kyphosis improved from 55 to 17 degrees and the lordosis improved from 50 to 40 degrees. She has shown no loss in correction since the brace was discontinued six months ago. (From Bradford, D. S., Moe, J. H., and Winter, R. B.: Kyphosis and postural roundback deformity in children and adolescents. Minn. Med. *56*:114–120, 1973, with permission of Minn. Med.)

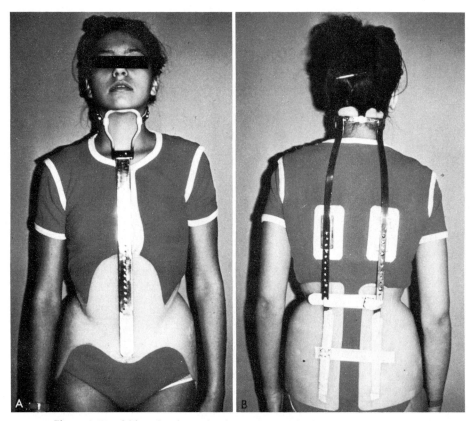

Figure 6–72. Milwaukee brace for the treatment of Scheuermann's kyphosis.

rected within one year. Once the kyphosis and wedging have been reversed, the patient may be gradually weaned from the brace. If significant loss of correction occurs during the weaning period, the time out of the brace should be decreased accordingly. All patients do not necessarily require full-time brace wear until skeletal maturation or closure of the ring apophysis of the vertebra. In contrast to patients undergoing brace treatment for adolescent idiopathic scoliosis, patients with juvenile kyphosis may be corrected and show stability of correction long before skeletal maturation.

Factors that may limit the degree of correction obtained in the brace are more severe degrees of kyphosis (greater than 70 to 80 degrees), severe vertebral wedging (greater than 10 to 15 degrees), or skeletal maturation as noted by closure of the iliac apophysis at the time of initial treatment. It should be remembered that correction is still possible even though the iliac apophysis may be closed as long as the ring apophyses of the vertebral bodies are still open (Fig. 6–70).

OPERATIVE TREATMENT. As a general rule, surgery should be reserved for those patients who present in the adult period with severe kyphosis, disabling back pain unresponsive to conservative management, neurologic signs and symptoms secondary to the kyphosis, or a combination of these manifestations (Fig. 6–74). Posterior spinal fusion alone for kyphosis greater than 70 degrees is usually associated with significant complications and loss of correction with instrumentation failure.[37] This can be expected in light of the problems of obtaining a solid posterior fusion over any kyphosis in which the fusion mass is under tension rather than compression. The technique we have found most useful for correcting kyphotic deformities secondary to Scheuermann's disease is a two-stage procedure.[36] The first stage consists of halo application with a transthoracic spinal fusion, dividing the anterior longitudinal ligament over the apical six or seven vertebrae and completely removing the intervertebral disc. Iliac bone graft along with rib bone graft is used to pack the interspace. The anterior fusion should be

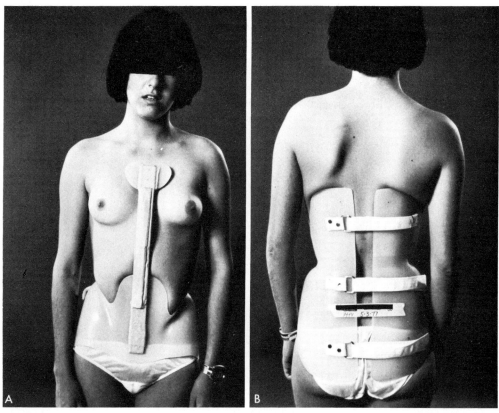

Figure 6–73. An underarm brace for the treatment of Scheuermann's kyphosis with the apex below T10.

carried out over the apical five to seven verte-bral levels or the most rigid portion of the kyphosis to be fused. Halo traction is then carried out for a two week period while the thoracotomy incision heals. Two weeks after the anterior procedure, a posterior spinal fusion and Harrington instrumentation using a Harrington compression assembly is carried out. The fusion must extend from the upper level to the lower level of the kyphosis in order to prevent too short a fusion mass. Otherwise correction may be lost. One week after the posterior arthrodesis, the patient is placed in a plaster cast and is encouraged to walk. The cast is worn for a total period of nine to twelve months with the cast being changed at approximately six months (Fig. 6–75).[28, 36]

In summary, one should carefully evaluate the magnitude of the problem, the natural history if not treated, and the risk, expense, and complications of treatment. Certainly in the juvenile and adolescent period, the treatment plan as outlined appears to be a rational one. In our experience, patients who wear a brace will get complete correction of the abnormal kyphosis usually within a year with little risk or complications.[38] Those who are not treated appear to run a greater risk of increased back pain and disability in the adult period. Treatment of deformity with back pain in the adult period requires considerable thought and analysis. In our experience, the results from a combined anterior and posterior fusion for patients with severe deformity unresponsive to the brace or for patients during the adult period with deformity and pain has been associated with relief of back pain in all cases and a significant improvement in the kyphosis.[36] Complications may occur and would consist of pseudarthrosis, progressive kyphosis, rod failure, and infection. Paraplegia remains a possibility but has not occurred in any of our patients to date. Finally, in those patients presenting with kyphosis and paraplegia as a result of Scheuermann's disease, surgery is the treatment of choice and would consist of anterior decompression and fusion followed by posterior fusion and Harrington instrumentation. In these cases, the benefit of operative treatment far outweighs the risks.

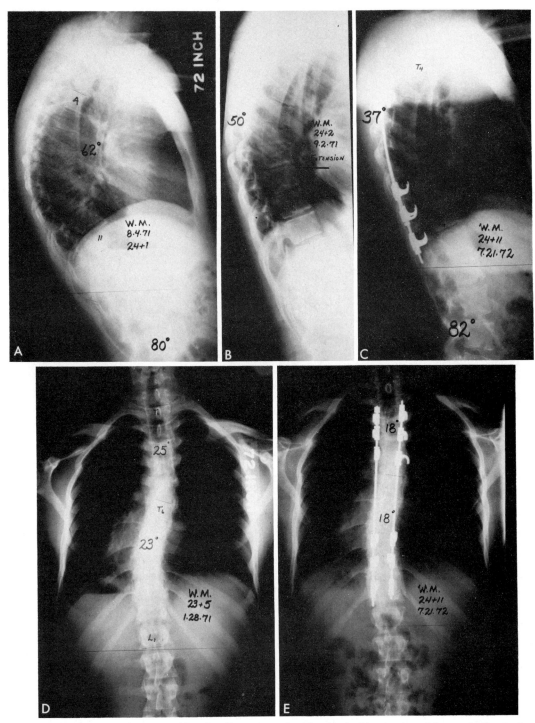

Figure 6–74. *A,* Twenty-four-year-old male who presented with a marked kyphosis and incapacitating back pain that was unresponsive to conservative management. His kyphosis was quite rigid, as noted by the hyperextension roentgenogram. (*B*). *C,* following spine fusion and Harrington rod instrumentation his deformity was improved and his back pain alleviated. He obtained an excellent correction of his deformity. He was kept supine for three months in a cast and ambulated for six months in an antigravity cast. He has shown no loss of correction since his cast was removed one year ago. *D* and *E,* His scoliotic curvature likewise showed great improvement following surgery. (From Bradford, D. S., Moe, J. H., and Winter, R. B.: Kyphosis and postural roundback deformity in children and adolescents. Minn. Med. *56*:114–120, 1973, with permission of Minn. Med.)

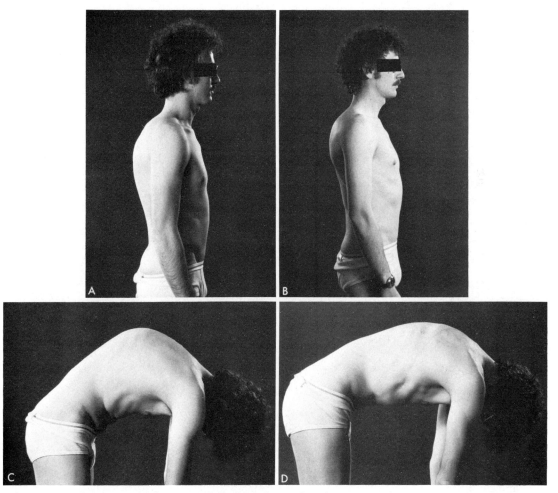

Figure 6–75.   Treatment of Scheuermann's kyphosis by combined anterior and posterior approach. *A* and *C*, preoperative appearance; *B* and *D*, postoperative appearance one year later.

Illustration continued on following page.

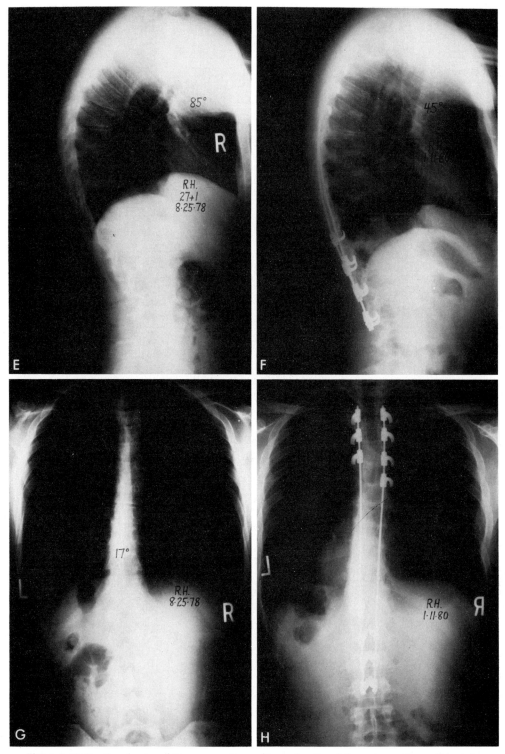

Figure 6–75 *Continued.* *E* and *G*, preoperative radiographs; *F* and *H*, postoperative radiographs.

SCOLIOSIS IN THE ADULT[65, 199, 249, 264]

Unfortunately, a significant number of patients with scoliosis in childhood receive inadequate treatment and present in adult life with complications and problems related to their curvatures. The most common complaint is pain, with less frequent complaints being dyspnea, neurologic deficit, and cosmetic malacceptance.

The nonoperative treatment of these problems is at best difficult and frequently unrewarding. Pain is best treated by immobilization in braces and corsets. Attempts to increase mobility of the curves by physical therapy usually result in increased rather than decreased pain.

Surgical correction and fusion have become an accepted form of treatment for the adult scoliotic. Careful preoperative evaluation is critical, both in general medical evaluation as well as in detailed evaluation of the curve itself, the area of pain, and the cardiopulmonary reserve.

Patients with severe curvatures and marked pulmonary deficits are a complex problem. Results at our center with a small number of patients have indicated that if a significant improvement in vital capacity and blood gases can be obtained by preoperative halo-wheelchair traction, the surgical stabilization of the curve in the corrected position is highly worthwhile. If, however, no improvement is obtained by traction, then surgical treatment is futile.

Pain has been more frequently associated with thoracolumbar and lumbar curves but also can be seen with thoracic curves.

For pain problems, stabilization has been more important than correction. Posterior fusion with instrumentation has been the procedure of choice, but certain large lumbar curves have been managed best with both anterior fusion and instrumentation as well as posterior fusion with Harrington rods (Fig. 6–76).

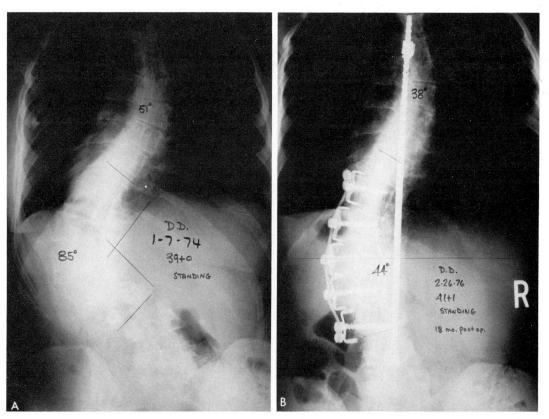

Figure 6–76. *A,* D.D., a 39-year-old female with progressive and painful idiopathic curvatures. The lumbar curve was the more progressive and more painful of the two curves. *B,* The same patient, 18 months after anterior Dwyer instrumentation, followed by fusion of the lumbar curve, posterior Harrington instrumentation, and fusion of both curves. Almost all her pain is gone.

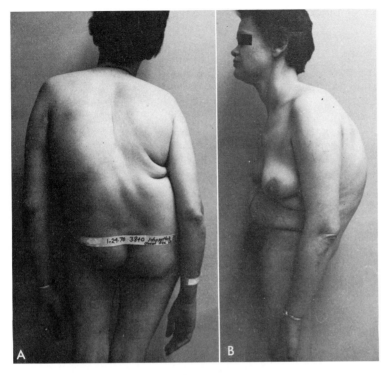

Figure 6–77. This 38-year-old female came with severely disabling back pain. She had an unsuccessful fusion of her lower back in her adolescent years.

Purely thoracic curves in younger adults are usually operated on because of continued progression during early adult life. These respond to the same type of posterior surgery used for adolescents.

Complications are far more frequent in adults, increasing with advancing age. Pseudarthrosis is directly related to age and is especially common if fusion is carried to the sacrum (Figs. 6–77 and 6–78).

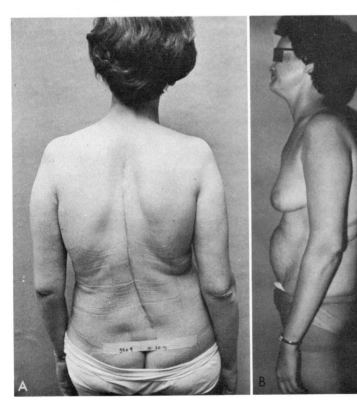

Figure 6–78. Same patient as in Figure 6–77. Treatment consisted of halofemoral distraction, multiple osteotomies of the fusion and final insertion of a Harrington distraction bar and fusion. There were no complications. The patient was relieved of her pain and the cosmetic result was excellent.

COMPLICATIONS OF UNTREATED SCOLIOSIS AND KYPHOSIS

The Natural History of Untreated Spine Deformity[11]

Untreated scoliosis may be associated with severe cosmetic deformity, major disability, and even death. It is our desire to prevent these complications that guides our recommendations to the patient and family regarding treatment of the child with bracing or surgery and treatment of the younger adult with surgery. Disability can be defined as the inability to function as a normal individual. Scoliosis may produce disability in several ways. The most common in our experience is pain, especially in the adult, but it may occur even in the adolescent. The pain may be mild or severe and may prevent successful pursuit of normal occupations. The pain appears to arise from degenerative changes in the facet joints and vertebral discs. The quantity of pain arising from the discs is not known, but most definitely pain does arise from the facet joints.

Respiratory insufficiency may produce severe disability and may reduce work power, athletic endeavor, and even employment possibilities (Fig. 6–79). Paraplegia is a major disability, of course, and can always be prevented by early adequate treatment of the curvature.

Death is a very real problem in spine deformity. Death usually occurs from respiratory insufficiency and right heart failure, although it may occur from pneumonia. There has been a tragic communication gap between the orthopaedist who treats the child with spine deformity, discharging her or him from care at age 18 "cured of the problem" and the internist who sees this patient in right heart failure at age 50.

Several authors have made significant contributions to our knowledge of the natural history of scoliosis. James[129] reviewed the course of a large number of children with untreated idiopathic scoliosis. He noted the marked tendency to progression, especially in

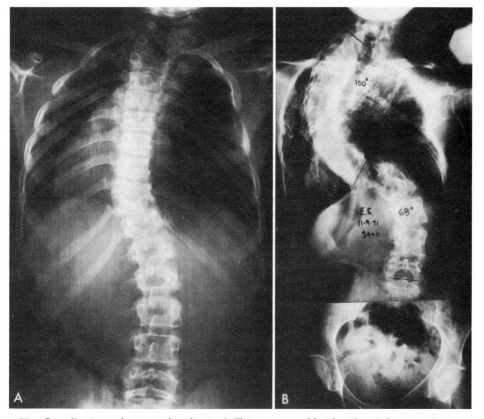

Figure 6–79. Complications of untreated scoliosis. *A,* Thirteen-year-old girl with a 47 degree scoliosis secondary to congenital anomalies of the thoracic spine. Fusion was recommended, but refused by her family. *B,* Age 35, 22 years after the previous roentgenogram. She presented at this time in early right heart failure. Life expectancy, even with medical treatment, is less than two years. The early death is directly due to the scoliosis.

infantile idiopathic scoliosis. One hundred per cent of these patients subsequently developed thoracic curvatures greater than 70 degrees. Marked progression of untreated thoracic adolescent scoliosis was also noted; 59 per cent of patients had curves of 70 degrees or more at maturity. James noted pain to be a frequent complaint in both lumbar and thoracolumbar curves.

Ponsetti and Friedman did a very similar study of untreated idiopathic scoliosis in 394 patients at the University of Iowa.[200] They noted marked progression of thoracic scoliosis with 80 per cent of the curvatures reaching 60 degrees or more. This is quite significant in that pulmonary function consistently shows a decrease in curves above 60 degrees. The amount of decrease in pulmonary function is directly related to the degree of curvature.[260] Double structural and lumbar curves are also noted to progress but in lesser amounts. The earlier the onset of the curve, the worse the prognosis. In 1969, Collis and Ponsetti reviewed the same series of patients, now some 20 years older.[60] Unfortunately, they were able to examine only 105, or 27 per cent of the original 394 patients. Collis and Ponsetti noted that thoracic curves of 60 to 80 degrees at the end of growth had progressed an average of 28 degrees. Thus, a patient with a 70 degree thoracic curve at age 18 had a 100 degree curve at age 38. Most curves were found to increase after skeletal maturity. In their study, lumbar curves appeared to progress to a lesser degree, and those less than 30 degrees did not progress, although those greater than 30 degrees progressed an average of 18 degrees. The authors did not feel that there was an increased mortality rate or an increase in the amount of back disability in adult scoliosis. Vital capacity was decreased in all thoracic curves over 85 degrees. Forty per cent of the patients noted shortness of breath. Figure 6–73 shows a patient of the original 1950 Iowa study group whose curve progressed from 65 degrees at age 17 to 101 degrees at age 38 with severe lumbar pain.

The most reliable statistics have come from Sweden, where a relatively small and nonmobile population combined with excellent data collecting has provided two superb long-term studies. Nachemson in 1969 presented an analysis of 130 nontreated patients with scoliosis of all types.[185] Of these, 117, or 90 per cent, were reviewed, and the average follow-up period was 35 years. The overall mortality was twice the normal population, and if only thoracic curves were considered, the mortality was four times the normal. There was a marked increase in death and disability at age 40. The deaths were predominantly from cardiorespiratory causes (80 per cent). Back pain was noted to be a "relatively constant" symptom in 39 of the 97 surviving patients. Twenty-five of the 97 reported constant use of a back brace or corset.

Nilsonne and Lundgren, in 1968, reviewed 117 patients with idiopathic scoliosis with a maximal follow-up time of 50 years.[190] Their retrieval rate was also 90 per cent. They also noted a 2.2 times increase of mortality, with deaths predominantly occurring from cardiorespiratory causes. The mean age of death was 46 plus 6 years. They also noted that 76 per cent of the females did not marry (probably an expression of the cosmetic deformity). Thirty per cent of the patients still alive were on disability pension because of their spine problems. An additional 17 per cent were unable to work because of spinal conditions but were not on pension. This classic article is highly recommended to anyone interested in the natural history of idiopathic scoliosis.

The relationship between lumbar scoliosis and adult low back pain is a controversial subject. An interesting contribution to this question was made by Ghavamian, who analyzed the curves in 3050 adult patients presenting with pain in the back.[91] Minor scoliosis (less than 15 degrees) was present in 852. Sixty per cent of the symptomatic curves were in the lumbar spine, and 24 per cent were cervical. Pain usually began after age 30 and seemed to be related to disc changes at the apex of the curve. Those with double curves tended to have problems at the junction of the two curves. It was the author's opinion that even small curves can produce back pain.

Except for the study by Ghavamian, the previous studies all dealt with curvatures that were already of a significant degree at the time they were originally detected, that is, curves greater than 30 degrees.

What is the natural history of curves less than 30 degrees? Studies from France on curvatures less than 30 degrees in children prior to completion of growth have indicated that many curves are not progressive. In that study, right thoracic curves and double structural curves (right thoracic and left lumbar) were more likely to progress than single lum-

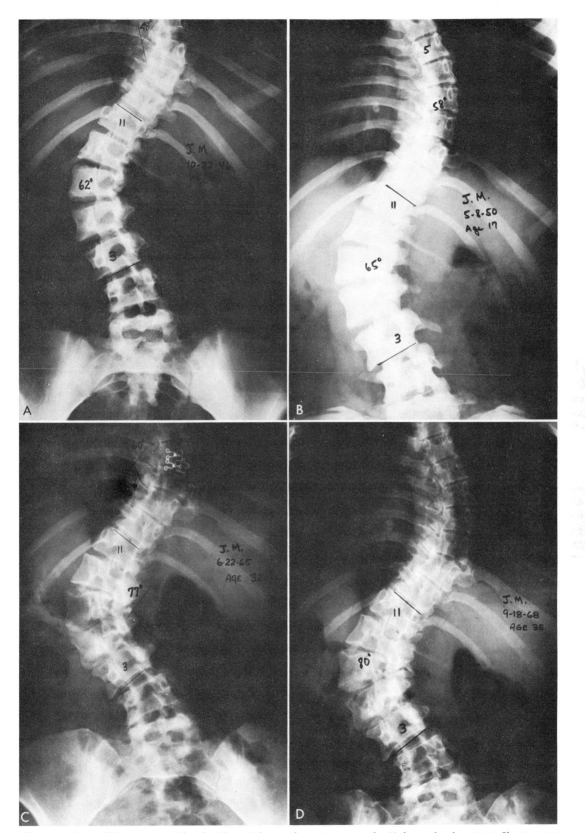

Figure 6–80. *A,* Thirteen-year-old girl with a 48 degree thoracic curve and a 62 degree lumbar curve. She was seen elsewhere and no treatment was given. *B,* Age 17, thoracic curve 58 degrees, lumbar 65 degrees. She was discharged from follow-up at this time. *C,* Age 32. She now has a 60 degree thoracic curve, and a 77 degree lumbar curve. Back pain began at about age 30. *D,* Age 35, now an 80 degree lumbar curve. Pain continues.

Illustration continued on following page.

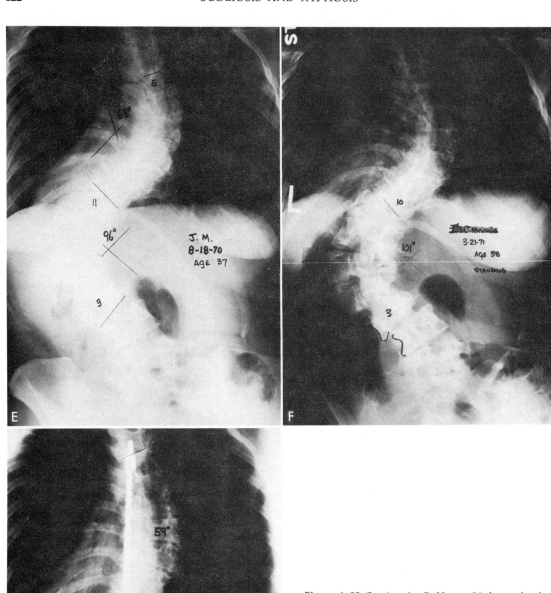

Figure 6–80 *Continued. E,* Now a 96 degree lumbar curve with increasing low back pain. *F,* The thoracic curve is 75 degrees, but the lumbar curve is 101 degrees. She not only has low back pain, but also has developed radicular pain. *G,* Age 39, one year after correction and fusion. She was fused from T5 to S1 after preliminary correction in halofemoral traction.

bar or thoracolumbar curves. The beginning of menses has marked the point at which most curves cease to progress.

Recent studies at our own institution, observing large numbers of patients detected through school screening programs, have indicated that most curvatures under 20 degrees in growing children are not progressive. A curvature of 15 degrees in a 12 year old child may spontaneously get better, may spontaneously get worse, or may remain unchanged. Approximately 70 per cent of our patients remained unchanged, only 15 per cent got worse, and 15 per cent improved spontaneously.

This spontaneous improvement has tended to indicate to some people that manipulative treatment, nighttime traction, or intermittent bracing has given improved results. One must know the natural history of these small curves before attributing therapeutic benefit to any type of treatment.

From these many reports and our own experience, the natural history of untreated spinal deformities is gradually emerging. Generally speaking, lumbar curves do not result in respiratory compromise, but, if symptomatic in the adult, the most common presenting symptom is pain. Lumbar curves seem to be more likely to progress than thoracic curves, perhaps because of the stability provided by the thoracic rib cage (Fig. 6–80).

With symptomatic thoracic curves, on the other hand, the major symptom is more likely to be respiratory insufficiency but sometimes may also be pain. Respiratory insufficiency is sometimes directly related to the curve on an AP roentgenogram, but the three-dimensional nature of scoliosis makes it imperative to evaluate the spine in a three-dimensional sense. Patients with thoracic lordosis have a much greater degree of respiratory distress than those patients with thoracic kyphosis and scoliosis.

Those patients progressing to respiratory insufficiency with right heart failure have a very poor prognosis. Salvage of the patient at this stage is nearly (but not entirely) impossible. (See section on adult scoliosis.) Death usually occurs between six months to three years from the onset of right heart failure. The right heart failure is very refractory to digitalis and other cardiac medications. The only answer to this problem is adequate and early treatment of scoliosis in the growing child.

Pain is the most frequent complaint in the adult scoliotic. This is most commonly noted in the lumbar spine or thoracolumbar junction and less commonly in the thoracic spine. The pain is a frequent indication for fusion in the adult scoliotic. It is quite common for us to see a patient, usually female, between 30 and 40 with a left lumbar scoliosis who noticed the onset of pain around age 30. She has noted a loss of height of 2 to 8 cm. after the age of 30. This is usually accompanied by an increase in the visible deformity. The pain is usually in the curve itself and not lumbosacral. Radicular pain is uncommon. The pain is alleviated by rest and is aggravated by physical activity. The pain is poorly responsive to conventional orthopaedic nonoperative measures, and when it is significantly disabling, fusion is indicated. (See section on adult scoliosis.) Finally, paraplegia is a complication that obviously produces a severe disability. It is infrequent but has been seen at this center in 50 patients. It does not occur in patients with scoliosis only regardless of the severity of the curve except in extremely rare circumstances, usually congenital scoliosis. Kyphosis, however, more frequently produces paraplegia. At our center, the most common cause was congenital kyphosis, followed by neurofibromatosis, kyphoscoliosis, a history of tuberculosis, postlaminectomy kyphosis, and other less common causes.

COMPLICATIONS OF SCOLIOSIS AND KYPHOSIS TREATMENT

Corrective spine surgery is a major undertaking and one of the most complex of orthopaedic procedures. All major operations carry a certain amount of risk, and scoliosis surgery is no exception. The complication inherent in such surgery may be divided into intraoperative, early postoperative, and late postoperative categories.

Intraoperative Complications

CARDIAC ARREST. Hypoxia is the most frequent cause of cardiac arrest. An adequate endotracheal airway must be present and securely fastened so that it will not come out while the patient is prone. Too deep insertion of the endotracheal tube may cause it to go into one main bronchus. Cardiac arrest also may be due to hypovolemia. Scoliosis surgery, if not done with great care, can result in substantial blood loss. The loss must be minimized with careful technique and must be accurately measured by laying sponges and calculated suction drainage. Blood replacement must be neither excessive nor inadequate. Too much blood will raise the venous pressure, resulting in cardiac decompensation and pulmonary edema. Inadequate blood replacement leads to hypovolemia, cardiac arrest, and brain ischemia. Blood should always be warmed before using.

Some surgeons prefer to use hypotensive anesthesia, but others prefer normotensive anesthesia because of the fear of lowered blood flow in the spinal cord by the hypotensive technique. Paraplegia due to this cause, however, has not been reported using hypotensive anesthesia.

SPINAL CORD INJURY. This may result from a direct injury to the spinal cord by surgical instrumentation or from excessive traction on the cord. Direct injury should be preventable by good surgical technique. In more than 3000 spinal fusions we have only experienced one partial paralysis due to a direct injury. This occurred in a patient with an unsuspected laminar defect due to dural ectasia of neurofibromatosis.

Cord injury due to traction is always a great fear of the scoliosis surgeon. Traction-related paraplegia was almost nonexistent in the days of plaster cast correction. Since the advent of Harrington instrumentation, halofemoral traction, and halo traction, paraplegia has been, unfortunately, more commonly reported. This is especially tragic since most of these cases occur in patients with severe curves and are, therefore, indirectly due to failure of early adequate treatment. Paraplegia is most frequent in congenital scoliosis, probably owing to the relatively common cord tethering by spinal dysraphism or bony spurs, fibrous bands, or tight filum terminale. In correcting congenital scoliosis, it is preferable to obtain the correction by traction or casting, and if Harrington rods are to be used, they should be inserted only as devices to maintain correction and not to obtain correction (Fig. 6–81).

The technique developed by Stagnara and colleagues of Lyon, France has been most helpful in our experience to assess spinal cord function in the operating room. It consists of partial awakening of the anesthetized patient after insertion of the Harrington distraction rod.[244] The patient is then requested to move the fingers and then the toes. If the toes move voluntarily, then one knows the cord is functioning at that moment. If the hands move to voluntary request but the feet do not, the rods should be loosened immediately or preferably removed, and the test should be repeated. The patient usually does not remember this episode. More sophisticated methods of electronic cord monitoring are being developed at this time but are not widespread or practical for everyday use.

All patients should be monitored carefully during the postoperative period. Patients may awaken from surgery without neurologic deficit but develop paralysis anywhere from four hours to three days later. If paralysis develops, the patient must be *immediately* returned to surgery, and the rods and all traction must be removed. Laminectomy appears to be unnecessary unless there is specific reason to suspect the presence of a fragment of bone or hematoma in the spinal canal. The patient who awakens from surgery completely paraplegic also should be instantly returned to the operating room, and rods and traction should be removed. The prognosis, however, seems to be much worse in those patients who wake up with paraplegia compared to those who develop paraplegia a few hours later.

PNEUMOTHORAX. Pneumothorax can occur during surgery for one of three primary reasons. Two of our patients have developed a tension pneumothorax secondary to a malfunctioning respirator. The spontaneous rupture of a pulmonary bleb may also lead to a tension pneumothorax. Finally, a pneumothorax without tension may develop from direct puncture of the pleura during some phase of the scoliosis surgery. This is particularly true when rib resection is being carried out as part of the operative procedure. Whenever pneumothorax occurs, regardless of the cause, chest tubes should be inserted and connected to closed underwater drainage.

HEMOTHORAX. Hemothorax may occur from rupture of an artery, either an intercostal along the rib or an intercostal branch around the vertebral bodies or transverse processes, which usually results from penetration by an instrument, resulting in laceration of a vessel. Blood loss may go undetected until severe hypotension, cardiac arrest, or both develop. In the presence of progressive hemothorax, the chest must be immediately opened, the bleeder ligated, and a chest tube inserted.

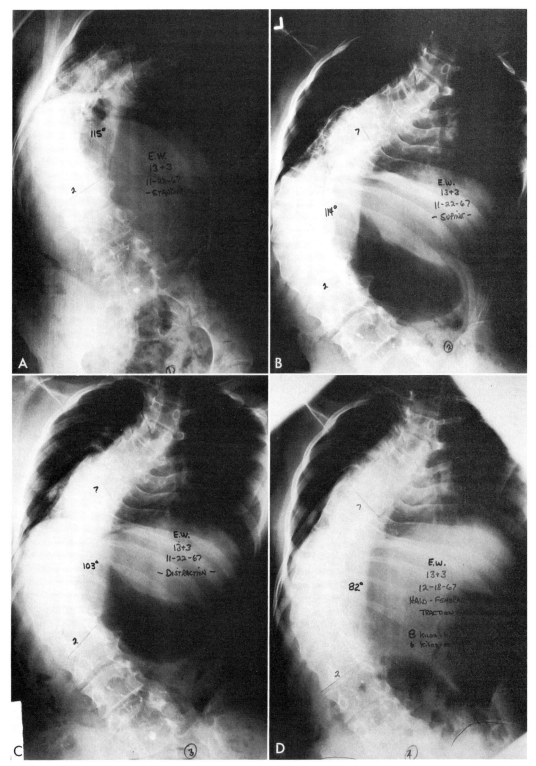

Figure 6–81. Complications in treated scoliosis. *A,* Thirteen-year-old female with a 115 degree congenital scoliosis. It is tragic that a patient be allowed to reach such a severe deformity. She had a mid-lumbar hair patch on the back and a mild cavus of the right foot. *B,* Supine roentgenogram showing no improvement in the curve. *C,* Distraction roentgenogram also showing little curve improvement. This amount of rigidity is typical of the patient with congenital scoliosis. *D,* Correction from 115 degrees to 82 degrees in halofemoral traction.

Illustration continued on following page.

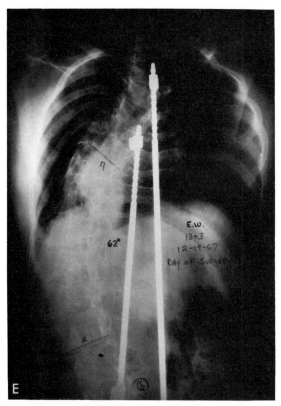

Figure 6–81 *Continued.* *E,* Additional correction from 82 degrees to 62 degrees was obtained in surgery with Harrington instrumentation. Unfortunately, the patient awoke with a paraplegia. The rods were removed and she experienced 75 to 80 per cent recovery, but lost the correction of the scoliosis. Correction greater than that obtained by halofemoral traction should not be attempted.

Postoperative Complications (Early)

RESPIRATORY DISTRESS. Respiratory distress is a major postoperative problem that is of concern in all patients undergoing scoliosis surgery, but it is of particular concern in those patients who already have a respiratory deficit. For this reason, preoperative evaluation of pulmonary function is routinely employed in our center and certainly should be employed for all patients in whom there is any suspicion whatsoever that there may be a deficit of pulmonary function. The knowledge that such a deficit is present will enable one to better plan for complications. Preoperative instructions in respiratory exercises and practical training on the IPPB machine are helpful measures. Patients with severe respiratory deficits (less than 25 per cent vital capacity,

reversal of blood gases, or both) may require preoperative tracheostomy or postoperative management on a respirator with nasotracheal intubation.

The patient who develops atelectasis during the postoperative period will usually have some restlessness, elevation of temperature, and increased respiratory rate. Whenever possible, the lungs should be cleaned out by vigorous coughing and suctioning. In some cases, lavage of the intratracheal tree will be necessary. Antibiotic therapy should be given at this time. A frank pneumonitis may pose major problems.

One patient expired of a fulminating pneumonia four days postoperatively despite all medical measures to control it. Pneumonia is most common in those patients who have respiratory deficits. Frequent turning of the patient is necessary as is the avoidance of excessive sedation. Patients with ineffective cough mechanisms should be suctioned by the nursing staff frequently. In high-risk patients, the insertion of a nasotracheal tube at the time of surgery and maintenance on a respiratory machine to allow adequate ventilation as well as a route for suctioning is important. Usually the nasotracheal tube can be removed in 24 to 48 hours as soon as the major pain and need for narcotics have subsided. If necessary, patients can be maintained on nasotracheal tubes as long as seven days, but if additional time is needed, a tracheostomy should be done. We have had to do only one tracheostomy for such respiratory support in the last seven years at this center.

GENITOURINARY TRACT INFECTIONS. Urinary tract infections are problems for any patient that has had a major operative procedure and can almost always be prevented if catheterization can be avoided. The patients are not catheterized routinely. Intermittent catheterization is preferable to indwelling catheterization. Narcotics such as morphine that depress bladder function should be avoided.

GASTROINTESTINAL TRACT PROBLEMS. With the avoidance of morphine, ileus has been very infrequent in our service. It is quite customary for the bowel sounds to be present on the evening of surgery and almost always on the following day. Clear liquid customarily can be started the day following surgery if the bowel sounds are present. The most difficult gastrointestinal problem is vascular obstruction of the duodenum.[78] Vascular obstruction of the duodenum, previously called the "cast syndrome," is the obstruction of the third portion of the duodenum by the superior mesenteric artery. It appears to occur as a result of the correction of the curve and narrowing of the angle between the superior mesenteric artery and the aorta. It presents as a high intestinal obstruction, with vomiting and epigastric discomfort but minimal bowel distention. The stomach may enlarge dramatically (Fig. 6–82).

The treatment for vascular obstruction of the duodenum is quick recognition and insertion of a nasogastric tube and the use of nasogastric suction and intravenous fluids for two to three days. Usually by this time the problem has spontaneously regressed. The tube can be removed and oral liquids begun. One should then progress to soft foods and then to a regular diet. Procrastination may

lead to an intractable obstruction requiring surgery. If surgery is necessary, a side-to-side duodenojejunostomy appears preferable. On occasions, mobilization of the ligamentum of Treitz can alleviate the problem. The need for surgery has been markedly reduced within the last five years by prompt recognition and early treatment. The patient with repeated vomiting, epigastric distress, and no distention of the small or large bowel but a large gastric distention should be suspected of having this problem. The diagnosis can be confirmed by contrast study, which shows the obstruction of the third part of the duodenum. Usually there is dilation of the proximal duodenum and if viewed under fluoroscopy there will be "writhing" of the duodenum owing to its attempts to pass material beyond the obstruction. Untreated obstruction may result in death from gastric rupture or electrolyte imbalance.

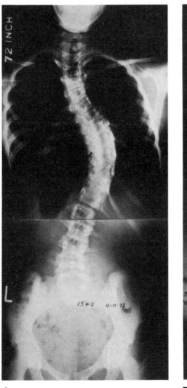
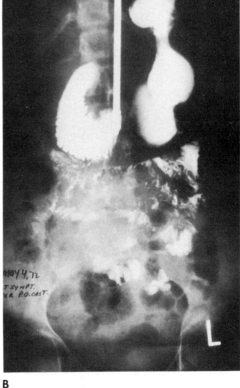

A   **B**

Figure 6–82. *A,* Thirteen-year-old girl with idiopathic scoliosis. There is a 60 degree T5-T12 right thoracic curve. Surgery was recommended. *B,* Barium study 10 days after surgery shows a nearly complete obstruction of the duodenum. Note the dilatation of the duodenum. Her symptoms were persistent vomiting and epigastric tenderness. She responded to four days of nasogastric suction. Abdominal surgery was not required.

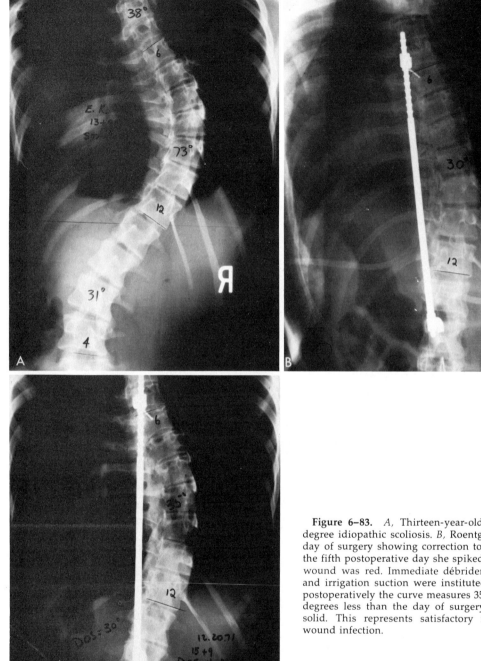

Figure 6–83. *A,* Thirteen-year-old girl with a 73 degree idiopathic scoliosis. *B,* Roentgenogram on the day of surgery showing correction to 30 degrees. On the fifth postoperative day she spiked a fever and the wound was red. Immediate débridement, irrigation, and irrigation suction were instituted. *C,* Two years postoperatively the curve measures 35 degrees, only 5 degrees less than the day of surgery. The fusion is solid. This represents satisfactory management of wound infection.

This complication may arise late and has resulted in the death of two of our patients, one at six weeks postoperatively and the other at three months postoperatively. Both of these occurred at home, were not recognized by the family physicians, and the patients were not referred soon enough back to our center.

WOUND INFECTION.   Wound infection is a significant potential problem owing to the large area of the wound and the relatively longer period of surgery time compared to some orthopaedic operations. Local trauma and hematoma also may predispose to infection. The incidence of infection may be markedly decreased by (1) delicate but brisk operative technique, minimizing muscle damage and the length of the surgical exposure, (2) proper operating room technique and avoidance of excessive traffic and talking along with maintenance of proper prepping and draping routines, and (3) use of prophylactic antibiotics. Prior to the routine use of prophylactic antibiotics at our main hospital, we were experiencing 5.3 per cent infection rate in scoliosis patients with Harrington instrumentation. After institution of routine prophylactic antibiotics using a cephalosporin intravenously during surgery and for 48 hours after surgery, the infection rate has been reduced to less than 1 per cent. Similar results have been reported by other authors. We do not feel that antibiotics given earlier than the morning of surgery or later than 48 hours after surgery are of any benefit.

If an infection develops, prompt diagnosis and immediate treatment are mandatory. It is tempting to "sit on the problem" and to start antibiotics and wait for a culture report. This is not correct management. The treatment of choice is to recognize the possibility of wound infection, to obtain a culture, and then to immediately take the patient to surgery. Under general anesthesia the patient is prepped and draped for sterile surgery, and the *entire* wound is opened. Further cultures are obtained from deep tissues. All sutures are removed down to the fusion mass, and the wound is thoroughly irrigated. Any dead or necrotic tissues are debrided. The wound is then irrigated with an antibiotic solution. The wound is closed over the suction-irrigation tubes. Closure should be done in a conventional cosmetic manner. Heavy retention sutures should be avoided. The suction and irrigation system is continued for five to seven days. At that time, if the patient is afebrile and the wound appears clean, the irrigation is discontinued, and the suction is discontinued 24 hours later. We no longer feel that culturing of the suction tube is of any value and that treatment of the wound by this technique for longer than five to seven days is of no value. Antibiotics are, of course, given in large doses intravenously during surgery and during the week after surgery, followed by oral antibiotics for approximately six weeks.

At surgery, the bone graft and the rods are not disturbed or removed. This is important to avoid compromising the scoliosis fusion. Under this program, infections have been handled with extremely good results (Fig. 6–83).

Postoperative Complications (Late)

"ADDING ON".   "Adding on" is a problem wherein the curvature is longer than it was originally, that is, there are vertebrae in the curve that were initially not part of the curve. It may be a problem of improper selection of the fusion area, or it can occur even though the proper area was selected, particularly in children with many years of growth remaining. We feel that all vertebrae that are rotated in the same direction as the vertebra at the apex of the curve should be included in the fusion area. This would mean that the curve ending at T12 may have rotation of L1 and L2 or even L3 in the same direction of the apical vertebra, in which case the fusion would include all rotated vertebrae. It is preferable to go one further, that is, to the furthest nonrotated vertebra. This will avoid "adding on" in many cases.

"Adding on" may also occur even though the proper fusion area was selected. This is particularly true of those patients undergoing fusion before the adolescent growth spurt. The problem sometimes can be prevented by the continual use of a Milwaukee brace following fusions in young children but may occur despite this preventive measure. If "adding on" occurs, then the fusion should be extended to include the additional vertebrae (Fig. 6–84).

BENDING OF THE FUSION.   The fusion mass may bend. This is particularly true of those patients undergoing fusion while quite young. Sometimes patients have both "adding on" and bending of the primary curve. Bend-

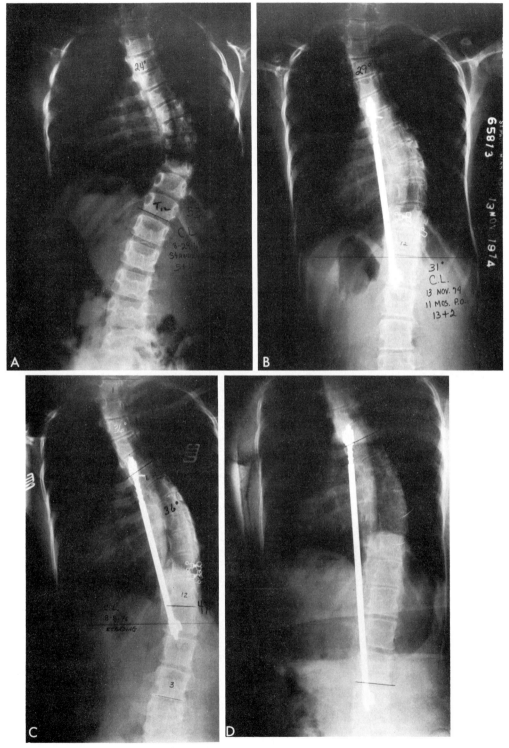

Figure 6–84. This patient underwent spinal fusion and Harrington rod instrumentation from T5 to L1. However, the fusion was too short, and "adding on" resulted. This required extension of the fusion to L4 (*D*).

ing is apparently due to continuous stresses placed upon the fusion mass with absorption of bone in some areas and deposition of bone in others. Bending is best prevented by the creation of a large, thick fusion mass at the time of the original surgery. This is less likely to bend than a thin fusion mass. In some patients it is best to go anteriorly and do a convex interbody fusion, which will eliminate the growth plate anteriorly and add a greater degree of mass to the fusion area. If bending of the fusion mass is produced in excessive loss of correction, it can be solved by osteotomy of the fusion mass at multiple levels to redirect the fusion.

PSEUDARTHROSIS. Pseudarthrosis is an accepted complication of scoliosis surgery. Advanced surgical technique over the past 20 years, particularly the use of facet joint fusion and abundant autogenous cancellous bone graft, have lowered the pseudarthrosis rate from levels as high as 50 per cent 20 years ago to about 5 per cent today. Most centers doing large volumes of surgery for idiopathic scoliosis experience pseudarthrosis rates of less than 1 per cent in adolescents. The recognition of the pseudarthrosis is most important.

We routinely take oblique roentgenograms of the fusion mass at the time the cast is removed. If pseudarthrosis is noted at this time, an exploration graft is carried out, and the pseudarthrosis is repaired even if there has been no loss of correction. We would prefer to prevent a loss of correction rather than the need for recorrection by early and aggressive pseudarthrosis repair.

If a pseudarthrosis has been missed and the patient is allowed to go without a cast, loss of correction will usually occur. Eventually the Harrington rod will break. A broken Harrington rod should be viewed as an indicator of pseudarthrosis and not as any failure of the metallic implant. At reexploration a pseudarthrosis may not be easy to see. In some cases it is necessary to remove the rods and decorticate the entire fusion mass before the pseudarthrosis will be evident. New instruments should be inserted, and one or more compression rods should be added. It appears that the pseudarthrosis will heal better with the compressive force applied across it. Adequate bone graft should also be added to the pseudarthrosis area. Often this can be obtained by shaving from the solid portion of the fusion, but if the remainder of the fusion mass is poor or if the pseudarthrosis is quite loose, additional iliac bone may be desirable.

Pseudarthrosis is more likely to occur in the lumbar than the thoracic spine. It is more common in paralytic curves than in idiopathic or congenital curves. It is especially common in patients in whom fusion extends to the sacrum. It is also age-related in that the older the individual, the greater the likelihood of pseudarthrosis. Patients with neurofibromatosis and dystrophic curves also have a high incidence of pseudarthrosis.

For patients with particularly high likelihood of pseudarthrosis due to one or more of the factors just mentioned, it can be a wise plan to routinely explore the fusion mass at six months and either repair the pseudarthrosis if present or, if not, augment the fusion by the addition of further bone and maintenance of the cast for an additional four to six months.

LATE INFECTION. Late infections are those making their appearance after the patient is discharged from the hospital. This may become evident in only a few days to even years after the surgery. It usually presents as a small draining sinus. The patient is usually afebrile, and the wound demonstrates little reaction. The treatment is the same as for acute infection, that is, the wound is opened in its entirety and all necrotic, dead material is debrided. The rods should be removed in order to make a better debridement, but if the fusion is not yet solid, the rods should be reinserted. If, however, the fusion mass is completely solid and weeks or months have elapsed since the time of surgery, the rods can be permanently removed and the wound can be closed over suction irrigation.

It is dangerous and only a procrastinating procedure merely to administer antibiotics or to place a drain in the wound. A complete and thorough debridement is mandatory.

LOSS OF LUMBAR LORDOSIS. One of the most disturbing complications of fusion of the lumbar spine is elimination of lumbar lordosis. This rarely occurred prior to the use of Harrington instrumentation and has only recently been recognized as a specific complication. The problem arises when the Harrington distraction rod is inserted from L5 or the sacrum to T12 or above. This distraction effect removes the normal lumbar lordosis, tending to produce a fixed forward leaning of the patient. The patient must compensate by hyperextending the thoracic spine or the hips or bending the knees. All these compensatory mechanisms, however, become fatiguing and are cosmetically unsightly. The gait pattern becomes quite abnormal.

Treatment consists of rod removal and a closing wedge osteotomy of the lumbar spine, attempting to gain lumbar lordosis. This is a difficult procedure, and great care must be taken not to compress any of the nerve roots. At least two heavy compression rods should be used to stabilize this osteotomy.

The problem is better prevented than treated. If a fusion is necessary to the sacrum, the rods must be bent into a significant degree of lordosis using a rod bender. Compression instrumentation on the convex side of the curve can also foster a certain degree of lordosis and prevent some of the loss of lumbar lordosis. When using bent rods in the lumbar spine only, one must use square-ended rods with square-hole hooks in order to prevent rotation of the rods. An alternative is using regular rods but wiring the rods to the apex of the lumbar lordosis by heavy wire under the laminae and around the rod.

STUNTING OF TRUNK LENGTH. An extensive fusion at a young age will, of course, produce a shortening of trunk height. The fusion mass does not elongate with growth. Long-term follow-up studies by Moe and Sundberg of patients undergoing fusion earlier than age ten reveal the average lengthening of the fusion mass to be only 1 mm. in five years.[263] These studies were done by inserting metal markers at the top and bottom of the fusion area and measuring them by standardized roentgenograms at yearly intervals. Similar studies have been done by other authors.

There are situations, such as congenital scoliosis, in which it is absolutely necessary to do a fusion in a young child because the abnormal area would not grow anyway; there is no loss of trunk height due to the fusion. There are other situations in which fusion at a young age is absolutely necessary, and the ultimate goal of a short, straight trunk will be better than a short, severely crooked trunk, a good example being a dystrophic curve of neurofibromatosis.

There are, however, many situations in which the fusion can be avoided or at least delayed until significant growth has taken place. Milwaukee brace treatment of juvenile idiopathic scoliosis has proved extremely beneficial in delaying and even totally preventing the need for fusion.

A recent development designed to maintain trunk growth and curve control has been the use of the Harrington rod subcutaneously anchored to the bone in the usual manner but without exposure of the vertebrae except at the points of hook insertion. The rod is protected externally by some type of orthosis at all times. At intervals of six to twelve months, the rod is lengthened or replaced. The curve can be controlled while growth is being maintained. Ultimately, of course, a fusion will be necessary, but often five or six years of growth can be obtained by this technique.

LORDOSIS IN THE FUSED AREA. Lordosis in the fused area can be caused by the effect of the posterior epiphysiodesis of an early fusion with continued anterior growth. This problem is most evident in patients with paralytic curvatures having a long fusion at a young age. Because of the lack of bone graft material, the fusion mass tends to be very thin. The growth plates anteriorly seem to be able to bend the thin fusion mass posteriorly. In our experience, also noted in a study by Moe and Sundberg,[180] this complication is relatively infrequent. It seems that the thicker the fusion mass is posteriorly, the less likely it is to be bent. Present treatment of early curvatures with the Milwaukee brace has lessened the need for extension fusion in the young patient; therefore, this problem is less frequently seen than in previous years. If for any reason lordosis is becoming a significant problem, anterior epiphysiodesis and arthrodesis may have to be done to arrest the deformity.

Sometimes the lordosis is not due to the fusion but rather to the inherent deformity, which obviously would be determined by preoperative lateral roentgenograms. Sometimes it also can be due to the position the patient was placed in at the time of the surgery. Localizers, which push upward from behind while the patient lies on his back on the casting table, may produce lordosis if the spine is sufficiently flexible. Harrington compression instruments are a helpful adjunct to surgery, but if tightened considerably, they may produce lordosis and should be avoided in patients who are already lordotic.

References

1. Adelstein, L. J.: Spinal extradural cyst associated with kyphosis dorsalis juvenilis. J. Bone Joint Surg. 23:93–101, 1941.
2. Akbarnia, B., Winter, R. B., Moe, J. H., Bradford, D. S., and Lonstein, J. E.: Surgical treatment of spine deformity in cerebral palsy. Ottawa, Scoliosis Research Society, 1976.
3. Albanese, A.: Le cifosi dell'adolescenze. Zrch. di ortho. 52:189–268, 1936.
4. Albee, F. H.: A report of bone transplantation and

osteoplasty in the treatment of Pott's disease of spine. New York Med. J. *95*:469, 1912.

5. Anderson, M., Hwang, S. C., and Green, W. T.: Growth of the normal trunk in boys and girls during the second decade of life. J. Bone Joint Surg. *47A*:1554, 1965.

6. Anderson, S., and Bradford, D. S.: Low profile halo. Clin. Orthop. *103*:72, 1974.

7. Barr, J. S., and Buschenfeldt, K.: Turnbuckle brace. J. Bone Joint Surg. *18*:760, 1936.

8. Becker, K.: Uber die Behandlung jugendlicher Kyphosen mit einem aktiven bzw. einem Kombinierten zweiteiligen aktiv-passiven Reklinationskorsett. Ztschr. Orthop. *89*:464–475, 1958.

9. Bergofsky, E. H., Turino, G. M., and Fishman, A. P.: Cardiorespiratory failure in kyphoscoliosis. Medicine *38*:263, 1959.

10. Bick, E. M., and Copel, J. W.: Ring apophysis of human vertebra; contribution to human osteogeny. J. Bone Joint Surg. *33A*:783–787, 1951.

11. Bjure, J., and Nachemson, A.: Non-treated scoliosis. Clin. Orthop. *93*:44–52, 1973.

12. Bjure, J., Grimby, G., Kasalicky, J., Lindh, M., and Nachemson, A.: Respiratory impairment and airway closure in patients with untreated idiopathic scoliosis. Thorax *25*:451, 1970.

13. Block, A. J., Wexler, J., and McDonnell, E. J.: Cardiopulmonary failure of the hunchback: A possible therapeutic approach. J.A.M.A. *212*:1520, 1970.

14. Blount, W. P.: Congenital Scoliosis, pp. 748–762. In Huitieme Congres de la Societe International de Chirurgie Orthopedique et de Traumatologie. New York, 4–9 September, 1960. Brussells, Imprimerie des Sciences, 1961.

15. Blount, W. P.: Physical therapy in the nonoperative treatment of scoliosis. Phys. Ther. *47*:919–925, 1967.

16. Blount, W. P.: Early recognition and prompt evaluation of spinal deformity. J. Iowa Med. Soc. *59*:1015–1025, 1969.

17. Blount, W. P.: Use of the Milwaukee brace. Orthop. Clin North Am. *3*:3–16, 1972.

18. Blount, W. P.: Bracing for scoliosis. Orthotics etcetera, B617–92. L617. pp. 306–332, 1966.

19. Blount, W. P., and Moe, J. H.: The Milwaukee Brace. Baltimore, The Williams & Wilkins Co., 1973.

20. Blount, W. P., Schmidt, A. C., and Bidwell, R. G.: Making the Milwaukee brace. J. Bone Joint Surg. *40A*:523–528, 1958.

21. Blount, W. P., Schmidt, A. C., Kevver, D., and Leonard, E. L.: The Milwaukee brace in the operative treatment of scoliosis. J. Bone Joint Surg. *40A*:511, 1958.

22. Blount, W. P., Schmidt, A. C., Kevver, D., and Leonard, E. L.: The Milwaukee brace in nonoperative scoliosis treatment. Acta Orthop. Scand. *33*:399, 1963.

23. Bonnett, C., Brown, J., and Brooks, H. L.: Anterior spine fusion with Dwyer instrumentation for lumbar scoliosis in cerebral palsy. J. Bone Joint Surg. *55A*:425, 1973.

24. Bonnett, C., Brown, J., and Grow, T.: Thoracolumbar scoliosis in cerebral palsy — results of surgical treatment. J. Bone Joint Surg. *58-A*:328–336, 1976.

25. Bonnett, C., Brown, J., Perry, J., Nickel, V., Walinski, T., Brooks, H. L., Hoffer, M., Stiles, C., and Brooks, R.: The evolution of treatment of paralytic scoliosis at Rancho Los Amigos Hospital. J. Bone Joint Surg. *57A*:206–215, 1975.

26. Boyer, A.: Étude de la restriction ventilatoire des scolioses adultes avant et après traitment chirurgical. M.D. Thesis, Claude Bernard University, Lyon, 1973.

27. Bradford, D. S.: Neurological complications in Scheuermann's disease. J. Bone Joint Surg. *51A*:567–572, 1969.

28. Bradford, D. S.: Juvenile kyphosis. Clin. Orthop. *128*:45, 1977.

29. Bradford, D. S. (guest ed.): Kyphosis symposia. Clin. Orthop. *128*:2, 1977.

30. Bradford, D. S.: Anterior spinal surgery in the management of scoliosis: Indications, techniques, results. Orthop. Clin. North Am. *10*:4, 1979.

31. Bradford, D. S., and Moe, J. H.: Scheuermann's juvenile kyphosis: A histologic study. Clin. Orthop. *110*:45, 1975.

32. Bradford, D. S., and Moe, J. H.: Scheuermann's juvenile kyphosis: A histologic study. Clin. Orthop. *110*:45, 1975.

33. Bradford, D. S., Moe, J. H., and Winter, R. B.: Kyphosis and postural roundback deformity in children and adolescents. Minn. Med. *56*:114–120, 1973.

34. Bradford, D. S., Moe, J. H., Montalvo, F. J., and Winter, R. B.: Scheuermann's kyphosis and roundback deformity — results of Milwaukee brace treatment. J. Bone Joint Surg. *56A*:740–758, 1974.

35. Bradford, D. S., Moe, J. H., Winter, R. B. and Montalvo, F. J.: Scheuermann's kyphosis. Results of surgical treatment by posterior spine arthrodesis in 22 patients. J. Bone Joint Surg. *57A*:439, 1975.

36. Bradford, D. S., Ahmed, K. B., Moe, J. H., Winter, R. B., and Lonstein, J. E.: The surgical management of patients with Scheuermann's disease. A review of 24 patients managed by combined anterior and posterior spine fusion. J. Bone Joint Surg. *62A*:705–712; 1980.

37. Bradford, D. S., Moe, J. H., Winter, R. B., and Montalvo, F. J.: Scheuermann's kyphosis: Results of surgical treatment by posterior spine arthrodesis in 22 patients. J. Bone Joint Surg. *57A*:439, 1975.

38. Bradford, D. S., Montalvo, F. J., Winter, R. B., and Moe, J. H.: Scheuermann's kyphosis and roundback deformity: Results of Milwaukee brace treatment. J. Bone Joint Surg. *56A*:740, 1974.

39. Bradford, D. S., Winter, R. B., Lonstein, J. E., and Moe, J. H.: Techniques of anterior spine surgery for the management of kyphosis. Clin. Orthop. *128*:129, 1977.

40. Bradford, D. S., Brown, D. M., Moe, J. H., Winter, R. B., and Jowsey, J.: Scheuermann's kyphosis: A form of osteoporosis? Clin. Orthop. *118*:10, 1976.

41. Bradford, D. S., Ganjavian, S., Antonious, D., Winter, R. B., Lonstein, J. E., and Moe, J. H.: Anterior strut grafting for the treatment of kyphosis, Spine; in press.

42. Brocher, J. E. W.: Die Scheuermannsche Krankheit und ihre Differentialdiagnose. Basel. B. Schwabe & Co., 1946.

43. Brocher, J. E. W.: Die Wirbelsaulentuberkulose und Ihre Differentialdiagnose. Stuttgurt, G. Thieme, 1953.

44. Brooks, H. L., Azen, S. P., Gerberg, E., Brooks, R., and Chan, L.: Scoliosis: A prospective epidemiologic study. J. Bone Joint Surg. 57A:968–972, 1975.

45. Brooks, L., Gerberg, E., Mazur, H., Brooks, R., and Nickel, V. L.: The epidemiology of scoliosis—a prospective study, Orthop. Rev. 1:17, 1972.

46. Brown, D. M., Jowsey, J., and Bradford, D. S.: Osteoporosis in ovarian dysgenesis. J. Pediatr. 84:816, 1974.

47. Bunch, W. H.: In Bunch, W. H., Cassl, A. S., Bernsman, A. S., and Long, D. M. (eds): Modern Management of Myelomeningocoele. St. Louis, W. H. Green, Inc., 1972. pp. 121–167.

48. Bunch, W. H.: The Milwaukee Brace in paralytic scoliosis. Clin. Orthop. 110:63–68, 1975.

49. Bunnell, W. P., and MacEwen, G. D.: Use of orthoplast jacket in the nonoperative treatment of scoliosis; presented at Annual Meeting of Scoliosis Research Society, Louisville, Kentucky, 1975. J. Bone Joint Surg., 58A:156, 1976.

50. Bunnell, W. P., and MacEwen, G. D.: Nonoperative treatment of scoliosis in cerebral palsy: Preliminary report on the use of a plastic jacket. Devel. Med. Child Neurol. 19:45–49, 1977.

51. Butler, R. W.: The nature and significance of vertebral osteochondritis. Proc. R. Soc. Med. (Section of Orthopedics) 48:895, 1955.

52. Caro, C. G., and DuBois, A. B.: Pulmonary function in kyphoscoliosis. Thorax 16:282, 1961.

53. Carr, W. A., and Moe, J. H.: Treatment of idiopathic scoliosis in the Milwaukee brace: Long-term results. J. Bone Joint Surg. 62A:599–612, 1980.

54. Chapman, E. M., Dill, D. B., and Graybill, A.: The decrease in functional capacity of the lungs and heart resulting from deformities of the chest: Pulmonocardiac failure. Medicine 18:167, 1939.

55. Clarisse, P.: Pronostic evolutif des scolioses idiopathiques mineures de 10° à 29° en periode de croissance. Thesis, Univ. Claude-Bernard, Lyon, September 20, 1974.

56. Cloward, R. B., and Bucy, P. C.: Spinal extradural cyst and kyphosis dorsalis juvenilis. Am. J. Roentgenol. 38:681–706, 1937.

57. Cobb, J. R.: Outline for the Study of Scoliosis. Instructional Course Lectures, and American Academy of Orthopaedic Surgeons, 5:261. Ann Arbor, J.W. Edwards, 1948.

58. Cobb, J. R.: Spine arthrodesis in the treatment of scoliosis. Bull. Hosp. Jt. Dis. 19:187, 1958.

59. Cockrell, R., and Risser, J.: Plastic body jacket in the treatment of scoliosis. Exhibit at the annual meeting of the American Academy of Orthopaedic Surgeons, Las Vegas, Nevada, 1973.

60. Collis, D. K., and Ponseti, I. V.: Long-term follow-up of patients with idiopathic scoliosis not treated surgically. J. Bone Joint Surg. 51A:425–445, 1969.

61. Cook, C. D., Barrie, H., Deforest, S. A., and Helliesen, P. J.: Pulmonary physiology in children. III. Lung volumes, mechanics of respiration and respiratory muscle strength in scoliosis. J. Pediatr. 25:766, 1960.

62. Cotrel, Y.: La scoliose idiopathique (Fr.). Acta Orthop. Belg. 31:796–810, 1975.

63. Cotrel, Y.: La technique de L'E.D.F. dans la correction des scolioses. Rev. Chir. Orthop. 50:59–75, 1964.

64. Cowell, H. R., Hall, J. N., and MacEwen, G. D.: Genetic aspects of idiopathic scoliosis. Clin. Orthop. 86:121–132, 1972.

65. Cummine, J., Lonstein, J., Moe, J., Winter, R., and Bradford, D.: Reconstructive surgery in the adult for failed scoliosis fusion. J. Bone Joint. Surg. 61A:1151–1161, 1979.

66. Dameron, T. B., and Gulledge, W. H.: Adolescent kyphosis. U. S. Armed Forces Med. J. 4:871–875, 1953.

67. Dawson, E., Moe, J. H., and Winter, R. B.: Surgical treatment of scoliosis in the adult. In Preparation.

68. Dayman, H.: The expiratory spirogram. Am. Rev. Resp. Dis. 83:842, 1961.

69. DeWald, R. L., and Ray, R. D.: Skeletal traction for treatment of severe scoliosis. The University of Illinois halo-hoop apparatus. J. Bone Joint Surg. 52A:233–238, 1970.

70. Dollery, C. T., Gillam, P. M. S., Hugh-Jones, P., and Zorab, P. A.: Regional lung function in kyphoscoliosis. Thorax 20:175, 1965.

71. Drummond, D., Rogala, E., and Gurr, J.: School screening, a community project. Paper presented at the Quebec Scoliosis Society Meeting, Montreal, June, 1976.

72. Duval-Beaupere, G.: Pathogenic relationship between scoliosis and growth. In Zorab, P. A., (ed.): Scoliosis and Growth. London, Churchill Livingstone, 1971, pp. 58–64.

73. Dwyer, A.: An anterior approach to scoliosis. A preliminary report. Clin. Orthop. 62:192–202, 1969.

74. Dwyer, A. F.: Experience of anterior correction of scoliosis. Clin. Orthop. 93:191–206, 1973.

75. Edgren, W.: Osteochondrosis juvenilis lumbalis. Acta Chir. Scand. Suppl. 227:1–47, 1957.

76. Elsberg, C. A., Dyke, C. G., and Brewer, E. D.: The symptoms and diagnosis of extradural cysts. Bull Neurol. Inst. 3:395–417, 1934.

77. Erkkila, J. C., Warwick, W. J., and Bradford D. S.: Spine deformities and cystic fibrosis. Clin. Orthop. 131:146, 1978.

78. Evarts, C. M., Winter, R. B., and Hall, J. E.: Vascular compression of the duodenum associated with the treatment of scoliosis. Review of the literature and report of 18 cases. J. Bone Joint Surg. 53A:431–444, 1971.

79. Ferguson, A. B., Jr.: Etiology of pre-adolescent kyphosis. J. Bone Joint Surg. 38A:149–157, 1956.

80. Ferguson, A. B., Jr.: Round back in children. J. Med. Assoc. Georgia 45:458–460, 1956.

81. Fishman, A. P.: Pulmonary aspects of scoliosis. In Zorab, P. A. (ed.): Proceedings of a Symposium on Scoliosis. National Fund for Research into Poliomyelitis and Other Crippling Diseases. London, Vincent House, p. 52.

82. Fisk, J., Winter, R. B., and Moe, J. H.: The lumbosacral articulation and its relationship to scoliosis. Scoliosis Research Society Eighth Annual Meeting, Goteburg, Sweden, 1973.

83. Flagstad, A. E., and Kollman, S.: Vital capacity and muscle study in one hundred cases of scoliosis. J. Bone Joint Surg. 10:724, 1928.

84. Freyschuss, U., Nilsonne, U., and Lundgren, K. D.: Idiopathic scoliosis in old age. Acta Med. Scand. 184:365, 1968.

85. Fry, D. L., and Hyatt, R. E.: Pulmonary mechanics: An amplified analysis of the relationship between pressure, volume, and gas flow in the lungs of normal and diseased human subjects. Am. J. Med. 29:672, 1960.

86. Gardemin, H., and Herbst, W.: Wirbeldeformierung bei der Adoleszentenkyphose und Osteoporose. Arch. Orthop. Unfallchir. 59:134, 1966.

87. Garrett, A. L.: Stabilization of the collapsing spine. J. Bone Joint Surg. 42A:883, 1960.

88. Garrett, A., Perry, J., and Nickel, V.: Stabilization of the collapsing spine. J. Bone Joint Surg. 43A:4, 1961.

89. Gazioglu, K., Goldstein, L. A., Femi-Pearse, D., and Yu, P. N.: Pulmonary function in idiopathic scoliosis. J. Bone Joint Surg. 50A:1391, 1968.

90. George, K. A.: Comparative study of the two popular methods of measuring scoliotic deformity of the spine. J. Bone Joint Surg. 43A:809–818, 1961.

91. Ghavamian, T.: The future of minor scoliotic curves of the spine. Exhibit, Am. Acad. Orthop. Surg. Washington D. C., 1972.

92. Godfrey, S.: Respiratory and cardiovascular consequences of scoliosis. Respiration 27:67, 1970.

93. Goldstein, L. A.: Result in the treatment of scoliosis with turnbuckle cast correction and fusion. J. Bone Joint Surg. 41A:321, 1959.

94. Goldstein, L. A.: The surgical management of scoliosis. Clin. Orthop. 35:95–115, 1964.

95. Goldstein, L. A.: Further experiences with the treatment of scoliosis by cast correction and spine fusion with fresh autogenous iliac bone grafts. J. Bone Joint Surg. 48A:962–966, 1966.

96. Goldstein, L. A.: Terminology Committee Report. Scoliosis Research Society. Fourth Annual Meeting. Los Angeles, 1969.

97. Goldstein, L. A.: Treatment of idiopathic scoliosis by Harrington instrumentation and fusion. J. Bone Joint Surg. 51A:209–222, 1969.

98. Goldstein, L. A.: The surgical treatment of idiopathic scoliosis. Clin. Orthop. 93:131–157, 1973.

99. Goldstein, L. A., and Waugh, T. R.: Classification and terminology of scoliosis. Clin. Orthop. 93:10–22, 1973.

100. Greulich, W. W., and Pyle, S. I.: Radiographic Atlas of Skeletal Development of the Hand and Wrist. 2nd ed. Stanford University Press, 1959.

101. Grobler, L. J., Moe, J. H., Winter, R. B., et al.: Surgically produced loss of lumbar lordosis —Its treatment and prevention. Clin. Orthop.; in press.

102. Grospic, F.: Kyphosis dorsalis adolescentium. Zentralbl. Chir. 551:61, 1928.

103. Gschwend, N., and Muller, G. P.: Ergebnisse einer aktivpassiven Behandlungsmethods fixierter juveniler Thorakalkyphosen. Arch. Orthop. Unfall-Chir. 61:55–65, 1967.

104. Gue, L., Savini, R., Vicenzi, G., and Ponzo, L.: Surgical treatment of poliomyelitic scoliosis. Ital. J. Orthop. Traum. 2:191–205, 1976.

105. Guntz, E.: Kyphosis juvenilis sive adolescentium. Beilage-heft zur Ztschr. Orthop. 67:53–75, 1937.

106. Guntz, E.: Gedanken zur Begutachtung von Wirbelsaulenschaden nach orthopadischen Gesichtspunkten. Arch. Orthop. Unfall-Chir. 47:558–572, 1955.

107. Hafner, R. H.: Localized osteochondritis. Scheuermann's disease. J. Bone Joint Surg. 34B:38–40, 1952.

108. Hall, J.: Remarks on spine deformity in myelomeningocoele. Scoliosis Research Society, 1972, Wilmington, Delaware.

109. Hall, J. E.: The anterior approach to spinal deformities. Orthop. Clin. North Am. 3:81–98, 1972.

110. Hardy, J. H. (ed.): Spinal Deformity in Neurological and Muscular Disorders. St. Louis, The C. V. Mosby Co., 1974.

111. Hare, S.: Practical Observations on the Prevention, Causes, and Treatment of Curvatures of the Spine. London, Churchill, 1849.

112. Harrington, P. R.: Treatment of scoliosis — correction and internal fixation by spine instrumentation. J. Bone Joint Surg. 44A:591, 1962.

113. Harrington, P. R.: The management of scoliosis by spine instrumentation: An evaluation of more than 200 cases. So. Med. J. 56:1367–1377, 1963.

114. Harrington, P. R.: An eleven-year clinical investigation of Harrington instrumentation, a preliminary report on 578 cases. Orthop. Clin. North Am. 3:113–130, 1972.

115. Harrington, P. R.: Technical details in relation to the successful use of instrumentation in scoliosis. Orthop. Clin. North Am. 3:49–68, 1972.

116. Harrington, P. R.: The history and development of Harrington instrumentation. Orthop. Clin. North Am. 3:110–112, 1972.

117. Henche, H. R., Morscher, E., and Weisser, K.: The effects of the Harrington instrumentation on pulmonary functions in the treatment of scoliosis. In Operative Treatment of Scoliosis. Fourth International Symposium, Nymegen, Netherlands. Stuttgart, Georg Thieme, 1973, p. 89.

118. Hensinger, R. N., and MacEwen, G. D.: Spinal deformity associated with heritable neurologic conditions: Spinal muscular atrophy. Freidreich's ataxia, familial dysautonomia, and Charcot-Marie-Tooth disease. J. Bone Joint Surg. 58A:13–23, 1976.

119. Hepper, N. G. G., Black, L. F., and Fowler, W. S.: Relationships of lung volume to height and arm span in normal subjects and in patients with spine deformity. Am. Rev. Resp. Dis. 91:356, 1965.

120. Hessing, F., and Hasslauer, L.: Orthopadische Therapie. Berlin. Urban and Schwarzenburg, 1903.

121. Hibbs, R. A.: An operation for progressive spinal deformities. New York Med. J. 93:1013, 1911.

122. Hibbs, R. A.: A report of 59 cases of scoliosis treated by the fusion operation. J. Bone Joint Surg. 6:3–37, 1924.

123. Hibbs, R. A.: Scoliosis treated by fusion operation — study of 365 cases. J. Bone Joint Surg. 13:91, 1931.

124. Hippocrates: On the articulations: In The Genuine Works of Hippocrates. Vol. 2. Translated by Francis Adams, London, Sudenham Society, 1849.

125. Hodgson, A. R.: Correction of fixed spinal curves. A preliminary communication. J. Bone Joint Surg. 47A:1221–1227, 1965.

126. Hodgson, A. R., and Stack, F. E.: Anterior spine fusion. Br. J. Surg. 44:266, 1956.

127. Hoffa, A.: Lehrbuch der Orthopadischen Chirurgie. Stuttgart, Verlag von Ferdinand Enke, 1898.

128. James, C. C. M., and Lassman, L. T.: Two curve patterns in idiopathic structural scoliosis. J. Bone Joint Surg. *33B*:399, 1951.

129. James, J. I. P.: Idiopathic scoliosis, the prognosis, diagnosis, and operative indications related to curve patterns and the age of onset. J. Bone Joint Surg. *36B*:36–49, 1954.

130. James, J. I. P.: Kyphoscoliosis. J. Bone Joint Surg. *37B*:414–426, 1955.

131. James, J. I. P.: Infantile idiopathic scoliosis. Clin. Orthop. *21*:106–116, 1961.

132. James, J. I. P.: Scoliosis. Edinburgh, E. & S. Livingstone, 1967.

133. James, J. I. P.: Idiopathic scoliosis. Clin. Orthop. *77*:57–72, 1971.

134. James, J. I. P.: Infantile idiopathic scoliosis. Clin. Orthop. J. *77*:57, 1971.

135. Johnson, B. E., and Westgate, H. D.: Methods of predicting vital capacity in patients with thoracic scoliosis. J. Bone Joint Surg. *52A*:1433, 1970.

136. Junghanns, H.: Für Atiologie, Prognose und Therapie des M. Scheuermann. Medizinische *1*:300, 1955.

137. Keller, R. B., and Pappase, A. M.: Infection after spinal fusion using internal fixation instrumentation. Orthop. Clin. North Am. *3*:99–111, 1972.

138. Kemp, F. H., and Wilson, D. C.: A further report on factors in the etiology of osteochondritis of the spine. Br. J. Radiol. *21*:449–451, 1948.

139. Kemp, F. H., and Wilson, D. C.: Social and nutritional factors in adolescent osteochondritis of the spine. Br. J. Soc. Med. *2*:66–70, 1948.

140. Kilfoyle, R. M., Foley, J. J., and Norton, P. L.: Spine and pelvic deformity in childhood and adolescent paraplegia. A study of 104 cases. J. Bone Joint Surg. *47A*:659–682, 1965.

141. Knutson, F.: Observations on the growth of the vertebral body in Scheuermann's disease. Acta Radiol. *30*:97–104, 1948.

142. Kostuik, J. P., Israel, J., and Hall, J. E.: Scoliosis surgery in adults. Clin. Orthop. *93*:225–234, 1973.

143. Lambrinudi, L.: Adolescent and senile kyphosis. Br. Med. J. *2*:800–804, 1934.

144. Larsen, E. H., and Nordentaft, E. L.: Growth of the epiphyses and vertebrae. Acta Orthop. Scand. *32*:210–217, 1962.

145. Leatherman, K. D.: Resection of vertebral bodies. J. Bone Joint Surg. *51A*:206, 1969.

146. Leatherman, K.: Operative treatment of congenital scoliosis. Paper presented at the Scoliosis Research Society, Wilmington, Delaware, Sept. 1972.

147. Leatherman, K. D.: The management of rigid spinal curves. Clin. Orthop. *93*:215–224, 1973.

148. Leatherman, K. D., and Dickson, R. A.: Two-stage corrective surgery for congenital deformities of the spine. J. Bone Joint Surg. *61B*:324–328, 1979.

149. Leider, L. L., Moe, J. H., and Winter, R. B.: Early ambulation after the surgical treatment of idiopathic scoliosis. J. Bone Joint Surg. *54A*:1792, 1972.

150. Lindh, M., and Bjure, J.: Lung volumes in scoliosis before and after correction by the Harrington instrumentation method. Acta Orthop. Scand. *46*:934, 1975.

151. Lindseth, R. E., and Stelzer, L.: Vertebral excision for kyphosis in children with myelomeningocoele. J. Bone Joint Surg. *61A*:699–703, 1979.

152. Littler, W. A., Brown, I. K., and Roaf, R.: Regional lung function in scoliosis. Thorax *27*:420, 1972.

153. Lloyd-Roberts, G. C., and Pilcher, M. F.: Structural idiopathic scoliosis in infancy — a study of the natural history of 100 patients. J. Bone Joint Surg. *47B*:520, 1965.

154. Lonsdale, E. F.: Observations on the treatment of lateral curvature of the spine. London, J. Churchill, 1847.

155. Lonstein, J., Winter, R., Bradford, D., Moe, J., and Bianco, A.: Post laminectomy spine deformity. Spine (1980 — to be published) J. Bone Joint Surg. *58A*:727, 1976.

156. Lonstein, J., Winter, R. B., Moe, J. H., and Gaines, D.: Wound infection with Harrington instrumentation and spine fusion for scoliosis. Clin. Orthop. *96*:222–233, 1973.

157. Lonstein, J. E., Winter, R. B., Moe, J. H., Chou, S., and Pinto, W. C.: Spinal cord compression due to spine deformity. Spine, accepted for publication.

158. Lyon, M.: Krankheiten der Wirbelkorperepiphyse. Fortschr. Geb. Rontgenstr. Nuklear Med. *44*:498, 1931.

159. MacEwen, G. D.: Report of the Morbidity Committee, Scoliosis Research Society, Hartford, Conn., Sept 1971.

160. MacEwen, G. D.: Operative treatment of scoliosis in cerebral palsy. Reconstr. Surg. Traumatol. *13*:58–67, 1972.

161. MacEwen, G. D., Conway, J. J., and Miller, W. T.: Congenital scoliosis with a unilateral bar. Radiol. *90*:711–715, 1968.

162. MacEwen, G. D., Winter, R. B., and Hardy, J. H.: Evaluation of kidney anomalies in congenital scoliosis. J. Bone Joint Surg. *54A*:1451–1554, 1972.

163. Makley, J. T., Herndon, C. H., Inkley, S., Doershuk, C., Matthews, L. W., Post, R. H., and Littell, A. S.: Pulmonary function in paralytic and non-paralytic scoliosis before and after treatment: A study of sixty-three cases. J. Bone Joint Surg. *50A*:1379, 1968.

164. Mankin, H. J., Graha, J. J., and Schack, J.: Cardiopulmonary function in mild and moderate idiopathic scoliosis. J. Bone Joint Surg. *46A*:53, 1964.

165. Manning, C.: Use of halo-pelvic distraction in preoperative reduction of scoliosis. Scoliosis Research Society, Eighth Annual Meeting. Goteborg, Sweden, 1973.

166. Mayfield, J. K., Riseborough, E. J., and Jaffee, N.: Irradiation effect on the axial skeleton following treatment for neuroblastoma. Orthop. Trans. *3*, Div. I, p. 49, 1979.

167. Mehta, M. H.: The rib-vertebra angle in the early diagnosis between resolving and progressive infantile scoliosis. J. Bone Joint Surg. *54B*:230–244, 1972.

168. Meister, R., and Heiner, J.: Vergleichende Untersuchungen der Lungenfunktion bei jugendlichen Skoliosepatienten vor und nach der Operation nach Harrington. Z Orthop. *111*:749, 1973.

169. Michelle, A. A.: Osteochondrosis deformans juvenilis dorsi. New York J. Med. *61*:98–101, 1961.

170. Moe, J. H.: Management of idiopathic scoliosis. Clin. Orthop. *9*:169–184, 1957.

171. Moe, J. H.: A critical analysis of methods of fusion for scoliosis. An evaluation in 266 patients. J. Bone Joint Surg. *40A*:529–554, 1958.

172. Moe, J. H.: Fundamentals of the scoliosis problem

for the general practitioner. Post-Grad. Med. *23*:518–532, 1958.

173. Moe, J. H.: Treatment of scoliosis. Results in 196 patients treated by cast correction and fusion. J. Bone Joint Surg. *46A*:293–312, 1964.

174. Moe, J. H.: Treatment of adolescent kyphosis by non-operative and operative methods. Manitoba Med. Rev. *45*:481–484, 1965.

175. Moe, J. H.: Complications of scoliosis treatment. Clin. Orthop. *53*:21–30, 1967.

176. Moe, J. H.: The Milwaukee brace in the treatment of scoliosis. Clin. Orthop. *77*:18–31, 1971.

177. Moe, J. H.: Methods of correction and surgical techniques in scoliosis. Orthop. Clin. North Am. *3*:17–48, 1972.

178. Moe, J. H.: Indications for Milwaukee brace nonoperative treatment in idiopathic scoliosis. Clin. Orthop. *93*:38–43, 1973.

179. Moe, J. H., and Kettleson, D. N.: Idiopathic scoliosis — analysis of curve patterns and the preliminary results of Milwaukee brace treatment in 196 patients. J. Bone Joint Surg. *52A*:1509–1533, 1970.

180. Moe, J. H., and Sunderberg, B.: A clinical study of spine fusion in the growing child. J. Bone Joint Surg. *46B*:784, 1964.

181. Moe, J. H., Winter, R. B., Bradford, D. S., and Lonstein, J. E.: Scoliosis and Related Spine Deformities. Philadelphia, W. B. Saunders Co., 1978.

182. Monnet, J. C.: Osteochondritis deformans. J. Okla. St. Med. Assn. *52*:376–386, 1959.

183. Muhlbach, von R., Hahnel, H., and Cohn, H.: Zur Bedeutung biochemischer Parameter bei der Beurteilung der Scheurmannschenkrankheit. Medizin und Sport *10*:331, 1970.

184. Muller, G., and Gschwend, N.: Endocrine Storungen und Morbus Scheuermann. Arch. Orthop. Unfall-Chir. *65*:357, 1969.

185. Nachemson, A.: A long-term follow-up study of non-treated scoliosis. Acta Orthop. Scand. *39*:466–476, 1968.

186. Nasca, R. J., Stelling, F. H., and Steel, H. H.: Progression of congenital scoliosis due to hemivertebrae and hemivertebrae with bars. J. Bone Joint Surg. *57A*:456–466, 1975.

187. Nash, C. L., and Moe, J. H.: A study of vertebral rotation: J. Bone Joint Surg. *51A*:223–229, 1969.

188. Nathan, L., and Kuhns, J. G.: Epiphysitis of spine. J. Bone Joint Surg. *22*:55–62, 1940.

189. Nicod, L.: Traitement de la maladie de Scheuermann et des dystrophies rachidiennes de croissance. Praxis *46*:1619–1627, 1968.

190. Nilsonne, U., and Lundgren, K. D.: Long-term prognosis in idiopathic scoliosis. Acta Orthop. Scand. *39*:456–465, 1968.

191. O'Brien, J. P.: Halo pelvic traction. J. Bone Joint Surg. *53B*:217–229, 1971.

192. O'Brien, J. P.: Anterior and posterior correction and fusion for paralytic scoliosis. Clin. Orthop. *86*:151–153, 1972.

192a. O'Brien, J. P., Yau, A., and Hodgson, A.: Halo pelvic traction: A technic for severe spinal deformities. Clin. Orthop. *93*:179–190, 1973.

193. Ollier, M.: Technique des platres et corsets de scolioses. *In* Corset Lyonnais, Masson et Cie, 1971, p. 87.

194. Outland, T., and Snedden, H. E.: Juvenile dorsal kyphosis. Clin. Orthop. *5*:155–163, 1955.

195. Overgaard, K.: Prolapses of nucleus pulposus and Scheuermann's disease. Nord. Med. *5*:593–603, 1940.

196. Paré, A.: Opera Ambrosii Parie. Paris, Apud Jocabum Du-Puys, 1582.

197. Peon, H., Winter, R. B., and Moe, J. H.: Nonoperative treatment of congenital scoliosis with the Milwaukee brace. Unpublished data.

198. Perry, J.: The halo in spinal abnormalities: Practical factors and avoidance of complications. Orthop. Clin. North Am. *3*:69–80, 1972.

199. Ponder, R., Dickson, J., Harrington, P., and Erwin, W.: Results of Harrington instrumentation and fusion in the adult idiopathic scoliosis patient. J. Bone Joint Surg. *57A*:797–801, 1975.

200. Ponseti, I. V., and Friedman, B.: Prognosis in idiopathic scoliosis. J. Bone Joint Surg *32A*:381–395, 1950.

201. Raisman, V.: Adolescent round back deformity — a late result of poliomyelitis. Bull. Hosp. Joint Dis. N.Y. *16*:94–102, 1955.

202. Rathke, F. W.: Pathogenese und Therapie der juvenilen Kyphose. Z. Orthop. *102*:16–31, 1966.

203. Raycroft, J. H., and Curtis, B. H.: Spinal curvature in myelomeningocoele: Natural history and etiology. *In* American Academy of Orthopaedic Surgeons Symposium on Myelomeningocoele, Hartford, Conn., Nov. 1970. St. Louis, C. V. Mosby Co., 1972.

204. Riseborough, E. J.: The anterior approach to the spine for correction of deformities of the axial skeleton. Clin. Orthop. *93*:207–214, 1973.

205. Riseborough, E. J., and Shannon, D. C.: The effects of scoliosis on pulmonary function and the changes occurring in the lungs following surgical correction of idiopathic scoliosis. *In* Keim, H. A. (ed.): Post-Graduate Course on the Management and Care of the Scoliosis Patient. New York Orthopedic Hospital, 1970.

206. Riseborough, E. J., Grobian, S., Burton, R., and Jaffee, N.: Skeletal alterations following irradiation for Wilm's tumor with particular reference to scoliosis and kyphosis. J. Bone Joint Surg. *58A*:526, 1976.

207. Risser, J. C.: The application of body casts for the correction of scoliosis. Am. Acad. Orthop. Surg. Instruct. Course Lect. *12*:255, 1955.

208. Risser, J. C.: A follow-up study of the treatment of scoliosis. J. Bone Joint Surg. *40A*:555–569, 1958.

209. Risser, J. C.: The iliac apophysis: An invaluable sign in the management of scoliosis. Clin. Orthop. *11*:111–119, 1958.

210. Risser, J. C.: Treatment of scoliosis during the past 50 years. Clin. Orthop. *44*:109–113, 1966.

211. Risser, J. C., Lauder, C. H., Norquist, D. M., and Craig. W. A.: Three types of body casts. American Academy of Orthopaedic Surgeons. Instructional Course Lectures *10*:131–142, 1953.

212. Roaf, R.: Vertebral growth and its mechanical control. J. Bone Joint Surg. *42B*:40–59, 1960.

213. Robin, G. C.: Scoliosis in childhood muscular dystrophy. J. Bone Joint Surg. *53A*:466–476, 1971.

214. Robin, G. C.: Treatment of the paralytic collapsing spine. A. African J. Surg. *9*:173–182, 1971.

215. Robin, G. C.: Scoliosis and Neurologic Disease. Jerusalem, Israel Universities Press, 1975.

216. Robins, R. R., Moe, J., and Winter, R.: Scoliosis in Marfan's syndrome. Its characteristics and results of treatment in 35 patients. J. Bone Joint Surg. *57A*:358–368, 1975.

217. Romer, V.: Behandlung des Morbus Scheuermann. Schweiz. Med. Wschr. *97*:1615–1617, 1967.

218. Rutt, A.: Zur Therapie der Scheuermannschen Krankheit. Beitr. Orthop. *13*:731–735, 1966.

219. Sayre, L. A.: Spinal Disease and Spinal Curvature. London, Smith-Elder & Co., 1877.

220. Scheuermann, H. W.: Kyfosis dorsalis juvenilis. Ugesk. Iaeger *82*:385–393, 1920.

221. Scheuermann, H. W.: Kyphosis juvenilis (Scheuermanns Krankheit). Fortschr. Geb Röntgens. *53*:1–16, 1936.

222. Schildback, J.: Die Entwicklung der juvenilen Kyphose. Zentralbl. Chir. *64*:2086–2104, 1937.

223. Schmidt, A. C.: Fundamental principles and treatment of scoliosis. Instruct. Course Lect. Am. Acad. Orthop. Surg. *16*:184, 1959.

224. Schmorl, G.: Die Pathogenese der juvenilen Kyphose. Fortschr. Geb Röntgen. *41*:359–383, 1930.

225. Schmorl, G., and Junghanns, R.: The Human Spine in Health and Disease. New York, Grune and Stratton, 1971.

226. Schwentker, E. P., and Gibson, D. A.: The orthopaedic aspects of spinal muscular atrophy. J. Bone Joint Surg. *58A*:32–38, 1976.

227. Scott, J. C.: Scoliosis and neurofibromatosis. J. Bone Joint Surg. *47B*:524–525, 1965.

228. Scott, J. C., and Morgan, T. H.: Natural history and prognosis of infantile idiopathic scoliosis. J. Bone Joint Surg. *37B*:400, 1955.

229. Shannon, D. C., Riseborough, E. J., and Kazemi, H.: Ventilation perfusion relationship following correction of kyphoscoliosis. J. Bone Joint Surg. *53A*:195, 1971.

230. Shannon, D. C., Riseborough, E. J., Valenca, L. M., and Kazemi, H.: The distribution of abnormal lung function in kyphoscoliosis. J. Bone Joint Surg. *52A*:131, 1970.

231. Sharrard, W. J. W.: Spinal osteotomy for congenital kyphosis in myelomeningocoele. J. Bone Joint Surg. *50B*:466–471, 1968.

232. Sharrard, W. J. W.: The kyphotic and lordotic spine in myelomeningocoele. *In* American Academy of Orthopedic Surgeons Symposium on Myelomeningocoele. Hartford, Conn., Nov. 1970. St. Louis, C. V. Mosby Co., 1972, pp. 202–218.

233. Shurtleff, D. B., Goiney, R., Gordon, L. H., and Livermore, N.: Myelodysplasia: The natural history of kyphosis and scoliosis. A preliminary report. Dev. Med. Child Neurol. *18*(Suppl. 37):126–133, 1976.

234. Siegel, I. M.: Scoliosis in muscular dystrophy. Clin. Orthop. *93*:235–238, 1973.

235. Simmons, E. H.: Observations on the technique and indications for wedge resection of the spine. J. Bone Joint Surg. *50A*:847–848, 1968.

236. Simon, R. S.: Diagnosis and treatment of kyphosis dorsalis juvenilis (Scheuermann's kyphosis) in early stage. J. Bone Joint Surg. *24*:681–683, 1942.

237. Sinha, R., and Bergofsky, E. H.: Prolonged alteration of lung mechanics in kyphoscoliosis by positive pressure hyperinflation. Am. Rev. Resp. Dis. *106*:47, 1972.

238. Slabaugh, P. B., Lonstein, J. E., Winter, R. E., and Moe, J. H.: Lumbosacral hemivertebrae: A review of 24 pts. with excision in eight. Spine *5*(3). May/June, 1980.

239. Sørensen, K. H.: Scheuermann's Juvenile Kyphosis. Copenhagen, Munksgaard, 1964.

240. Spitzy, H.: Scoliosis. *In* Fritz Lange's Lehrbuch der Orthopädie. Jena, G. Fischer, 1928.

241. Stagnara, P.: Personal communication.

242. Stagnara, P., and Perdriolle, R.: Elongation vertebralé continue par platres a tendeurs. Possibilities therapeutiques. Rev. Chir. Orthop. *44*:57–74, 1958.

243. Stagnara, P., du Peloux, J., and Fauchet, R.: Traitement orthopedique ambulatoire de la maladie de Scheuermann en periode d'evolution. Rev. Chir. Orthop. *52*:585–600, 1966.

244. Stagnara, P., Vauzelle, C., and Jouvinroux, P.: Functional monitoring of spinal cord activity during spinal surgery. Presented at the Scoliosis Research Society, Wilmington, Delaware. September, 1972.

245. Stein, H., and von Zahn, L.: Zur Pathogenese, Fruhdiagnose und Prophylaxe des Morbus Scheuermann. Deutsche Wchnschr. *81*:200–202, 1956.

246. Steindler, A.: Diseases and Deformities of the Spine and Thorax. St. Louis, C. V. Mosby Co., 1929.

247. Steindler, A.: Post-graduate Lectures on Orthopedic Diagnosis and Indications. Springfield, C. C. Thomas, 1952, p. 276.

248. Stracker, O.: Zur Behandlung der Kyphosis adolescentium-Scheuermann. Wein. Med. Wchnschr. *99*:48, 1949.

249. Swank, S., Lonstein, J., Moe, J., Winter, R., and Bradford, D.: The surgical treatment of adult scoliosis. Orthop. Trans. *3*(1):46, 1979.

250. Tachdjian, M. O.: Orthopedic aspects of intraspinal tumors in infants and children. J. Bone Joint Surg. *47A*:223–248, 1965.

251. Ting, E. Y., and Lyons, H. A.: The relation of pressure and volume of the total respiratory system and its components in kyphoscoliosis. Am. Rev. Resp. Dis. *89*:379, 1964.

252. Vallbona, C., Harrington, P. R., Harrison, G. M., Freire, R. M., and Reese, W. O.: Pitfalls in the interpretation of pulmonary function studies in scoliosis patients. Arch. Phys. Med. Rehab. *50*:68, 1969.

253. Vitko, R. J., Cass, A. S., and Winter, R. B.: Anomalies of the genitourinary tract associated with congenital scoliosis and congenital kyphosis. J. Urol. *108*:655–659, 1972.

254. Wassman, K.: Kyphosis juvenilis Scheuermann. Acta Orthop. Scand. *21*:65–74, 1951.

255. Watermann, H.: Die Kyphosis Adolescentium und die Notwendigkeit ihrer Erkenntnis in der Unfallbegutachtung. Arch. Orthop. Unfall-Chir. *24*:179–188, 1927.

256. Waugh, T. R.: Terminology Committee Report, Scoliosis Research Society, Seventh Annual Meeting, Wilmington, Delaware, 1972.

257. Westgate, H. D.: Hemi-lung ventilation and perfusion changes secondary to thoracic scoliosis. J. Bone Joint Surg. *50A*:845, 1968.

258. Westgate, H. D.: Pulmonary function in thoracic scoliosis: before and after corrective surgery. Minn. Med. *53*:839, 1970.

259. Westgate, H. D., and Johnson, B. E.: Pre-operative pulmonary evaluation and post-operative respiratory management of patients with severe thoracic scoliosis. J. Bone Joint Surg. *53A*:195, 1971.

260. Westgate, H. D., and Moe, J. H.: Pulmonary function in kyphoscoliosis before and after correction by the Harrington instrumentation method. J. Bone Joint Surg. *51A*:935–946, 1969.

261. Williams, E. R.: Observations on the differential diagnosis and sequelae of juvenile vertebral osteochondrosis. Acta Radiol. Suppl. *116*:293–299, 1954.

262. Winter, R. B.: Anterior fusion of the spine for difficult curvature problems. J. Bone Joint Surg. *52A*:833–834, 1970.

263. Winter, R. B.: The effects of early fusion on spine growth. *In* Zorab. P. A. (ed.): Scoliosis and Growth, London, Churchill Livingstone, 1971, pp. 98–104

264. Winter, R. B.: Combined Dwyer and Harrington instrumentation and fusion in the treatment of selected patients with painful adult idiopathic scoliosis, Spine *3*:135–141, 1978.

265. Winter, R. B., and Moe, J. H.: Idiopathic scoliosis. Minn. Med. *55*:529–535, 1972.

266. Winter, R. B., Lovell, W., and Moe, J. H.: Excessive thoracic lordosis and loss of pulmonary function in patients with idiopathic scoliosis. J. Bone Joint Surg., *57A*:972, 1975.

267. Winter, R. B., Moe, J. H., and Bradford, D. S.: Congenital thoracic lordosis, J. Bone Joint Surg. *60A*:806–810, 1978.

268. Winter, R. B., Moe, J. H., and Eilers, V. E.: Congenital scoliosis. A study of 234 patients treated and untreated. J. Bone Joint Surg. *50A*:1, 1968.

269. Winter, R. B., Moe, J. H., and Eilers, V. E.: Terminology Committee Report, Scoliosis Research Society, Sixth Annual Meeting, Hartford, Connecticut, 1971.

270. Winter, R. B., Moe, J. H., and Wang, J. F.: Congenital kyphosis, its natural history and treatment as observed in a study of 130 patients. J. Bone Joint Surg. *55A*:223–256, 1973.

271. Winter, R. B., Haven, J., Moe, J. H., and Lagaard, S. M.: Diastematomyelia and congenital spine deformities. J. Bone Joint Surg. *56A*:27–39, 1974.

272. Winter, R. B., Moe, J. H., MacEwen, G. D., and Peon-Vidales, H.: The Milwaukee brace in the non-operative treatment of congenital scoliosis. Spine *1*:33–49, 1976.

273. Winter, R. B., Moe, J. H., Bradford, D. S., Lonstein, J. E., Pedras, C. V., and Weber, A. H.: Spine deformity in neurofibromatosis, A review of 102 patients. J. Bone Joint Surg. *61A*:677–694, 1979.

274. Wullstein, L., and Schulthess, W.: Die Skoliose in ihrer Behandlung und Entstehung nach klinischen und experimentellen Studien. Zeitschr. Ortho. Chir. *10*:178, 1902.

275. Wynne-Davies, R.: Familial (idiopathic) scoliosis. J. Bone Joint Surg. *48B*:583, 1966.

276. Wynne-Davies, R.: Genetic and environmental aspects. J. Bone Joint Surg. *50B*:24–30, 1968.

277. Yong-Hing, K., Kalamchi, A., and MacEwen, A. D.: Cervical spine abnormalities in neurofibromatosis. J. Bone Joint Surg. *61A*:695–698, 1979.

278. Zorab, P. A., and Prime, F. J.: Estimation of height from tibial length. Lancet *1*:195, 1963.

CHAPTER 7

Cervical Disc Disease

FREDERICK A. SIMEONE, M.D.

RICHARD H. ROTHMAN, M.D., Ph.D.

Pennsylvania Hospital and the University of Pennsylvania

Patients who are symptomatic from cervical disc degeneration usually suffer from compression of a nearby nerve root or the spinal cord. Acute herniation of degenerated disc material which produces such compression in principle resembles acute lumbar disc herniation. The various syndromes related to chronic disc degeneration, with subsequent herniation and subluxation, make this entity deceptive in its clinical presentation. Typical of the confusion surrounding the problem of chronic disc degeneration are its many partial synonyms: osteoarthritis, chronic herniated disc, chondroma, spur formation, and others. Recently, the term "cervical spondylosis" has gained favor, and in this chapter may be used interchangeably for "chronic cervical disc degeneration."

Key, in 1838, probably gave the first actual pathologic description of a spondylotic "bar" as a possible cause of spinal cord compression.[54] Definitive surgical therapy for cervical disc degeneration with spinal cord compression was probably not performed until the twentieth century, but in 1892, Taylor and Collier reported that Horseley had decompressed the spinal cord of a young man who had developed progressive weakness in all of his extremities several months after a fall.[92] Gowers, in 1892, implied that both spinal cord and nerve roots could be compressed by "vertebral exostosis."[37] However, not until the middle of the present century was a large series of patients with symptomatic cervical disc degeneration reported. Brain, Northfield, and Wilkinson, in 1952, described 45 cases of chronic disc degeneration, of which 38 had myelopathy and 7, radiculopathy.[8] These authors also delineated the focal features of acute disc herniation, as compared with chronic disc degeneration. Although acute and chronic cervical disc degeneration are likely to be stages in the same degenerative process, they must be handled separately in clinical discussion.

PATHOLOGY

Chemical Pathology

MARK BROWN, M.D.

The source of pain stimulus as the result of abnormality of the intervertebral joint is a complex problem. Although much is known concerning the biochemistry, biomechanics, and pathologic anatomy of the degeneration of the intervertebral joint, certain basic questions remain to be answered. It is not known why the disc between the fifth and sixth cervical vertebrae and the fourth and fifth lumbar vertebrae are the most commonly symptomatic intervertebral joints in the human spine. Since aging changes occur at a similar rate in the connective tissue matrix of all the discs, biomechanical factors are felt to be the primary cause of pathologic changes in the susceptible discs. However, the specific biomechanical stress centered upon these discs still has not been defined.

It is classically accepted that disc protrusion is a source of pain owing to the distortion of the free nerve endings in the region of the peripheral anulus fibrosus and the longitudinal ligaments, and that radicular pain is due to mechanical compression and distortion of the spinal nerves and nerve roots. However, clinical experience and certain scientific observations lead us to believe that other factors play an important role in pain production that may be unique to the degenerated intervertebral joint.

Mechanical insufficiency secondary to degeneration of the disc leading to susceptibility to repeated sprains has been implicated as the culprit of neck and back pain by many serious students of the spine. Yet the most experienced clinicians and scientists who have studied the intervertebral joint have difficulty defining the mechanically unstable symptomatic joint.

Roentgenographic signs of degenerative changes in the spine show an increasing incidence with aging but no correlation with the incidence of symptoms. With our present stage of knowledge, we are just beginning to learn the basic biomechanics and pathophysiology of the intervertebral joint, particularly with respect to pain production.

It is naive, in light of our present stage of knowledge, to consider disc degeneration simply as a mechanical process. Many fundamental biochemical alterations occur during the disease process, and indeed, it appears that the chemical changes precede the structural changes. These chemical changes may be in fact the most important source of pain stimulation with mechanical factors occurring later in the degenerative process and of much less importance with respect to frequency of symptom production. Our basic fund of knowledge of cellular function in biochemical and biophysical terms has not progressed to the point at which reasonable and testable mechanisms can be proposed and evaluated.

Biologic changes associated with aging and pathologic processes should be differentiated. The term pathology implies a deviation from normal that is associated with a disease process. In attempting to establish an accurate definition of degenerative disc disease, it seems reasonable to state that this is a deteriorative process productive of pain. The changes in the bone and soft tissue structures of the spine are so ubiquitous that without the presence of symptoms, one hesitates to include them under the heading of a disease process. Indeed, the tenuous link between the structural changes and the production of symptoms is one of the great problems of this area, both diagnostically and therapeutically.

The concept of aging is not simply defined. A reasonable definition is that proposed by Comfort: "Senescence is a deteriorative process. What is being measured when we measure it is a decrease in viability and an increase in vulnerability."[20] The individual is rendered progressively more likely to die from accidental causes. The term "accidental" is used in its broadest sense, implying that no death is completely natural and that no one dies from the burden of years alone. It should be pointed out that in the broad biologic realm, aging and natural death are not universal. Natural death as such does not occur until the metazoan species of development is reached. The unicellular organism has the potential, like the gods of ancient Greece, to live forever. We can name many species in which there is only a minimally increased mortality as a function of age. The family of birds — particularly the parrot — the fish — particularly the sturgeon—and certain reptiles, such as the box turtle, give good evidence that certain species are free from the ravages of senescence. It is the hope, of course, of investigators concerned with gerontology that by a more complete understanding, other processes of aging can be controlled and eventually prevented.

It is necessary to consider briefly the three basic theories that are evolving today regarding the cause of age-related changes. These three theories are the developmental theory and its basic concept, a failure in the basic mechanism of embryonic tissue and cellular development. A second theory is based on intercellular relationships, with particular emphasis on immunologic competition between cells, and a third theory is based on instability of certain cellular structures caused by a failure of the genetic coding and readout machinery, which results in a failure of steady-state energy maintenance. In addition to the three basic theories that are evolving today regarding the cause of age-related changes, one must consider an additional theory of aging that has arisen out of the study of the intervertebral disc.[11] This theory is that the cell loses control over the surrounding matrix that it has produced and through which its nutrients and wastes must pass. This theory states that avascular tissues are subject to degeneration because of the natural process of cross-linking of macromolecules. The process is similar to that which we have observed with aging plastics, which become brittle and discolored and crack as they get older.

Having introduced the theories of aging, we shall turn to the various aspects of the degeneration of the highly avascular intervertebral disc. Although the cervical disc is being considered in this chapter, we should consider the basic pathologic process as it occurs in all the discs throughout the spine. The consequences of disc degeneration in the cervical spine will be considered in this chapter, whereas those in the lumbar spine will be considered in Chapter 9. The following processes are basic processes common to all disc degeneration and subsequent symptom production.

BIOCHEMICAL CHANGES IN AGING AND DISEASE

CHANGES IN HYDRATION. The efficient functioning of an intervertebral disc depends largely on the physical properties of the nucleus pulposus, which, in turn, are closely related to its water-binding capacity. It has been repeatedly demonstrated that there occurs a progressive lowering in the degree of hydration of the intervertebral disc from early life, at which time the water content approaches 88 per cent, to a level of 69 per cent in the eighth decade of life.[72] These changes are grossly obvious during the examination of fresh human specimens. In children, the nucleus is a thick gel. With the passage of time, the consistency becomes increasingly firm until ultimately it is not unlike that of the anulus.

A basic question must be posed: What is the mechanism whereby water is retained by the disc? Two possibilities exist: (1) osmotic pressure exerted by the individual molecules or (2) imbibition pressure exerted by the protein-polysaccharide gel. Many theoretical difficulties prevent the acceptance of osmosis as the source of hydrophilia of the nucleus. These are outlined in detail by Hendry.[42] It is more likely that the hydration of the nucleus is predominantly due to imbibition pressure of the gel. The imbibition characteristics of normal and pathologic specimens have been found to be markedly different. The imbibition index, which is a measure of the water-binding capacity of the disc, was found to be markedly

depressed in degenerated discs. Not only were they less hydrophilic than the normal discs, but they also showed a greater than normal susceptibility to changes in pressure.

Several results may derive from this reduction in the imbibition pressure of the nucleus. Mainly, a greater percentage of the total strain will be transmitted to the anulus; the normal pattern of alternating tension and compression on the anulus will be modified on continued compression, and, finally, a pathologic disc that has imbibed fluid may be unable to retain the nucleus when stressed. The former factors could lead directly to injury to the anulus; the latter may lead to a herniation.

The nucleus pulposus functions as a hydraulic ball-bearing within the confines of the anulus fibrosus. The hydraulic properties of the nucleus pulposus have been observed by direct intradiscal measurements. With third-degree degenerative changes, characterized by loss of distinction between the nucleus and the anulus, intradiscal pressure measurements show a loss in the hydraulic properties of the nucleus pulposus.[12]

A recent compilation of the biomechanical data that were available in the literature has shown that with repeated loading and egress of fluids from the nucleus pulposus, there occurs a slight narrowing of the intervertebral disc and a change in the angle of origin and insertion of the collagen fibers within the lamellae of the anulus fibrosus. Existing biomechanical data based on measurement of the tensile strength of the various components of the intervertebral disc show that with normal physiologic loading after egress of fluids and change in the angle of origin of the collagen fibers in the anulus, one may experience tears in the anulus fibrosus with failure in torsion.[22]

These two scientific observations have substantiated the classic teaching that the basic mechanism of degenerative changes in the intervertebral disc begins with a loss of water-binding capacity of the nucleus, and this results in susceptibility of the disc to torsional stress rather than compressive load.

COLLAGEN. Collagen is the main structural component of the intervertebral disc. It possesses great tensile strength, and, through its configuration of alternating sheets, one set at an angle to another, compressive forces applied to the spine are absorbed. The highly ordered structure on the anulus produces the great tensile strength in containment while the random distribution of collagen within the nucleus allows for flexibility and resistance to distortion. Aging is accompanied by a number of changes in the collagen of the human intervertebral disc.[38] Roentgenographic crystallographic studies and hydroxyproline determinations performed by Naylor show that degeneration of the disc is associated with an increase in collagen of the nucleus pulposus as well as an increase in its crystallinity and orientation.[70] The relationship between the acid amino glycans and the collagen with aging has been seen under the scanning electron microscope.[47] The typical 640 angstrom unit banding seen in collagen fibers becomes more apparent in the aged nucleus pulposus. This is true because the binding of the acid amino glycans to the collagen fibers in the youthful nucleus pulposus obscures this typical banding. With aging, there is a decrease in the association between the amino-sugar polymers and the collagen fibers; thus, the bands become visible. It has also been noted by electron microscopy that the collagen fibers increase in diameter in the nucleus pulposus with aging. The reason for these changes in collagen and the changes in relationship of the collagen to ground substance is not known. In addition, the relationship of these changes to the pathologic processes of disc degeneration and to the production of pain is not known.

ACID AMINO GLYCANS. The high water content and hydrostatic properties of the nucleus pulposus of the disc are directly attributable to the acid amino glycans, formerly called mucopolysaccharides, of the nucleus pulposus. These macromolecules are responsible for the bulk of the substance of the avascular connective tissue matrix of the disc. A gradual decrease in hydration of both nucleus and anulus with aging directly correlates with a decrease in the relative and absolute amount of acid amino glycans within the disc. Although the acid amino glycans are not as plentiful in the anulus, they are specifically distributed between the thick lamellar layers of collagen. Diffusion studies have shown that these seams of amino sugar polymers are the pathways by which nutrients diffuse through the anulus into the nucleus. The macromolecular acid amino glycans are polymers composed of noncollagenous protein cores to which are attached polysaccharide side chains chondroitin 4 sulfate, chondroitin 6 sulfate, and keratosulfate. There is a decrease in the

absolute amount of chondroitin-4 and chondroitin-6 sulfates with aging and a relative increase in keratosulfate. These changes occur with an absolute increase in the noncollagenous protein of the aged intervertebral disc. The hydrostatic properties of the gel-like nucleus pulposus are directly dependent upon the imbibition of water by functioning macromolecular acid amino glycans of the nucleus pulposus. With gradual loss in the imbibition power of the acid amino glycans with aging, there is an overall decrease in the hydration of the intervertebral disc. Marked changes in the macromolecular structure of the acid amino glycans lead to a loss of hydration and degeneration of the connective tissue matrix of the disc.

The work of Mitchell and colleagues suggests that biochemical differences in regard to acid amino glycans are much more striking when normal and pathologic discs are compared rather than young and aged discs.[66] It is his theory that a rapid breakdown in the structure of the acid amino glycans is the underlying process of the nucleus pulposus that eventually leads to disc herniation and prolapse.

It is the rapid breakdown of acid amino glycans that allows for a change in the imbibition characteristics of the nucleus pulposus, thus causing abnormal weight-bearing, uneven distribution of pressure, and subsequent tears in the anulus fibrosus. Tears in the anulus fibrosus are accompanied by prolapse of the nucleus in a self-sealing mechanism.[34]

The biochemical changes in the disc matrix with aging and degeneration are only a small part of the overall pathophysiologic processes in the intervertebral joint that eventually lead to symptoms. More important than these static observations are the cellular events that precede them. More recent investigations have been directed toward the study of connective matrix of the discs as a living cellular structure. But before turning to this subject, let us make one final observation concerning the breakdown products of mucopolysaccharides or acid amino glycans. It has been noted in peripheral joints that these breakdown products, when injected, can cause a synovitis and effusion typical of the findings noted during a painful stage of joint inflammation from osteoarthritis.[34] Our theory is that radial cracks and fissures in the anulus fibrosus may provide pathways of diffusion of partial breakdown products of acid amino glycans into the region of the free nerve endings of the posterior longitudinal ligament or to the region of the spinal nerves, or both. These breakdown products incite a marked inflammatory response that may be responsible for prolonged chronic intermittent pain production, which is unique for degenerative disc disease.

GENETIC FACTORS IN INTERVERTEBRAL DISC DEGENERATION

Few investigations of the genetic factors in human intervertebral disc degeneration have been performed. Bull and colleagues tried to establish a genetic basis for disc degeneration through the study of roentgenograms of the human cervical spine.[13] He found that elderly twins had very similar degrees of cervical disc degeneration. He also noted that in a small group of siblings of elderly patients free of cervical disc degeneration, there was also a striking absence of these degenerative changes.

Berry has demonstrated that in certain genetic mutations in mice, the intervertebral disc will show greatly accelerated age changes.[6] He demonstrated that the effect of this abnormal change was a reduction in the mitotic rate of the notochord in gestation. It was his feeling that the greatly accelerated age changes in the abnormal discs of the mice were a direct consequence of their reduced size.

The embryologic anlage of the nucleus pulposus is the notochord remnant containing notochord cells, which produce a gel-like nucleus pulposus similar to that of Wharton's jelly in the umbilical cord. It has been noted in canine species that are predisposed to disc degeneration that these notochord cells are prematurely lost as compared to normal canine species that are not predisposed to develop degenerative discs.[41] Human discs are devoid of notochord cells by the end of the first decade,[38] around the time of onset of the first degenerative changes in the nucleus and the anulus fibrosus. One could speculate that the entire human species has a genetic predisposition to premature disc degeneration.

Since the notochord cells are sequestered in an avascular nucleus pulposus prior to the development of competent immunologic mechanisms by the fetus, theoretically the nucleus pulposus is a sequestered antigen that could be seen as a foreign antigen when exposed to the vascular system in adult life. Therefore, an autoimmune theory of disc degeneration has been proposed. Although several studies have attempted to substantiate this etiology of disc degeneration, none have been convincing.

AUTOIMMUNE PHENOMENON

The autoimmune etiology of the degeneration of the intervertebral disc has been proposed by Bobechko and colleagues.[7] The totally avascular nucleus pulposus is formed during fetal life prior to the development of competent immunologic defense mechanisms. Subsequently, nucleus pulposus, as it is exposed to the vascular system, may theoretically incite an autoimmune response in the mature lymphatic system. Bobechko performed a study in which he placed rabbit nucleus pulposus subcutaneously and then studied the regional lymph nodes. These lymph nodes showed an increase in pyronine-staining lymphatic cells. This nonspecific indicator of an increase in RNA content of the lymphoid cells was interpreted as evidence for an autoimmune response. Naylor examined sera from patients with prolapsed intervertebral discs and found that there was no increase in gamma globulin.[70] However, Elves and his associates showed an in vitro inhibition of leukocyte migration in patients with prolapsed intervertebral discs, which they interpreted as evidence for an autoimmune response.[27] Gertzbein and associates could not demonstrate humoral antibody against nucleus pulposus.[35] However, they felt that they did demonstrate the presence of a cellular immune response in patients whose discs were found to be sequestered at the time of surgery through the leukocyte migration-inhibition test. None of these studies are conclusive. However, there is enough circumstantial evidence to suggest that in certain patients who form marked hypertrophic fibrosis following disc excision, an autoimmune mechanism may be responsible.

POSTURE AND PATHOLOGY

Erectness of the trunk can be regarded as an essential primate characteristic. Along with this truncal erectness, there is a marked tendency of the forelimbs to assume a dominant role. Many primates engage in standing, walking, and running. However, humans alone stand with knees extended and indulge in prolonged standing.[90] Fossil evidence suggests that this erect bipedal type of posture had its beginnings approximately 12 million years ago in the early Pliocene era. It is evident that humans have imperfectly adapted to this upright posture, shown not only by degenerative intervertebral disc disease but also by varicose veins, hemorrhoids, and hernias. The structural shortness of the quadriped skeleton was transformed into an erect bipedal posture, the evolution of which has been beautifully demonstrated by Yamada.[102] He amputated the forelegs and tails of rats in the first postnatal week. Subsequently, those rats that survived assumed an upright bipedal posture. Histologic examination of the intervertebral discs revealed changes typical of intervertebral disc disease in humans. However, the conclusive biomechanical data concerning the incidence of disc degeneration and subsequent herniation have only recently been demonstrated to show that torsional stresses rather than axial loading are the important component of stress by which failure leads to displacement of the disc.

SUMMARY

One must explain herniation of the nucleus pulposus on the basis of either an extraordinarily high pressure in the nucleus or a weakening in the anulus, or both. In the authors' opinion, the most realistic explanation of this protrusion is that a series of biochemical changes occurs through which the nucleus loses its gel-like behavior and its ability to distribute stress evenly. Thus, the nucleus will transmit high pressures to certain areas of the anulus. It has also been demonstrated that certain pathologic biochemical changes occur in the anulus with structural changes that allow radial tears and fissures in the anulus and subsequent migration and prolapse of the nucleus to occur. The relationship between biochemical changes and structural stress is not entirely clear. However, it has recently been shown that repeated loading of the disc with egress of fluids changes the angle of insertion of the anulus fibrosus collagen fibers and, through physiologically normal torsional stresses, may, with this change in angulation, allow for radial tears. The first phenomenon that must occur is a loss of the weight-bearing capacity of the disc through a loss of its ability to imbibe fluids. Thus, biochemical abnormalities that lead to a loss in hydration in the disc are the primary processes that weaken the structure of the anulus fibrosus and allow for decompensation under mechanical stress.

Histologic Changes in the Intervertebral Disc

In a sequential histologic and histochemical examination of the anulus fibrosus from childhood to old age, it has been found that histochemical changes make their first appearance in the third decade of life.[93] The innermost lamellae of the anulus fibrosus show an irregular distribution of the PAS-positive and Alcian blue–positive polysaccharides. There is a loss of homogeneity and enrichment of the polysaccharides in the pericellular areas and a loss of the regularity of the fibrous pattern with tears and holes in certain areas. The appearance of groups of typical cartilage cells can also be noted. In later age groups, the distinction between the nucleus pulposus and anulus fibrosus becomes increasingly obscure. Whether these changes are due to accumulative mechanical stresses or to a metabolic disease is as yet unclear.

The nucleus pulposus shows considerable structural changes with aging. At birth the nucleus is a well-defined structure, clearly demarcated from the anulus. It consists of a loose network of primitive mesenchymal cells. By the second and third decades of life, the border between the nucleus and the anulus becomes less well-defined, the cellular content becomes sparser and the fibrous components more prominent. In the fourth and fifth decades, evidence of cavitation and desiccation in the center of the nucleus may be noted, with nests of cartilage cells scattered throughout the nucleus pulposus. As yet it is not possible to say which of these changes may be classified as characteristic of aging and which as definitely pathologic.

Descriptive Pathology of the Cervical Spine

In discussing disc lesions and degeneration in the cervical spine, one must be precise in terminology. There is an acute type of pathology of the intervertebral disc that consists of nuclear herniations, and another, more diffuse type with anular bulging or protrusion. In nuclear herniation, a circumscribed mass is formed by the extrusion of nuclear material through a tear in the anulus. This is a lesion found in young people, and is frequently associated with trauma.[99] Middle-aged and elderly people are more vulnerable to anular protrusion. When using these terms we are speaking primarily of a problem of the intervertebral disc itself. Both of these lesions may with time develop into a diffuse degeneration of the disc and its associated ligamentous and osseous structures, termed chronic cervical disc degeneration or "cervical spondylosis."[63] The term "degenerative arthritis" is restricted to arthritis of synovial joints and, therefore, should be applied only to degeneration of the apophyseal joints.

The acute disc protrusions may be classified as dorsal, intraforaminal, lateral, or ventral. Most investigators today agree that there is an intimate relationship between intervertebral disc degeneration and cervical spondylosis. Narrowing of the intervertebral discs allows close approximation of the bodies of the adjacent vertebrae, which in turn leads to the deformation of the uncus and to the formation of osteophytes along the superior margins of the distal vertebrae and the inferior margins of the proximal vertebrae. Ridge formation also develops on the anterior wall of the spinal canal, with varying degrees of occlusion of the intervertebral foramen.

DePalma and Rothman studied in detail 70 cervical spines, ranging in age from 38 to 95 years, obtained from the anatomic laboratory.[24] The spines were studied grossly, microscopically, and radiographically. Degeneration of the cervical intervertebral discs was seen not as an isolated process but as one that affected the entire structure of the cervical spine. Degeneration of the cervical discs was found to be closely associated with aging. The majority of spines after the fourth decade showed implication of one or more discs, and after the fifth decade, a sharp rise in the severity of the degenerative process occurred. Of the specimens over the age of 70, 72 per cent had severe abnormalities. Those discs that were most frequently implicated also showed the most severe alterations. In general, the discs below the C3-C4 level exhibited a higher incidence of involvement and more severe changes. The C5-C6 level was most frequently involved; the next most frequently altered disc was at the C6-C7 level. The disc at the C2-C3 level was least often affected (Table 7-1).

When several discs are involved, changes in their configuration and decrease in their height produce alterations in the adjacent vertebral bodies and in the normal alignment of the cervical column. The anterosuperior sur-

TABLE 7-1. INCIDENCE OF DISC DEGENERATION (IN PER CENT)

Level	Severity of Change	
	Mild	Advanced
C2-C3	40	16
C3-C4	70	22
C4-C5	70	38
C5-C6	86	48
C6-C7	75	38
C7-T1	66	14

face of the bodies may become rounded and the bodies may be elongated. The height of the cervical column is reduced, and the normal lordotic curve may be decreased, straightened, or even reversed (Fig. 7-1). Fissures in the central portion of the discs frequently extended in a lateral direction and became continuous with fissures in the joints of Luschka. Nuclear material was found to be extruded under the longitudinal ligament laterally into the joints of Luschka, and superiorly or inferiorly through the cartilaginous plates into the adjacent vertebral bodies (Fig. 7-2). Extrusions of nuclear material under the longitudinal ligament were thought to be of particular significance because they are capable of exerting pressure on the anterior surface of the spinal cord and the adjacent nerve rootlets. This was particularly true when the protrusions were associated with large, marginal osteophytes arising from the posterior surface of the vertebral body (Fig. 7-3). Disc degeneration results in close proximity of adjacent vertebral bodies. This, in turn, is followed by a reactive process producing osteophytes at the superior and inferior peripheral attachments of the discs to the vertebral bodies. A high statistical correlation was noted between disc degeneration and posterior formation of osteophytes. The level most frequently involved in posterior osteophyte formation was C6-C7. These posterior osteophytes were capable of decreasing the anteroposterior diameter of the spinal canal and of exerting pressure on the spinal cord and nerve roots. They also narrowed the intervertebral foramina (Fig. 7-4).

Anterior osteophyte formation differed from posterior osteophyte formation in that it was not as closely related to disc degenerations. It was felt that ligamentous stress played a greater role in initiating the reactive

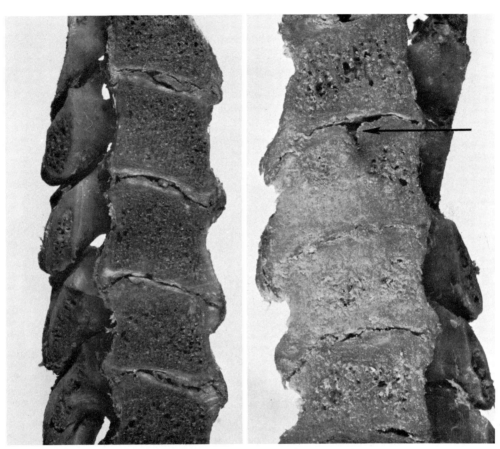

Fig. 7–1   Fig. 7–2

Figure 7–1. Marked multilevel disc degeneration in the cervical spine with drying and loss of substance of the intervertebral disc, collapse of the disc space, and osteophyte formation. (From DePalma, A. F., and Rothman, R. H.: The Intervertebral Disc. Philadelphia, W. B. Saunders Co., 1970.)

Figure 7–2. Herniation of the nucleus into the body of the adjacent cervical vertebra as indicated by the arrow. Note also the marked disc degeneration at other levels in the cervical spine. (From DePalma, A. F., and Rothman, R. H.: The Intervertebral Disc. Philadelphia, W. B. Saunders Co., 1970.)

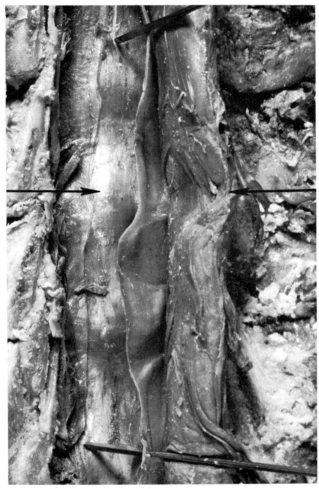

Figure 7–3. Photograph illustrating pressure of posterior osteophyte (arrow on left) which has indented the cervical cord (arrow on right). This type of cervical disc pathology is a frequent cause of myelopathy. (From DePalma, A. F., and Rothman, R. H.: The Intervertebral Disc. Philadelphia, W. B. Saunders Co., 1970.)

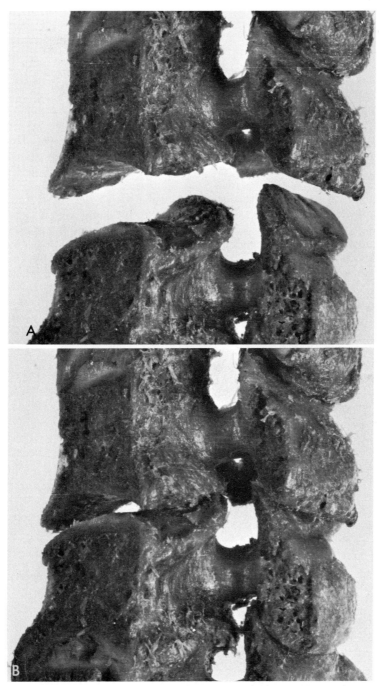

Figure 7–4. These photographs illustrate marked posterior osteophyte formation in the cervical spine. Viewed with vertebrae separated, *A,* and vertebrae opposed, *B.* Note encroachment of the intervertebral foramen by these posterior osteophytes. (From DePalma, A. F., and Rothman, R. H.: The Intervertebral Disc. Philadelphia, W. B. Saunders Co., 1970.)

process involved in anterior osteophyte formation. The anterior osteophytes were noted to be more prominent than their posterior counterparts and to be most frequent below the fourth cervical vertebra (Figs. 7–5 and 7–6).

Reactive changes in the region of the joints of Luschka also appeared to be closely related to disc degeneration. Severe alterations in the joints of Luschka were most often encountered in the lower three levels of the cervical spine, the highest incidence being at the C5-C6 level.

The frequency of severity of changes in the apophyseal joints showed a progression commensurate with aging. However, these articulations are not frequently involved, and the changes are rarely severe. Subluxation of the facets of the apophyseal joint was noted frequently with advanced disc degeneration. This is of significance because it may cause constriction of the adjacent intervertebral

foramina, particularly when associated with osteophyte formation about the facets (Figs. 7–7 and 7–8).

Changes in the various components of the cervical spine are of particular significance if they decrease the lumina of the intervertebral foramina and thereby compress their contents. When compromised intervertebral foramina were evaluated, it was found that the joints of Luschka were involved in 79 per cent, the discs in 78 per cent, and the apophyseal joints in 79 per cent. It is thus apparent that all three areas can play a major role in producing narrowing of the intervertebral foramina. The most frequently involved foramina were at the C3-C4, C4-C5, and C5-C6 levels (Fig. 7–9).

Bony ankylosis between two adjacent vertebrae is invariably associated with resorption of the osteophytes surrounding the foramina. The correlation between the gross anatomic and roentgenographic findings when

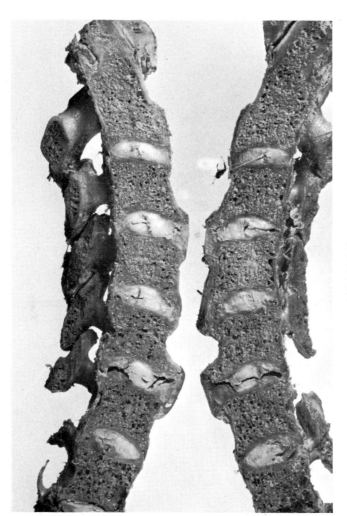

Figure 7–5. Photograph of sagittal section of a cervical spine illustrating multilevel disc degeneration with marked anterior osteophyte formation. These osteophytes may produce in the neck. (From DePalma, A. F., and Rothman, R. H.: The Intervertebral Disc. Philadelphia, W. B. Saunders Co., 1970.)

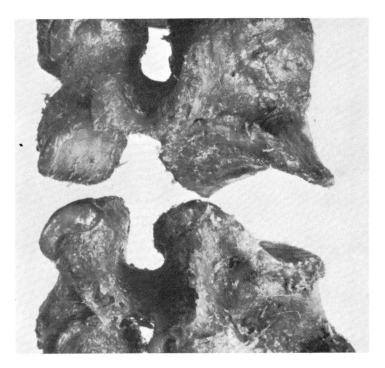

Figure 7–6. Photograph of the osseous changes in cervical spondylosis with osteophyte formation circumferentially about the entire vertebra. In routine roentgenograms we would describe these as anterior and posterior osteophytes, although in actuality they are frequently present about the entire circumference of the vertebral body. (From DePalma, A. F., and Rothman, R. H.: The Intervertebral Disc. Philadelphia, W. B. Saunders Co., 1970.)

applied to the discs and intervertebral foramina was found to be extremely high. The findings just reported agree in general terms with other pathologic descriptions noted in the literature.[30, 44, 73, 83]

The prominent anterior osteophytes have been reported to cause pressure symptoms not only on the esophagus but also on the trachea. They do not commonly occur to this extent, but should be considered in obscure cases of esophageal and tracheal compromise.

From C3 through C7 the average meas-

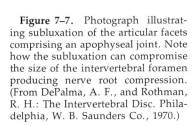
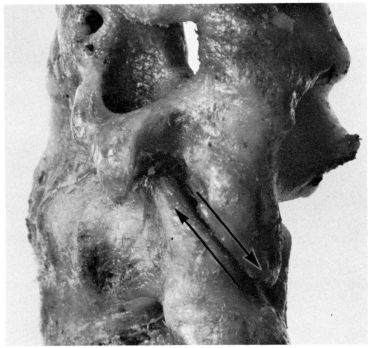

Figure 7–7. Photograph illustrating subluxation of the articular facets comprising an apophyseal joint. Note how the subluxation can compromise the size of the intervertebral foramen producing nerve root compression. (From DePalma, A. F., and Rothman, R. H.: The Intervertebral Disc. Philadelphia, W. B. Saunders Co., 1970.)

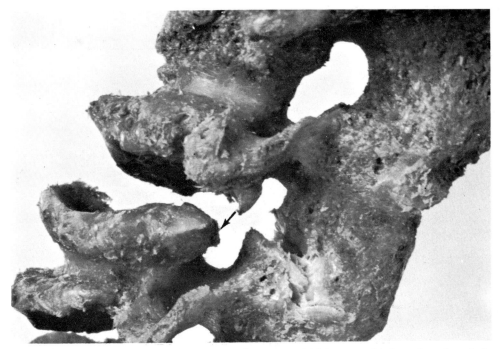

Figure 7–8. Illustration of apophyseal joint degenerative changes in which hypertrophic facets have intruded upon the intervertebral foramen. (From DePalma, A. F., and Rothman, R. H.: The Intervertebral Disc. Philadelphia, W. B. Saunders Co., 1970.)

urement of the cervical canal is 17 mm.[73] It is generally agreed that spinal cord compression will occur only if this figure is reduced to 11 mm. or less.[99] In cervical spondylosis some reduction will usually take place in the anteroposterior diameter of the spinal canal and, when associated with a canal that was initially small, myelopathy can occur. It should be noted that the cervical cord is oval, whereas the canal is roughly triangular in shape, producing the recess to the anterolateral direction. Because of the presence of this canal,

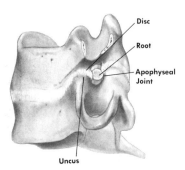

Figure 7–9. This figure illustrates the various components of the motor unit which can compress the nerve root as it courses through the intervertebral foramen. The disc and the uncinate process anteriorly, as well as the apophyseal joint posteriorly, can compromise the nerve root. The anterior-posterior diameter is usually more critical than the superior-inferior diameter.

some reduction of canal size can occur in a lateral direction without resultant cord compression; also, when the cord is compressed in the midline this recess may remain open to serve as a pathway for cerebrospinal fluid.

The work of Friedenberg and Miller is helpful in attempting to correlate changes seen on roentgenograms with patient symptomatology.[30] They evaluated two large groups of patients, one symptomatic and the other asymptomatic in regard to the cervical spine. Patients were evaluated radiographically with roentgenograms of the cervical columns of the anteroposterior, lateral, and oblique projections. It is striking to note that in the asymptomatic group, 25 per cent of patients in the fifth decade of life exhibited degenerative changes, and in the seventh decade 75 per cent showed degenerative changes. In both the symptomatic and asymptomatic groups the highest incidence of abnormalities was noted between the fifth and sixth and sixth and seventh vertebral bodies. It is significant that the incidence of narrowing of the interspaces between the fifth and sixth and the sixth and seventh cervical vertebrae was higher in the symptomatic than in the asymptomatic group. No differences were noted between these two groups in incidence of changes at the joints of Luschka, the intervertebral foramina, or the posterior articular processes. These studies should give the clinician some cause for hesitation before deciding that the changes noted on routine roentgenograms of the cervical spine are causing a particular patient's clinical syndrome. It is felt that over-reliance on routine roentgenograms as a guide to operative intervention has often resulted in the incorrect disc being removed, with a resultant surgical failure. It has been pointed out by Robinson that after surgical fusion osteophyte resorption can take place.[81] This may explain the mechanism of relief of radicular pain in cervical spondylosis after interbody fusion, even when the osteophytes are not removed.

In addition to the common type of chronic disc degeneration previously described, there is a group of cervical intervertebral disc lesions associated with major trauma to the cervical spine with or without fractures and dislocations. Disc injury can be indirectly surmised radiographically in fractures and dislocations when there is either a decreased height of the intervertebral disc space or an abnormal increased width of the intervertebral disc space when the neck is subjected to traction.[2]

In flexion-type fracture dislocations, there is frequently an avulsion of the disc from its attachment to the superior vertebra and less frequently from its inferior vertebra. The line of disruption is most frequently at the junction of the disc and the cartilaginous plate. In hyperextension injuries where there is a teardrop type of fracture, the nucleus may herniate into the fracture site itself.[2] It has been the authors' experience that in certain patients with extensive laminectomy, particularly when the articular facets have been implicated, a degree of instability may result that will subsequently lead to intervertebral disc degeneration. This is particularly true in individuals with weak cervical musculature who cannot compensate for loss of the posterior stabilizing structures. Relief in these individuals can be obtained only by cervical fusion, preferably through the anterior route.[77]

CLINICAL SYNDROME OF CERVICAL DISC DISEASE

The clinical syndrome of acute cervical disc herniation with nerve root compression differs principally from chronic cervical disc degeneration in the mode of presentation and acuity of the initial symptoms. The patient

with acute cervical disc herniation can often date the onset of his or her symptoms to a specific traumatic incident. In the absence of such history, there still is a rather specific point in time that can be recalled as the onset of the condition. With chronic disc degeneration, however, the nerve root and spinal cord compression symptoms develop insidiously, and their time of onset is usually blurred. Acute cervical disc herniation with myelopathy is rare and is usually associated with forceful hyperextension injury to the neck.

In general, the syndrome of acute cervical disc herniation is attended by severe pain that leads to voluntary immobilization of the neck. In contrast, the pain of chronic disc degeneration, though at times severe, may wax and wane sufficiently to allow those affected to maintain a relatively normal activity schedule. Beyond these peculiarities, acute and chronic disc degeneration can be considered together.

AXIAL PAIN. The patient often will present predominantly with a painful and stiff neck. Pain is usually appreciated in the middle of the upper part of the neck, and it can radiate to the suboccipital region along the distribution of the greater occipital nerves. It may, then, be termed a headache by the unwary patient. Most frequently, the discomfort will spread across the shoulders, where it may seem to emanate from the levator scapulae muscles. It is usually aggravated by motion, particularly extension, and is relieved by rest or immobilization with a collar. The discomfort may be particularly severe at the end of an active day or when the patient has been unable to wear the collar. Many patients, however, will awaken with severe neck pain, probably because of awkward neck positions during sleep. The painful neck in cervical disc degeneration is frequently tender when pressure is applied to the spinous processes or deep cervical muscles.

The headache of cervical disc degeneration can be the principal or only symptom. The mechanism of the headache is mysterious. It may be reasonable to assume that involvement of the greater occipital nerve, whose roots of origin are C2, C3, and C4, would be responsible for such headache. Lower cervical disc degeneration, however, is equally liable to produce this symptom. Often the discomfort will radiate along the temple to the forehead, where the occipital nerve distribution meets the sensory dermatome of the first division of the trigeminal nerve. Occasionally the patient experiences a discomfort deep behind the eye. Interestingly, similar retro-orbital pain is reproduced on stimulation of the C2 nerve root during surgery. Langfitt and Elliot described low back and leg pain in cases of cervical cord compression from disc degeneration.[56]

RADICULAR PAIN AND NUMBNESS. Discomfort in the shoulder, chest, arm, or hand, with or without associated weakness, can be the only symptom of chronic disc degeneration.

Though the pathologic entity is chronic and progressive, the onset of discomfort may be more acute. Since there is usually only one root affected at the onset, the discomfort will be restricted to a portion of the neck, chest, or extremities. The pain is often related to neck position and can be significantly worsened by rotation, lateral flexion, or extension of the head. The patient usually prefers to lie with the neck in mid-position. Occasionally, in the most severe cases, the patient may present with a torticollis-like deviation of the head.

The following is a tabulated summary of the site of numbness and discomfort with each individual root.

Nerve Root	Disc Level	Symptoms
C3	C2-C3	Pain and numbness in back of neck, particularly around mastoid process and pinna of ear.
C4	C3-C4	Pain and numbness in back of neck, radiating along levator scapulae muscle and occasionally down anterior chest.
C5	C4-C5	Pain radiating from side of neck to shoulder top; numbness over middle of body of deltoid muscle (axillary nerve distribution).
C6	C5-C6	Pain radiating down lateral side of arm and forearm, often into thumb and index fingers; numbness of tip of thumb or on dorsum of hand over first dorsal interosseous muscle.
C7	C6-C7	Pain radiating down middle of forearm, usually to middle finger, though index and ring finger may be involved.
C8	C7-T1	Pain down medial aspect of forearm to ring and small finger; numbness can involve small finger and medial portion of ring finger. Numbness rarely extends above wrist.

At times only numbness will develop, with a virtual absence of pain. There may be a few days or weeks of low-grade, aching discomfort that subsides, leaving in its wake a persistently numb finger or arm.

The symptoms are frequently misdiagnosed as bursitis or tennis elbow. As time goes on, the discomfort may remain relatively stable or may become gradually progressive. The annoying, unrelenting nature of these symptoms encourages the patient to seek medical attention. Often roentgenograms of the wrist, elbow, or shoulder are obtained, with normal results. The patient is frequently unwilling to admit that the hand symptoms emanate from a problem in the neck, particularly when there have been no cervical symptoms. Chronic radiculopathy is frequently unaffected by neck position or motion, unlike acute symptomatic disc degeneration.

MOTOR DEFICIT. Occasionally one may see the development of a motor radiculopathy in the absence of significant pain or even numbness. Usually, however, there is concurrent discomfort in the hand and numbness appropriate to the motor deficit. With the exception of acute motor radiculopathies, seen only in acute cervical disc degeneration, the patient is amazed to find, on formal testing, that the weakness is greater than expected. Usually the deficit affects a single root and can evolve so slowly that the patient is able to adjust with other muscles for the specific loss of strength.

As before, the motor symptoms and signs (including reflexes) can be tabulated.

Nerve Root	Disc Level	Weakness; Reflex Change
C3	C2-C3	No readily detectable weakness or reflex change except by EMG.
C4	C3-C4	No readily detectable weakness or reflex change except by EMG.
C5	C4-C5	Weakness of extension of arm and shoulder, particularly above 90°; atrophy of deltoid muscle; no reflex change.
C6	C5-C6	Weakness of biceps muscle; depression of biceps reflex.
C7	C6-C7	Weakness of triceps muscle; depression of triceps reflex.
C8	C7-T1	Weakness of triceps and small muscles of the hand; no reflex change.

Monoradiculopathies can be associated with detectable weakness of shoulder rotators, pronators, supinators, wrist flexors, and extensors. These functions are subserved by several muscles, however, so testing can mislead the examiner. Restriction to a careful, symmetric assessment of deltoid, biceps, triceps, and intrinsic hand muscle strength will detect the majority of common radiculopathies associated with weakness. When possible, simultaneous testing of the same function in each extremity should be attempted in order to rule out emotionally or artificially induced weakness.

With progressive chronic disc degeneration and nerve root compression, particularly at multiple levels, the patient with little insight may present only with atrophy. If the C8 nerve root is affected, the atrophy is particularly noticeable, since it involves the small muscles of the hand. Unilateral or bilateral multiple level involvement with atrophy is often seen in older patients in the guise of other neurologic disease (see Chapter 3).

MYELOPATHY. Chronic disc degeneration with posterior osteophyte formation is the commonest cause of spinal cord dysfunction in patients over 55. The characteristic stooped, wide-based, or somewhat jerky gait of the aged summarizes the effects of cervical myelopathy. For years this condition was unrecognized, and the diffuse arm and leg weakness or gait disorders of the elderly were attributed to a natural process of aging.

A small number of patients with chronic disc degeneration will present with a fairly acute myelopathy. The reason for this is not certain, though involvement of the anterior spinal artery and its branches by direct compression has been considered. A flexion or extension injury to a spinal canal compromised by osteophytic spurs can initiate acute myelopathy.

The more common syndrome evolves from a gradual compression of the spinal cord. Because the osteophytes may be single, or at several different levels, a standard clinical syndrome cannot be presented. In general, however, chronic myelopathy follows this course:

Over a period of months the patient may notice a peculiar sensation in the hands, associated with clumsiness and weakness. The lower limbs may precede or follow the arms in the development of these symptoms. The patient has greater difficulty in walking at night, because of reduced proprioceptive impulses

from his or her legs. The leg weakness is fairly symmetric, though the upper extremity weakness may favor one side. With further disuse there may be wasting in the lower extremities and, somewhat mysteriously, fasciculations may develop. The mechanism for these is unclear, though lumbar spondylosis may be implicated. Wasting and atrophy of the upper extremities with appropriate reflex changes is present according to the severity of foraminal encroachment. Reflexes in the lower extremities are almost invariably brisk, and clonus at the ankle is frequent.

Reflexes in the upper extremities are variable because foraminal encroachment may depress the reflex arc at the root level. Hyperreflexia is more common in reflexes mediated by lower cervical segments (the triceps reflex) than by upper segments, particularly when an isolated spur at C5-C6 is the culprit. Extremely brisk Hoffmann's signs, which characteristically involve all of the fingers when the extended middle finger is flicked, are further evidence of diffuse hyperreflexia.

Selective involvement of the fifth cervical segment will produce an "inverted radial reflex." Below this point the extrapyramidal systems in the cord are involved. On percussion of the lower end of the radius, one finds that the normal radial reflex is much diminished owing to C6 nerve root compression. The stimulus to the spinal cord, however, readily elicits a reflex flexion of the digits which are enervated by disinhibited nerve roots below the site of compression.

The abdominal reflexes are usually diminished. Whereas spasticity of the lower extremities with markedly exaggerated knee jerks and ankle jerks is common the plantar reflexes are commonly flexor. One may expect an extensor plantar response (Babinski sign), however, when the myelopathy is relatively severe.

Sensory examination can be somewhat complicated and is a less reliable index of spinal cord involvement. This is because the sensory system is involved at three levels: (1) The spinothalamic tract, in the anterolateral portion of the spinal cord, which mediates pain and temperature sensation on the contralateral side of the body below; (2) the posterior columns, which are involved with the mediation of position and vibratory sense on the ipsilateral side of the body below; and (3) the dorsal division of the nerve root, which, though not a part of myelopathy, is commonly involved and will produce a confusing dermatomal diminution of several sensory modalities in the extremities. Severe cases will reduce appreciation of pain and temperature below the level of spinal cord compression. The level of involvement is variable. It may extend only below the knees or thighs. The most severe cases can affect these modalities throughout the body below T3 or T4. Because pain and temperature fibers ascend for a few segments prior to entering the spinothalamic tract, the sensory level is always well below the compression. Because touch sensation is preserved, the patient is frequently unaware that pain and temperature appreciation are blunted. He does not feel "numbness" with spinal cord compression as might occur with nerve root compression, in which touch sensation is impaired. He may note, however, that he can no longer test the warmth of his bath water with his toes. Serious injury because of loss of pain sensation is rarely seen. Proprioceptive involvement, which is far more common in the lower extremities, is in part responsible for the wide-based gait. Because proprioceptive fibers, which run mainly in the posterior columns, can no longer inform the brain as to where the feet are in space, the patient must look at his feet for this information. Loss of this function is confirmed by vibratory testing with a low-frequency tuning fork. Vibratory sensation is commonly lost at the ankle in older patients, so it should be followed to the knees and iliac crests as well. Only in the most severe cases does one find impairment of appreciation of joint position sense or passive motion at the fingers or toes. Similarly, despite other signs of advanced spinal cord compression, loss of sphincter control is not common.

VERTEBRAL ARTERY COMPRESSION. Vertebral artery compression from acute disc herniation has not been described, though a few cases of traumatic occlusion of this vessel secondary to subluxation or disc distractions have been reported. Most of these cases resulted from severe neck trauma or forceful movements induced by chiropractic manipulation.

The vertebral arteries may be compressed in chronic cervical disc disease by three mechanisms that are obvious when one considers the anatomic confines of the foramen transversarium in vertebrae C2 through C6, through which the vertebral artery passes (Fig. 7–10). These are (1) osteophytes from the lateral portion of the disc margin; (2) osteophytes

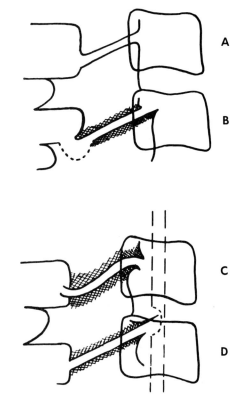

Figure 7–10. Schematic representation of zygapophyseal joint. *A,* Normal; *B,* posterior slip of superior facet with lamina erosion; *C,* locking of joint by hooked osteophytes; *D,* vertebral artery compression by anterior osteophyte. (From Brain, Lord, and Wilkinson, M.: Cervical Spondylosis. Philadelphia, W. B. Saunders Co., 1967.)

extending anteriorly from the zygapophyseal joint; and (3) compression by the inferior articular facet from posterior subluxation with scissoring action by the adjacent superior articulating facet. Most authors feel that narrowing of the foramen transversarium is rarely symptomatic unless associated with atheromatous disease of the vertebral artery. Flow in the vertebral artery is compromised somewhat when the head is turned to the opposite side. Consequently, the symptoms of dizziness and unsteadiness (even to loss of consciousness) may be associated with rotary head movements in patients with a combination of severe lateral osteophyte formation and vertebral artery sclerosis.

The symptoms are rarely incapacitating and usually are not associated with persistent neurologic deficit. Rarely a strokelike syndrome in the distribution of the posterior inferior cerebellar artery is seen. As time progresses, however, patients may find that their lives are limited because of inability to rotate the head.

Most patients will respond to reassurance and a warning that rapid extreme head turning must be avoided. Occasionally, individuals will require a cervical collar, which may be worn for an indefinite interval. Rarely, the symptoms are severe enough to warrant surgical decompression, prior to which vertebral angiography with head rotation is advised.

VISCERAL PRESSURE SYMPTOMS. On rare occasions, proliferative changes secondary to chronic disc degeneration may press the adjacent structures of the throat and present primarily with dysphagia. Figure 7–11 demonstrates a huge spondylotic formation that developed in a 78-year-old man who also had congenital fusion (Klippel-Feil) of the cervical vertebrae below. He was unable to swallow solid foods comfortably and was ultimately restricted to a liquid and soft diet. In those

rare instances in which symptoms become excessively uncomfortable or dangerous, removal of the mass by the anterior cervical approach should be considered.

"SYMPATHETIC" SYMPTOMS IN CERVICAL DISC DISEASE. Many patients with evidence of acute or chronic cervical disc disease will present a variety of vague and indefinite symptoms, which must be considered valid because of their stereotyped description from patient to patient. These include migratory headaches, dizziness, visual blurring, alteration in auditory perception, and feelings of separation from the environment. Some will describe a sensation of constriction in the neck, difficulty with swallowing, or even change in the character of the voice.[4]

The explanation for these symptoms remains obscure. Many patients have associated features of hysteria, but others are well motivated, without psychological disorder, and

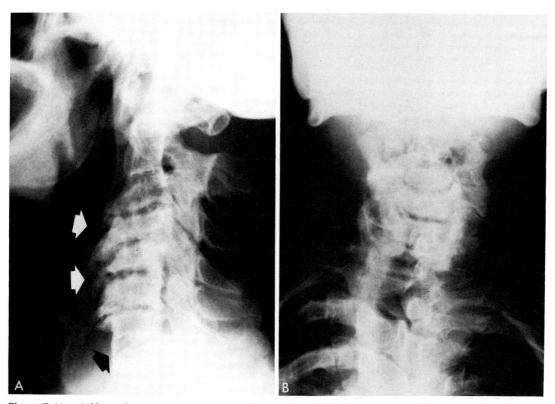

Figure 7–11. *A*, Visceral pressure symptoms secondary to chronic disc degeneration and huge osteophyte formation. The lower (black) arrow indicates a congenital fusion of C7-T1 which has participated in the development of this condition. There is extensive disc degeneration of cervical vertebrae 3 through 7. The vertebrae in addition have collapsed, and marked anterior bony projections protrude into the retropharyngeal space. The white arrows outline the pharyngeal air shadow, which is deviated markedly anteriorly and thus responsible for difficulty with swallowing solid foods.

B, The same cervical spine in the anterior-posterior view indicating similar distortion and collapse of the normal vertebral anatomic relationships.

are not interested in litigation or compensation. Barré thought that these symptoms were related to compression of the nervous plexus around the wall of the vertebral artery.[4] It is known that various ill-described pains in the face can result from injury to the sympathetic plexus about the carotid artery (carotidynia). Perhaps vertebral artery compression produces analogous discomfort. Bartschi-Rochai considered this syndrome to be caused by intermittent disturbances in the vertebral artery flow, in conjunction with irritation of the periarterial plexus.[5] The pharyngeal symptoms (migraine pharyngee of Terracol) appear in the absence of roentgenographic evidence of a pharyngeal compression from cervical spondylosis.[94] The vague nature of the symptoms further adds to the mystery that surrounds their cause. In their excellent monograph on cervical spondylosis, Brain and Wilkinson give little attention to these symptoms.[10] The examiner should be aware, however, that in certain instances their presence does not invariably indicate psychological abnormality.

SYNDROME OF "SILENT" AND CENTRAL CERVICAL SOFT DISC HERNIATION. Central soft disc herniations, as opposed to chronic cervical disc degeneration, are an uncommon cause of myelopathy, and patients with this disease comprise only 1 to 2 per cent of all operations done for acute or chronic cervical disc degeneration. Lourie and colleagues summarized the literature and added six cases of progressive myelopathy secondary to midline herniations of disc material.[62] A significant factor in this entity is the surprisingly frequent absence of a history of antecedent trauma in the face of a subacute or chronic myelopathy characterized by spasticity, with or without weakness of the lower extremity, with variable involvement of the upper extremities. Several patients demonstrated partial loss of pain and temperature discrimination in the upper thoracic region. In some cases plain films of the cervical spine were normal, and degenerative changes, if present, did not indicate the offending interspace. In other instances, congenitally narrowed cervical spinal canal seemed to predispose to the early development of symptoms. These authors reported excellent results with anterior discectomy and fusion, a procedure that avoids dangerous retraction of the spinal cord, which would be necessary to remove a similar lesion by laminectomy.

ATYPICAL PRESENTATION OF CERVICAL DISC DISEASE. The neurologic differential in cervical disc disease, particularly slowly progressive spondylosis, is often complex. This common entity may affect the nervous system in a surprising variety of ways. The symptoms may be almost entirely motor, entirely sensory, or there may be pain in the absence of neurologic findings. Differential diagnosis is reviewed in more appropriate context in Chapter 3.

LABORATORY DATA

Plain Film Examination

Unlike lumbar disc disease, symptomatic cervical disc disease is rarely seen without some radiographic signs on plain film examination. Conversely, evidence of chronic disc degeneration is prominent in the middle-aged group and is virtually universal in elderly patients, even in the absence of signs or symptoms. Radiographic criteria, therefore, will have value only when combined with clinical details.

Routine cervical spine roentgenographic examination should include anteroposterior, lateral, and bilateral oblique projections. The atlas and axis can be visualized, as required, with open-mouth views. When clinically indicated in patients who experience neck or arm pain with head motion, lateral films of the neck in flexion and extension are valuable.

ACUTE DISC HERNIATION

NARROWING OF INTERSPACE. A single narrow cervical interspace, associated with appropriate clinical symptoms, suggests an acute soft disc herniation. Obviously, cervical disc degeneration may develop with protrusion of disc material that does not impinge on the nerve root, so narrowing of an interspace per se does not mean symptomatic disc disease. Although measurements may be helpful, significant disc narrowing is detectable on gross examination.

VACUUM DISC. Although it is a relatively rare finding, disc degeneration may be associated with the development of air in the disc space. This is seen with increased frequency in patients with symptomatic disease at that level, which suggests an acute degenerative process.

STRAIGHTENING OF SPINE; LOSS OF NORMAL LORDOTIC CURVE. Both acute discal and musculoskeletal cervical spine injuries may be associated with paravertebral spasm and straightening. This appearance can be voluntarily assumed by the patient, but more frequently it signals some degree of restricted motion secondary to neck pain.

CERVICAL INSTABILITY. Lateral views of the neck in flexion and extension can show excessive motion at the level of an acutely degenerated disc. This hypermobility is often associated with injury to supporting ligaments at the same level (see Chapter 4).

CHRONIC DISC DEGENERATION

The following are emphasized because they often correlate with specific signs and symptoms.

NARROWING OF ANTEROPOSTERIOR DIAMETER OF CERVICAL SPINAL CANAL. In the lateral cervical spine film, normally taken at a distance of 30 inches between x-ray tube and patient, the anteroposterior diameter of the spinal canal should not be less than 13 mm. at any point. Maximum diameter is usually considered to be 20 mm. Measurements taken opposite a "spur" of a chronic disc degeneration of less than 13 mm. suggest spinal cord compression. Many feel that an AP diameter of 11 mm. or less means definite spinal cord impingement. This measurement is reliable, and myelography will confirm spinal cord compression as predicted by these lateral films. Figure 7–12 shows an analysis by Wolfe and colleagues of this measurement in 200 adults.[101]

FORAMINAL ENCROACHMENT. In the oblique view, the intervertebral foramina should appear as oval structures, formed superiorly and laterally by the laminae and zygapophyseal joints, and anteriorly and medially by the vertebral body and intervertebral disc. Chronic cervical disc disease with proliferation will, therefore, encroach upon this foramen from its medial and slightly inferior aspect. The obliquity of projection is important, for both normal and diseased foramina seem foreshortened at certain angles.

CERVICAL INSTABILITY. Radiologic examination of the patient with unexplained neck or suboccipital pain (which may at times radiate to the forehead or behind the eye) is not complete without lateral views while the neck is in full flexion and full extension. Evidence of abnormal movement at one or more levels is frequently associated with such pain. The capsular ligaments about the intervertebral joints, the anterior and posterior spinal ligaments, and other musculature-supporting structures of the neck generally maintain an even distribution of vertebral motion. In flexion and extension, therefore, vertebrae should move proportionately, much in the fashion of a gooseneck lamp. Because the thoracic vertebrae are essentially immobilized by the ribs, and because the upper two vertebrae are designed for rotatory movement of the head, C3 through C7 will function principally in forward and backward head motion. Although these ligaments are commonly injured in acute trauma, apparently chronic disc degeneration, with associated proliferative involvement of the intervertebral joints, encourages laxity of the spinal supporting structures. This may occur at one level but, with chronic disc degeneration, multiple level involvement is sometimes observed. Figure 7–13 indicates

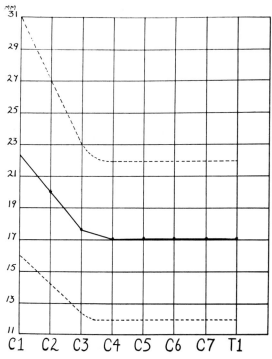

Figure 7–12. Mean sagittal diameter of spinal canal as measured on lateral roentgenograms taken at 30-inch tube-patient distance. The dotted lines represent standard deviation among 200 "normal" adults. (From Wolfe, B. S., Kilnani, M., and Malis, L.: The sagittal diameter of the bony cervical spinal canal and its significance in cervical spondylosis. J. Mt. Sinai Hosp. 23:283, 1965.)

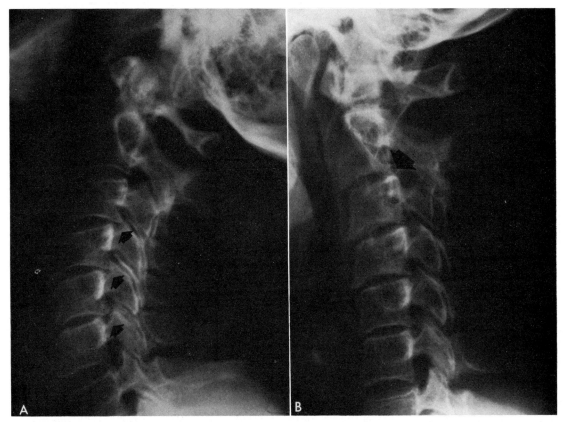

Figure 7–13. Neck and suboccipital pains secondary to multiple level subluxation in flexion and extension.

A, At the C3-4, C4-5 and C5-6, there was posterior overriding of the vertebral bodies in extension. At this time the patient experienced neck and shoulder top pain.

B, In flexion, there was good alignment of these vertebrae, but C2 subluxed anteriorly on C1, at which time the patient noted marked suboccipital pain. Stabilization in a cervical collar alleviated her symptoms.

the apparently small but clinically significant vertebral movement seen in a patient with persistent suboccipital pain aggravated by head flexion. Radiographically, abnormal motion of more than 3.5 mm. (subluxation) in flexion or extension must be considered significant.

NARROWING OF THE INTERSPACE. Disc degeneration, with subsequent prolapse of the interspace, precedes the formation of osteophytes. This finding, therefore, is extremely common in itself and does not suggest symptomatic disease as reliably as the three radiographic findings just described.

DEGENERATIVE CHANGES IN THE ZYGAPOPHYSEAL JOINTS. As a result of chronic disc degeneration and associated inflammatory changes in its synovial mechanism, the superior articular surface of the zygapophyseal joint tends to slip backward and can erode the lamina below. Various forms of spondylotic

changes in the zygapophyseal joint are shown in Figure 7–10, taken from Brain and Wilkinson.[10]

Lawrence and colleagues undertook an interesting radiologic survey in which lateral views of the cervical spine were taken in a general population and evaluated by disc degeneration and osteoarthritis of the zygapophyseal joints.[57] Among 279 males over the age of 55, 83.5 per cent demonstrated evidence of disc degeneration. Among 368 women over 55, 80.7 per cent also demonstrated disc degeneration. He discovered also that, although the incidence in the male and female population was similar, the men seemed to be more severely affected. Unlike lumbar disc disease, evidence of cervical disc degeneration was unrelated to occupation.

McRae examined patients over the age of 30 with and without symptoms of cervical spine disease.[65] Under the age of 40 there was fair correlation between radiologic changes and presence of symptoms. Over 40, however, one could not predict which patients were symptomatic on the basis of radiologic film review.

Positive Contrast Myelography

Positive contrast myelography is indicated in disc disease patients with evidence of spinal cord or nerve root compression when surgery is contemplated. In advanced or progressive myelopathy, this procedure is attended with certain risks. Indications for myelography in cervical disc disease when surgery is not planned are unusual.[45]

ACUTE DISC HERNIATION. The only significant myelographic change of acute disc herniation is an impression in the column of contrast material opposite an interspace. The indentation caused by an acute disc is greater than one would expect from bony spurs, which may or may not appear on the plain films at the same level (Fig. 7–14). Other myelographic changes resemble those of chronic disc degeneration. The latter, of course, frequently produces multiple level myelographic deformities, unlike acute disc degeneration, which develops at a single level.

CHRONIC DISC DEGENERATION. *Evidence of Spinal Cord Compression.* Spondylotic "spurs" may indent the subarachnoid space to varying degrees. In the lateral view the indentation may be readily apparent. In the anteroposterior view, severe compression appears as a lucent "bar." In more severe cases, a complete block is demonstrated. The cervical spinal cord may be flattened by the spur and, therefore, may appear wider than normal in the anteroposterior view. This appearance may be mistaken for an intramedullary spinal cord tumor. A lateral view, however, can usually make this distinction.

Evidence of Nerve Root Compression. Because the subarachnoid space extends only a short distance along each nerve root the myelographic contrast material does not flow well into the foramen. Compression of the nerve root by spurs of chronic degenerative disc disease may produce a relatively small defect in the column of contrast material at its visible portion. Relatively large spurs, grossly compressing and deviating the nerve root in the foramen, have been known to

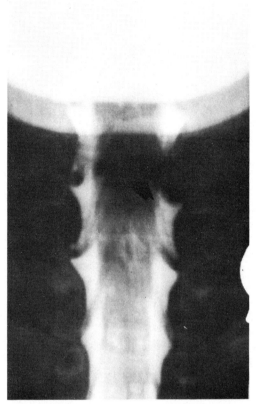

Figure 7–14. Typical findings of acute disc degeneration with herniation and nerve root compression.

The nerve root sleeves in this anterior-posterior myelographic view fill out in a normal pattern except for the C6 root, which is exiting between C5 and C6. The arrow indicates a large, laterally placed defect which is actually in contact with the spinal cord shadow. Above and below, contrast material in the subarachnoid space lateral to the spinal cord is clearly seen. The dural sleeve and its associated structures, however, are severely compressed by a huge extruded disc fragment. On other views it was possible to visualize distortion of the nerve root by this fragment.

produce only minimal myelographic changes, which ordinarily consist of notching of the normal root sleeve pattern. However, because the site of maximal compression occurs so far distally, this notched or amputated appearance of the root sleeve should be considered significant when at a level appropriate for the radicular symptoms.

Hypertrophy of Ligamentum Flavum. This entity can be appreciated only on myelography. Contrast material on the dorsal surface of the spinal cord is indented in a symmetric, washboard fashion. Dynamic myelography in the lateral view with the head in

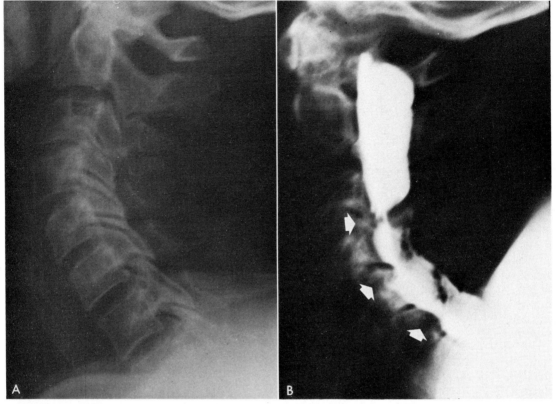

Figure 7–15. The clinical presentation suggested chronic disc degeneration with spinal cord compression. Plain lateral cervical spine films (A) surprisingly indicated little degenerative disc disease. At myelography, there was evidence of minor indentations of the opaque column opposite the mid-cervical interspaces (B). With the patient's neck in extension during the myelogram, however, extensive posterior compression of the spinal cord could be demonstrated which was secondary to hypertrophy and infolding of the ligamentum flavum.

various positions confirms Stoltman's and Blackwood's interesting studies on isolated cervical spine segments, in which extension further buckles these ligaments and significantly narrows the spinal canal (Fig. 7–15).[89]

Air Myelography

Positive contrast myelography will delineate compressive lesions of the spinal cord in most cases. Occasionally, however, the subarachnoid space around the spinal cord must be visualized. In some instances, such as in Figure 7–16B, the density of the contrast material is such that it can obscure the details of the compressing bar. Air myelography, when combined with tomography, has a distinct advantage in that it outlines the entire spinal cord and makes more obvious any compressing lesion. Disadvantages of this procedure, however, include greater discomfort to the patient, greater difficulty in the interpretation

of anteroposterior views, and failure to adequately outline the details in the lateral portions (nerve roots) of the spinal canal.

More recently, the study has been done with the patient in a lateral decubitus position, the head and shoulders elevated above the buttocks level. A water-filled bag is placed between the patient's neck and the tomogram table, so that the air density in this space does not obscure detail. While the patient is in this position a lumbar puncture is performed and air is injected in 10 cc. increments. When a patient experiences pain in the uppermost shoulder and neck, one ordinarily finds that air has begun to enter the cervical spinal canal. The exchange of further air initiates a suboccipital headache, at which time midline lateral tomograms are taken. Figure 7–16C indicates significant spinal cord compression, even though the positive contrast myelogram demonstrated in Figure 7–16B is far less impressive. This procedure has been made obsolete by advances in computed tomography.

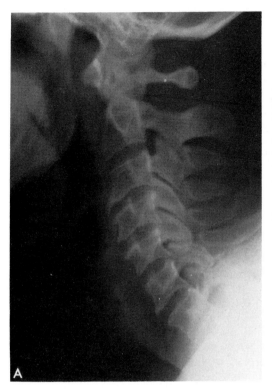

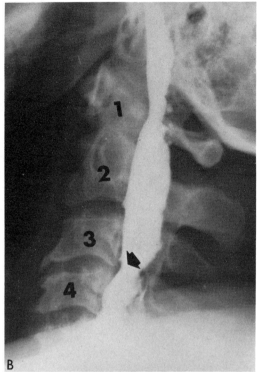

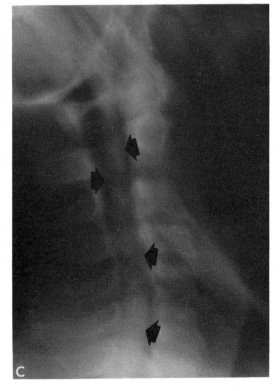

Figure 7–16. The value of air myelography and delineation in certain cases of spinal cord compression secondary to disease of the cervical spine. The lateral roentgenogram shown in *A* was taken of a 44-year-old man with evidence of high cervical cord compression. Neurologic examination demonstrated increased reflexes in the upper and lower extremities. There is evidence of chronic disc degeneration with compression deformities of the upper cervical vertebrae, perhaps due to old trauma.

B, At myelography, only a small indentation in the opaque column was demonstrable at the C3-4 level.

C, Air myelogram with tomographic slices through the center of the spinal canal. The upper arrows indicate air in front of and behind the cervical spinal cord. The two lower arrows indicate air along the anterior surface of the spinal cord. Opposite C3-C4 there is no air demonstrable and the posterior margins of the vertebral bodies at this level are in direct contact with the spinal cord. The spinal cord itself is deviated posteriorly and appears to be in contact with the lamina. Such delineation was not possible on positive contrast myelography because the density of the contrast material obscured the detail of the spinal cord itself. Contrast-enhanced computed tomography has replaced air myelography in those rare cases not clarified by oil or water-soluble myelography.

Cineradiography in Diagnosis of Cervical Instability

Lateral films of the cervical spine with the neck in extreme flexion and extension are usually sufficient to diagnose cervical instability. Occasionally, however, further elucidation of this problem in a dynamic sense may be required, and this can be done by a cineradiogram. This study is an ordinary lateral fluoroscopic view of the cervical spine in motion. Moving pictures taken from the fluoroscopic screen record the mechanics of mobility. At times there may be a sudden subluxation, often accompanied by reproduction of the patient's symptoms, during such motion. When this dramatic observation is recorded, further support for the concept of fusion at the appropriate level is afforded. This study is reserved for unusual cases, and it rarely reveals unexpected abnormal motion.

Cervical Discography and the Disc Distention Test

In 1948, Lindblom first described a technique by which the center of a disc could be visualized after injection of a radiopaque solution into its substance.[60] This technique, which has many enthusiastic supporters, has not reached general acceptance in the past 34 years. Some reasons for its unpopularity are fear of disc injury by needle puncture, accuracy of cervical myelography, discomfort associated with the procedure, fear of damage of the spinal cord by the needle, and reports that abnormal discograms are commonly seen in asymptomatic patients. Nonetheless, supporters of this technique can demonstrate instances in which discography clearly indicated a symptomatic abnormality despite a normal cervical myelogram. This technique requires continued evaluation and improvement. In particularly difficult cases, the surgeon should keep an open mind about its use and interpretation.

The procedure is carried out in the radiology department, with aseptic preparation of the anterior surface of the neck. The neck is hyperextended after the infiltration of local anesthesia. The larynx is displaced to the contralateral side of the neck by gentle digital retraction. With further downward pressure, the discographer's fingers can palpate the anterior cervical spine in a groove between the larynx and the carotid sheath. The skin is punctured with a 2-inch, 20-gauge needle, which will soon come in contact with the anterior surface of the bone at a 45 degree angle. The point of the needle is then stepped up or down lightly until soft disc is encountered. This is usually moderately uncomfortable. The needle is then inserted at a depth of about 2 mm., and a lateral roentgenogram checks its position. A 2½ inch, 25-gauge needle is then inserted through the previous needle. When properly placed, the point of this second needle will lie near the center of the disc. Via a tuberculin syringe, 0.5 ml. of radiopaque soluble solution is injected through the fine needle. A normal cervical disc will rarely accept more than 0.2 ml. This seldom induces pain in a normal disc. Pathologic discs will accept a larger quantity of solution, and the injection is usually associated with pain. The location and distribution of this pain is an important additional diagnostic clue. This procedure is sometimes termed the "disc distention test." Many feel that production of symptoms by an intradiscal injection is of greater significance than is the discogram itself; in fact, some simply perform the disc distention test with less toxic saline, without concern for radiographic demonstration. If the induced pain reproduces the patient's symptoms, the disc is implicated. If the symptoms are not reproduced, or if the discogram is normal, it may be wise to study another disc. When the appropriate disc is identified, a few drops of indigo carmine are injected into each needle as a surgical marker. The interspace elected for study depends, of course, on the patient's symptoms. Since the C5-C6, C6-C7, and C4-C5 discs are so commonly affected, they should be studied in that order if further investigation is required.

Axial Tomography

FREDIE P. GARGANO, M.D.

INTRODUCTION

The cervical vertebrae and spinal canal can be adequately visualized by routine radiographic techniques. The normal anatomy is well known, and the size and shape of the spinal canal can be ascertained by inspection of routine cervical spine studies and myelography. However, axial tomography portrays the cross-sectional anatomy in a manner not feasible by any other radiographic technique.[32, 33, 39]

Since the introduction of total body scanners, computed tomography has become an important tool in evaluating the spinal column. Computed tomography has been used in the diagnosis of spinal dysraphism,[49, 76, 97] spinal cord arteriovenous malformations,[26] spinal cord tumor,[40, 69] syringomyelia,[78] multiple sclerosis of the cervical cord,[18] spinal stenosis,[39] vertebral fractures,[19] vertebral metastases,[69] paraspinal masses,[69] spondylosis,[17] and herniated discs.[17] It has also been used in conjunction with myelography, especially with metrizamide.[17, 76]

The normal anatomy of the cervical spinal canal as demonstrated by axial tomography will be briefly reviewed. The configuration of the cervical canal changes at various levels. The shape of the craniocervical junction is round, conforming to the boundaries of the foramen magnum. At the C1 level the canal is formed dorsally by the semicircular arch of C1, laterally by the lateral masses of C1, and ventrally by the ligamentum-covered dens. Between the C1 and C2 dorsal arches exists the only probable level in the cervical canal where no dorsal bony boundary will be seen on axial tomography. The canal is more rectangular in outline, formed dorsally by the ligamenta flava, laterally by the pedicles of C2, and ventrally by the body of C2. At the level of the C2 dorsal arch, the canal is elliptical with the longer diameter transversely oriented. Posteriorly, the larger rounded elliptical shape is formed by the laminae. Ventrolaterally the contour is shaped by the medial aspect of the pedicles. Ventrally, the elliptical shape is flattened by the posterior aspect of the body of C2.

Caudal to the level of C2, the configuration of the cervical canal is altered by the anatomic changes in the pedicles and the laminae. The pedicles decrease in height, progressively changing the elliptical shape into a semicircle by decreasing the ventrolateral component. The laminae become flattened and meet at a more acute angle, resulting in a dorsal triangular shape. The shape of the spinal canal, the intervertebral foramina, the zygoapophyseal joints, the pedicles, the vertebral artery foramina, and the laminar configuration are shown to excellent advantage by this technique (Figs. 7–17 to 7–20). Persistent notochordal remnants may also be demonstrated.

With the noncomputed axial tomographic units, the spinal cord cannot be visualized unless tomography is performed in conjunction with contrast myelography. With the CAT scanners, the spinal cord cannot always be shown as a distinct structure. However,

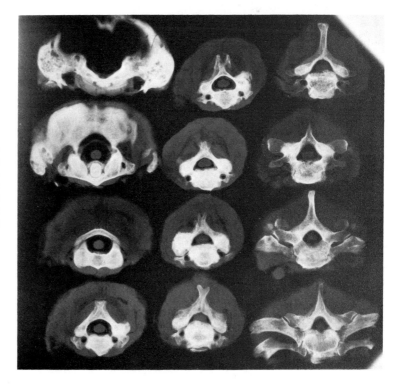

Figure 7–17. Axial sections through the cervical spine from the foramen magnum to the upper thoracic spine. Note the changing configuration of the spinal canal, the laminar and pediculate changes from above downward, and the changing cord:canal ratio.

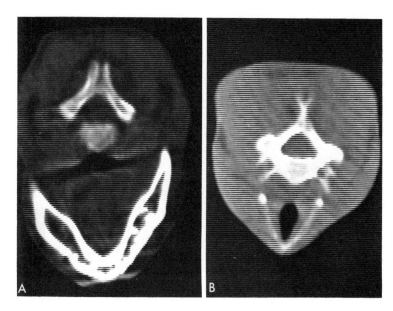

Figure 7–18. *A,* CAT section through the intervertebral foramina of C2-C3. *B,* CAT section through the C5 vertebral body.

abnormalities within the spinal cord may occasionally be seen on plain CAT scans or with enhancement. As resolution improves and as water-soluble contrast media become available, demonstration of the spinal cord by CAT scanning will become routine.

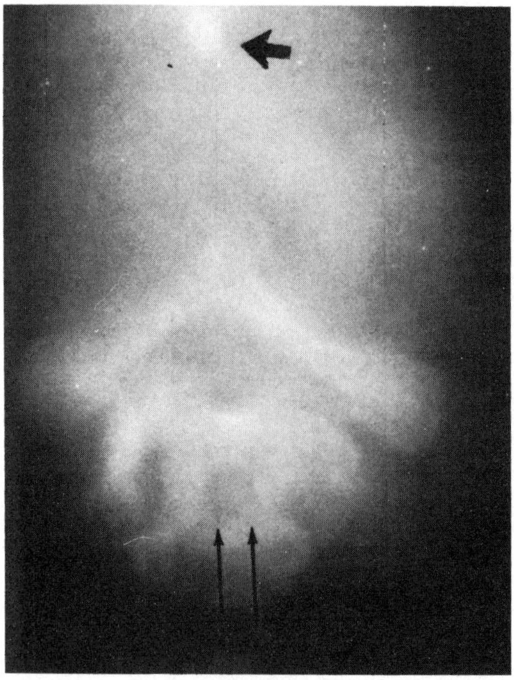

By tomography of anatomic specimens, the cord:canal ratio can be ascertained in the cervical canal. In the upper cervical area, the cord:canal ratio is low. As the cervical canal decreases in size caudally, the cord:canal ratio increases to the level of the cervical cord enlargement at C6. Below this level, the cord:canal ratio again decreases.

CERVICAL SPONDYLOSIS

This is a condition in which progressive degeneration of the intervertebral disc leads to changes in surrounding structures. With loss of disc substance, the anulus fibrosus may bulge into the spinal canal. If a tear develops in the anulus fibrosus, the nucleus pulposus may prolapse. The disc space narrows as well as the intervertebral foramina. Secondary changes develop in the apophyseal joints (degenerative arthritis) and in the joints of Luschka (spondylosis). Osteophytes develop, which encroach on the spinal canal and on the intervertebral and vertebral artery foramina. Secondary thickening of the ligamentum flavum occurs, which further compromises the spinal canal. Also, subluxation of the spine may occur. Grossly, the cervical spine shortens, and there is caudal displacement of the nerve roots.[100]

The cross-sectional area of the cervical spinal canal as well as its transverse and sagittal diameters are important. With compromise of the available space in the cervical

Figure 7–19. Axial tomogram through level of C4, showing persistent notochordal remnant (double arrows) and calcified ligamentum nuchae (short arrow).

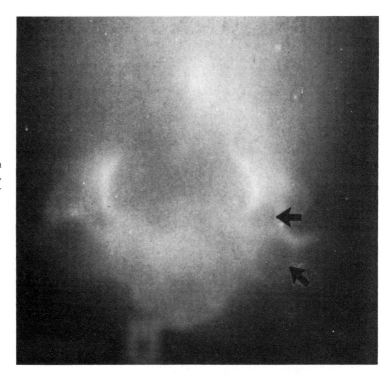

Figure 7–20. Axial tomogram through level of the C6 vertebral body, showing a double foramen transversarium (arrows) on one side.

canal, compression of the cervical cord can result. The normal sagittal diameter of the cervical spine from C3 to C7 is 12 mm. to 22 mm. The average sagittal diameter of the cervical cord is 10 mm. Thus, a patient with a normally smaller sagittal diameter of the canal will be more likely to develop cord compression with the same degree of spondylosis than another patient with a more generous-sized canal. Pallis, Jones, and Spillane[71] produced evidence that the canal is smaller in cases of cervical spondylosis. Payne and Spillane[73] measured the sagittal diameter of the cervical canal in 90 patients. Their series included three equal groups of patients: (1) 30 normal patients, (2) 30 patients with cervical spondylosis, and (3) 30 patients paraplegic from cervical spondylosis. They found the average sagittal diameter of the canal was smaller in paraplegic patients.

The plain film findings and myelographic abnormalities in cervical spondylosis are well known. However, there are patients who have radicular pain secondary to spondylosis who do not have significant osteophytes on the plain film or myelogram to explain their symptoms. Not infrequently we see patients with unilateral radicular pain with contralateral osteophytes. These patients may have significant osteophytes causing symptoms, but our present radiographic techniques are inade-

quate for their detection. When we see an osteophytic spur on the lateral film projection over the spinal canal, it is difficult to determine whether it is midline or lateral in position. We have to rely on the AP film to evaluate the joints of Luschka or the oblique films to evaluate the intervertebral foramina. It may be impossible at myelography to distinguish a midline osteophyte from a herniated midline cervical disc. Also, we see patients who have cervical spondylosis and myelopathy with sagittal canal measurements more than 10 mm. on the lateral myelographic study (from the back of the spur to the inner aspect of the neural spine). These patients may have a large midline spur that is indenting and compressing the cord but that cannot be ascertained because of the density of the myelographic contrast agent. Axial tomography can help in the proper evaluation of these patients (Figs. 7–21 to 7–23).

DISC DISEASE

At present, investigation has been limited, utilizing CAT scanning in conjunction with metrizamide myelography to evaluate for the presence of herniated cervical discs. Routine myelography remains the most accurate radiologic method to diagnose herniated cervical discs.

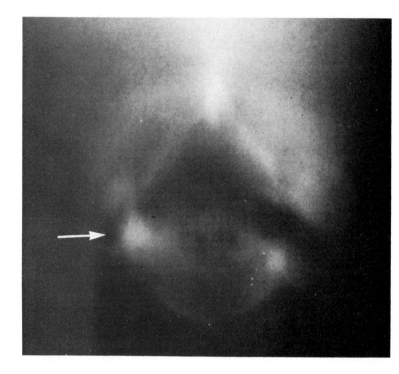

Figure 7–21. Axial tomogram showing an osteophyte obliterating the right C5-C6 intervertebral foramen (arrow).

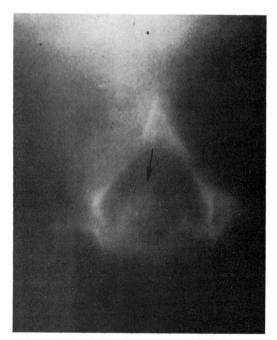

Figure 7–22. Axial tomogram at C6-C7 showing a large osteophyte (arrow) extending halfway to the neural spine.

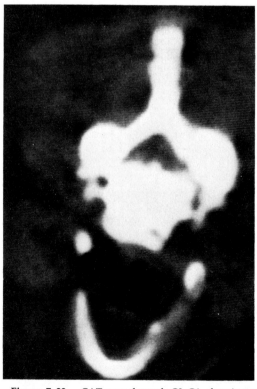

Figure 7–23. CAT scan through C3-C4, showing extensive spondylosis with neuroforaminal encroachment and a small midline spur.

CONGENITAL ABNORMALITIES

Abnormalities such as meningocele or spina bifida can be readily demonstrated with plain films as well as axial tomography.

Spinal dysraphism, which includes abnormalities such as diastematomyelia, neuroenteric cysts, dermoid cysts, teratomas, lipomas, and low spinal cord conus, have all been evaluated with CAT scanning with and without metrizamide myelography. Some of these abnormalities may also be demonstrated by TAT (Transverse Axial Tomography).

TUMORS

Ordinarily one relies on myelography for the detection and localization of intraspinal tumors. The enlargement of the canal (Figs. 7–24 and 7–25) and erosive change secondary to an intraspinal tumor (Fig. 7–26) can be readily seen on transverse axial tomography. Occasionally, one encounters a calcified tumor that can be detected on plain films (Fig. 7–27).

With the CAT scanner, more information is obtainable in patients with suspected intraspinal and paraspinal neoplasms. The presence, extent of the tumor, and degree of bone destruction with paraspinal neoplasms are more accurately delineated by CAT scanning. Intraspinal tumors such as meningiomas, neurofibromas, lipomas, osteoblastomas, astrocytomas, hemangioblastomas, and chordomas have been successfully demonstrated.

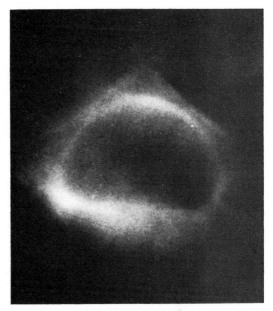

. **Figure 7–24.** Transverse axial tomogram at the C4 level. Expansion of the canal in all diameters is noted. Diagnosis: astrocytoma of the cervical spinal cord.

TRAUMA

Standard radiographic examinations are important in the management of cervical spine injury. These studies usually allow assessment of injury to the spinal cord and canal. However, obtaining routine radiographic examinations may be severely limited in patients with acute cervical spine injury. It is not difficult to obtain a CAT scan of the spine while the patient is in the supine position following

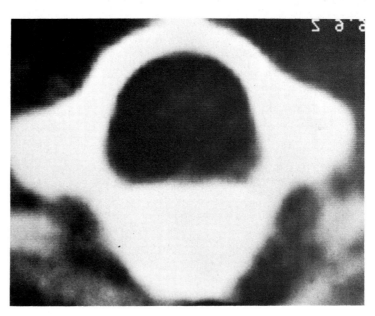

Figure 7–25. CAT scan at the C5 level. The uniformly expanded canal due to syringomyelia is well demonstrated.

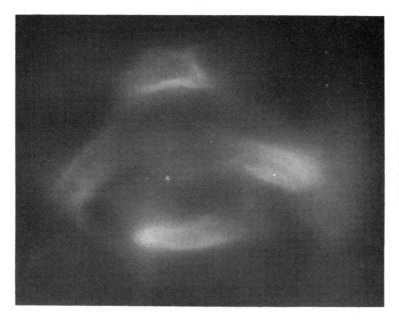

Figure 7–26. Axial tomogram through C3. Note marked erosive changes involving the laminae, dorsal arch, and posterior aspect of the vertebral body. The intervertebral foramina are widened. Diagnosis: intraspinal neurofibroma.

initial radiographs, thus avoiding unnecessary and dangerous manipulations. The CAT scanner can provide valuable additional information, allowing delineation of unsuspected or additional fractures, intraspinal fragments (Fig. 7–28), and secondary traumatic stenosis (Fig. 7–29). The CAT scan should be utilized as an adjunct to the standard radiographic techniques in the evaluation and management of serious injuries of the cervical spine.

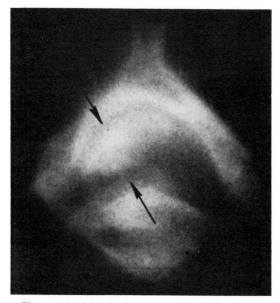

Figure 7–27. Transverse axial tomogram at the level of C3. Intraspinal location and extent of calcified mass (arrows) is well demarcated.

SUMMARY

On routine radiography, the configuration of the cervical canal cannot be completely assessed. Axial tomography gives an accurate cross-sectional view of the spinal canal. The bodies, intervertebral foramina, pedicles, lamina, and neural spines are well demarcated. The size and shape of the canal can be exactly demonstrated. The existence of midline spurs can be accurately determined. Small but significant spurs encroaching on the intervertebral foramina can be detected.

Axial tomography (both TAT and CAT) provides a new dimension in the evaluation of cervical spine disease. Correlation with other radiographic methods, such as plain films, tomography, myelography, and spinal cord angiography, is essential. Of the two types of axial tomography, the CAT scanner is definitely superior. The limitation of present CAT scanners is related to the inability of the equipment to demonstrate the normal anatomy of the intraspinal space (spinal cord, subarachnoid space, and cauda equina). As the resolution of the CAT scanners improves (Fig. 7–30) and as their use with water-soluble contrast myelography (Figs. 7–31 and 7–32) increases, more precise anatomic delineation will result. It is concluded that spinal CAT will have a major role in the diagnosis and management of spinal disorders because of its diagnostic capabilities and its noninvasive characteristics.

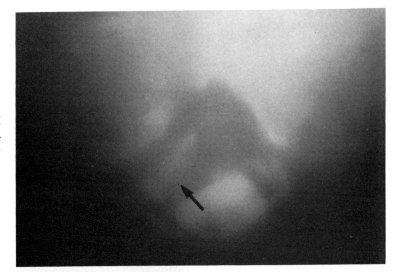

Figure 7–28. Axial tomogram through C6-C7. The displaced bony fragment (arrow) compromising the intervertebral foramen is well demonstrated.

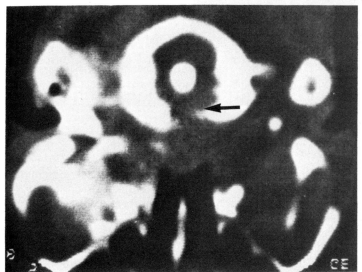

Figure 7–29. Rupture of the atlantoaxial ligament with posterior displacement of the odontoid with respect to the posterior margin (arrow) of the anterior arch of C1.

Figure 7–30. Plain CAT scan through C1-C2, showing the spinal cord.

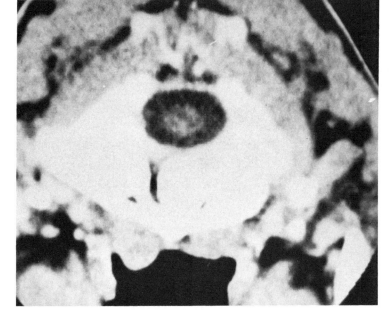

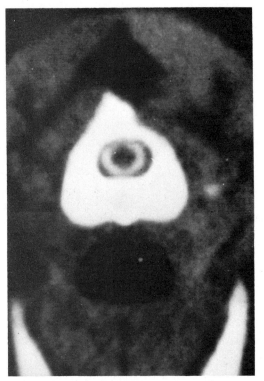

Figure 7–31. Metrizamide CAT scan showing the spinal cord outlined by contrast material at the C2 level.

Electromyography

The electromyogram rarely offers significant diagnostic information in evaluation of suspected cervical radiculopathy. After a variable period of time (usually six weeks) following destructive compression of an anterior root, the muscles supplied by this root will fibrillate. By inserting the needle into appropriate muscles, the electromyographer can determine whether this fibrillation follows the distribution of a nerve root, the brachial plexus, or the peripheral nerve itself. Electromyography, therefore, is reserved for those special situations in which differential diagnosis includes either radicular or peripheral nerve involvement. It is occasionally of some value when the decision to do myelography is borderline. Finally, in those instances in which organic syndrome cannot be separated from an emotional problem, the electromyogram, if positive, adds credence to the organicity of the symptoms. Unfortunately, the electromyogram can be normal in the presence of organic radicular pain, but it will likely be abnormal if chronic weakness is described in an organic radicular syndrome.

Spinal Fluid Examination

Biochemical and cytologic examination of spinal fluid is rarely of diagnostic value in disc disease. It is the authors' opinion that the only study worthy of consideration is the protein determination, which, if elevated over 100 mg./ml., suggests disc disease with complete spinal block, or a spinal cord tumor.[3]

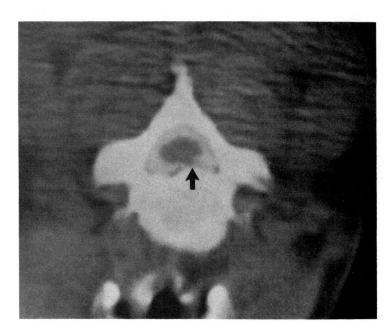

Figure 7–32. Metrizamide CAT scan at the C5-C6 level, showing a large posterior osteophyte (arrow) displacing the spinal cord.

TREATMENT

Nonoperative Treatment of Cervical Disc Disease

The majority of patients with cervical disc disease, either acute or chronic, respond to a conscientious program of conservative therapy. The success of this program is based in large measure on good doctor-patient rapport. The physician must possess complete understanding of the pathologic processes involved and must be able to translate this knowledge into a rational and pragmatic course of treatment. He must then educate the patient to understand the disease process and the reasons for a protracted course of therapy. Only with thorough understanding of the problem and strong confidence in the treating physician can the patient gain the necessary patience to persist with what may be a long and burdensome course of therapy.

IMMOBILIZATION

In both acute and chronic disc disease, immobilization of the cervical spine is the cornerstone of therapy. In acute cervical injuries, rest and immobilization allow for healing of torn and attenuated soft tissues, such as the anterior longitudinal ligament and the anulus fibrosus. In chronic disc degeneration, the purpose of immobilization is to reduce inflammation of the supporting soft tissues around the nerve roots in the cervical spine. Immobilization can be achieved through the use of various types of collars, braces, bedrest, and traction. It has been the authors'

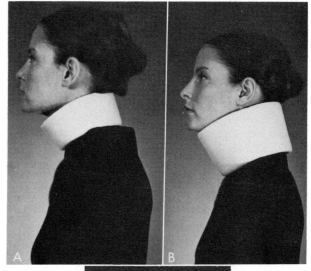

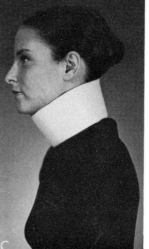

Figure 7–33. *A,* This photograph illustrates a soft cervical collar that is of insufficient height. It does not provide support or protection for the cervical spine. It does not accomplish its purpose.

B, A soft cervical collar that is excessively high. This collar forces the neck into hyperextension, which is uncomfortable for the patient.

C, The correct height of a cervical collar supports the neck in a neutral position.

experience that the use of a soft cervical collar that holds the head in a neutral or slightly flexed position is the method of choice. The more rigid and burdensome devices, such as plastic collars and metal braces, not only are less tolerable to the patient but also are less effective in the relief of pain. When the rigid devices are used for a prolonged period of time, they lead to marked soft tissue atrophy and stiffness, which are not found with the use of a soft collar. These collars are manufactured in various heights, from 2 to 4 inches, depending on the length of the patient's neck. The most commonly used height is 3½ inches.

The collar should be placed in such a way that the head is held in a position of slight to moderate flexion (Fig. 7–33). This is far more comfortable than the hyperextended position and allows for maximal opening of the intervertebral foramen. We have had many patients referred to our office to be evaluated for surgery because of failure of conservative treatment. In many instances, simply changing the position of immobilization from extension to flexion allowed a successful course of nonoperative treatment.

In acute cervical injuries the collar is worn on a full-time basis, night and day, for two to three weeks until the acute pain subsides and healing of the soft tissues has progressed well. If, at the end of this time, the patient is relatively free of symptoms, he may start on a course of cervical isometric exercises to strengthen the neck musculature in preparation for weaning from the cervical collar over the subsequent two to three weeks. It should be expected, and the patient should be warned, that a six-week recuperation period may be necessary in a significant cervical tissue injury. Patients should be aware of this at the onset of treatment so that the physician will not feel pressured to discontinue immobilization before the proper time. In the acute phase of a cervical syndrome, occasionally patients fail to attain adequate relief with ambulatory treatment; it may be necessary to place these people at bedrest, either at home or in the hospital. This will relieve the cervical spine from the burden of supporting the weight of the head. While at bedrest, these patients should be instructed to continue using their collar on a full-time basis. Cervical traction is rarely indicated in the treatment of soft tissue injuries and disc degeneration in the cervical spine. It is our feeling that traction serves as an irritant, and in many cases may

actually increase the patient's discomfort. It is no more logical to place an acutely injured cervical spine in traction than it is to manipulate an acute ligamentous injury of an ankle. The only apparent benefit of cervical traction is that it will help to enforce a regimen of confinement to bed. When used for this purpose, only minimal amounts of weight (4 to 6 lbs.) should be utilized, and the direction of pull should be in slight flexion. Traction in the neutral or hyperextended position is contraindicated for the same reason that collars which force the neck into an extended position are contraindicated.

DRUG THERAPY

Three groups of drugs have been found useful in the treatment of cervical disc disease — muscle relaxants, anti-inflammatory drugs, and analgesics. The use of one or more of these drugs is predicated upon the patient's particular requirement.

Acute injuries to the cervical discs and the supporting soft tissues of the spine frequently result in painful muscle spasm. A vicious cycle is established, whereby pain leads to muscle spasm, which leads to ischemia and a further increase in pain. Once the cycle is established, it tends to be self-perpetuating. An effective muscle relaxant frequently breaks this painful cycle and allows more comfort and an increased range of motion in the cervical spine. An excellent therapeutic effect has been noted with the use of carisoprodol (Soma), 350 mg. every eight hours. A strictly controlled double-blind trial by Shatwell confirms this impression.[86] A not infrequent side effect of this drug and other skeletal muscle relaxants is drowsiness, which may necessitate reduction in the dosage and the avoidance of hazardous occupations.

In addition to muscle relaxants, the authors have found it worthwhile to utilize anti-inflammatory drugs. The spectrum utilized varies from the more mild drugs such as aspirin to those in an intermediate category such as phenylbutazone (Butazolidin) and, at the most potent end of the spectrum, cortisone and its derivatives. The most commonly used regimen is phenylbutazone 100 mg. three times daily after meals. This drug is effective in many cases in which an inflammatory response is responsible for the symptoms.[75] Phenylbutazone has several serious side effects of which the physician and patient should be aware. Gastrointestinal irritation is the most common of these and may be prevented in some measure by taking the drug with food or an antacid. A history of ulcer disease or other gastrointestinal disorders must be carefully sought out and constitutes a relative contraindication to the use of this family of drugs. For those individuals unable to tolerate phenylbutazone, a less irritating derivative, oxyphenbutazone (Tandearil), can be used in an equivalent dosage. Periodic blood counts are recommended.

CERVICAL ISOMETRIC EXERCISES

Exercises for the cervical spine should be directed at strengthening the paravertebral musculature and not at increasing the range of motion. During the acute phase of a cervical injury the patient will be unable to tolerate exercises of any type, and it is not until the initial pain has subsided that an exercise program should be instituted. A typical cervical injury requires two to three weeks for the pain and muscle spasm to subside to a point at which an exercise program should be started. There is considerable variation in time as to when this point is reached. At this time, the patient should be instructed in the performance of cervical isometric exercises while still in the collar (Fig. 7–34). As strength and stability in the cervical spine increase, the patient may gradually be weaned from the

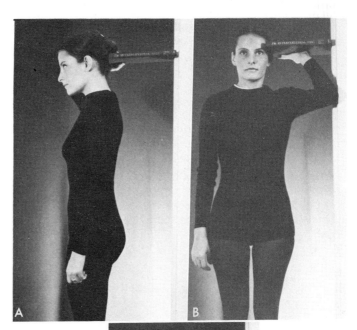

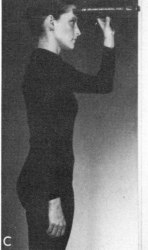

Figure 7–34. The correct position for performance of cervical isometric exercises. A maximum voluntary effort is exerted for five seconds, with 15 repetitions performed in each of the four directions. These are performed twice daily.

cervical collar, at first during the day and ultimately at night. For those patients who are unable to tolerate a program of isometric exercises, muscle strengthening can be achieved by carrying a weight, such as a book or a bean bag, balanced on the top of the head.

INFILTRATION OF TRIGGER POINTS

Localized tender areas in the paravertebral musculature and the trapezius muscles are found in many individuals with acute and chronic cervical disc degeneration. Marked relief of symptomatology often can be dramatically achieved by infiltration of the trigger points with 5 to 10 ml. of 1 per cent procaine (or "caine-like" derivative). The patient should, of course, be cautioned as to allergy to procaine and should be lying down or supported during the injection. The more localized the trigger point, the more effective this form of therapy will prove to be. This type of approach yields disappointing results in areas of diffuse tenderness that cannot be accurately localized. It is interesting to note that although the pharmacologic effects of these drugs may wear off in two to three hours, the relief may last for days or even weeks in many instances. These injections may be repeated at intervals of three days to several weeks. The effect may be entirely the result of psychological suggestion.

PHYSICAL THERAPY

Since muscle ischemia is one of the mechanisms of pain production in the cervical disc syndrome, modalities designed to increase blood flow to these muscles might be expected to be of benefit. Hot packs, diathermy, and ultrasound will accomplish this goal. It has been our experience that hot turkish towels applied for 10 to 20 minutes several times a day are the most effective and least expensive of the modalities mentioned. Light massage combined with the application of moist heat may also give a measure of temporary relief.

GENERAL MEASURES

A patient can take certain general measures that may hasten the recovery from a cervical syndrome and prevent recurrences. Sleep hygiene is one of the most important. The patient should be cautioned not to sleep in a prone position, which requires the head to be in a position of forced rotation. He may sleep on either his side or his back. Extreme flexion, such as that found when the head is propped on three to four pillows, should also be avoided. An ideal head support, described by Jackson, is a cylindrical pillow, 8 inches in diameter and approximately 18 inches in length, stuffed with a soft filler such as feathers or down.[48] This type of pillow has been demonstrated radiographically to keep the cervical spine in a neutral position regardless of whether the patient is sleeping supine or in a lateral posture.

The patient should be also informed of the deleterious effect of automobile riding during the acute phase of the syndrome, since vibration has a deleterious effect on the cervical spine. When long-distance travel is absolutely essential, air travel is preferable to either automobile or train.

Work areas should be arranged so that during performance of the patient's occupation it is not necessary for him to assume a position of extreme flexion, extension, or rotation. This may require a rearrangement of desk patterns, typewriters, or other frequently used equipment. Overhead work in which the patient is forced to hyperextend the spine is particularly detrimental to a patient with a disorder of the cervical spine. Drivers should be encouraged to learn to use rear-view and side-view mirrors rather than forced neck rotation when backing up.

Manipulation is mentioned only to be condemned in the treatment of acute or chronic cervical disc disorders. Many tragic sequelae have been described with the use of cervical manipulation, and it is our feeling that manipulation has no place in the treatment of cervical spine disorders of this type. It is true that patients with certain acute cervical syndromes enjoy a symptomatic response after cervical manipulation, but we feel the hazards are too great to warrant its use. An extensive clinical study by Livingston reveals that as high as 7 per cent of patients receiving spinal manipulation sustain a significant injury.[61] Injuries from manipulation include joint injury, nerve and spinal cord damage, vascular injury, and fracture-dislocation.

RESULTS OF NONOPERATIVE TREATMENT

The results to be expected from the plan of treatment just outlined are of interest. In a group of 225 patients treated this way for three months, complete relief was obtained in 29 per cent, partial relief in 49 per cent, and no improvement in 22 per cent.[24] Patients who failed to respond to conservative treatment were maintained with the various measures outlined for approximately one year before surgical intervention was recommended. Certain of these individuals who failed to respond to nonoperative treatment declined surgery and elected to "live with the disease." From this group of patients much interesting information was gleaned regarding the natural course of cervical disc disease.

Natural History

Of great importance to the authors is our attempt to outline the natural history of cervical disc disease so that we may intelligently discuss the future with patients who have this disorder; of greater importance, perhaps, is the necessity for a guideline to measure the effectiveness of cervical disc surgery. Those cases that were considered failures after conservative treatment at one year were followed for a total of five years, in an effort to determine the course of their symptoms and their ability to return to normal activities. At the time of follow-up only 45 per cent of the group had achieved a satisfactory level of pain relief and activity, and 55 per cent remained unsatisfactory, with significant pain and limitation of activity. Approximately one fourth of this group were never able to return to their original occupations.[25]

Certain other observations on patients in our conservative treatment group who have been followed have been noted. Those patients with hyperextension injuries and litigation tend to do more poorly than the group as a whole. These two factors, so often seen together, could not be evaluated separately in our studies. This tendency was not noted in our evaluation of patients who underwent surgery, and presumably the motivation was higher in these individuals. A second observation was that after a period of rapid improvement of symptoms, subsequent progress is slow and may extend for a period of years. It does not appear that cervical disc degeneration is a brief self-limiting disorder but rather a chronic disease, productive of significant pain and incapacity over an extended period of time.[58]

Surgical Treatment

SELECTION OF ANTERIOR OR POSTERIOR APPROACH TO THE CERVICAL SPINE

There is little unanimity among surgeons with reference to the desired route to specific cervical disc lesions. Often the surgeon will choose the procedure with which he is most comfortable, even though it may be more difficult in terms of eradicating the problem. Neurosurgeons may tend to favor the more familiar posterior approach, which they use in a wide variety of non-discogenic entities. Orthopedic surgeons frequently use the anterior route because of fear of damage to the underlying neural structures that may come into view during the posterior operation. There are, however, specific advantages and disadvantages that should be considered when one selects the type of operation.

ANTERIOR CERVICAL APPROACH

Advantages
1. Floor of the spinal canal can be reached without retraction of the spinal cord (as in a midline soft cervical disc protrusion).
2. Stability of the spine can be restored if the surgery or pathologic entity has weakened supporting ligaments.
3. Exposure of the spinal cord, and therefore possible damage to this structure, is reduced. If a postoperative hematoma develops, spinal cord compression is less likely than in a posterior approach.
4. Nerve root foramina can be opened by distraction of the vertebra and insertion of a plug of larger size.
5. Positioning and preparation of the patient is less complicated in that the operation is done in the supine rather than in more involved face-down or sitting-up positions.
6. In most patients the postoperative course may be less painful, with earlier ambulation and mobility.

Disadvantages
1. With time, instability and disc degeneration may develop above and below the fusion because of excess stress on these joints. This is particularly true where multiple anterior fusions have been done (Fig. 7–35).
2. With certain entities, such as soft disc herniation, there is poor visualization in the affected root, and fragments may be missed by the anterior approach.

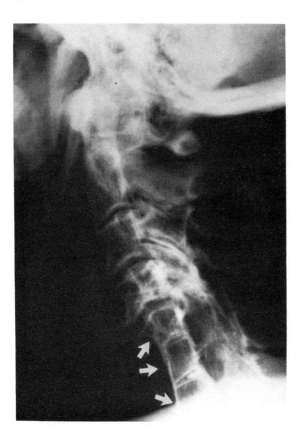

Figure 7–35. Late effects of fusion of cervical vertebrae. *A,* Lateral roentgenogram of a 55-year-old woman who has congenital fusion of the lower three cervical vertebrae (Klippel-Feil anomaly). These vertebrae did not participate in flexion and extension of her neck throughout life. Additional stress, therefore, was applied to the upper cervical vertebrae in these movements. At the level immediately adjacent to the fusion, C4-C5, there is extensive disc degeneration, with marked hypertrophic changes, producing both anterior and posterior osteophytes, which ultimately compressed the spinal cord.

3. Because the nerve root itself cannot be examined for an extensive length, intraoperative assessment of nerve root decompression is less accurate.
4. If multiple level decompression is necessary, as in advanced cervical disc degeneration with hypertrophic spur formation, extensive surgery and multiple fusions are required to decompress the spinal cord.
5. Decompression of the spinal cord itself is frequently less adequate in the anterior approach because the ligamentum flavum, which may be thickened and thereby become a source of spinal cord compression, remains intact (Fig. 7–15).
6. Though postoperative infections are very rare, osteomyelitis of the cervical spine is extremely difficult to treat and could lead to a variety of neural and visceral complications.
7. Although of no consequence to most patients, some prefer a scar on the back of the neck rather than one in the front and another at the donor site on the hip.

With the preceding description, one can easily determine the advantages and disadvantages of the posterior approach. It offers better visualization of the neural structures and it affords, in almost every instance, more generous decompression. Conversely, laminectomy can add to any preexisting spinal instability, and intraoperative misfortunes are more serious when the spinal cord is exposed (Fig. 7–36).

Following is a list of diseases of the cervical disc for which each approach is suggested. These impressions will vary with the skill and experience of the surgeon.

Definite Indications for Anterior Cervical Approach
1. Midline soft cervical disc herniation.
2. Cervical instability secondary to degenerative disease or trauma (fusion).

Definite Indications for Posterior Cervical Approach
1. Degenerative cervical disc disease with myelopathy and multiple areas of compression.
2. Compression of the spinal cord above C2-C3 or below C7-T1. These areas are inaccessible through the anterior cervical approach.

Lesions Which can be Reached Either Way, Depending upon the Facility of the Surgeon
1. Laterally placed acute disc herniation or hypertrophic chronic disc herniation.

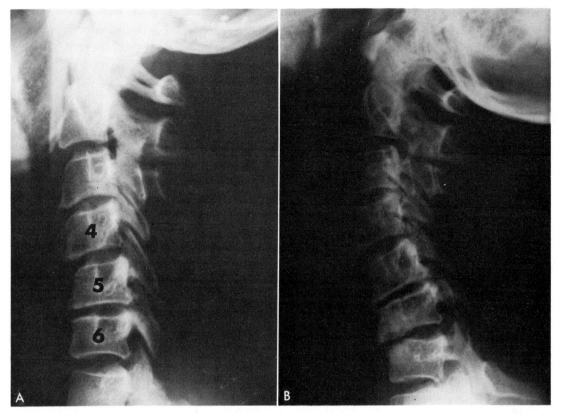

Figure 7–36. The effects of cervical laminectomy and multiple level facetectomy. *A,* Lateral cervical spine film taken one week after an extensive cervical laminectomy and facetectomy for multiple level spinal cord and nerve root compression secondary to chronic disc degeneration. Two years later, after the patient had experienced considerable neck and suboccipital pain, further roentgenograms *(B)* showed anterior subluxation of C6 on C7, with anterior compression deformities. In addition, there was separation of C4 from C5 and the combination of effects produced the so-called "swan neck" deformity.

2. Single and midline degeneration with hypertrophic spur formation and spinal cord compression.

OPERATIVE TECHNIQUE (See Chapter 4 for additional description of approaches and techniques.)

ANTERIOR DISC EXCISION AND INTERBODY FUSION. Two techniques for anterior disc excision and interbody fusion utilized by the authors are the Robinson technique with a horseshoe-type graft and the Cloward technique with a dowel graft.[15, 80] The primary advantage of the Robinson-type fusion is the higher immediate stability, while that of the Cloward technique is greater accessibility for the removal of osteophytes.[98] Unquestionably, both have been effective in the treatment of degenerative disc disease.

Robinson Technique. Although this operation can be performed using local anesthesia, it has been our experience that general anesthesia is more satisfactory. We routinely utilize an endotracheal tube and not uncommonly an esophageal stethoscope. Both devices allow for more certain recognition of the pertinent soft tissues during the approach to the spine. The anesthesiologist should be cautioned not to utilize extreme positions of either flexion or extension during intubation and positioning of the patient. Patients who have advanced disc degeneration with prominent osteophytes may sustain damage to the cord when extreme positions are utilized. Particular attention should be paid to care of the eyes, since draping of the neck may obscure the anesthesiologist's view of the face, and corneal abrasions may occur. The position of the anesthesiologist and his equipment should be such that he can rotate the patient's head and

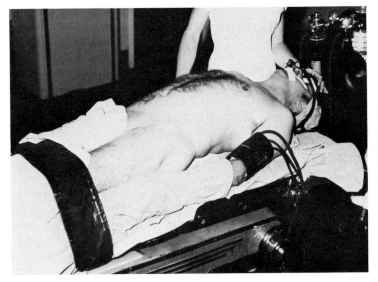

Figure 7–37. This photograph illustrates the correct position for an anterior cervical fusion using a left-sided approach to the cervical spine and a left iliac crest graft. Note that a folded sheet is placed beneath the scapula and also beneath the left iliac crest. Hair is covered with a sterile towel or cap.

neck during the surgical procedure and exert longitudinal traction if necessary as the operation proceeds.

The patient is placed in the supine position, with a folded sheet beneath the left iliac crest and a second sheet beneath the scapula to extend the neck slightly (see Fig. 7–37). The chin is tilted upward so as not to obscure the approach to the anterior spine and is turned slightly to the right. The hair is carefully covered with sterile towels or a sterile cap.

The anterior approach to the cervical spine can be through either a horizontal or an oblique incision. The horizontal incision will render a more cosmetically pleasing scar but is much more limited in area of spine exposed (Fig. 7–38). For a one-level fusion, we routinely use a horizontal approach, and for two or more levels the oblique incision is preferred. When any doubt occurs in the mind of a surgeon with limited experience in this type of surgery, an oblique incision should be utilized (see Fig. 7–39).

The transverse incision should begin in the midline and extend laterally 1 cm. beyond the anterior border of the sternocleidomastoid muscle. It should be at the level of the disc space to be entered, preferably in a skin

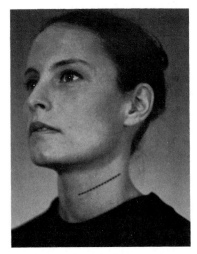

Figure 7–38. The horizontal incision for an anterior cervical fusion. This is usually cosmetically acceptable but is not an extensile approach.

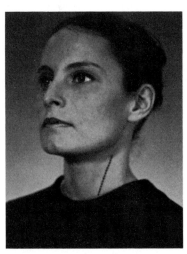

Figure 7–39. The oblique incision for an anterior cervical fusion. This produces a less satisfactory cosmetic appearance but is the more extensile approach.

crease. A landmark for this level can be obtained either through a prominent osteophyte, which can often be well palpated, or through the cricoid cartilage, which is usually located at the C5-C6 level.

An oblique incision has the advantage that, because it is extensile, errors in the level of the incision can easily be rectified. The incision is made along the anterior border of the sternocleidomastoid muscle and should be centered above the disc spaces to be fused.

The skin incision should be carried immediately down to the platysma muscle. Subsequent to this, absolute hemostasis should be obtained. The cardinal rule in conducting anterior cervical spine surgery is to obtain complete control of bleeding as one approaches the spine. If this rule is ignored, clear vision will be denied the surgeon, and this is an obvious invitation to surgical errors. The platysma muscle should then be divided between hemostats and cauterized throughout the entire length of the skin incision. After this muscle is divided, it should be gently retracted with small rake retractors. The anterior border of the sternocleidomastoid muscle should then be carefully delineated. The common error at this point is to enter through the mass of this muscle rather than along its anterior border. The surgeon should maintain as wide an exposure as possible at this point, being careful not to narrow down his incision to a small orifice. After the anterior margin of the sternocleidomastoid muscle is exposed, it may be gently retracted laterally. At this point the carotid artery sheath should be sought by finger palpation. When the carotid sheath has been located, the pretracheal fascia is incised longitudinally. The interval is defined between the carotid sheath laterally and the trachea and esophagus medially. The surgeon should stay close to the carotid sheath in order to maintain this plane. The proper interval can be assured by repeated palpation of the carotid laterally and of the anterior portion of the cervical spine, which should be directly in the plane of approach.

The prevertebral fascia is then seen as a smooth sheath covering the anterior portion of the vertebral bodies, the intervertebral disc, and the longus colli muscles. The omohyoid muscle may obscure a portion of the approach, depending on the level sought, and may be divided without hesitation. On occasion it may be impossible to retract near the middle or inferior thyroid vessels, and when this occurs they should be carefully divided

and ligated. Care must be taken not to injure the recurrent laryngeal nerve, which lies between the esophagus and the trachea, particularly in low approaches to the anterior cervical spine. The pretracheal fascia should be divided longitudinally in order to expose the spine itself. The fascia and paraspinal muscles can then be retracted laterally, to secure placement of retractors. Flat knee retractors or Cloward retractors are useful at this point (Fig. 7–40). The Keith straight needle is then inserted into a disc space, and a lateral film of the cervical spine is obtained. While the film is being developed, a full-thickness iliac crest graft is obtained in a routine manner.

After the appropriate interspace is identified, the paraspinal muscles are bluntly dissected away from the anterior portion of the spine well laterally. If this is not carefully done, retraction will be difficult, and the disc excision will be incomplete. The assistant who is holding the retractors must be careful not to allow his retractor to slide over the anterior portion of the muscle belly and possibly dam-

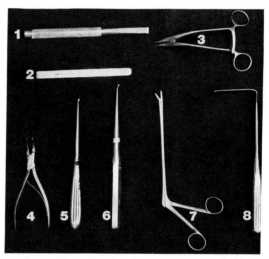

Figure 7–40. The various instruments found useful in the performance of the anterior cervical disc excision and fusion. Instruments 1 and 2 are round and flat impactors used for driving and then countersinking the graft. Number 3 is a small, self-retaining lamina spreader useful for completing the disc excision. Number 4 is a narrow rongeur useful for excising the anulus and anterior longitudinal ligament as well as prominent anterior osteophytes. Numbers 5 and 6 are small, curved curets useful for removing disc material, the cartilaginous end plates, and posterior bars and osteophytes. Number 7 is a narrow pituitary rongeur useful for removing disc material and small fragments of posteriorly extruded discs. Number 8 is a flat knee retractor useful for retraction of the esophagus, trachea, and carotid sheath.

age the sympathetic chain. After careful placement of the retractors, the transverse incision through the anterior longitudinal ligament and the anulus is performed, utilizing electrocautery. Again, careful attention is paid to hemostasis. This transverse incision is then completed, using a small scalpel. The anterior portion of the anulus should then be excised, using a narrow rongeur. A narrow straight curet is inserted into the disc space, and the disc is carefully curetted (Fig. 7–41).

Contact should always be maintained between the curet and the end plate of the vertebra so as not to inadvertently penetrate the posterior longitudinal ligament. Pressure may be exerted superiorly or inferiorly, but never in a posterior direction. The pituitary forceps and curets are used alternately to clean out the central portion of the disc.

After this is accomplished, the small self-retaining lamina spreader is then utilized to open the disc space widely. This is placed on one side of the disc space to allow complete clearing of the contralateral portion of the disc. It is important to meticulously excise the nucleus, the cartilaginous end plates, and the lateral portion of the disc, extending completely out to the uncus. Incomplete excision of disc material introduces the hazard that these fragments of disc material may be forced posteriorly or laterally with introduction of the graft. After one side of the disc space is completely clear, the lamina spreader is transferred to that side, allowing for final clearing of the entire disc space. At the termination of this portion of the procedure, both cartilaginous plates have been completely excised, and no soft disc material at all should remain. We do not routinely excise anterior osteophytes, as they will help to stabilize the graft. They should be removed, however, if esophageal pressure has been a problem.

We do not routinely remove posterior and lateral osteophytes unless cord compression or neurologic deficit secondary to nerve root compression has been demonstrated. The posterior longitudinal ligament is clearly demonstrable, and extruded fragments of disc material can be removed through rents in this ligament. The end plate may be perforated at scattered locations in order to aid rapid revascularization of the graft, but these perforations should be limited so that they do not sacrifice the integrity or strength of the end plate. At this point, the interspace is irrigated and ready to receive the graft.

Using the full-thickness iliac bone block previously removed, which is approximately 1 by 2 inches in size, a graft is fashioned, the height of which is approximately that of the normal disc space, and the depth of which is measured so that it will fill the disc space after being countersunk 1 to 2 mm. (Fig. 7–42). The graft will be wedge-shaped posteriorly, with

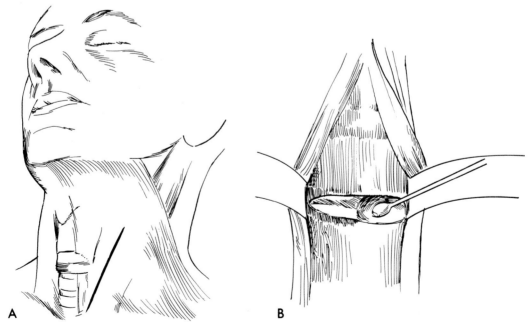

A   **B**

Figure 7–41. Curettage of the disc space after the anterior longitudinal ligament and anulus have been excised. Retractors are placed to both sides of the disc space to protect carotid sheath, trachea and esophagus. Care must be taken that these retractors do not lie on top of the paraspinal muscles, thereby injuring the sympathetic chain.

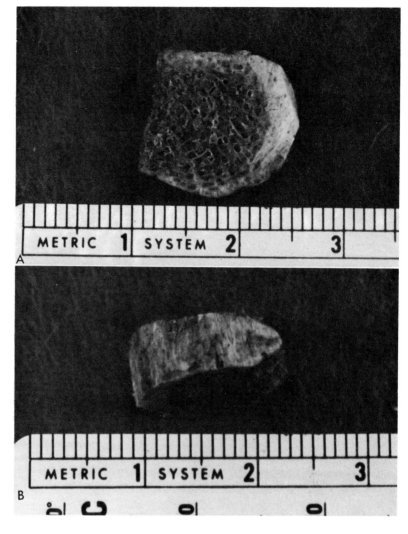

Figure 7–42. The shape of the horseshoe graft as seen from above. Note that it is bounded by cortical bone on three sides to support the disc space, while the central portion is cancellous bone which will rapidly fuse the adjacent vertebra. *B,* Lateral view of the graft illustrates the correct shape of the sides of the graft, with a slight bevel allowing easy introduction into the disc space.

cortical bone anteriorly and laterally. The height of the graft is a critical dimension. A graft of insufficient height will be insecure in its fit and will be prone to extrusion and delayed union or nonunion. Restoration of the size of the foramen will not occur. If the graft is too high, it will put excessive stress on the disc space above and below, although its fit may be exceedingly stable.

After the graft is fashioned the anesthesiologist or an assistant places traction on the neck, and the graft is introduced into the disc space and gently impacted into position so that the anterior surface of the graft is countersunk by 1 to 2 mm. (Fig. 7–43). If this is not done, the graft may extrude during the postoperative period. Retraction is then released and the stability of the graft is evaluated. The wound is then copiously irrigated. The platysma muscle is closed with a few interrupted chromic sutures, and the skin is closed with

interrupted fine nylon. The patient is then placed in a soft cervical collar of appropriate height and is returned to the recovery room.

The postoperative course with this type of surgery is usually benign. The patients are out of bed and walking as soon as they are comfortable, either on the night of surgery or on the following day. After the acute swelling and the danger of respiratory embarrassment has passed, the patient is fitted with a light cervical brace (Fig. 7–33) which is to be worn until the fusion is solid. When the fusion is healed, usually at six weeks, the patient is started on a course of cervical isometric exercises and placed in a soft collar. As the neck muscles strengthen, the patient is gradually weaned from the collar, and over a period of two to three weeks may be completely free of all external support.

Cloward Technique. In this operation the cervical spine is approached anteriorly, as

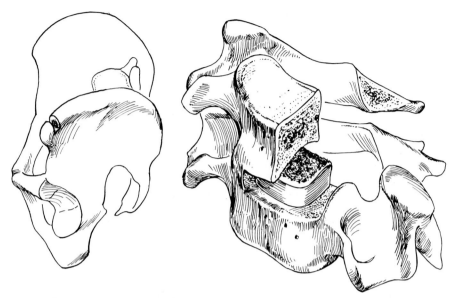

Figure 7–43. This drawing illustrates the correct position of the graft introduced into the disc space. Note that the graft is countersunk one to two millimeters posterior to the lip of the adjacent vertebra to prevent anterior extrusion. The graft should fit snugly into the disc space after release of traction.

described before. Instead of simply excising portions of the disc, however, Cloward has devised a series of instruments by use of which a cylindrical opening of 1 cm. or more in diameter can be made into the spinal canal.[16] This greater exposure facilitates the removal of osteophytes and disc fragments. In most instances, more definitive decompression of cervical nerve roots or the vertebral artery is possible. At the end of the procedure, a cylindrical bone graft taken from the patient's ilium (or from a bank of frozen cadaver

LAMINECTOMY

FACETECTOMY

ACCESS by ANTERIOR APPROACH
and FUSION

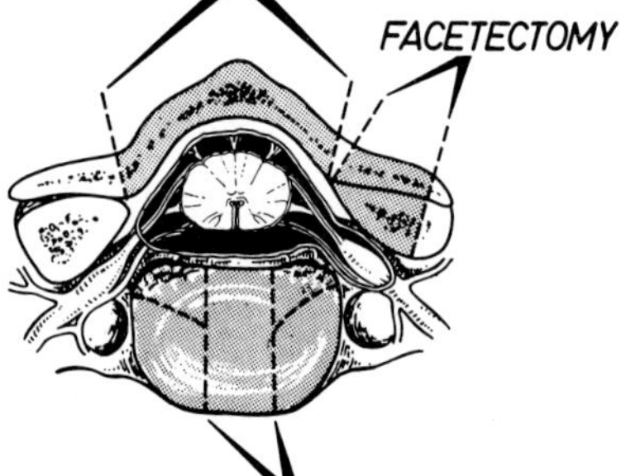

Figure 7–44. Removal of osteophytic spur through dowel (Cloward) anterior approach. Through the cylindrical interbody opening, instruments can enter the intervertebral foramen and remove significant portions of the spur and adjacent vertebral body. This is done prior to removal of the anterior longitudinal ligament by fine Kerrison rongeurs.

grafts) is fitted into the opening. The dowel-shaped graft is slightly larger than the cylindrical intervertebral hole, thus affording added stability in the immediate postoperative period. At times the author has advised the use of two smaller dowels for laterally placed symmetrical disc lesions. This technique is preferred when anterior osteophytes must be removed or when an extensive exploration of the spinal canal and foramina is required (Fig. 7–44).

Anterior Cervical Discectomy Without Bone Graft Fusion. Recently, Hirsch[43] and others[67, 79] have evaluated anterior cervical discectomy, particularly for soft cervical disc protrusions without bone graft fusion. The cartilaginous plates of the adjacent vertebrae are scraped and, in time, the vertebrae fuse spontaneously. Subsequent roentgenograms indicate that the two vertebrae become a single mass. Prolonged immobilization of the neck is apparently not necessary during the spontaneous fusion process.

POSTERIOR APPROACHES. *Posterior Foraminotomy and Disc Excision.* For isolated cervical nerve root compression, due to either herniation of disc material or chronic degeneration with osteophyte formation, the offending lesion may be approached from behind. With the pathology so well localized, and with accurate radiographic confirmation prior to making the incision, one need expose only the laminae of the vertebrae adjacent to the affected disc (Fig. 7–45).

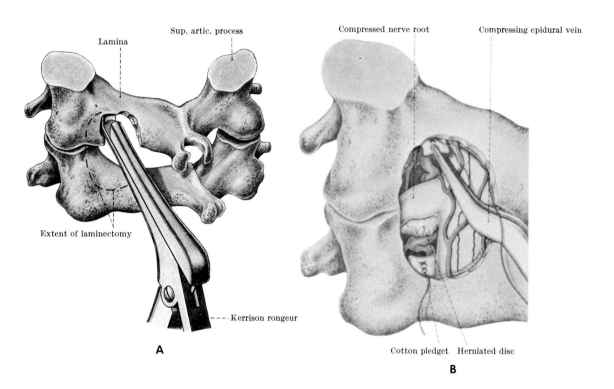

Lamina

Sup. artic. process

Extent of laminectomy

- - - - Kerrison rongeur

A

Compressed nerve root   Compressing epidural vein

Cotton pledget   Herniated disc

B

Figure 7–45. Posterior cervical partial laminectomy and discectomy. These illustrations indicate the steps in the removal of a soft cervical disc herniation.

A, The small, thumbnail-size laminotomy involving the inferior portion of the superior lamina and the superior portion of the inferior lamina. *B,* The important maneuver of collapse of epidural veins above and below the operative site with cotton pledgets. *C,* Removal of the disc herniation after incision of the posterior longitudinal ligament and general retraction of the affected nerve root.

(From Kempe, L.: Operative Neurosurgery. Springer-Verlag, 1972.)

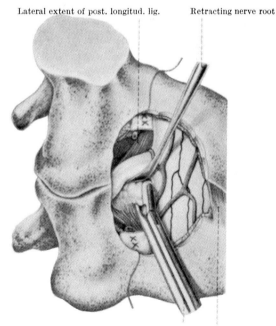

Lateral extent of post. longitud. lig.   Retracting nerve root

Removing herniated disc   Ligamentum flavum

C

The operation can be done in the prone or sitting position. The advantage of the sitting position is that the epidural veins are collapsed and there is less venous oozing. There are, however, complications which relate largely to anesthesia and positioning, and which render this approach potentially dangerous. We prefer, therefore, to use the prone position. When the patient is fixed firmly in place, the operating table can be angulated in a reversed Trendelenburg position, so that the neck is above the level of the right heart. In this way, venous oozing can be minimized. A needle is placed between the spinous processes of the suspected vertebrae for radiographic localization. When accurate localization is confirmed, the incision need cover only two spinous processes, the one above and the one below the affected disc. Paraspinous muscles are stripped away from the laminae only on the appropriate side and are held in place with a Taylor retractor. A small laminotomy is made laterally, involving the inferior margin of the superior lamina and the superior margin of the inferior lamina. Thereafter, the laminotomy can extend to, but not necessarily involve, the articulating facet. When there is a significant myelographic defect and appropriate symptoms, one always finds a tight nerve root, which must be retracted medially or laterally. If the nerve root is loose, the surgeon should reascertain the level of the laminotomy. While exposing the nerve root, one frequently enters a rather large, laterally placed vein, which travels in the anterolateral spinal canal. Bleeding from this vein can be controlled by placing small cotton patties above and below the nerve root. With the root gently retracted, soft disc material is removed piecemeal. If a hard spur is present, the bone overlying the nerve root is removed until the root moves freely. Often, more than 1 cm. of root is exposed to achieve this effect. When fully decompressed an angled dissector can pass freely along the nerve root beyond the confines of the foramen. The root is then covered with a thin layer of cellulose foam (Gelfoam), and the paraspinous muscles and skin are closed. Recovery is prompt, and the patient is usually discharged on the third postoperative day. No collar is required. Late follow-up roentgenograms to date have shown no tendency to subluxation at the operated levels, in contrast to those patients who are followed after bilateral laminectomy and foraminotomies.

Microsurgery in Cervical Disc Disease. Recently, excision of a lumbar disc with the aid of the operating microscope has attracted attention in the medical and lay press. Use of the operating microscope can avoid certain pitfalls in cervical disc surgery, and a brief mention is worthwhile.

Nerve root injury during posterior approach to a cervical disc has been described. Although relatively rare, this complication occurs because of the necessity to retract the nerve root to remove the herniated portion of the disc. Occasionally, the root is so attenuated over a bulging disc that to the naked eye, it is indistinguishable from the anulus fibrosus. It is possible mistakenly to section a portion of the root during the incision of the anulus under such circumstances. With the operating microscope, however, this distinction is quite clear because the margins of the nerve root can be defined clearly. Root retraction is minimized because a more defined approach to the exposed portion of the disc herniation is possible, particularly with the use of microinstruments. In addition, troublesome bleeding can be avoided because the large vein found in the lateral recess of the spinal canal can be coagulated under direct visualization. This vein may be difficult to see with the unaided eye or even with operating loupes.

Posterior Decompression of the Spinal Cord. Although posterior decompression has had a long history in the treatment of disc disease, the not infrequent aggravation of myelopathic symptoms subsequent to this operation have led some to prefer an anterior removal of spondylotic bars even at multiple levels. An uncomplicated, generous cervical laminectomy, however, affords an attractive way to relieve the spinal cord of its compressive forces. The surgeon really visualizes the extent of his decompression, and a true "feel" for the completeness of his efforts is afforded. Posterior laminectomy in patients with chronic cervical disc degeneration and secondary spinal cord compression does not involve removal of compressive forces anterior to the spinal cord. Removal of the neural arches and ligamenta flava is usually sufficient to free the spinal cord. Efforts to excise the protrusions anterior to the spinal cord may be dangerous or unnecessary. Even the most carefully performed posterior decompressions in patients with myelopathy are attended by a significant incidence of worsening of neurologic symptoms.

The patient may be positioned sitting or face down. The anesthetist must avoid hyperextension during the intubation, and the head is supported firmly in all positioning maneuvers. Only modest flexion or extension is permitted during any portion of the operative procedure. Laminae are removed from the inferiormost level first, because of their shingling effect.

It is preferable to begin the laminectomy at a level at which there is minimal myelographic evidence of spinal cord compression. The extent of the laminectomy remains undefined. Rogers indicated that all the cervical laminae must be removed to produce significant decompression of the spinal cord.[82] In addition, he sectioned all the dentate ligaments and left the dura mater open. Kahn and Rogers also favored sectioning the dentate ligaments.[52, 82] Recently, there has been a tendency to avoid opening of the dura, though a laminectomy that includes at least two laminae above and below the sites of significant compression is generally recommended. Recent demonstration of significant widening of the subarachnoid space after this procedure alone, as well as the fewer complications when the dura is left intact, may be responsible for this trend.[1] After extensive laminectomy, particularly when facetectomy is involved, cervical bracing for several weeks may be indicated. After the laminae have been removed, the cord should pulsate freely with changes in the patient's respiration. If this is not the case, laminectomy should be extended in an appropriate direction. As previously described, the issue of dural opening remains uncertain. A rule-of-thumb on which some surgeons rely involves observation of the spinal cord through the intact dura. If the cervical spinal cord has been pushed up against the dura for some time, one can see the surface vessels on the cord through the thinned, almost transparent, intact dura. Under these circum-stances, some surgeons feel that laminectomy alone does not afford adequate decompression, and they suggest careful dural incision throughout the entire extent of the laminectomy. This approach is probably more reasonable than those which dictate that the dura should "never" or "always" be opened.

COMBINED POSTERIOR DECOMPRESSION FOLLOWED BY ANTERIOR FUSION FOR MYELOPATHY. Verbiest has noted that secondary vertebral dislocation may occur many years after an extensive laminectomy.[95] He feels that if radiographic anterior angulation or abnormal movement is present after extensive laminectomy, an elective anterior fusion at the appropriate level should be performed early.

POSTERIOR FUSION. Posterior spinal fusion may be utilized in conjunction with a limited posterior laminectomy or for the repair of a nonunion of an anterior cervical spinal fusion. It is a dependable and easily performed procedure when the posterior elements of the spine are relatively intact. After an extensive posterior decompressive laminectomy, we prefer to perform an anterior spinal fusion at a later date rather than utilizing the more tenuous forms of lateral posterior spinal fusion, if at all possible.

The patient is placed on the operating table with the chin tucked down and the neck in a slightly flexed position. The head rests on a well-padded horseshoe headrest (Fig. 7–46). Meticulous attention should be paid to protection of the eyes, which should be taped shut after instillation of a protective ointment. The padding should be carefully checked to insure that no pressure is placed about the orbit and no points of localized pressure are placed upon the face.

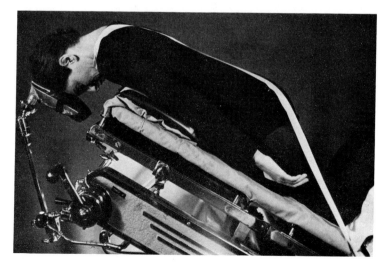

Figure 7–46. The proper position for posterior cervical fusions and laminectomy. Meticulous attention should be paid to protection of the eyes. The chin is in a slightly tucked and flexed position.

A midline incision from the tip of the spinous process is utilized, beginning one level above the fusion and ending one level below the fusion. After the skin incision is completed and hemostasis is obtained, the incision is deepened down to the spinous processes, using electrocautery, again obtaining hemostasis as the dissection proceeds. Identification of the appropriate vertebra is made, utilizing the easily palpable spinous process of the second vertebra, the bifid spinous process of the fifth vertebra, or the prominent spinous process of the sixth and seventh vertebrae. If any uncertainty remains, a needle should be placed in a spinous process and a lateral roentgenogram should be obtained.

Dissection of the paraspinal muscles should be performed, using a sharp periosteal elevator or scalpel, being careful to remain in a subperiosteal plane. Self-retaining retractors are inserted, and the posterior elements of the spine are cleaned of all soft tissues, utilizing sharp dissection and curets. After the lamina, which are to be included in the fusion, are clean, the surgeon is ready to proceed with wiring and stabilization of the spine.

A drill hole is made through the base of the spinous process of the upper vertebrae to be included in the fusion. This can be accomplished with a right angle dental burr or a strong towel clip. If only two levels are to be included in the fusion, the drill holes need be made only in the upper vertebra. If several levels are to be fused, drill holes are placed in all but the lower vertebra. A loop of #18 wire is then placed above the upper spinous process, and the end of the wire is introduced through the hole in the base of the spinous process in a transverse fashion (Fig. 7–47). The loop is then tightened, and the ends of the wire are brought beneath the spinous process of the inferior vertebra. The wire is then tightened, the edges are cut, and the wire is bent to lie flush with the spinous process. Subsequent to this, iliac cancellous graft material is obtained from a posterior iliac crest in a routine fashion and is cut into matchstick grafts. The cancellous bone is then carefully packed along the lamina of the involved vertebra (Fig. 7–48).

Decortication of the lamina is unnecessary. The cancellous graft will fuse satisfactorily to the lamina, while the wiring maintains initial stability.

The wound is tightly closed, utilizing heavy interrupted chromic suture material for the fascia, lighter chromic suture material for the subcutaneous tissues, and interrupted wire for the skin. The skin sutures are left in place for a full 10 days because of slow healing in this area.

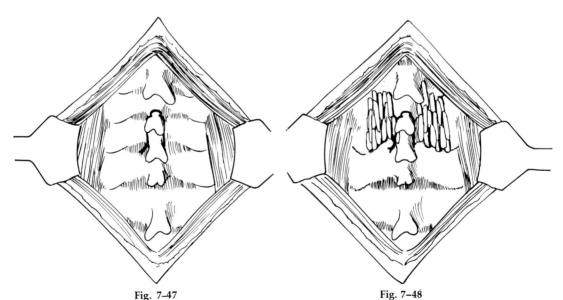

Fig. 7–47   **Fig. 7–48**

Figure 7–47. This drawing illustrates the technique of wiring adjacent vertebrae for a posterior cervical fusion. 18 gauge wire is utilized. The wire is looped through a drill hole in the superior vertebra and is tied beneath the spinous process of the inferior vertebra. This will produce rigid immobilization.

Figure 7–48. This drawing illustrates the correct placement of matchstick cancellous grafts bridging adjacent laminae.

After wound closure and dressing, a soft cervical collar is utilized for immobilization. The patient is allowed out of bed on the night of surgery or the following day. After the acute swelling has subsided, the soft collar is replaced with a firm, lightweight molded support and the patient is discharged after suture removal.

A brace is utilized until sound bone union has occurred and can be demonstrated radiographically. The patient is then started on cervical isometric exercises and is transferred to a soft cervical collar, which is worn for a further two to three weeks.

REPAIR OF PSEUDARTHROSIS. A nonunion of a cervical spinal fusion may be repaired through either the anterior or posterior approach. If the anterior approach is selected, the technique is similar to that for a Robinson fusion, described in the preceding section. In most instances, it is easier if the side opposite the original incision is utilized, as less scarring will be encountered during the approach to the spine. Once the site of nonunion is identified, the graft should be removed, utilizing small straight curets, and the disc space reconstructed. It is usually possible to identify the end plates, and these should be cleaned of any soft tissues or remaining cartilage. A definite effort should be made to perforate the bony end plates without completely sacrificing their integrity. A fresh graft should be inserted from the iliac crest, with careful attention to firm fixation. We have not had a failure of this technique of repair of nonunion.

If the posterior approach is utilized, the technique would be exactly as described under "Posterior Fusion."

It should be emphasized that prior to surgical intervention for a nonunion the entire clinical picture should be carefully reviewed in an effort to be certain that the nonunion is the cause of the patient's symptoms. One must be certain that another disc space or, indeed, another disease entity is not causing the symptoms with which the patient presents. We have encountered several patients with nonunions of cervical spinal fusions who are completely asymptomatic, and certainly in these individuals no further surgery is warranted.

LATERAL APPROACH TO THE CERVICAL SPINE. Although it had been recognized for some time that the vertebral artery could be reached through a posterolateral incision, it was not until 1963 that Jung recommended this route in cervical disc disease.[50] The technique has been amplified considerably by Verbiest, who favors a direct lateral approach for decompression of the vertebral artery and removal of laterally placed disc pathology.[96] The exposure can be extended anteriorly to relieve cord compression by chiseling posterior osteophytes.

The transverse processes are approached through a lateral incision between the sternocleidomastoid muscle and the carotid sheath on one side and the visceral compartment on the other. The anterior roots of the brachial plexus are exposed as they leave the transverse processes in the target area (which is identified by an intraoperative roentgenogram). The anterior tubercles of the appropriate transverse processes are removed and retracted, together with the attachments of the anterior scalene muscle. Then the longus capitis and longus colli muscles are divided and retracted medially. The foramina transversaria, which surround the vertebral artery, are now exposed, and their lateral margins are resected. The vertebral artery is separated from the surrounding fibrous connections and is retracted gently with tapes. The anterior rami of the brachial plexus can now be followed through the intervertebral foramina, after the important step of retracting the vertebral artery. Loose disc material, interforaminal spurs, and other effects of disc degeneration can be removed with the chisels or drills. For a more complete description of this procedure, the reader is referred to the recent descriptions of Verbiest and Jung.[51, 95]

RESULTS OF CERVICAL DISC SURGERY

The treating physician who would confidently advise a patient to undergo cervical disc excision must have at his command an accurate knowledge of (1) the quality of result that can be expected, (2) the complications that are possible and their incidence, and (3) the natural history of the disease process. The course and natural history of cervical disc degeneration when treated with conservative modalities has been discussed on page 473, under Nonoperative Treatment of Cervical Disc Degeneration. In the following sections an attempt will be made to outline the authors' and others' experience with the surgical treatment of disc degeneration. It should be clearly understood that the quality of result will vary with the type of pathology, i.e., acute protrusion with nerve root compression, chronic disc degeneration with neck and referred pain, or chronic disc degeneration with myelopathy. Each must be considered separately. In general, those individuals with acute protrusions, a strong component of radiculitis, and a well-defined neurologic deficit will respond well to nerve root decompression, whether from the anterior or posterior approach. Patients with chronic disc degeneration, a strong history of axial spine pain, and referred symptoms in their upper extremity without signs of nerve root compression yield less dependable results. The reason for this is not the inadequacy of surgical technique but, rather, the difficulty in ascertaining which cervical discs are responsible for the patient's symptoms. This is particularly true in multilevel disc degeneration.

RESULTS OF ANTERIOR DISC EXCISION AND FUSION. The technique of anterior cervical spinal fusion, as described by Robinson and Smith, has proved to be a relatively safe and effective treatment for patients with refractory neck and arm pain from cervical disc disease.[80] DePalma, Rothman, and colleagues have described results of anterior cervical disc excision and fusion in 281 patients. This information will be reviewed in some detail to demonstrate the quality of result that can be expected with this type of surgical procedure.[25]

Patient Material. 281 patients underwent anterior cervical disc excision and fusion utilizing the standard Robinson technique. Follow-up information was obtained on 229 patients. Two thirds of these individuals were reexamined and follow-up roentgenograms were performed. The average age of the patient was 43 years, and the average time of follow-up was five years.

Indications for Surgery. The criterion for operative intervention was the failure of an adequate trial of nonoperative therapy to relieve the symptoms of neck and arm pain secondary to cervical disc degeneration. The great majority of these patients did not have a neurologic deficit. Pain then, of an intractable and intolerable nature, was the factor that forced patients to surgery, and it is this factor that was most critically evaluated in terms of the quality of the result in these individuals. Treatment prior to surgery varied. One fourth of the patients had up to six months of nonoperative therapy, one fourth had six to 12 months, and one half had 12 months or more. The modalities of nonoperative therapy utilized have been previously described.

TABLE 7-2. LEVELS FUSED IN 229 PATIENTS

	Number of Fusions	Per Cent
C2-C3	1	0.4
C3-C4	15	7
C4-C5	150	65
C5-C6	194	85
C6-C7	77	34
C7-T1	5	2
Total	442	

Operative Procedures. In 229 patients 442 disc levels were fused. Thirty-two per cent of the patients had a one-level fusion, 53 per cent had a two-level fusion, and 15 per cent had a three-level fusion. C5-C6 was fused most frequently, C4-C5 and C6-C7 being next most common (Table 7-2).

Complications of Anterior Fusion. The most common problem seen postoperatively was a transient sore throat, hoarseness, or difficulty in swallowing. These symptoms, although of short duration, occurred in approximately one half of the patients. It should be noted, however, that these symptoms are frequently seen after endotracheal intubation and are not, strictly speaking, related to disc surgery itself. Complications of the anterior iliac crest incision were next most common. Hematomas, seratomas, persistent pain, and tenderness were not infrequent.

Neurologic complications occurred in three patients. In one individual, the neck was hyperextended and disc material was retropulsed into the spinal canal, with a subsequent Brown-Séquard syndrome that was permanent. The other neurologic complications were paresthesias in a radicular pattern, present for the first time postoperatively. These both cleared within several weeks of surgery.

Graft extrusion occurred in 3 per cent of patients and graft resorption in 7 per cent; a nonunion of the fusion occurred in 7 per cent of the levels fused and in 12 per cent of patients (see Table 7-3).

Quality of Result. Results were graded excellent through poor. An excellent result indicates complete freedom from symptoms and a return to full activity; a good result indicates occasional discomfort but full activity; a fair result indicates some pain, improved by surgery but with some persistent limitation of activity; and a poor result indicates no improvement with surgery. At the time of follow-up evaluation, 35 per cent of patients

TABLE 7–3. COMPLICATIONS OF ANTERIOR FUSION

	Per Cent	Number
Hoarseness, sore throat (see text)	49	112
Hematoma, iliac crest	9	20
Drainage, iliac crest	11	25
Pain over iliac crest scar	50	94
Temporary	14	32
Persisting	36	63
Hematoma, neck	0.4	1
Drainage, neck	1	3
Neurologic loss (see text)	1	3
Temporary	1	2
Persisting	0.4	1
Horner's Syndrome	3	8
Temporary	1	3
Persisting	2	5
Partial graft extrusion	3	6 (in 211 fusions)
Pseudarthroses (per fusion)	7	20 (of 283 fusions)
Pseudarthroses (per patient)	12	18 (of 150 patients)

TABLE 7–5. TIME FROM SURGERY TO RETURN TO FORMER EMPLOYMENT FULL TIME

Months Out of Work						
0–1	2–3	4–5	6–7	8–9	10–11	12 or more
4%	16%	21%	27%	8%	2%	22%
(7)	(28)	(37)	(48)	(14)	(4)	(39)

1st quartile (25th percentile) = 4.0 mos.
2nd quartile (median)   = 6.2 mos.
3rd quartile (75th percentile) = 9.4 mos.

achieved an excellent result, 28 per cent a good result, 29 per cent a fair result, and 8 per cent a poor result (Table 7–4). Restated, one can say that 92 per cent of these patients were improved by surgery, 63 per cent had unrestricted activities, and 34 per cent were completely free of symptoms. Eighty-eight per cent of these individuals considered their surgery worthwhile.

These patients were analyzed to determine if the length of follow-up evaluation affected the quality of result. There was no tendency for patients to deteriorate or improve with increased length of follow-up.

Employment records and work ability are a reasonable guide to the efficacy of surgery. The average time from surgical intervention through return to full-time employment was six months (Table 7–5). Seventy-six per cent of these individuals were able to return to their former positions full time, 15 per cent switched to lighter work or part-time work, and 9 per cent remained totally disabled (preoperatively 40 per cent worked full time, 25 per cent were partially disabled, and 35 per cent were totally disabled).

Follow-up roentgenograms showed further disc degeneration at adjacent levels in 81 per cent of the cases. The criteria utilized to diagnose disc degeneration were osteophyte formation, decrease in the height of the disc space, and rounding of the anterosuperior border of the vertebra below the disc. Disc degeneration was somewhat more common below a fusion mass than above. It is, of course, uncertain how many of these disc spaces would have undergone degenerative change without the presence of an adjacent fusion. It is interesting that there was no correlation with the quality of the result and the occurrence of this disc degeneration. Of the osteophytes present preoperatively, two thirds had resorbed by the time of follow-up examination. This phenomenon, which has been observed by many spine surgeons, speaks against the necessity of excision of these osteophytes when a neurologic deficit is not present.

The Effect of Multiple-Level Fusions. It is interesting to note that multiple fusions as a group did as well as single-level fusions. It is rare that a patient with a three-level spinal fusion does not develop disc degeneration above or below this fusion mass, but during the period of time under consideration, this did not show an apparent effect on the relief of symptoms (Table 7–6).

Pseudarthrosis. The development of a pseudarthrosis did not preclude a satisfactory result, and, indeed, 56 per cent of patients with a pseudarthrosis achieved an excellent or good result (Table 7–7). Although 64 per cent of

TABLE 7–4. RESULTS OF ANTERIOR DISC EXCISION AND FUSION USING ROBINSON TECHNIQUE

	Per Cent	Number of Patients
Excellent	35	81
Good	28	64
Fair	29	66
Poor	8	18
Total	100	229

TABLE 7–6. NUMBER OF LEVELS FUSED
VS. RESULTS

	Number of Levels Fused		
	1	*2*	*3 or more*
Excellent and good	62% (42)	66% (78)	60% (25)
Fair and poor	38% (26)	34% (41)	40% (17)

nu = 2
$X^2 = 0.58$
$p > 50\%$

TABLE 7–8. SYMPATHETIC SYMPTOMS
VS. RESULTS

Results	Preoperative Sympathetic Symptoms	No Preoperative Sympathetic Symptoms
Excellent	29% (29)	41% (53)
Good	37% (37)	21% (27)
Fair	28% (28)	29% (37)
Poor	6% (6)	9% (12)

nu = 3
$X^2 = 8.29$
$5\% > p > 2.5\%$

patients with a solid fusion achieved an excellent or good result, the difference between these two groups is not statistically significant. This would imply either that a stable fibrous union develops at the site of the disc excision or that the performance of an interbody fusion is not essential at the time of disc excision for relief of pain. For this reason, the authors advise a prolonged period of observation before reoperation for pseudarthrosis is undertaken, and a careful reevaluation to be certain which disc is causing the patient's symptoms and if, indeed, disc disease is the causative agent.

Miscellaneous Factors. Patients with preoperative sympathetic symptoms tended to have less excellent results (Table 7–8). It has also been the authors' experience that patients who demonstrate vasomotor instability of their hands, with color and temperature change, tend to do poorly. This is also true of patients with excessively mobile ligaments and joints.

Comparison with Other Techniques of Anterior Fusion. Several other techniques of anterior cervical disc excision and fusion have been reported.[31] In many instances, it is difficult to compare various series because of dissimilarity in methods of evaluation. Cloward, in describing his dowel technique, reported

that approximately 90 per cent of his series of 310 patients have been totally relieved of all symptoms.[16] However, an independent report by authors utilizing the same technique failed to substantiate this high level of satisfactory results. Stuck, reporting a series of 151 patients, found only 22 per cent completely relieved of symptoms, with 6 per cent showing no improvement whatsoever.[91] Simmons and colleagues reported the technique of anterior fusion using a Keystone graft.[87] In a series of 68 patients, they found excellent or good results in 81 per cent, fair results in 15 per cent, and poor results in 4 per cent.

RESULTS OF ANTERIOR REMOVAL OF CERVICAL DISC WITHOUT FUSION. Robertson reported on 93 patients who underwent anterior removal of a cervical disc.[79] Fifty-three had a fusion at the time of surgery, and 40 did not. All cases with simple anterior discectomy went on to spontaneous fusion or marked settling of the interspace, with no evidence of movement of the affected joint. There was no difference in the stability of the cervical spine with either technique. Robertson feels that the added morbidity of bone grafting is avoided by his technique. Murphy and Gado, however, reported one case in which subsequent reoperation, with insertion of an interbody graft, was necessary.[67]

RESULTS OF POSTERIOR DECOMPRESSION FOR MYELOPATHY. Between 1956 and 1965 at least five series, of greater than 30 cases each, were reported in which myelopathy was treated by cervical decompression. Variability in results was remarkable. The fewest complications (6 per cent) were reported by Peserico, whereas the earlier paper of Clarke and Robinson (1956) acknowledged that 45 per cent of their patients who survived surgery had an accentuation of their myelopathic symptoms.[14, 74] All of Clarke and Robinson's cases,

TABLE 7–7. RESULTS IN PATIENTS
WITH PSEUDARTHROSES

	Pseudarthroses	No Pseudarthroses
Excellent and good	56% (10)	64% (84)
Fair and poor	44% (8)	36% (48)

nu = 1
$X^2 = 0.450$
$p > 50\%$

however, were operated on after a period of extensive medical treatment. Some of the recent improvement in results of this operation, however, undoubtedly derive from the great respect that neurosurgeons now extend to the compromised cervical spinal cord. Nevertheless, a significant number of patients remain unchanged after the surgery. This suggests that once myelopathy has advanced, there is a combination of compressive and ischemic symptomatology, the latter of which is not benefited by relief of pressure. Over all, in a series of 177 cases reported by several authors, 56 per cent were improved after cervical laminectomy, 25 per cent were unchanged, and the remaining 19 per cent were worsened. The role of dural and dentate ligament section cannot be derived from these papers.[9]

RESULTS OF POSTERIOR DECOMPRESSION FOR RADICULOPATHY. In contrast to results of the posterior approach for decompression of the compromised cervical spinal cord, results of posterior operations for relief of spinal root compression are uniformly favorable among authors and are excellent in duration. In 1965, Scoville quoted a 97 per cent success rate in 702 cases.[85] Both Knight and Spurling achieved similar results in their smaller series.[55, 88] These initial reports did not indicate problems with subsequent mobility of the spine after single or multiple-level posterior operations around the nerve roots. Nonetheless, acute or chronic disc protrusion with radiculopathy remains one of the most favorable conditions a spine surgeon treats. Results are usually excellent and recurrence rate is extremely small. Permanent complications are uncommon. Afforded the advantage of being able to demonstrate the "tight" nerve root and to persist until this structure is loose, the surgeon has reason to predict satisfying results after posterior foraminotomy.

To determine the effectiveness of the posterior approach to soft lateral disc protrusion, 50 patients from the author's series (FAS) were randomly selected for review. The follow-up period was one to seven years. Forty-four per cent were followed for more than six years. The patients were operated on by the same neurosurgeon, and they were personally interviewed and examined in detail by an orthopaedic surgeon. All patients had myelographically proven lesions. The results were as follows: 88 per cent were rated excellent, and 8 per cent good. Two patients were clinically improved but later were declared psychologically disabled.

At this point, it is significant to mention that the author does not treat patients involved in litigation and compensation unless forced by progressive neurologic deficit, a treatment approach that must be considered a primary factor influencing the quality of these results. Of interest in this group is the observation that only 16 per cent related the onset of their problem directly to trauma. Eighty per cent of the patients reported awakening to the onset of pain in the neck or arm.

LATE COMPLICATIONS OF POSTERIOR DECOMPRESSION. The neurologic complications of posterior decompression have been discussed with results of the surgical procedures, in the preceding pages. Non-neurologic complications include infection, hematoma formation, respiratory difficulty due to immobilization, and a variety of problems that are both individually and aggregately uncommon. As time goes on, however, surgeons are revisited by patients who have undergone extensive posterior decompression and who complain several years later of increasing neck and suboccipital pain. Roentgenograms exhibit minor degrees of subluxation of the laminectomized vertebrae, progressive proliferative degenerate disc disease, and even collapse of the anteriormost portion of the vertebrae, with forward angulation (swan-neck) deformity. Figure 7–36 shows roentgenograms taken after bilateral foraminotomy at C5-C6 and C6-C7 was performed. Some three years later, the patient returned with neck pain aggravated by head motion. Roentgenograms demonstrated the ravages of excessive mobility and a swan-neck deformity. Although her symptoms responded to a cervical collar, at age 43 she could not face a life with this appliance, and dowel-type anterior fusions of the lower cervical vertebra were performed. Since then she has been symptom-free.

REASONS FOR FAILURE OF CERVICAL DISC SURGERY

Psychosocial Factors

Within the spectrum of patients whose cervical or lumbar disc surgery is considered a failure, there exist several identifiable groups in whom such failure seems preordained. Despite deftly performed surgery, the symptoms can persist, and the patient seeks further medical attention.

THE SYNDROME

Certain characteristics are common to all patients with this syndrome, and others occur with such frequency that they are worthy of mention.

PAIN. This is the principal symptom. Rarely does the patient with neurologic deficit as the main problem complain a great deal and seek other opinions. It is pain that prompted surgeons to operate, and persistent pain after surgery is the hallmark of failure.

DISABILITY. The pain is sufficient to prevent the patient from engaging in his normal activities, most notably work. If the patient is a housewife, she cannot tend to her daily chores. In certain cases, the pain may be just sufficient to allow the patient to perform sedentary aspects of his job, but the more vigorous tasks are impossible because of some form of discomfort. The patient can exhibit reasonable mobility about the house, but as soon as he returns to work, certain job requirements induce incapacitating pain.

ABSENCE OF LOCALIZED NEUROLOGIC FINDINGS. Preoperatively, deep tendon reflex asymmetry is usually absent. Focal motor weakness is likely not present, and if it is, it may appear only when the extremity is tested separately. Double simultaneous testing of wrist extension, for instance, may demonstrate that the weak extensor has now become stronger. Sensory abnormalities, if they exist at all, do not occur in an anatomic distribution. The majority of patients with failed disc surgery did not have convincing neurologic deficit preoperatively.

ABSENCE OF RADIOGRAPHIC ABNORMALITIES. As mentioned previously, radiographic signs of chronic disc degeneration in the adult population are so common that they are not of diagnostic value in the absence of localized neurologic deficit. Myelography is often normal in patients who are subjected to unsuccessful cervical disc surgery.

Any experienced spine surgeon would not be surprised that the above-mentioned group would represent a high risk for surgical cure. Certainly those patients with pain as the primary symptom, with disability secondary to pain, and with no myelographic or neurologic abnormalities are at high risk to fail when compared to those patients who have convincing abnormalities. The patient's insistence, however, often forces the surgeon to perform an operation that is undertaken in the hope of relieving the pain despite the paucity of objective criteria.

It is well known that not every patient with a painful disc herniation has neurologic deficit or myelographic abnormality. In certain cases, surgery that may be loosely considered "exploratory" has been successful, but the results will depend largely on the patient's psychosocial environment. If there are factors that require him to continue to complain of pain, the operation will fail. In the absence of these factors, the result might be rewarding.

The surgeon's failure to recognize the psychosocial factors that surround the patient with a disappointing result continues to give spine surgery a bad name. There exists a group of individuals who must continue to complain of pain independently of whatever form of therapy is used. These individuals are often vocal because of their need to complain, and the failure of their operation may convince their friends and colleagues that disc surgery is fruitless.

Armed with the characteristics of the clinical syndrome just described, a list of surgical failures, which subdivide into six categories, follows:

COMPENSATION. Among those individuals who perceive that neck and arm pain is the result of an injury sustained at work, the potential for quick relief of their symptoms remains poor. Frequently these symptoms will persist inordinately, well beyond what one might expect from a single injury. Response to nonoperative treatment, if there is any response at all, is delayed. If surgery is performed, recovery is prolonged, and the postoperative symptoms (which ordinarily should last a few weeks) may persist indefinitely. This individual usually begins his history by indicating that he was well until he hurt himself at work. Quite frequently the injury and the forces involved seem trivial compared to the prolonged disability that follows. The patient continues to complain of this pain until he is laid off from work, and then he continues to resist attempts to be reemployed. This process may continue month after month, or year after year. If the symptoms become established, it is nearly impossible to rehabilitate the individual to a pain-free working life, even though his compensation payments may have run out. At some point, the patient becomes truly convinced that he has been permanently damaged, that nothing can be done for his pain, and that he will never be able to work again.

The frustration in dealing with these patients is known to all mature spine surgeons, although surprisingly little advice appears in the medical literature for those who must treat this large group of unfortunate individuals. This syndrome has been called "compensation neurosis" by some. Not all the patients are neurotic. Some of them seem sociopathic in their refusal to cooperate and return to a socially acceptable way of life. Most do not appear to be malingerers. They all seem to have a reason to have some pain initially, despite how trivial the injury, but the degree and duration of symptoms far exceed what one would expect.

LITIGATION. A similar sequence may be seen in patients who perceive that their neck symptoms are related to a single injury that is the reason for litigation. Again, the typical patient has no neurologic deficit or myelographic findings. He dates all difficulties to a single accident. The accident is invariably described as the fault of the defendant in the case. One is impressed that those individuals who sustain substantial neck injury in a car accident usually tend to respond much more promptly if there is no issue of negligence in the accident. This peculiarity has led to the term "litigation neurosis," but these individuals are not invariably neurotic.

These clients tend to have neck pain rather than arm pain. They believe that all their symptoms are a result of the accident, and, surprisingly, many of the general and specialist physicians they see concur with this. The remarkable result is that the patient may ultimately believe that he truly will experience disabling neck pain for an indefinite interval, perhaps the rest of his life, as the result of a single mild injury. The patient's attorney participates in this unusual misconception by citing similar cases in patients who were never able to work and who had chronic pain after such an injury.

In an effort to explain persistent and disabling pain in the absence of any objective criteria, physicians in the United States often use such terms as "cervical sprain" or "cervical strain." These are ill-defined diagnoses, and the terms may simply reflect the physician's frustration as he treats a patient who long since should have recovered from his injury. Even the terms "strain" and "sprain" suggest spontaneous recovery, yet they are used even though the injury may be several years old. Cases are being adjudicated regularly and awards are indeed based on the anticipation of permanent pain and disability. It seems that experts are willing to testify of such permanency even in the absence of path-

ologic findings. Another preconception that is often erroneous is that a patient's symptoms will subside after the litigation is settled. Although this is frequently true, patients who undergo surgery for neck conditions that they feel are the result of an accident fare significantly worse than similar individuals not involved in litigation, even after the case is settled. The reason for this is unknown. Certainly the process of continued visits to physicians, frequently those chosen by his attorney, rehashing of the trauma, emphasis of the culpability of the defendant, and the process of calculation of damages must reinforce the concept that substantial injury occurred, independent of the actual tissue damage. In fact, the greatest injustice done in this whole process may not be to the hapless defendant but rather to the patient/plaintiff who has been encouraged to believe that his pain will forever prevent him from competing socially. The physician who is willing to "help" his patient by testifying to the severity and permanency of his patient's injuries may in fact be participating in the plaintiff's social destruction.

ADDICTION. The complaint of pain is most frequently handled by the administration of an analgesic medication. The severity of the pain frequently dictates the drug, and narcotics are used for those individuals who complain most severely. Narcotic medications have the capacity to quiet these complaints, while the prescribing physician anticipates spontaneous resolution of symptoms. By a mechanism as yet undefined (though modern endorphin theories are evolving), "liberal" narcotic administration can prolong the symptoms beyond the expected interval of spontaneous recovery. The narcotic is incorporated in the patient's metabolism, and it seems as though he is conditioned to have pain in order to receive the medicine. The pain seems to be a memory engram, and it will frequently retain the characteristics of the original and purely organic discomfort. It may follow a classic radicular pattern. In other instances, treatment of the pain while the patient is still addicted may alleviate the original discomfort, but it will be replaced soon by another pain that requires a narcotic medication.

Patients who have this form of addiction exhibit certain characteristics. They will awaken regularly in the middle of the night with pain, and they can get more rest only after taking another dose of narcotics. It is not typical of purely organic pain to awaken a patient from sleep at specific times. In particular, these patients awaken regularly three to six hours after they fall asleep; this interval being related to the frequency of the narcotic administration during waking hours. It seems when blood narcotic level drops to its lowest during sleep, mechanisms by which the body becomes dependent are sufficient to produce awakening. Surprisingly, many patients will claim that the narcotic really "doesn't work," but it provides some relief by taking the "edge" off the pain. Patients frequently take narcotics in anticipation of pain and claim that it works better before the pain becomes really severe. Many of them will require increasing doses as the addiction progresses, although others have a surprisingly fixed addiction that lasts for many years. Those individuals who take self-administered narcotics for long intervals eventually realize that they are in fact addicted, and they will often continue the narcotic use while complaining of pain that is no longer terribly distressing. Short-temperedness, insomnia, jitteriness, and nightmares are seen with much greater frequency in this group of patients than any other. They may be related to intervals when the blood narcotic level becomes low. Patients who are chronically addicted are often manipulative, demanding, and tend to develop panicky exacerbations of their symptoms.

A frequent misconception is that there is a set dosage and frequency of administration below which addiction cannot be assumed. Although this may apply in street usage of narcotics, when pain is the reason for administration, such may not be the case. Examples of addiction-dependent pain have been seen with patients who take two or three 60 mg. codeine tablets daily. Frequently these patients have been taking a small dose for a long interval, and it seems that the cumulative amount of narcotics administered plays some role in the addiction independent of the duration over which the drugs have been administered. In the absence of specific education about this subject, many physicians misconceive that a patient's pain cannot be based on addiction because he or she only takes a few tablets every day.

Fewer therapeutic exercises are more difficult yet rewarding than the observation of dramatic relief of pain after the narcotic has been withdrawn. During a period of abstinence the pain will increase, and the patient will become unruly and perhaps hallucinatory, but after a week or two the "ghosts" of the original discomfort will gradually resolve. The patient may complain of nondisabling residua for some time, and occasional "flashbacks" will trouble him.

Individuals who are otherwise psychologically healthy and who have sound emotional support systems at home can undergo withdrawal without hospitalization. The more severely affected may require inpatient care until the physicians are convinced that the addiction has subsided. The withdrawal period may be eased by the administration of liberal amounts of hydroxyzine pamoate (Vistaril), antidepressant drugs, and other non-narcotic analgesics.

DEPRESSION. Reactive depression can occur with any chronic pain syndrome. When pain and depression occur concurrently, the patient and his family, if they are willing to admit that the depression exists at all, will invariably believe that the depression is a natural result of pain. Although this may be true, depression frequently precedes the development of pain. Patients suffer a great resistance to the concept that the pain is a symptom of depression. The types of individuals in whom depressive illness may result in chronic complaints of pain are usually those with a long-standing history of preexisting depression. A history of psychotherapy or hospitalization for shock treatment in early life, particularly when associated with chronic recurrent attacks of pain, is often seen in the older patient who now has persistent neck pain.

Involutional depression in the absence of depressive illness in earlier years frequently precedes the development of chronic neck pain. Pain in these older patients seems to respond better to the administration of tricyclic antidepressants than the pain seen in the chronically depressed. In both groups, antidepressant medication used for prolonged intervals and in liberal amounts is the hallmark of therapy. The treating physician may have difficulty in finding a psychiatrist who is willing to accept the interdependence of pain and depression, and he must not let the psychiatric opinion force him into an operation that he does not believe will effect pain relief.

Accurate statistics on the incidence of each of these high-risk-for-failure groups are unavailable because the problems do not lend themselves to statistical analysis. The broad overview of patients with failed cervical disc surgery certainly indicates that the following are true.

1. Surgery was performed for pain, and the failure is based on lack of pain relief.
2. The pain is more likely to be in the neck than in the arm.
3. Compensation, litigation, preexisting depression, or narcotic addiction, singularly or in tandem, complicate the case preoperatively.

Improperly Performed Surgery

Improperly performed surgery, which one might think would be common among a group of failures, seems to be the exception. Failures are far less frequent in cervical than in lumbar disc surgery, even when the relative frequency of the operation is taken into account. (The ratio of lumbar to cervical symptomatic disc disease is about four to one.) The fact that anterior and posterior approaches for bona fide cervical disc lesions are about equally effective and that satisfactory results may be expected in over 95 per cent of patients when the previously mentioned psychosocial factors are not involved suggests a generally favorable outlook on the level of technical competence of cervical disc surgeons. When patients with these psychosocial factors have been excluded and when it has been ascertained that a technically satisfactory operation has been performed, the remaining numbers in the failed category are few. Some of them may have causes for the pain in other structures of the neck or arm. Still others may have a psychiatric illness that does not conveniently fall into these categories.

References

1. Aboulker, J.: Les myelopathies cervicales d'origine rachidienne. Neurochirurgie *11*:89–198, 1965.
2. Bailey, R. W.: Observations of intervertebral disc lesions in fracture and dislocation. J. Bone Joint Surg. *45A*:461–470, 1963.
3. Baker, A. B.: Clinical Neurology. New York, Hoeber-Harper, 1962, p. 1610.
4. Barré, J. A.: Le syndrome sympathique posterieur. Rev. Neurol. (Paris) *33*:248–249, 1926.
5. Bartschi-Rochaix, W.: Migraine cervicale, das encephale Syndrom nach Halswirbeltrauma. Bern, Huber Verlag, 1949.
6. Berry, R.: Genetically controlled degeneration of the nucleus pulposus in the mouse. J. Bone Joint Surg. *47B*:574–580, 1965.
7. Bobechko, W., et al.: Auto-immune response to nucleus pulposus in the rabbit. J. Bone Joint Surg. *47B*:574, 1965.
8. Brain, W. R., Northfield, D. W. C., and Wilkinson, M.: Neurological manifestations of cervical spondylosis. Brain *75*:187, 1952.
9. Brain, Lord: Some unsolved problems of cervical spondylosis. Br. Med. J., *5333*:771–777, 1963.
10. Brain, Lord, and Wilkinson, M.: Cervical Spondylosis. Philadelphia, W. B. Saunders Co. 1967, p. 154.
11. Broden, H.: Paths of nutrition in articular cartilage and intervertebral discs. Acta Orthop. Scand. *124*:177–183, 1954–55.
12. Brown, M. D.: The pathophysiology of the intervertebral disc. Anatomical, physiological and biochemical considerations. Ph.D. thesis, Thomas Jefferson University, 1969.
13. Bull, J., Gammal, T., and Popham, M.: A possible genetic factor in cervical spondylosis. Br. J. Radiol. *42*:9–16, 1969.
14. Clarke, E., and Robinson, P. K.: Cervical myelopathy: Complication of cervical spondylosis. Brain *79*:483, 1956.
15. Cloward R. B.: New method of diagnosis and treatment of cervical disc disease. Clin. Neurosurg. *8*:93–132, 1962.
16. Cloward, R. B.: Lesions of the intervertebral disc and their treatment by interbody fusion methods. Clin. Orthop. *27*:51–77, 1963.
17. Coin, C. G., Chan, Y., Keranen, V., and Pennink, M.: Computer assisted myelography in disc disease. J. CAT *1*:398–404, 1977.
18. Coin, C. G., and Hucks-Folliss, A.: Cervical computed tomography in multiple sclerosis with spinal cord involvement. J. CAT *3*:421–422, 1979.
19. Coin, C. G., Pennink, M., Ahmad, W. D., and Keranen, V. J.: Diving-type injury to the cervical spine: Contribution of computed tomography to management. J. CAT *3*:362–372, 1979.
20. Comfort, A.: The Biology of Senescence, New York, Rinehart, 1956.
21. Coppen, A.: Mineral metabolism in melancholia. Br. Med. J. *2*:1439, 1963.
22. Coventry, M. B., Ghormley, R. K., and Kernohan, J. W.: The intervertebral disc: Its microscopic anatomy and pathology. I. Anatomy, development, and physiology. J. Bone Joint Surg. *27*:105–112, 1945.
23. Davidson, E., et al.: Biochemical alterations in herniated intervertebral discs. J. Biol. Chem. *234*:2951, 1959.
24. DePalma, A., and Rothman, R.: The Intervertebral Disc. Philadelphia, W. B. Saunders Co., 1970.
25. DePalma, A., Rothman, R., Lewinnek, G., and Canale, S.: Anterior interbody fusion for severe cervical disc degeneration. Surg. Gynecol. Obstet. *134*:755–758, 1972.
26. DiChiro, G., Doppman, J. L., and Wener, L.: Computed Tomography of Spinal Cord Arteriovenous Malformations. Radiology *123*:351–354, 1975.
27. Elves, M. W., Bucknill, T., and Sullivan, M. F.: In vitro inhibition of leukocyte migration in patients with intervertebral disc lesions. Orthop. Clin. North Am. *6*:59–65, 1975.
28. Eyring, E.: The biochemistry and physiology of the intervertebral disc. Clin. Orthop. *67*:16–28, 1968.
29. Franklin, L., and Hull, E. W.: Lipid content of the human intervertebral disc. Clin. Chem. *12*:253–257, 1966.

30. Friedenberg, Z., and Miller, W.: Degenerative disc disease of the cervical spine. J. Bone Joint Surg. *45A*:1171–1178, 1963.
31. Gallera, R., and Tovi, D.: Anterior disc excision with interbody fusion in cervical spondylotic myelopathy and rhizopathy. J. Neurosurg. *28*:305–310, 1968.
32. Gargano, F. P.: Transverse axial tomography of the spine. Crit. Rev. Clin. Radiol. Nucl. Med. *8*(3):279–328, 1976.
33. Gargano, F. P., Meyer, J., Houdek, P. V., and Charyulu, K.: Transverse axial tomography of the cervical spine. Radiology, *113*(2):363, 1974.
34. George, R. C., and Chrisman, O. D.: The role of cartilage polysaccharides in osteoarthritis. Clin. Orthop. *57*:259–265, 1968.
35. Gertzbein, S. D., Tile, M., Gross, A., and Falk, R.: Autoimmunity in degenerative disc disease of the lumbar spine. Orthop. Clin. North Am. *6*:67–73, 1975.
36. Gower, W., and Pedrini, V.: Age related variations in protein polysaccharides. J. Bone Joint Surg. *51A*:1154–1162, 1969.
37. Gowers, W. R.: Diseases of the Nervous System, 2nd ed. London, Churchill, 1892, p. 260.
38. Hallen, A.: The collagen and ground substance of the human intervertebral disc at different ages. Acta Chim. Scand. *16*:705, 1962.
39. Hammerschlag, S. B., Wolpert, S. M., and Carter, B. L.: Computed tomography of the spinal canal. Radiology *121*:361–367, 1976.
40. Handel, S., Grossman, R., and Sarwar, M.: Computed tomography in the diagnosis of spinal cord astrocytoma. J. CAT *2*:226–228, 1978.
41. Hansen, H. J.: Comparative views on the pathology of disc degeneration in animals. Lab. Invest. *8*:1242–1265, 1969.
42. Hendry, N.: The hydration of the nucleus pulposus. J. Bone Joint Surg. *40B*:132–144, 1968.
43. Hirsch, C.: Cervical disc rupture: Diagnosis and therapy. Acta Orthop. Scand. *30*:172–186, 1960.
44. Hirsch, C., Schajowicz, F., and Galante, J.: Structural changes in the cervical spine. Acta Orthop. Scand. Suppl. *109*:1967.
45. Hitselberger, W. E., and Witten, R.: Abnormal myelograms in asymptomatic patients. J. Neurosurg. *28*:204–206, 1968.
46. Hukins, D., and Hickey, D.: Relationship between the structure of the annulus fibrosus and the function and failure of the intervertebral disc. Volvo Award-winning paper in Biomechanics, International Society for the Study of the Lumbar Spine, Göteborg, Sweden, June, 1979.
47. Inou, H., and Hashizume, H.: Three dimensional architecture of lumbar intervertebral discs. Presented at the International Society for the Study of the Lumbar Spine, Göteborg, Sweden, June, 1979.
48. Jackson, R.: The Cervical Syndrome. Springfield, Ill., Charles C Thomas Co., 1966.
49. James, H. E., and Oliff, M.: Computed tomography in spinal dysraphism. J. CAT *1*:391–397, 1977.
50. Jung, A.: Resection de l'articulation unco-vertebrale et ouverture du trou de conjugaison par voie anterieure dans le traitement de la neuralgie cervicobrachiale. Technique operatoire. Mem. Acad. Chir. (Paris), *89*:361–368, 1963.
51. Jung A., and Vierling, J. P.: Nouveau resultats et complement de technique de l'uncusectomie dans le traitement des complications radiculaires et arteriovertebrales des cervicarthroses. Rev. Chir. Orthop. *51*:605–618, 1965.
52. Kahn, E. A.: Role of dentate ligaments in spinal cord compression and syndrome of lateral sclerosis. J. Neurosurg. *4*:191–199, 1947.
53. Kempe, L.: Operative Neurosurgery, New York, Springer-Verlag, Vol. 2 1970, pp. 254–255.
54. Key, C. A.: Guy's Hosp. Rep. *3*:17, 1838.
55. Knight, G. C.: Neurosurgical treatment of cervical spondylosis. Proc. R. Soc. Med. *57*:165–168, 1964.
56. Langfitt, T., and Elliot, F.: Pain in the back and legs caused by cervical spinal cord compression. J.A.M.A. *200*:112–116, 1967.
57. Lawrence, J. S., Bremner, J. M., and Bier, F.: Osteoarthrosis: Prevalence in the population and relationship between symptoms and x-ray changes. Ann. Rheum. Dis. *25*:1, 1966.
58. Lees, F., and Turner, J.: Natural history and prognosis of cervical spondylosis. Br. Med. J. *2*:1607–1610, 1963.
59. Leone, M. E.: Depression, back pain, and disc protrusion. Dis. of Nerv. Syst., *32*:41–45, 1971.
60. Lindblom, K.: Technique and results in myelography and disc puncture. Acta Radiol. Stockh. *34*:321, 1950.
61. Livingston, M.: Spinal manipulation causing injury. Clin. Orthop. *81*:82–86, 1971.
62. Lourie, H., Shende, N., and Stewart, D.: The syndrome of central cervical disc herniation. J.A.M.A. *226*:302–305, 1973.
63. MacNab, I.: The traction spur. J. Bone Joint Surg. *53A*:663–670, 1971.
64. Markolf, K. L., and Morris, J. M.: The structural components of the intervertebral disc. J. Bone Joint Surg. *56A*:675–687, 1974.
65. McRae, D. L.: The significance of abnormalities of the cervical spine. Am. J. Roentgenol. *84*:3, 1960.
66. Mitchell, P. E., Hendry, N. G., and Billewicz, W. F.: The chemical background of intervertebral disc prolapse. J. Bone Joint Surg. *43B*:141–151, 1961.
67. Murphy, M. G., and Gado, M.: Anterior cervical discectomy without interbody bone graft. J. Neurosurg. *37*:71–74, 1972.
68. Nachemson, A.: Towards a better understanding of low back pain: A review of the mechanics of the lumbar disc. Rheumatol. Rehabil. *14*:129–143, 1975.
69. Nagagawa, H., Huang, Y. P., Malis, L. I., and Wolf, B. S.: Computed tomography of intraspinal and paraspinal neoplasms. J. CAT *1*:377–390, 1977.
70. Naylor, A.: The biochemical changes in the human intervertebral disc in degeneration and nuclear prolapse. Orthop. Clin. North Am. *2*:343–358, 1971.
71. Pallis, C., Jones, A. M., and Spillane, J. D.: Cervical spondylosis: Incidence and implications. Brain *77*:274–289, 1954.
72. Paschal, J.: Beitr. Path. Anct. *84*:123–130, 1930.
73. Payne, E. E., et al: The Cervical Spine. Brain *80*:571–596, 1957.
74. Peserico, L., Uihlein, A., and Baker, G. S.: Surgical

treatment of cervical myelopathy associated with cervical spondylosis. Acta Neurochir. *10*:365–375, 1962.

75. Radin, E., and Bryan, R.: Phenylbutazone for prolapsed discs. Lancet *2*:736, 1968.

76. Resjo, I. M., Harwood-Nash, D. C., Fitz, C. R., and Chuang, S.: Computed tomographic metrizamide myelography in spinal dysraphism in infants and children. J. CAT *2*:549–558, 1978.

77. Riley, L.: Cervical disc surgery: Its role and indications. Orthop. Clin. North Am. *2*:443–452, 1971.

78. Rinaldi. I., Kopp, J. E., Harris, W. O., Regan, T. J., and Murphy, D.: Computer assisted tomography in syringomyelia. J. CAT *2*:633–636, 1978.

79. Robertson, J. T.: Anterior cervical disc removal with and without fusion. Presented at the 33rd Annual Meeting of the American Academy of Neurological Surgery, Lake Tahoe, Nevada, September 29, 1971.

80. Robinson, R. A., and Smith, G. W.: The treatment of certain cervical-spine disorders by anterior removal of the intervertebral disc and interbody fusion. J. Bone Joint Surg. *40A*:607, 1958.

81. Robinson, R. A.: The results of anterior interbody fusion of the cervical spine. J. Bone Joint Surg. *44A*:1569–1586, 1962.

82. Rogers, L.: The treatment of cervical spondylitic myelopathy by mobilisation of the cervical cord into an enlarged spinal canal. J. Neurosurg. *18*:490, 1961.

83. Saunders, J., and Inman, V.: Pathology of the intervertebral disc. Arch. Surg. *40*:389–416, 1940.

84. Scott, J.: Stress factor in the disc syndrome. J. Bone Joint Surg. *37B*:107, 1955.

85. Scoville, W. B.: Cervical spondylosis treated by bilateral facetectomy and laminectomy. Neurosurg., *18*:423–428, 1961.

86. Shatwell, G.: Carisoprodol compared with aspirin in the treatment of cervical spondylosis. Br. J. Clin. Pract. *20*:303–307, 1966.

87. Simmons, E., et al.: Anterior cervical discectomy and fusion. J. Bone Joint Surg. *51*:225, 1969.

88. Spurling, R. G.: Lesions of the Cervical Interverte-bral Disc. Springfield, Charles C Thomas Co., 1956.

89. Stoltman, H. F., and Blackwood, W.: The role of ligamenta flava in the pathogenesis of myelopathy in cervical spondylosis. Brain *87*:45, 1964.

90. Straus, W.: Fossil evidence of the evolution of the erect bipedal posture. Clin. Orthop. *25*:9–19, 1962.

91. Stuck, R. M.: Anterior cervical disc excision and fusion: Report of 200 consecutive cases. Rocky Mtn. Med. J. *60*:25–30, 1963.

92. Taylor, A. R., and Collier, J.: Brain *24*:532, 1901.

93. Taylor, T. K., et al.: Calcification in the intervertebral disc. Nature *199*:612–613, 1963.

94. Terracol, J.: Les troubles segmentaires sensitifs et trophiques du pharynx et l'osteoarthrite deformante de la colonne cervicale. Arch. Int. Laryngol. *33*:1025–1047, 1927.

95. Verbiest, H., and Paz y Geuse, H. D.: Anterolateral surgery for cervical spondylosis in cases of myelopathy or nerve-root compression. J. Neurosurg. *25*:611–622, 1966.

96. Verbiest, H.: A lateral approach to the cervical spine: Technique and indications. J. Neurosurg. *28*:191–203, 1968.

97. Weinstein, M. A., Rothner, A. D., Duchesneau, P., and Dohn, D. F.: Computed tomography in diastomyelia. Radiology *117*:609–611, 1975.

98. White, A., and Hirsch, C.: An experimental study of the immediate load bearing capacity of some commonly used iliac bone grafts. Acta Orthop. Scand. *42*:482–490, 1971.

99. Wilkinson, M.: The anatomy and pathology of cervical spondylosis. Proc. R. Soc. Med. *57*:159–162, 1964.

100. Wilkinson, M.: Cervical Spondylosis. Philadelphia, W. B. Saunders Co., 1971.

101. Wolfe, B. S., Kilnani, M., and Malis, L.: The sagittal diameter of the bony cervical spinal canal and its significance in cervical spondylosis. J. Mt. Sinai Hosp. *23*:283, 1965.

102. Yamada, K.: The dynamics of experimental posture. Clin. Orthop. *25*:20–31, 1962.

CHAPTER 8

Thoracic Disc Disease

M. VALLO BENJAMIN, M.D.

JOSEPH RANSOHOFF, M.D.
New York University

HISTORICAL BACKGROUND

Gowers, in 1892, under the heading "vertebral exostosis," described protuberances growing from the bodies of the vertebrae into the spinal canal that could compress the spinal cord or nerves.[17] He claimed that they were exceedingly rare, and that their chief characteristic was extreme chronicity. The symptoms might be those of slow compression of the cord or of irritation expressed chiefly by pain. He concluded that exostosis constituted a more promising field for the surgeon than other kinds of vertebral tumors. Many were so placed that their removal was feasible and, if situated in front of the cord, the division of some nerve roots, at least in the thoracic region, might permit access to the growth.[8]

Bailey and Casamajor, in 1911, discussed osteoarthritis of the spine as a cause of compression of the spinal cord and its roots.[5] They noted that osteoarthritis of the spinal column was extremely common in persons past middle age. In the same year, Middleton and Teacher reported the case of a young man who after lifting a heavy plate could not straighten up and rapidly became paraplegic.[27] He died 16 days later, and postmortem examination revealed protrusion of the twelfth thoracic disc, with thrombosis of the underlying vessels and destruction of the spinal cord. Stooky, in 1928, attributed compression of the spinal cord to ventral extradural chondromas.[36] The misconception of chondroma was sustained by other authors.[14, 18] Peet and Echols, in 1932, made the first suggestion that

the so called "chondromas" or "ecchondrosis" were in reality protrusions of the intervertebral disc.[31] In 1934, Mixter and Barr reported four patients with thoracic disc protrusions.[28] After surgery three patients became paraplegic.

As clinical experience accumulated and neurosurgeons became familiar with diseases of the disc, the conventional laminectomy was used exclusively to deal with thoracic discs. Disappointing results, with a high incidence of paraplegia, were reported by Hawk, Logue, Love and Kiefer, Muller, and Tovi and Strang.[18, 22, 24, 29, 37]

In 1960, Hulme gave the first account of a lateral approach to the posterior protrusions of the thoracic discs.[19] He reported six cases in which this approach was used without an incidence of paraplegia.

In 1969, Perot and Munro, and Ransohoff and coworkers reported on transthoracic removal of thoracic discs, with similar encouraging results.[32, 33]

INCIDENCE

It is difficult to assess the frequency of symptomatic thoracic disc disease. However, certain inferences can be drawn from the few reports in the literature. Love and Kiefer reported 17 cases in 5500, and Arseni and Nash reported 12 thoracic discs out of 2544 in patients who underwent surgery for disc disease.[3, 4, 24] An incidence of one to six cases per 1000 seems to be reasonable. Thoracic disc degeneration appears predominantly in males, with those in their fifth decade being most often affected. However, it has also been reported in children.[30] Tovi and Strang report that approximately one fourth of their cases occurred at the eleventh space, and more than half of all protrusions have involved the ninth, tenth, and eleventh spaces.[37] The eleventh interspace appears to be the most commonly involved.[15]

CLINICAL PRESENTATION

History

The patients' complaints and histories might vary greatly, according to the location, size, and duration of the disc disease. Thoracic disc herniations can be divided into central, central-lateral, and lateral locations. The clinical history and neurologic findings seem to correlate fairly accurately with the strategic locations of the disc herniation. A history of trauma is quite rare; however, a vague history of minor trauma can be elicited in roughly one third of the patients.[11]

The most common presenting symptom is pain, which occurs in central-lateral or lateral herniations. Localized spontaneous pain at the site of the lesion is not uncommon. This may be unilateral or bilateral, with girdle-like midline distribution. In unilateral lesions this history is long-standing and chronic. Patients with bilateral radicular pain, on the other hand, tend to have a shorter history and show more evidence of spinal cord compression. We have seen a patient with a 27-year history of pain related to a lateral thoracic disc herniation. An average history of one to three years is given by most patients. In lower thoracic segments the pain might radiate to the abdominal viscera, epigastric region, kidney, and groin.

Sensory complaints in the distribution of the nerve roots of corresponding spinal cord segments are not infrequent. Segmental dysesthesia or numbness may be seen. In central-lateral lesions the numbness will usually start in one or both lower extremities and gradually take an ascending course.

In centrally located herniations the patient's history may be strictly one of spastic paraparesis without any sensory complaints. The progression may vary in speed, affecting one or both lower extremities, and may at times follow a stepwise course.

Sphincteric symptoms related to bowel, bladder, and sexual function usually appear in later stages of the disease but may be seen in more acute herniations.

Physical Findings

Essentially, there are no specific physical findings to direct one's attention to the correct diagnosis. Local tenderness on percussion of the spine may be present. Basically, there are signs of compression of the spinal cord with spastic paraparesis, increased deep tendon reflexes, and a Babinski sign. Not infrequently, a Brown-Séquard syndrome might be found with central-lateral disc protrusions.[22, 23] Segmental loss of the superficial abdominal reflexes may aid in localization of the lesion.[20, 29]

Sensory findings are quite common. Tovi reported an incidence of findings in 90 per cent of his patients.[37]

Disturbances of bowel, bladder, and sexual functions appear quite late in most instances. In the lower thoracic and upper lumbar lesions compressing the conus medullaris, early sphincter involvement is commonly seen. Radicular pain and some signs of spinal cord dysfunction appear to be the most common clinical symptoms.

Radiologic Findings

Plain radiographs of the thoracic spine are of little help in reaching an accurate diagnosis of thoracic disc protrusion. Backer reported calcified protruded disc fragments visible within the spinal canal in only five of 43 cases.[6] Focal narrowing of the intervertebral disc space, calcification of the nucleus pulposus, sclerotic changes, and degenerative spondylosis are quite nonspecific findings. Notwithstanding extensive focal calcification of the posterior aspect of the intervertebral space, corresponding to the clinical level of radicular pain and sensory findings should increase the suspicion of thoracic disc protrusion.

Tomography may more adequately define the extent and position of the calcified disc.

Positive contrast myelography is the most important and decisive diagnostic tool. Since it is difficult to keep the contrast fluid in the thoracic region, it is recommended that at least 25 to 30 ml. of contrast medium be used.

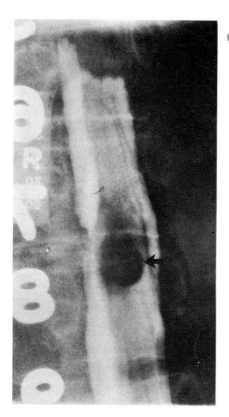

Figure 8–1. Anterior-posterior view of T7-T8 central filling defect (arrow) secondary to disc protrusion.

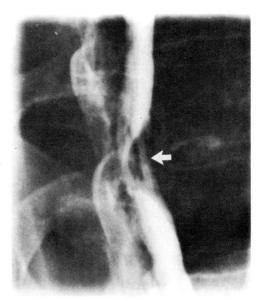

Figure 8–2. Lateral projection of T7-T8, with ventral extradural defect (arrow) at the level of disc space.

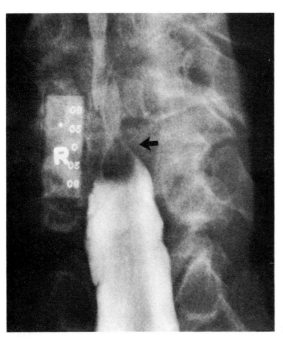

Figure 8–3. Anterior-posterior projection showing the inferior aspect of the extradural disc lesion (arrow).

If anterior-posterior and lateral views do not reveal the lesion well, bilateral decubitus and oblique views are obtained to exclude lateral defects. It is most important to realize that routine anterior-posterior views will show widening of the spinal cord, which can be distinguished from an intramedullary tumor on only the lateral and decubitus films (Figs. 8–1 and 8–2). When a lesion is found 0.5 ml. of methylene blue is injected into the skin to determine the approximate level at the time of surgical intervention.

There appear to be two different myelographic pictures. One is associated with central protrusion, which is quite characteristic. The anterior-posterior view may be confused with that of an intra- or extramedullary tumor. However, on the lateral projection, the posterior extradural displacement of the dye column, opposite the disc space, will establish the diagnosis (Figs. 8–3, 8–4, and 8–5). In lateral disc protrusion the AP and lateral myelographic views may be normal. In such cases the oblique and lateral decubitus films are diagnostic.

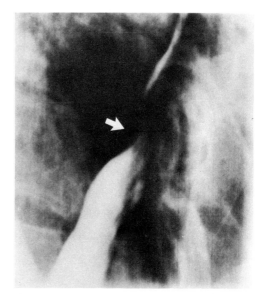

Figure 8–5. Lateral projection of the extradural disc defect (arrow) of the same patient as in Figures 8–3 and 8–4.

Computed Tomography

With the advent of computed tomography of the spine, thoracic disc lesions that protrude into the spinal canal can be demonstrated readily. This technique requires accurate localization of the tomographic section. It is likely that the newer generation of CAT scanners will provide precise diagnostic information without the need for myelography.

Angiography

Selective spinal angiography will be necessary if the lesion is below the T8 level, to determine the point of entry of the "arteria radicularis anterior magna" of Adamkievich, which supplies the anterior two thirds of the spinal cord. This vessel is usually single and arises on the left side in 80 per cent of individuals. In 85 per cent of cases it reaches the cord with a nerve root between T9 and L2, 75 per cent between T9 and T12, and 10 per cent between L1 and L2.[12] Since the majority of disc protrusions involve T9, T10, and T11, one may assume that some of the disastrous results after laminectomy are due to obliteration of this vessel during rhizotomy. Based on this information, it would be wiser for the surgeon to operate from the opposite side of the entry of this artery to spare the blood supply of the spinal cord (Fig. 8–6).

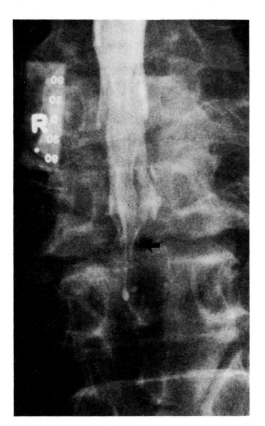

Figure 8–4. The pantopaque from above, outlining the upper aspect of the disc lesion (arrow), in the same patient as in Figure 8–3.

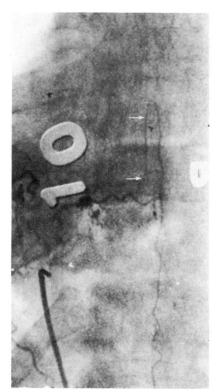

Figure 8–6. Selective spinal angiography performed prior to surgery, showing the Adamkievich artery (arrows) entering the spinal canal at T10-T11 on the left side.

Diagnosis

Symptomatic thoracic disc protrusions are notoriously difficult to diagnose. When the clinical presentation is limited to pain, the disease may remain a puzzle for many years. It might be mistaken for costovertebral joint syndrome, early stages of ankylosing spondylitis, metastatic tumors, neurofibromas, chronic duodenal ulcers, "intercostal neuralgia," disc space infections, herpes zoster, or many other abdominal diseases.[11]

On the other hand, signs and symptoms of spinal cord dysfunction may appear that may mimic any disease of the spinal cord, such as intra- and extramedullary tumors and demyelinating diseases of the spinal cord. As was mentioned previously, there should be a high index of suspicion in thoracic disc protrusion in the presence of local thoracic pain, radicular pain, or any manifestation of spinal cord disease that is not easily explained. Ultimately, myelography is the only means of making a correct diagnosis. In our experience, lumbar puncture and manometric studies have no specific diagnostic value in these patients.

Electromyography may be of value in isolated cases, particularly when there is severe radicular involvement without myelopathy.[25]

SURGICAL THERAPY

Symptomatic thoracic discs, unlike cervical and lumbar discs, are treated only by surgical intervention. When the diagnosis is suspected on clinical grounds and confirmed with myelography, the patient should be operated as soon as possible. Delay in surgery not only will make the operation more difficult and hazardous but also might decrease the chances of spinal cord recovery. The surgical results of thoracic disc protrusions, again unlike cervical and lumbar discs, have been quite poor in the past. Aside from the difficulty in diagnosing these lesions, the pitfalls of surgery lie in the pathologic anatomy and strategic location of the disc. First, the thoracic spinal canal is quite narrow and there is very little room for manipulation of the spinal cord. Second, the lesion is located ventral to the dura. In the past, most of these lesions have been attacked posteriorly through a laminectomy, and this makes the problem doubly difficult. Third, the problem of interrupting the main blood supply of the spinal cord by way of the Adamkievich artery has not been appreciated until recently.

The literature is replete with disappointing results of laminectomy in the treatment of these lesions. In their 1969 publication, Perot and Munro summarized from the literature the results of laminectomy in a large group of patients.[32] Of a total of 91 patients with lateral, central-lateral, and central disc lesions who had surgery, 18 did not improve, 16 became paralytic, and 6 died. In centrally located lesions in 57 patients, 12 did not improve, 15 became paraplegic, and 5 died. These dismal results in a benign disease are difficult to accept.

Hulme, in 1960, for the first time reported an alternative approach to laminectomy.[19] This approach was basically an extension of Menard's costotransversectomy.[6] This operation was first performed by N. Carpenter and reported by Alexander and Seddon.[2, 35] Dott, in 1947, gave further accounts of this operation.[13]

Chesterman and Crafoord each reported one case utilizing the same approach recommended by Hulme.[9, 10, 19] Perot and Ransohoff, in 1969, reported on variations of this operation for anterior disc protrusions.[32, 33]

The favorable results so far reported with the transthoracic or translateral approaches make laminectomy an undesirable and risky operation. If the preoperative diagnosis is well established with myelography, laminectomy certainly is contraindicated. However, in rare situations, a surgeon does a laminectomy under the assumption of the existence of a tumor and, after the exposure, finds that he is faced with a centrally located disc or ridge. The surgeon should make no attempt to remove the lesion; rather, after the patient has recovered from the laminectomy, or soon thereafter, the disc should be approached translaterally. We have surgically treated seven patients with thoracic discs, two patients with kyphoscoliosis, two patients with fractures, one patient with an anterior bullet, and three patients with tumors located anterior to the dural tube without an incident of paraplegia or death. Only one patient with thoracic disc has not improved. This was due to inadequate removal of the lesion. Postoperative myelography revealed the persistence of the preoperative defect in this patient.

Position and Incision

The patient is placed in a prone or three fourths prone position, supported by two chest rolls, in order to avoid pressure on the abdomen and to allow proper chest expansion.

A 15 to 20 cm. long paramedian incision, centered at the methylene blue marker, is made. The incision should be at least 20 cm. from the midline in order to expose the angle of the rib (Fig. 8–7). The lateral extent of the exposure should be parallel to the plane of the anterior aspect of the dura (Fig. 8–8). If too small a portion of the rib is removed, the

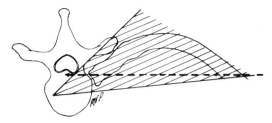

Figure 8–8.

visualization of the anterior dura becomes difficult, and, consequently, the removal of the defect will be done blindly (Fig. 8–9). For this reason, a transverse incision over the corresponding rib is preferred in a one-level disc protrusion.

Exposure

The incision is deepened to the fascia, and the muscles are incised at the lateral border of the longitudinal paravertebral muscles. The paravertebral muscles are retracted medially, and the flat muscles are reflected laterally, until the ribs are seen. A marker is left on the rib, and a radiograph is obtained for exact determination of the affected disc level. The rib to be removed is that attached to the lower vertebra of the intervertebral disc (for exposure of T7-T8 the rib is removed). After subperiosteal dissection, that portion of the rib between the neck and the angle is removed. The transverse process of the vertebra and the neck and head of the rib are removed with rongeurs and are then disarticulated. The articulation of the head of the rib to the vertebra is used as a landmark for identification of the intervertebral disc space.

The intercostal neurovascular bundle is another landmark that leads the surgeon to the intervertebral foramen (Fig. 8–10). The use of magnification techniques (microscope or four-

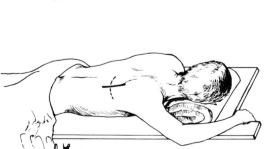

Figure 8–7.

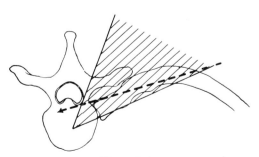

Figure 8–9.

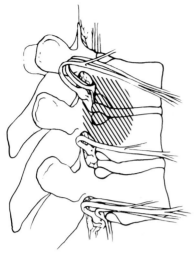

Figure 8–10.

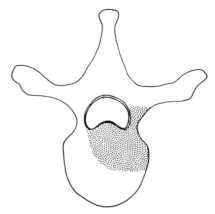

Figure 8–12.

power loupes) is helpful in the latter stages of the approach and ridge removal. The intercostal nerve is dissected and divided to prevent postoperative pain. The pedicle of the lower vertebra is freed from the muscle. The parietal pleura is gently pushed away from the lateral aspect of the vertebral bodies. With a periosteal elevator, the costal capitis ligament and anterior longitudinal ligament are dissected clear of the vertebral bodies. At this point, the anulus fibrosus is brought into view. The pedicle of the lower vertebra is removed with a high speed drill, and the lateral aspect of the dura is seen (Fig. 8–11). With a blunt dissector, the anterior aspect of the dura is dissected cautiously.

Removal of Bone

After incision of the anulus fibrosus and removal of a portion of the disc, the posterior third of the upper and lower vertebrae are drilled. This leaves a thin shell of bone over the anterior dura. After the drilling is well past the midline, and using an angled curet, the central disc protrusion and spondylosis is withdrawn from the dura into the cavity drilled in the bone (Fig. 8–12). In rare instances, when the lesion is adherent to the dura, a section of the dura can be resected.

The closure is routine, and there is no need for spinal fusion after this operation. If the pleura is opened, or if a transpleural approach is used, a chest tube, through a separate incision, to a water-sealed bottle is left.

In summary, it is clear that the clinical diagnosis of thoracic disc protrusions is difficult. There must be a high index of suspicion in the presence of radicular pain and some signs of spinal cord dysfunction. Positive contrast myelography is essential for the diagnosis. Selective spinal cord angiography is recommended for visualization of the Adamkievich artery in the lower segments. The classical laminectomy for these lesions has been universally unsuccessful. The lateral extra- or transpleural approaches offer a superior alternative for the surgery of the thoracic discs.

References

1. Abbott, K. H., and Retter, R. H.: Protrusions of thoracic intervertebral discs. Neurology, Minneap., 6:1–10, 1956.

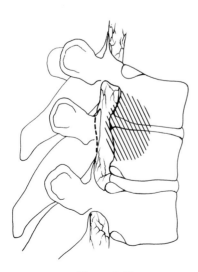

Figure 8–11.

2. Alexander, G. L.: Neurological complications of spinal tuberculosis. Proc. R. Soc. Med. *39*:730, 1946.

3. Arseni, C., and Nash, F.: Thoracic intervertebral disc protrusions. A clinical study. J. Neurosurg. *17*:419–430, 1960.

4. Arseni, C., and Nash, F.: Protrusion of thoracic intervertebral disc. Acta Neurochirurg. *11*:1–33, 1963.

5. Bailey, P., and Casamajor, L.: Osteo-arthritis of the spine as a cause of compression of the spinal cord and its roots. J. Nerv. Ment. Dis. *38*:588, 1911.

6. Baker, H. L., Jr., Love, J. C., and Uhlein, A.: Roentgenologic features of protruded thoracic intervertebral discs. Radiology *84*:1059–1065, 1965.

7. Bradford, F. K., and Spurling, R. G.: The intervertebral disc. With specific reference to rupture of the annulus fibrosus with herniation of the nucleus pulposus. 2nd ed. Springfield, Charles C Thomas Co., 1945.

8. Brain, W. R., and Wilkinson, M.: Cervical Spondylosis and Other Disorders of the Cervical Spine. Philadelphia, W. B. Saunders Co., 1967, p. 3.

9. Chesterman, P. J.: Spastic paraplegia caused by sequestrated thoracic intervertebral disc. Proc. R. Soc. Med. *57*:87–88, 1964.

10. Crafoord, C., Hiertonn, T., Lindblom, K., and Olsson, S. E.: Spinal cord compression caused by a protruded thoracic disc. Report of a case treated with antero-lateral fenestration of the disc. Acta Orthop. Scand. *28*:103–107, 1958.

11. De Palma, A. F., and Rothman, R. H.: The Intervertebral Disc. Philadelphia, W. B. Saunders Co., 1970, pp. 171–180.

12. Djindjian, R., Hurth, M., and Houdart, R. (English text by Kricheff, I.): Angiography of the Spinal Cord. Baltimore, University Park Press, 1970, pp. 7–8.

13. Dott, N. M.: Skeletal traction and anterior decompression in the management of Pott's paraplegia. Edinb. Med. J., *54*:620–627, 1947.

14. Elsberg, C. A.: The extradural ventral chondromas (ecchondroses), their favorite sites, the spinal cord and root symptoms they produce, and their surgical treatment. Bull. Neurol. Inst. N.Y. *1*:350–388, 1931.

15. Epstein, J. A.: The syndrome of herniation of the lower thoracic intervertebral discs with nerve root and spinal cord compression. A presentation of four cases with a review of the literature, methods of diagnosis and treatment. J. Neurosurg. *11*:525–538, 1954.

16. Feiring, E. H.: Extruded thoracic intervertebral disc. Arch. Surg. Chicago *95*:135–137, 1967.

17. Gowers, W. R.: Diseases of the Nervous System. 2nd ed. London, Churchill, 1892, Vol. 1, p. 260.

18. Hawk, W. A.: Spinal compression caused by ecchondrosis of the intervertebral fibrocartilage: with a review of the recent literature. Brain, *59*:204–224, 1936.

19. Hulme, A.: The surgical approach to thoracic intervertebral disc protrusions. J. Neurol. Neurosurg. Psychiat. *23*:133–137, 1960.

20. Joung, J. H.: Cervical and thoracic intervertebral disc disease. Med. J. Aust. *2*:833–838, 1946.

21. Lazorthes, G., Poulhes, J., Bastide, G., Chancholle, A. R., and Zadeh, O.: La Vascularisation de la Moele Epiniere. Pathologie Vasculaire de la Moelle. XXV Reunion Neurologique Internationale, Paris, Masson et cie, 1962. p. 5–27.

22. Logue, V.: Thoracic intervertebral disc prolapse with spinal cord compression. J. Neurol. Neurosurg. Psychiat. *15*:227–241, 1952.

23. Love, J. G., and Walsh, M. N.: Protruded intervertebral disc. Report of one hundred cases in which operation was performed. J.A.M.A. *111*:396–400, 1938.

24. Love, J. G., and Kiefer, E. J.: Root pain and paraplegia due to protrusions of thoracic intervertebral discs. J. Neurosurg. *7*:62–69, 1950.

25. Marinacci, A. A.: Applied Electromyography, Philadelphia, Lea and Febiger, 1968.

26. Menard, V.: Etude Pratique sur le Mal de Pott. Paris, 1900.

27. Middleton, G. S., and Teacher, J. H.: Injury of the spinal cord due to rupture of an intervertebral disc during muscular effort. Glasgow Med. J. *76*:1–6, 1911.

28. Mixter, W. J., and Barr, J. S.: Rupture of the intervertebral disc with involvement of the spinal canal. N. Engl. J. Med. *211*:210–215, 1934.

29. Muller, R.: Protrusion of thoracic intervertebral discs with compression of the spinal cord. Acta Med. Scand. *139*:99–104, 1951.

30. Peck, F. C., Jr.: A calcified thoracic intervertebral disc with herniation and spinal cord compression in a child. Case report. J. Neurosurg. *14*:105–109, 1957.

31. Peet, M. M., and Echols, D. H.: Herniation of the nucleus pulposus: A cause of compression of the spinal cord. Arch. Neurol. Psychiat. Chicago *32*:924–932, 1934.

32. Perot, P., and Munro, D. D.: Transthoracic removal of midline thoracic disc protrusions causing spinal cord compression. J. Neurosurg. *31*:452–458, 1969.

33. Ransohoff, J., Spencer, F., Siew, F., and Gage, L.: Transthoracic disc protrusions causing spinal cord compression. J. Neurosurg. *31*:459–461, 1969.

34. Reeves, D. L., and Brown, H. A.: Thoracic intervertebral disc protrusion with spinal cord compression. J. Neurosurg. *28*:24–28, 1968.

35. Seddon, H. J.: Pott's paraplegia: Prognosis and treatment. Br. J. Surg. *22*:769–799, 1936.

36. Stooky, B.: Compression of the spinal cord due to ventral extradural cervical chondromas. Arch. Neurol. Psychiat. *20*:275–291, 1928.

37. Tovi, D., and Strang, R. R.: Thoracic intervertebral disc protrusions. Acta Chir. Scand. (Suppl. 267), 41, 1960.

CHAPTER 9

Lumbar Disc Disease

RICHARD H. ROTHMAN, M.D. Ph.D.

FREDERICK A. SIMEONE, M.D.

PHILIP M. BERNINI, M.D.

Pennsylvania Hospital and The University of Pennsylvania

INTRODUCTION

Back pain has plagued humans for many thousands of years. Descriptions of lumbago and sciatica are described in the Bible and in the writings of Hippocrates. Despite the long history of awareness of this problem, a reasonable and scientific explanation of the source of low back and leg pain did not emerge until 1934 with the publication of the classic paper by Mixter and Barr.[10] These investigators for the first time delineated prolapse of the intervertebral disc as the etiologic agent in the production of these symptoms. It is commonly acknowledged today that derangements of the intervertebral disc represent the great majority of cases of back pain and sciatica.

Human disease assumes importance as a cause of either death or disability. Degenerative disease of the spine for all intents and purposes is a nonlethal entity, and its priority must rest on determination of its prevalence in the population and its impact on this population in terms of pain and disability.

INCIDENCE

The frequently ill-defined and multifaceted causes of postural low back and leg pain have prevented accurate evaluation of the epidemiology of low back pain syndromes. Estimation of the problem has been made, but these reported figures have been derived primarily from the industrial compensation setting.

In Sweden, each member of the National Health Insurance, in order to receive compensation, reports his or her illnesses by telephone to a central bureau. Thus, excellent statistics are readily available in terms of population analysis. Back pain has been reported in 53 per cent of persons engaged in light physical activity and in 64 per cent of those involved in heavy labor.[5]

The disability of endemic proportions resulting from the painful low back can be better appreciated in terms of its economic impact. Benn and Wood[1] reviewed various medical statistics from the National Insurance in the United Kingdom and found that more than 13 million days are lost annually owing to a painful back. This ranked third behind chronic and acute pulmonary disease and atherosclerotic coronary vessel disease and was responsible for more working time lost than labor strikes in the United Kingdom in 1970.

Nachemson[11] has estimated that at some time during our adult life 80 per cent of us will experience back pain to a significant extent. An extensive investigation by Horal[4] showed that low back pain of a significant degree begins in the younger age groups with a mean age of onset of 35 years. Kelsey[7, 8] found a similar age onset in males with low back pain due to disc disease but found that females averaged nearly a decade of delay in the development of significant symptomatology. In Horal's study of the individuals complaining of low back pain, only 35 per cent developed sciatica. After subsidence of the original attack of low back pain, 90 per cent had a future recurrence.

While Kelsey found that males underwent surgery for low back pain and sciatica due to disc disease significantly more often than females, the male predominance was not as evident in the overall sample of low back pain sufferers. Furthermore, there were no racial differences in the incidence of low back pain and sciatica due to disc disease.

NATURAL HISTORY

Intelligent treatment of lumbar disc degeneration must be predicated on a thorough knowledge of the natural history of this disorder. If this information is not available to the treating physician and to the patient, they will be unable to honestly and effectively make the decisions necessary for the management of this disorder. All too often, decisions either for or against surgical intervention are based on distorted concepts of disc disease.

Back pain can be expected to precede the onset of radicular symptoms by approximately 6 to 10 years.[9, 13] The initial low back pain episode will usually be of acute onset, whereas the subsequent recurrences[2, 13] will tend to surface insidiously. The radicular component will usually originate insidiously and will recur in a similar fashion.[13]

A group of 583 patients were studied at the Karolinska Institute after their first attack of sciatica. Surgery was undertaken in 28 per cent of the group, and patients who had undergone surgery as well as those who had not were followed for an average of seven years.[3] The results of this study indicated that the acute episodes of sciatica ran a relatively brief course in most cases, regardless of whether the treatment was conservative or surgical. However, the subacute or chronic symptoms secondary to disc degeneration, although less dramatic, were prolonged and had a profound effect on the patients' lives. At the end of the follow-up period, approximately 15 per cent of the conservatively treated group continued to have a reduced work capacity, restriction in leisure activities, and regular sleep disturbances. Twenty per cent of the conservatively treated group continued to have pronounced residual sciatica.

Weber[13] conducted a carefully controlled, well-documented prospective study of 280 patients with low lumbar disc herniations. All herniations were myelographically proved. All patients were initially treated with 14 days of conservative management in the hospital. At the completion of this treatment regimen, the study group with relative indications for surgery were assigned randomly into either a conservative or surgical treatment group. Those who improved were dropped from the study. Those with a sphincter disorder or progressive neurologic deficit were treated surgically and dropped from the study. At the one year follow-up examination of the randomized study group, surgery was found to be superior to the conservative regimen in regard to low back pain and the radicular component caused by the disc herniation. After four years, however, while the conservatively treated group improved, the tendency for better results following surgery prevailed, but the differences as to the efficacy of treatment were no longer significant. Similar long-term results of nonoperative treatment reported earlier[12] had also suggested the longer morbidity involved, the slow but definite improvement realized, and acceptable but less than ideal results.

It is important to note that in Weber's study, there was no loss of quality of surgical result by a three month period of observation. Therefore, in the absence of urgent indications for surgery (cauda equina syndrome or a progressive neurologic deficit), one can allow this period of time to pass so that the symptoms can resolve, and so that certain patients can be spared a needless operation. Beyond this three month period, however, the quality of surgical results begins to deteriorate.

Disability from lumbar disc disease must be considered in terms of back and leg pain with its attendant limitation of function. Although neurologic deficits, including motor weakness, are helpful diagnostically, they are not necessarily compelling surgical factors since residual weakness is not markedly different in patients treated operatively or conservatively.[3] Bowel or bladder dysfunction affects a relatively small percentage of patients but assumes greater significance in terms of surgical urgency.

With this background, the treating physician and the patient must make their decision for the role of surgery. If, after careful diagnostic evaluation, a firm diagnosis can be established and a course of conservative treatment has failed and the treating surgeon feels that operative intervention would with certainty shorten the disease process, then surgery can be recommended.

References

1. Benn, R. T., and Wood, P. H. N.: Pain in the back: An attempt to estimate the size of the problem. Rheumatol. Rehabil. *14*(3):121–128, 1975.
2. Gulliver, J.: Acute low back pain in industry. Acta Orthop. Scand. (Suppl.) *170*:9–17, 1977.
3. Hakelius, A.: Prognosis in sciatica. Acta Orthop. Scand. *129*:6–76, 1970.
4. Horal, J.: The clinical appearance of low back disorders. Acta Orthop. Scand. (Suppl.) *118*:7–109, 1969.
5. Hult, L.: The Munkfors investigation. Acta Orthop. Scand. (Suppl.)*16*:5–102, 1954.
6. Kelsey, J. L.: An epidemiological study of acute herniated lumbar intervertebral discs. Rheumatol. Rehab. *14*:144–159, 1975.
7. Kelsey, J. L.: An epidemiological study of the relationship between occupations and acute herniated lumbar intervertebral discs. Int. J. Epidemiol. *4*(3):197–205, 1975.
8. Kelsey, J. L.: Demographic characteristics of persons with acute herniated lumbar intervertebral disc. J. Chron. Dis. *28*:37–50, 1975.
9. Lassoner, E. M., Alho, A., Karalarju, E. O., and Paavilaimen, T.: Short term prognosis in sciatica. Ann. Chir. Gynaecol. *66*:47–51, 1977.
10. Mixter, W. J., and Barr, J. S.: Ruptures of the intervertebral disc with involvement of the spinal canal. N. Eng. J. Med. *211*:210–215, 1934.
11. Nachemson, A. L.: The lumbar spine: An orthopaedic challenge. Spine, *1*:59–71, 1976.
12. Pearce, J., and Moll, J.: Conservative treatment and natural history of acute lumbar disc lesions. J. Neurol. Neurosurg. Psychiatry *30*:13–17, 1967.
13. Weber, H.: Lumbar disc herniations: A prospective study of prognostic factors including a controlled trial. J. Oslo City Hosp. *28*:33–64, 89–120, 1978.

THE PATHOLOGY OF LUMBAR DISC DISEASE

MARK BROWN, M.D., Ph.D.*

*Department of Orthopedic Surgery, University of Miami School of Medicine

Ballooned Discs

Ballooning of the intervertebral disc is characteristically seen in association with diseases that weaken the body of the vertebra itself. Classically, osteoporosis, more accurately termed osteopenia, will weaken the vertebral body sufficiently to allow expansion of the intervertebral disc into the upper and lower end plates of the body (Fig. 9–1). This occurs because of the imbibition characteristics of the nucleus pulposus conferred by the acid aminoglycans. For this ballooning to

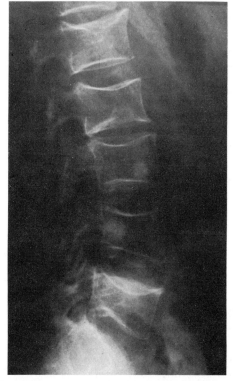

Figure 9–1. Radiograph of the lumbar spine revealing severe osteoporosis with ballooning of multiple discs into the softened adjacent vertebral body.

occur, the disc must still have its elastic gelatinous nucleus pulposus.[17] It is interesting to note that many people who suffer from osteopenia of the skeleton and ballooning of the disc do not exhibit disc degeneration. This is a curious observation that needs to be studied further. If the disc has lost its integrity, collapse and wedging of the vertebrae will occur rather than ballooning. This is probably due to the fact that the disc has lost its cushioning ability and the already weakened vertebral body must sustain abnormal loads. Malignant processes, such as multiple myeloma, will produce weakness of the vertebral body sufficient to allow ballooning to take place. This disease process must be considered in the differential diagnosis of osteopenia when first encountering a patient with the roentgenographic changes of osteopenia. An interesting observation is that astronauts on return from space will have gained height. Their discs balloon when allowed to expand without the constraints of constant gravity. The discs gradually return to normal height, as do the astronauts themselves, on return from their celestial pursuits. This is just another example of the balance between imbibition, gravity, and ligamentous and muscular constraint on the nucleus pulposus.

Intraspongy Nuclear Herniations

(Schmorl's Node)

It has been noted for over 100 years that the intervertebral disc can herniate through the cartilaginous end plate into the cancellous bone of the vertebral body. This herniation of disc material takes place through a defect in the cartilaginous plate, which may represent the point of passage of blood vessels from the body of the vertebrae to the disc during early life. These herniations are of irregular size and shape and alternately will be surrounded by a rim of bony sclerosis. These defects are seen thoughout adult life. The adjacent disc space frequently exhibits thinning (Fig. 9–2).

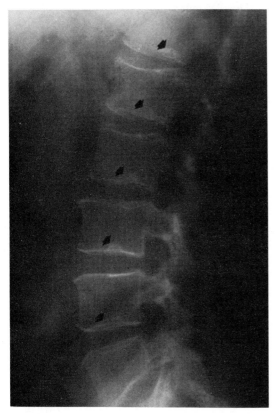

Figure 9–2. Radiograph of the lumbar spine illustrating multiple intra-spongy nuclear herniations into the central portion of the adjacent end plate of the vertebral body.

Osteophyte Formation

Peripheral osteophyte formations anteriorly and laterally and to a lesser extent posteriorly are often found on the bodies of the lumbar vertebrae associated with disc degeneration. These osteophytes represent pathologic stimulation of new bone formation at the attachment of the longitudinal ligaments or the anulus fibrosus to the vertebral bodies. Recent electron microscopic studies of the collagen fibers within the anulus fibrosus show strong attachments between the peripheral one third of the anulus and the vertebral body. The collagen fibers of the longitudinal ligaments also communicate with those of the periosteum of the vertebral body. The abnormal motion and abnormal distribution of stresses on the anular ligaments as the result of disc degeneration stimulate traction spurs (osteophytes). Macnab differentiated the traction spur from other osteophytes.[11] It is horizontally directed and arises 2 mm. away from the distal border of the anterior and lateral surfaces of the vertebral body (Fig. 9–3A). He feels that it denotes "segmental instability." We have noted Macnab's traction spurs more commonly in discs in the upper and middle lumbar spine. We have not noted a particular predisposition toward mechanical symptoms in patients who have this roentgenographic finding. The decreased incidence of posterior osteophytes compared to those of the anterior and lateral position may be explained by the absence of strong attachments of the posterior longitudinal ligament to the bone. Osteophyte formation in association with disc degeneration has often been termed lumbar spondylosis, which has its counterpart in cervical spondylosis.

Osteophytes secondary to degenerative disc disease must be differentiated from syndesmophytes, more commonly associated with rheumatic inflammatory disorders. Marie-Strümpell's ankylosing spondylitis and ankylosing hyperostosis are two conditions of the spine that most commonly are associated with syndesmophytes. These diseases, termed enthesopathies by Ball,[2] have their primary pathologic process based upon chronic round cell inflammatory infiltrates in the enthesis or points of strong attachments of ligaments to bone. First a round cell inflammatory process occurs, followed by new fibrous bone production. The syndesmophytes tend to be vertically oriented (Fig. 9–3B) rather than horizon-

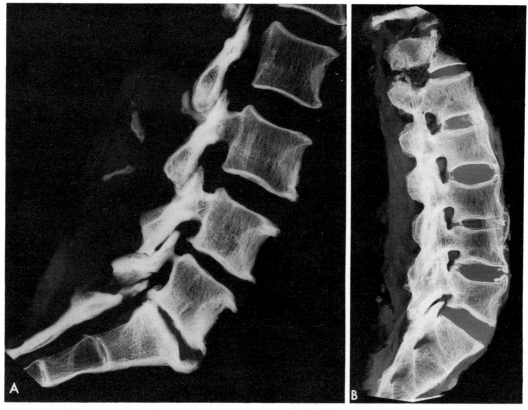

Figure 9–3. *A,* Lateral roentgenogram thin slice pathologic section of the lumbar spine. Note the narrowing of the L4 disc associated with typical "traction spurs" (osteophytes). *B,* Lateral roentgenogram thin slice pathologic section of the lumbar spine. Note maintenance of L4 disc height with vertically oriented syndesmophytes.

tally oriented like osteophytes and tend to fuse with one another without a corresponding decrease in disc height. On the other hand, disc degeneration results in disc narrowing and osteophytes that are more apt to be horizontally oriented. This fine distinction helps one in the roentgenographic differentiation in inflammatory processes versus degenerative processes involving the intervertebral joint.

Thinned Discs

Three distinct situations are present that may be associated with thinning of the disc. The first situation occurs in the presence of transitional fifth lumbar vertebrae (Fig. 9–4). Between the transitional vertebrae and the sacrum a vestigial disc is often found, which is devoid of nucleus pulposus. This narrow disc is not the result of disc degeneration but is, in fact, a developmentally small disc. When the transverse process of the transitional vertebra is incompletely sacralized to one side and

is normal on the other, it is possible that the caudal intervertebral disc may be degenerated. More often there is a broad sacralization of the transverse processes, either unilaterally or bilaterally. In these situations one looks for disc degeneration above the transitional vertebrae rather than below it. These transitional segments are usually asymptomatic, stable, and may predispose to pseudospondylolisthesis secondary to disc degeneration at the level above.

A second group of thinned intervertebral discs is associated with degeneration of the nucleus pulposus without herniation. One must assume that the loss of nucleus pulposus in these discs and this form of disc degeneration occur by way of depolymerization of the macromolecules of the nucleus pulposus and diffusion into the subchondral vascular channels. There may be cracks and fissures produced in the bony end plate of the vertebral body and direct invasion of granulation tissue with dissolution of the nucleus pulposus by humoral enzymes. One may see such a

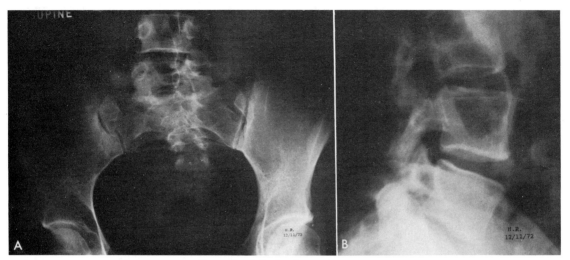

Figure 9–4. *A*, Anterior-posterior radiograph of the lumbar spine reveals a transitional fifth lumbar vertebra. *B*, Lateral view of the same patient reveals loss of height of the disc space between the transitional vertebra and the sacrum. This is not due to disc degeneration but rather to the congenital variation of the transitional vertebra.

marked disc resorption in this process that only a gas shadow is left (Knuttson's sign).[9] This occurs with disc narrowing and abnormal weight distribution, and a vacuum phenomenon may be seen. Not infrequently, the vacu-um phenomenon occurs with stress films in standing and flexion and extension lateral views (Fig. 9–5*A*). Crock has termed this process isolated disc resorption where it occurs most commonly at the L5 level, al-

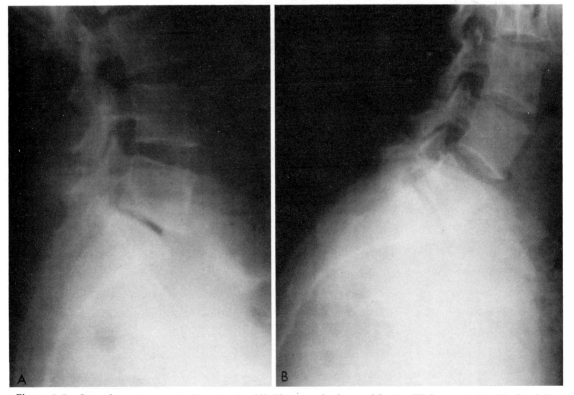

Figure 9–5. Lateral roentgenograms in extension (*A*). Note gas shadow and flexion (*B*) demonstrating "isolated disc resorption" at L5.

Illustration continued on following page

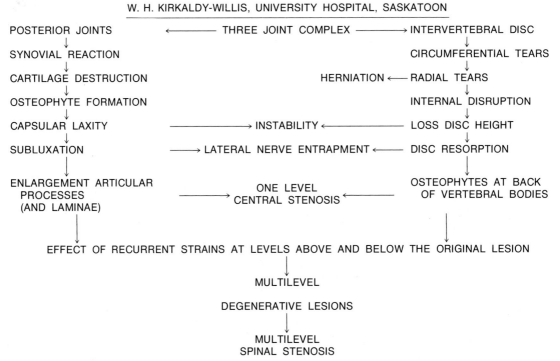

Figure 9–5. *Continued   C,* Degenerative lesions in the lumbar spine. (Reproduced from Kirkaldy-Willis, W. H., Wedge, I. H., Yong-Hing, K., and Reilly, J.: Pathology and pathogenesis of lumbar spondylosis and stenosis. Spine, 3:320, 1978.)

Illustration continued on opposite page

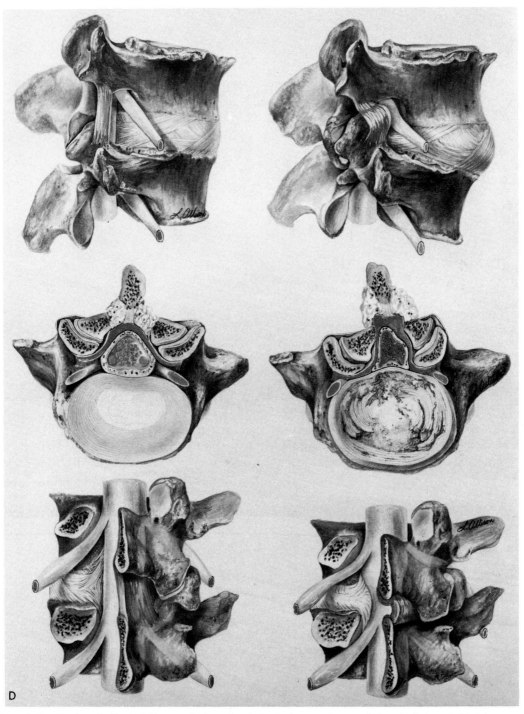

Figure 9–5. *Continued D,* Artist's compilation of pathologic changes that result in spinal stenosis (right) compared to three normal views of the L4–5 intervertebral joint (left).

Illustration continued on following page

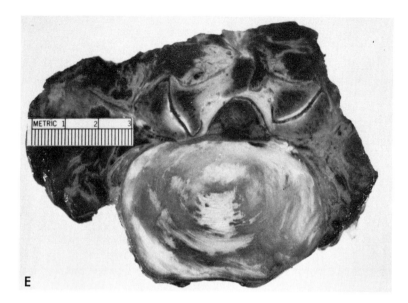

Figure 9–5. *Continued E,* Transverse section pathologic specimen L4 intervertebral joint demonstrates severe disc degeneration associated with subluxation and degeneration of the facet joints and the medial displacement of the L5 nerve roots.

though the process may occur at any level of the spine. It is most common in the lower lumbar spine and in the lower cervical spine. Crock's terminology "isolated disc resorption" is confusing, in that this is not a pathologic process that is limited to the L5-S1 intervertebral disc.[4]

Finally, disc narrowing or thinning can occur secondary to a disc space infection with resorption of the nucleus pulposus. This process is discussed in depth in Chapter 12.

Disc Protrusion

The process of nuclear herniation and anular protrusion is caused by a combination of biomechanical factors previously discussed, chronic degenerative structural changes, and superimposed mechanical stress. The pathologic cycle has been described in detail by Armstrong.[1] Prior to actual displacement of disc material, the nucleus and anulus undergo certain well-defined structural changes. Radiating cracks in the anulus fibrosus develop in the most centrally situated lamellae and extend outward toward the periphery.[8] These radiating clefts in the anulus weaken its resistance to nuclear herniation. If they are subject to persistent mechanical pressure by a turgid nucleus, herniation may ensue. Herniation is a much greater threat in the younger individual, between the ages of 30

and 50, having good turgor in the nucleus, than in the elderly, in whom the nucleus is desiccated and fibrotic. In the older individual the degenerated, thinned disc will often develop without any of the signs and symptoms of acute nerve root compression. This may explain the predominance of acute disc syndromes in the middle-aged population and their rarity in the elderly.

Posterior displacement of the nucleus pulposus may occur in a variety of ways (Fig. 9–6). In an extreme circumstance, there may be a massive nuclear retropulsion, in which a large volume of disc material is suddenly thrust into the spinal canal, producing a profound neurologic catastrophe. More commonly, the extrusion is a gradual and intermittent process. The nucleus progressively bulges through the rent in the anulus, being retained in position by the posterior longitudinal ligament. This ligament, which may be stretched and detached by the herniating nuclear material as it forces its way relentlessly backward to the spinal canal, may rupture, with the formation of a free sequestrum into the spinal canal. This disc fragment may then migrate cephalad or caudad or laterally into the intervertebral foramen. It is not only the size of the nuclear herniation that determines its clinical significance but also the direction in which this herniation takes place. In addition, the shape of the spinal canal is shown to be of great importance. Failure to recognize the variety of

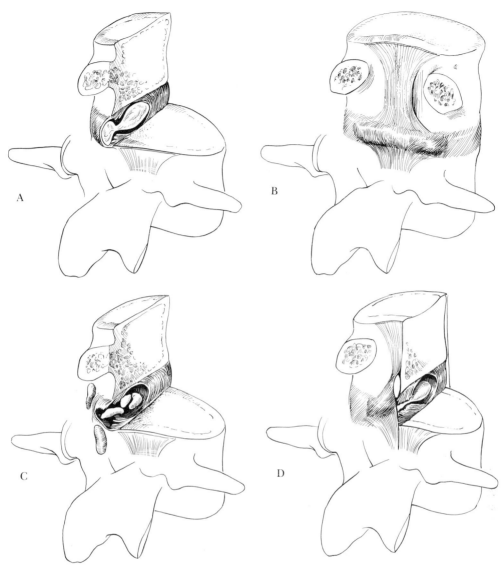

Figure 9–6. *A,* Herniation of a lumbar disc beneath the posterior longitudinal ligament in the common lateral position. *B,* Herniation of a lumbar disc in the less frequent central position beneath the strong portion of the posterior longitudinal ligament. *C,* Complete herniation of a lumbar disc through a rupture in the anulus and the posterior longitudinal ligament, with free fragments in the neural canal. These fragments may migrate cranially, caudally or into the intervertebral foramen. *D,* Herniation of a lumbar disc, with upward migration of the disc fragments, beneath the posterior longitudinal ligaments. These fragments may go unnoticed unless specific exploration in these areas in undertaken. (From DePalma, A. F., and Rothman, R. H.: The Intervertebral Disc. Philadelphia, W. B. Saunders Co., 1970.)

types of disc pathology having significant spatial relationships will lead to inadequate surgical treatment of these problems. It should also be pointed out that posterior protrusion of disc material may often occur at some site other than that of an obviously thin disc.[3]

Subsequent to the loss of the integrity of the anulus fibrosus, there may be invasion of the disc by granulation material, either through rents in the anulus or through cracks in the cartilaginous end plate. The role of this granulation tissue in regard to the production of pain is as yet unclear.

It should be emphasized that as the process of disc herniation occurs, biochemical as well as mechanical irritation of the nerve root must be considered. The clinical symptoms that are produced are in all likelihood closely related to biochemical irritation of the nearby nerve root by degradation products of the degenerating disc. It has been dramatically demonstrated by Falconer that myelographic defects are unchanged after successful conservative treatment of sciatica.[5] Thus, mechanical factors alone are insufficient explanations for nerve root symptomatology.

Spinal Stenosis

The recent classic studies give us an excellent synopsis of the overall understanding of the evolution of spinal stenosis. Porter and colleagues have shown that those individuals who suffer from back pain are more apt to have small spinal canals than patients who have been asymptomatic.[13] Our clinical observations at the time of surgery have led the authors to conclude that this scientific observation holds up in clinical circumstances. We hardly ever encounter a normal spinal canal while doing a simple disc excision or unroofing a stenotic spine.

The natural evolution of disc degeneration and the pathologic changes that occur in the intervertebral joint lead to a subsequent stiffening of the intervertebral joint, through the natural healing processes of osteophyte formation (spondylosis). This can be seen in population studies in which the changes consistent with spondylosis and degenerative disc disease increase with aging radiographically, although the back pain symptoms peak between the ages of 30 and 50 and subside as one gets older. We frequently tell our patients that they will get better as they get older. But a certain minority of patients will go on to develop symptoms of spinal stenosis over the age of 60. The natural evolution of this process has been eloquently summarized by Kirkaldy-Willis and coworkers[9] (Fig. 9–5C). We have endeavored to summarize the pathologic processes that occur in the intervertebral joint late in the aging process and that account for entrapment in the lateral recess and spinal foramen, as well as the spinal canal itself. Three views of the spine (Fig. 9–5D), showing the lateral, transverse axial, and posterior views in both the normal and abnormal spine, have been drawn from a compilation of pathologic findings in over 100 autopsy specimens.

The universal failure that occurs in the intervertebral joint, subsequently leading to central stenosis or foraminal entrapment, is disc space narrowing. The disc narrows as the result of loss of hydration of the nucleus pulposus. The narrowing may occur with or without mechanical instability, and the narrowing may occur in a disc attached to a normal size or a small spinal canal. Disc space narrowing causes laxity of the anulus fibrosus, and subsequent anular tears may result in failure to obtain normal healing of the ligament. The subsequent hypermobility of the intervertebral joint will lead to marginal osteophyte formation, bulging of the anulus fibrosus, and narrowing of the intervertebral disc. The consequence of narrowing of the disc will be subluxation of the facet joints. The tripod joint complex, composed of the intervertebral disc and two facet joints, must be visualized in order to understand the pathophysiology of stenosis. The articular facets sublux in the axial, sagittal, and frontal planes, and the disc tends to narrow more in the posterior half as compared to the anterior half. This leads to a rotation of the superior facet anteriorly toward the posterior lateral corner of the adjacent vertebra. With subluxation of the facet joint, both in an axial plane and a sagittal plane, joint erosion, recurrent joint effusion, and degenerative changes with osteophyte formation occur. These diarthrodial joints are subject to all the changes that can occur in a peripheral joint. Rotational subluxation affects the inferior facet on one side and the superior facet on the contralateral side, causing them to protrude into the spinal canal (Fig. 9–5E). The ligamentum flavum, a passive elastic ligament, shortens with narrowing of the disc and subluxation of the facet joint. As a consequence of this shortening, the elastic ligament thickens. The thickened ligament is passively pushed into the neural space by the subluxation of the facet joint. These changes are best seen in the transverse view of the intervertebral joint.

The consequences of an anvil effect of the bulging anulus fibrosus with its marginal osteophytes pushed up against the anterior subluxating superior facet joints is that it takes up the room lateral to the nerve roots, which are just anterior and medial to the superior facet. For example, if the intervertebral joint depicted in Figure 9–5C is the L4-5 disc, then the L5 nerve roots are displaced by this anvil effect of the superior facet of L5 against the bulging L4 disc. The L5 roots are displaced medially. Note also the rotation of the left inferior facet and the right superior facet into the spinal canal. Note the degenerative changes in the joint in the marginal osteophyte formation. The ligamentum flavum has thickened and has been passively displaced into the neural space by the subluxed hypertrophied facet joints. From a posterior view, one can appreciate the natural consequences of central stenosis and the passive constriction of the dura silhouetted beneath the narrowed interspace. The relationship of the L4 nerve root taking a serpiginous course above the subluxed and rotated superior facet can also be seen in this diagram. These are all permutations of nerve root entrapment as a result of disc narrowing and facet joint subluxation. If these changes occur gradually and in the absence of anular tears, pain may not occur until late in the disease process, when ischemia of the vasonervosum occurs. However, usually the patient complains of chronic intermittent back pain, which can be attributed to minor flares of osteoarthritis of the facet joint as a consequence of degenerative changes. The patient may also complain of a component of mechanical back pain, increased by stress as a consequence of disc degeneration and laxity of the anulus fibrosus and longitudinal ligaments. The most common clinical findings correlated with the pathologic condition is that the patient has had nondisabling backache for a number of years. The patient then complains that over a period of two or three years

claudicant-type pain of a radicular nature has developed. What has happened is that the spinal nerves become progressively entrapped within a smaller space. With ambulation, mechanical irritation, poor excursion of the spinal nerves owing to entrapment, edema, and ischemia as the result of compromise of a vasonervosum of the cauda equina occurs. This produces the pseudoclaudicant type of pain typical of central or foraminal encroachment. Whether the markedly degenerated intervertebral joint with foraminal or central stenosis is mechanically unstable or not cannot be determined with accuracy until the time of surgical decompression. All these joints fail through disc narrowing and rotation. As a consequence of narrowing and rotation, the intervertebral disc may remain lax or it may stiffen. If it stiffens, one may decompress the neural canal with impunity. However, if the disc remains floppy or mechanically unstable, then in the process of properly decompressing the neural elements, further instability is produced. Future research on how to predetermine mechanical insufficiency prior to decompression is of great importance (Figs. 9–7, 9–8, 9–9).

One final note concerning the evolution of spinal stenosis should be the role that the pedicle plays when there is failure in rotation,

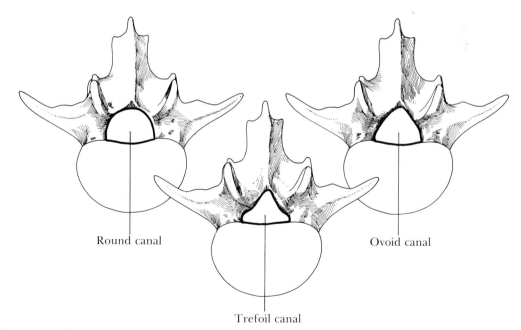

Figure 9–7. The three variations of the spinal canal: round, ovoid and trefoil. The lateral recesses of the trefoil canal render the lumbar roots particularly vulnerable to compression by extruded disc material (From DePalma, A. F., and Rothman, R. H.: The Intervertebral Disc. Philadelphia, W. B. Saunders Co., 1970.)

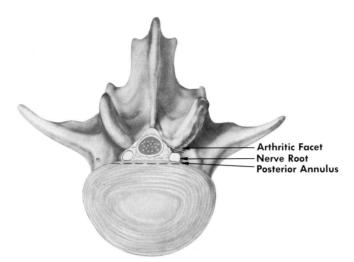

Arthritic Facet
Nerve Root
Posterior Annulus

Figure 9–8. This drawing illustrates entrapment of a lumbar nerve root in a lateral narrow recess secondary to degenerative changes. Note how posterior buckling of the anulus and arthritic changes in the facet joints can compromise the nerve root in the anterior-posterior direction. Failure to decompress this recess will result in persistent sciatica after surgery.

Figure 9–9. Foraminal encroachment secondary to chronic disc degeneration. The nerve root exiting the foramen will be compressed by the arthritic facet joint posteriorly, the relative descent of the pedicle superiorly and the posterior bulge of the anulus or disc extrusion anteriorly. The surgeon must satisfy himself that the nerve root is entirely free throughout the entire course of the foramen when the nerve root is decompressed.

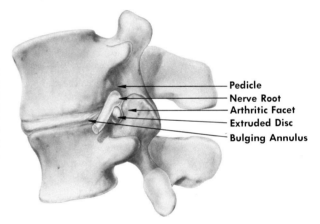

Pedicle
Nerve Root
Arthritic Facet
Extruded Disc
Bulging Annulus

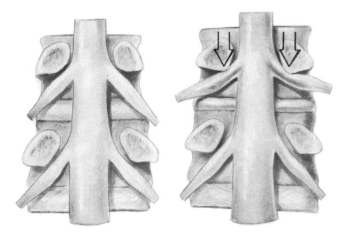

Figure 9–10. These drawings illustrate the relative caudal migration of the pedicles during disc degeneration which may tether the nerve roots. During exploration of a nerve root it must be ascertained that the root is free not only of compression but also of tension. If the root is tethered about the pedicle, excision of the offending pedicle must be undertaken.

as pointed out so eloquently by Farfan.[6] A few degrees of rotation with disc narrowing will greatly stretch and distort the nerve root, just medial to the pedicle. Also, narrowing of the disc with displacement of the pedicle in an axial direction will kink the nerve root, according to Macnab.[11] The most common nerve root to be affected as a consequence of these changes is L5, in our experience (Fig. 9–10).

One final change that we have noted, which we feel accounts for entrapment of the nerve root in the lateral recess, is the consequence of the inferior facet subluxing into the axilla between the lamina and the margin of the superior facet. When this occurs, the inferior facet forms a false fossa, which causes hypertrophy of bone anteriorly at the point of the lateral recess. It is most important to observe this pathologic finding, because in the process of spinal decompression one must be certain to inspect the medial aspect of the superior facet, particularly at the junction with the lamina and pedicle.

One should note on the posterior view in a diagrammatic representation of spinal stenosis that the ligamentum flavum may bulge posteriorly between the lamina and the narrowed intervertebral joint. This often gives the false appearance of a thickening of the ligamentum flavum or hypertrophy at the time of surgical exposure. We have also noted that lamina may overlap one another and that the major weight-bearing characteristics of the spine may shift posteriorly onto the subluxed hypertrophied facets and shingled lamina in the central stenosis syndromes. Keeping in mind these overall changes in the intervertebral joint that lead to spinal stenosis will help us to understand diagnostic tests, such as CT scanning and myelography, as well as to plan for more thorough surgical exploration and stabilization in the symptomatic patient with canal stenosis.

References

1. Armstrong, J. R.: Lumbar Disc Lesions. Baltimore, The Williams & Wilkins Co., 1965.
2. Ball, J.: Enthesopathy of rheumatoid and ankylosing spondylitis. Ann. Rheum. Dis. *30*:213–223. 1971.
3. Coventry, M. B., et al.: The intervertebral disc, its microscopic anatomy and pathology. J. Bone Joint Surg. *27*:460, 1945.
4. Crock, H. V.: Isolated lumbar disc resorption as a cause of nerve root canal stenosis. Clin. Orthop. *115*:109–115, 1975.
5. Falconer, M. A., et al.: Observations on the causes and mechanics of symptom production in low back pain and sciatica. J. Neurol. Neurosurg. Psychiatry *11*:13–26, 1948.
6. Farfan, H. F.: A reorientation in the surgical approach to degenerative lumbar intervertebral joint disease. Orthop. Clin. North Am. *8*:9–21, 1977.
7. Fitzpatrick, J. A. W., and Newman, P. H.: Degenerative spondylolisthesis. J. Bone Joint Surg. *58B*:184–192, 1976.
8. Hirsch, C., and Schajowicz, F.: Studies on structural changes in the lumbar anulus fibrosus. Acta Orthop. Scand. *22*:184–231, 1952.
9. Kirkaldy-Willis, W. H., Wedge, J. H., Yong-Hing, K., and Reilly, J.: Pathology and pathogenesis of lumbar spondylosis and stenosis. Spine *3*:319–328, 1978.
10. Knuttson, F.: The instability associated with disc degeneration in the lumbar spine. Acta Radiol. *25*:593–609, 1944.
11. Macnab, I.: Negative disc exploration: An analysis of the causes of nerve root involvement in sixty-eight patients. J. Bone Joint Surg. *53A*:891–903, 1971.
12. Macnab, I.: The traction spur. J. Bone Joint Surg. *53A*:663–670, 1971.
13. Porter, P. W., Hibbert, C. S., and Wicks, M.: The spinal canal in symptomatic lumbar disc disease. J. Bone Joint Surg. *60B*:485–487, 1978.

CLINICAL SYNDROME OF LUMBAR DISC DISEASE

Lumbar disc degeneration represents the most common cause of back and leg pain. It is a multifaceted syndrome and must be recognized as such if the diagnosis is to be correct and the treatment effective. One sees with disturbing regularity missed diagnoses of herniated lumbar discs that present in an atypical fashion, unfamiliar to the practitioner. It is equally precarious, however, to polarize one's thinking at the opposite extreme and attribute all cases of back and leg pain to abnormalities of the intervertebral disc. A wide variety of vascular, infectious, and space-occupying lesions can mimic the herniated lumbar disc. An attempt will be made in this section to outline the classic picture of the lumbar disc syndrome, as well as the more common variants.

It is important from the outset to recognize that the clinical syndromes discussed represent manifestations of the sequential spectrum of degeneration that affects the "three joint complex."[14] That is, the clinical presentation ranging from backache with and without referred pain through radicular pain to neurogenic claudication is a reflection of the totality of degeneration of the intervertebral disc and the facet joints. Furthermore, symptoms can be conveyed over well-defined but frequently simultaneously stimulated pain pathways (the sinovertebral nerves to the anulus and theca, the spinal nerves, and the medial and lateral branches of the posterior rami). Systematic analysis of these pathways will allow a more exact therapeutic solution.

History

BACK PAIN

The majority of patients with degenerative disc disease in the lumbar spine have low back pain as the earliest symptom. Spangfort's computerized analysis of 2504 disc operations demonstrated a mean duration of low back pain of 5.6 years prior to surgery, and this temporal disability preceded the onset of complaints of leg pain by nearly two years.[39] Weber's[43] excellent prospective study of lumbar disc herniation suggested that in greater than 90 per cent of patients studied there were nearly 10 years of episodic low back pain prior to the insidious onset of a radicular component. The patient recalls that after periods of demanding physical activity or after periods of seemingly benign but prolonged postures, pain appears in the lumbosacral area. The pain may last a few days and usually subsides with limitation of activity and bedrest. The pain pattern at this time is me-

chanical in nature in the sense that it is made worse by standing, lifting, and prolonged sitting and is relieved by rest.

It is the authors' feeling that pain at this stage is due to early degeneration of the anulus fibrosus and desiccation of the nucleus pulposus. Since the nucleus no longer functions as a perfect gel with viscoelastic properties, it will, therefore, transmit forces in a nonlinear and asymmetric fashion[23] (Fig. 9–11).

Disc degeneration, with its dorsally situated sinovertebral sensory nerve involvement, can reasonably be implicated in this pain syndrome. The initial onset of low back pain in the late twenties and early thirties coincides with the obliteration of vascular supply to the nucleus pulposus and all but the most peripheral aspects of the anulus fibrosus. The subsequent age-related defective defusion mechanism at the vertebral end plate–anular interface[8, 27] provides a basis for the loss of structural integrity of the disc at this time in the axial skeleton's aging process. The mechanical intensification and relief seen in this clinical syndrome can also be attributed to disc degeneration and easily understood in light of Nachemson's[31, 32] landmark *in vivo* determination of disc pressure in various postures (Fig. 9–12).

It should be reemphasized that at this early stage, disc degeneration cannot be clear-

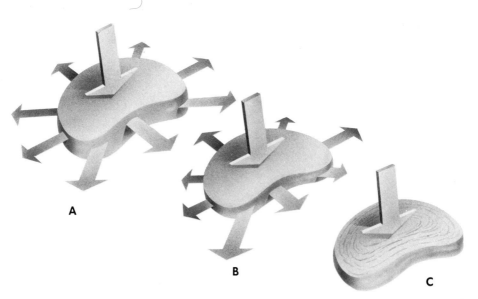

Figure 9–11. Distribution of forces in the normal and abnormal disc. *A*, When the disc functions normally, as in the early decades of life, the nucleus distributes the forces of compression and tension equally to all parts of the anulus. *B*, With degeneration, the nucleus no longer functions as a perfect gel and the forces transmitted to the anulus are unequal. *C*, With advanced degeneration of the nucleus, the distribution of forces to the anulus from within is completely lost since the nucleus now acts as a solid rather than a liquid. For this reason, disc herniation is unusual in the elderly.

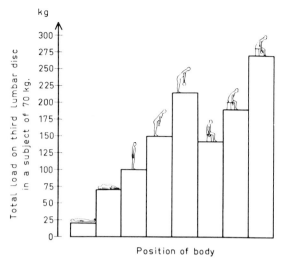

kg

Total load on third lumbar disc in a subject of 70 kg.

300
275
250
225
200
175
150
125
100
75
50
25
0

Position of body

Figure 9–12. This figure illustrates the total load on the third lumbar disc in a subject weighing 70 kg. (From Nachemson, A.: In vivo discometry in lumbar discs with irregular nucleograms. Acta Orthop. Scand. 36:426, 1965.)

ly differentiated from certain other common causes of low back pain, such as neural arch defects, postural strain, and unstable lumbosacral mechanisms.

With the passage of time, these episodes may become more frequent and intense and may lead to more disability. Between acute episodes of back pain, the patient usually describes a sense of stiffness, weakness, or instability that is present at a low but noticeable level. Indeed, these are probable manifestations of adverse motion segment (vertebral body, disc, and facet joint) behavior alter-

ations, which Kulak and others[23] have appreciated in their mathematical and two-dimensional finite element models. These defined changes occur in disc geometry, anular structural integrity, and in the way the disc nucleus is pressurized prior to load. Discogenic pain usually has the definite mechanical quality of being accentuated with prolonged sitting and standing. There is a clinical correlation of increased load with increased symptoms. Pain that is accentuated while the patient is in bed at night is more suggestive of a neoplastic process. An intermittent character of the pain is also characteristic of disc degeneration, and one should be wary when the patient states that from the onset the pain has been unrelenting and progressive, as in infectious or neoplastic states.

Injury is frequently noted by the patient at some time during the clinical course, and in many instances, spine pain to a greater or lesser degree was present prior to injury. Weber's[43] study revealed precipitating events for the first episode of low back pain in 55 per cent of patients who eventually developed disc herniations. The trauma reported, however, ranged from a falling episode through lifting and heavy work activity to nothing more serious than an abrupt movement. It is interesting that these incidents of pain usually occur during the early hours of the day after an extended supine position in sleep, when the turgor (function of increased hydration) of the nucleus pulposus is at its maximum[32] (Fig. 9–13).

Our current concepts of the pathophysiology of symptomatic disc disease show trauma to be a precipitating rather than a causative

Experimental flow of fluid in autopsy discs.

Figure 9–13. Theoretical calculation on the hydration-dehydration points as obtained experimentally by Kramer combined with the findings of intradiscal pressure measurements by Nachemson. (From Nachemson, A.: Toward a better understanding of low-back pain: A review of the mechanics of the lumbar disc. Rheumatol. Rehabil. 14(3):129, 1975.)

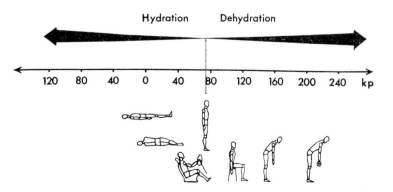

Hydration   Dehydration

120   80   40   0   40   80   120   160   200   240   kp

factor. Jayson and others[19] subjected 78 cadaver intervertebral discs to discography and
roentgenographically classified their nuclear
morphology. When subjected to compressive
loads, bursting most commonly occurred into
the adjacent vertebral bodies and not posteriorly. When nuclear herniation was realized
posterolaterally and directly posterior, it occurred in discs that were previously noted to
have posterolateral, direct posterior, or degenerative nuclear morphology. While the
discs were subject to compressive forces only,
the obvious importance of the premorbid nuclear and anular status is apparent.

Excessive stress applied to a young,
healthy spine will fracture the osseous elements of the vertebra before the disc is ruptured. When disc herniation occurs in young
healthy spines not yet subject to disc degeneration, the herniation will also likely follow
areas of premorbid structural weakness,
namely residual indentations in the cartilaginous end plate left as a result of notochord or
embryologic vascular regression, yielding
Schmorl's nodes.[36] The other premorbid area
of relative structural weakness persists at the
interface between the cartilaginous end plate
and the ossified portion of the vertebral body.
Keller[21] reported two cases of disc and vertebral rim prolapse in adolescents that were
confirmed by myelography with significant
spinal canal compromise and symptoms.

REFERRED PAIN

When certain of the mesodermal structures, such as ligaments, periosteum, joint
capsule, and the anulus, are subjected to abnormal stimuli, such as excessive stretching or
injection of hypertonic saline, a deep, ill-
defined, dull, aching discomfort is noted that
may be referred into the areas of the lumbosacral joint, sacroiliac joint, the buttocks, or the
legs[22, 29]; (Fig. 9–14). The pattern of referral is
to the area designated the sclerotome, which
has the same embryonic origin as the mesodermal tissues stimulated. While this peripheral pathway can explain this referred pattern,
the significant individual variations encountered must include consideration of central
neural pathways. Indeed, Kellgren[22] has concluded that the referred distribution of pain
depends not only on segmental innervation
but also on the severity of pain and the extent
to which an individual is cognizant of the
stimulated components of the axial skeleton.

Pain of this type can often present concurrently with radicular pain from nerve root
tension. The deeper, boring pain is classically
attributed to distribution along myotome and
sclerotomes, and the sharper and better localized superficial pain is conveyed via the dermatomes.[10] The two may be easily confused.
Moreover, sympathetic dystrophic signs and
symptoms due to nerve root encroachment
can further confuse the presentation, since the

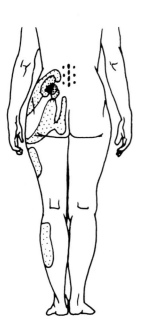

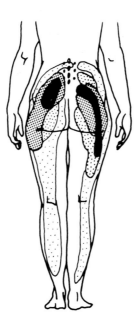

Figure 9–14. Pain referral pattern for asymptomatic and symptomatic subjects. This confirms that the
pain referral pattern from stimulation of the lumbar
facet joint is in the typical locations of lumbago. (From
Mooney, V., and Robertson, J.: The facet syndrome.
Clin. Orthop. *115*:149, 1976.)

NORMAL   ABNORMAL

causalgia may exist with or without the more classic complaints associated with radiculopathy.[3]

RADICULAR SYMPTOMS

Pressure on an inflamed nerve root by a disc fragment, bulging anulus, or compromised lateral recess may produce pain and motor or sensory signs and symptoms in the lower extremities. It had been first suggested by Smythe and Wright in 1958[40] and later demonstrated by Macnab[25] that nonpathologic nerve roots subjected to a compression will produce paresthesias, whereas nerves that are inflamed will yield a painful response to manipulation.

The etiologic role of mechanical tension on the nerve root yielding radicular pain is generally accepted, but whether there is damage to the intrinsic structure of the neural tissue, its accompanying vasculature, or both is uncertain.[30] The production of pain with straight leg raising or cross leg raising for the L5 and S1 spinal nerves and reverse straight leg raising for an L4 radiculopathy reflects the mechanical inability of the nerve root to yield to tension in and around the neural foramina.

The inflammatory component of the radicular syndrome is likewise of significance, but again the causative agents are uncertain. With the evolution of anular rents, the avascular nucleus pulposus may evoke an autoimmune response and act as a causative factor. This conclusion has been theorized owing to the susceptibility of the nerve roots to inflammatory agents and owing to an enhanced immune cellular response to homogenized disc material in both animals and humans.[5, 12] Furthermore, a humoral mechanism has been suggested since significant increases of IgM and IgG antibodies have been found in patients with disc prolapse.[4, 33] As yet, no immunoglobulins have been found in the disc tissue removed at the time of surgery.

The interaction of mechanical and inflammatory components yielding signs and symptoms of the various lumbar disc syndromes is obvious, but specific information concerning the dynamics of that interaction at this time remains hypothetical.

LEG PAIN

The patient notes a sharp, lancinating pain, usually starting in the proximal portion of the leg and ultimately progressing distally in a pattern typical of a dermatome. The L5 and S1 spinal nerves are most frequently involved, reflecting the greatest number of disc herniations occurring at L4-5 and L5-S1, respectively.[35, 39] While the onset of leg pain may be insidious or extremely dramatic and associated with a tearing or snapping sensation in the spine, the former presentation will be more usual for both the first sciatic attacks or those that precipitated the surgical intervention.[43]

At the time of onset of the sciatica, the back pain may suddenly abate. The mechanical explanation of this is that once the anulus has ruptured, it is no longer placed under tension and there is no longer a stimulus for pain in the lower back.

When the sciatic pain is acute, the patient or family of the patient may note that he is listing, usually away from the side of the sciatica. Occasionally, if the disc herniation is axillary or central in position, the patient may list toward the side of the sciatica. Both maneuvers obviously tend to decrease tension on the compromised nerve root.

The pain is frequently made worse by any maneuver that increases intraspinal pressures, such as the Valsalva maneuver, coughing, sneezing, and bearing down during defecation, a clinical correlate better understood with Nachemson's *in vivo* disc pressure studies.

The patient may be aware of a marked limitation of motion in the spine, and he often states that his back is "locked." This is particularly true in adolescents with disc herniations.[6, 7] In extreme cases, the pain may prevent any stress from being placed on the back or leg, and the patient may lie helpless on the floor or in bed with the feeling that he is "paralyzed," while in reality the limiting factor is pain. In high disc lesions affecting the fourth lumbar spinal nerves, the pain may be isolated to the area of the knee, and the patient may protest vigorously that the difficulty is confined only to the knee joint and may discourage any examination of the lumbar spine. When the clinical course has progressed to motor weakness involving the quadriceps muscle, the patient may complain of buckling of the knee in addition to the knee pain, which makes the situation still more confusing.

MOTOR SYMPTOMS

Infrequently, the patient may present with weakness in the lower extremities as the outstanding sign, which may disable without symptomatology or clinically appreciated sphincter disturbances. This is particularly true in lesions affecting the fourth and fifth anterior roots.

If the fifth nerve is compromised, the patient may note weakness on dorsiflexion of the foot and toes and occasionally a complete foot drop. Furthermore, the hip abductors may likewise be affected, yielding an abductor lurch with an associated positive Trendelenburg sign. Hakelius[18] found an equal number of disc herniations in patients with isolated dorsiflexion weakness compared to patients who also had other neurologic signs. Nonetheless, a *relatively painless* monoradicular or particularly multiradicular paresis must include a differential diagnosis of a metabolic or infectious neuropathy or space-occupying lesion of the cord itself.

DISC SYNDROMES

SCIATIC PAIN. It is not uncommon with the acute extrusion of a fragment of nuclear material against a nerve root to have the sudden onset of sciatica without concomitant back pain. The diagnosis of discogenic disease is suggested by accentuation of this leg pain by the Valsalva maneuver — a clinical correlate of increased intradiscal pressure and neural irritation. This, of course, would not be present in leg pain caused by pathologic conditions of the joints of the lower extremities or lesions of the sciatic nerve itself. Although the patient may be free of back pain, he may have a marked list, muscle spasm, and limitation of motion in the lumbar spine. This is particularly true of extreme lateral lumbar disc herniations.[2] The limited lumbar mobility is not purely a defensive and learned reaction to discogenic and radicular pain but may be a manifestation of an intrinsic neuromuscular pathologic state. Indeed, Fidler and others[15] found that when biopsies of the multifidus muscles from patients with positive root signs were subjected to histologic studies designed to differentiate slow fibers (low levels of myosin-ATPase activity), which primarily function in a postural role, from fast fibers, which function more dynamically, there was a higher ratio of slow to fast fibers than normally found. The cross-sectional area of the fast fibers was also increased. These findings, different from the pattern usually found in nor-

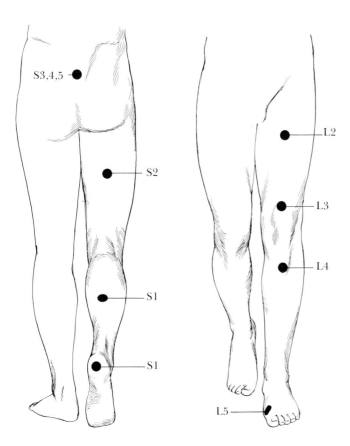

Figure 9–15. Pain may radiate to small, isolated, specific areas along the course of a dermatome.

mal individuals and with aging, were interpreted as reflecting a selective injury to fast fiber motor neurons as a result of either ischemia or mechanical injury at the anterior root of the involved spinal nerve.

It should be pointed out that in certain individuals, isolated areas of pain in the lower extremities are noted by the patient rather than the typical pattern of dermatome involvement. The primary complaint may be pain of the knee, calf, ankle, or heel in these individuals (Fig. 9–15). In studying pain and spinal root lesions, Friis and others[16] have found that approximately 10 per cent of patients with L5 or S1 lesions in particular had asymptomatic areas of a dermatome between painful foci. The unwary examiner who fails to instruct the patient to completely undress and who does not perform a meticulously thorough examination can obviously be led astray in these instances.

BACK PAIN ALONE. It has been pointed out that most patients with discogenic pain have intermittent episodes of back pain at the onset of their clinical course. Many of these individuals may proceed through the entire natural history of their disease and never experience sciatica. During acute exacerbation, pain will be accentuated by the Valsalva maneuver, and they will have typical findings in the lumbar area noted with degenerative disc disease. It is in this group of patients that great judgment must be utilized before surgical intervention is elected. It is far too easy to place patients with lumbar pain into this category without careful diagnostic evaluation. The treating physician must discipline himself to rule out other causes of back pain, such as tumor, infection, and intra-abdominal disease, before this diagnostic category is utilized.

NEUROGENIC CLAUDICATION

With increased awareness of this syndrome, first appreciated by Verbiest[41] in 1954, many more patients are benefiting from a correct diagnosis of the cause of their leg pain. Vague leg pain, dysesthesias, and paresthesias distributed over the anterior and posterior thighs and calves are classically brought on by spinal postures that mechanically compromise the neural canal and the neural foramina. Less often this syndrome is precipitated by the increased metabolic and vascular demands of the lower extremities, causing a compromise of neural blood flow,[13, 45] although a combined mechanism is feasible.

Ischemia to the cauda equina is most probably the final pathway of the syndrome, but it is the postural type of neurogenic claudication that has been best defined and differentiated from the claudication due to muscle ischemia secondary to aortofemoral disease.

The clinical presentation is well documented.[12, 46] Patients of either sex, usually not before their fifth decade, will first appreciate vague pains, dysesthesia, and paresthesias with ambulation and will get excellent relief of their symptoms with sitting or a supine posture. The increased lordotic stance assumed with walking and particularly while walking down grades is most likely causative. This symptomatic relationship to posture has been verified with the "bicycle test" of van Gelderan,[9] in which claudication symptoms are not produced while on the bicycle since there is a reduction of the lumbar lordosis and a subsequent increase in the central sagittal and foraminal dimensions of the canal. In contrast, muscle claudication symptoms will be produced with ambulation up grades, which increases metabolic demands and is not avoided by stress on the bicycle. The absence of pulses below the hips and rubor and pallor changes with elevation are classic for muscle claudication but not neurogenic claudication. In cases in which the diagnosis is uncertain, arteriography may be indicated.

With the maturation of the syndrome, symptoms at rest will occur, and muscle weakness and atrophy and asymmetrical reflex changes may then be appreciated, but as long as the symptoms are only aggravated dynamically, abnormal neurologic findings may only be found after stressing the patient.

The clinical syndrome has been associated with lumbar spinal stenosis and nerve root entrapment syndromes. An internationally accepted classification of the anatomic syndrome (Fig. 9–16) has been defined, and the production of symptoms has been attributed to those changes occurring locally, segmentally, or generalized in affecting osseous and soft tissue. It is, however, important to realize that structural changes in the spinal and foraminal canals exaggerated with posture are, as noted by Verbiest, "conditions, but not absolute determinants of intermittent claudication."[42] Indeed, the symptoms manifested may vary significantly among individuals with similar pathomorphologic changes owing to the temporal framework within which the

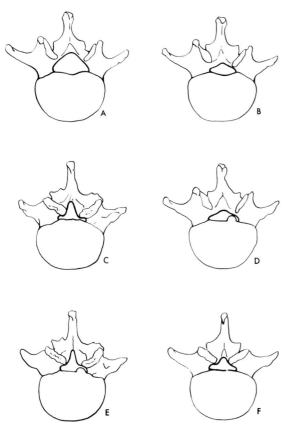

Figure 9–16. Types of lumbar spinal stenosis. *A*, Normal canal; *B*, Congenital/developmental stenosis; *C*, Degenerative stenosis; *D*, Congenital/developmental stenosis with disc herniation; *E*, Degenerative stenosis with disc herniation; *F*, Congenital/developmental stenosis with superimposed degenerative stenosis. (From Arnoldi, C. C., et al.: Lumbar spinal stenosis and nerve root entrapment syndromes. Clin. Orthop. *115*:4, 1976.)

neural compression has occurred, the individual susceptibility of the nerves involved, and the unique functional demands and pain tolerance of the patient.

THE CAUDA EQUINA SYNDROME

Occasionally, a large midline disc herniation may compress several roots of the cauda equina. Raaf[35] reported an incidence of 2 per cent of 624 patients with protruded discs, and Spangfort[39] reported 1.2 per cent of 2500 cases, and his review of the literature found a total incidence of approximately 2.4 per cent. He further found no noticeable differences in sex distribution or age and found L4 and L5 discs the most common offending herniations but with a significantly larger number of high lumbar herniations contributing than found in

other disc syndromes. Peyser and Harari[34] reviewed the literature and found an extremely high occurrence (11 of 17 cases) of cauda equina syndrome when there was an intradural rupture of the intervertebral disc. These herniations occur predominantly in the high lumbar areas and fortunately have a very low incidence of only approximately 0.2 per cent of all disc herniations.

If the lesion reaches a large size, it may mimic an intraspinal tumor, particularly if it has been slowly progressing. Often, back or perianal pain will predominate, and radicular symptoms may be masked. Difficulty with urination, consisting of frequency or overflow incontinence, may develop relatively early. In males a history of recent impotence may be elicited by the probing examiner. If leg pain develops, this may be followed by numbness of the feet and difficulty in walking. The large midline disc lesions, which ordinarily produce a complete myelographic block when associated with these symptoms, compress several spinal nerve roots. When compromised, the centrally placed sacral fibers to the lower abdominal viscera produce symptoms that characterize cauda equina compression. Perianal numbness and a loss of the anal reflex or bulbocavernosus reflex characterizes an advanced cauda equina syndrome. Sensory deficit is usual and frequently situated higher than the motor level.

Confusion as to the exact definition of the lesion will be encountered because the lesion will frequently be incomplete in evolving. It has been reported presenting infrequently as a lower motor neuron lesion or more frequently with abnormal radicular signs with normal or upper motor neuron lesion activity.[28] This latter lesion can be explained only on a vascular basis, but the specific mechanism in cases reported was purely speculative.

The significance of this entity is that it must be considered a reason for prompt surgical intervention since spontaneous neurologic recovery has not been observed. If incontinence is present, only prompt surgery can offer a chance to lessen the hazards of possible future urinary drainage problems. Similarly, sudden severe paresis or paraplegia merits prompt and generous decompression. When the symptoms are florid, a careful preoperative myelogram for level identification with insertion of only a small amount of contrast medium is indicated, since a complete block can be anticipated (Fig. 9–17).

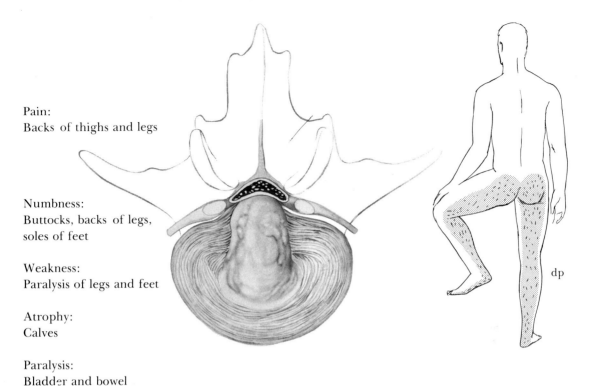

Pain:
Backs of thighs and legs

Numbness:
Buttocks, backs of legs,
soles of feet

Weakness:
Paralysis of legs and feet

Atrophy:
Calves

Paralysis:
Bladder and bowel

dp

Figure 9–17. Massive herniation at the level of the third, fourth or fifth disc may cause severe compression of the cauda equina. Pain is confined chiefly to the buttocks and the back of the thighs and legs. Numbness is widespread from the buttocks to the soles of the feet. Motor weakness or loss is present in the legs and feet with loss of muscle mass in the calves. The bladder and bowels are paralyzed. (From DePalma, A. F., and Rothman, R. H.: The Intervertebral Disc. Philadelphia, W. B. Saunders Co., 1970.)

BLADDER SYMPTOMS

It has been recently recognized that disc protrusions may present as an abnormality of bowel and bladder function in patients with minimal or absent back pain and sciatica. It has been well documented by Emmett and Love[11] and by Ross and Jackson[37] that disc disease should be ruled out in young or middle-aged patients who develop problems of urinary retention, vesical irritability, or incontinence. This is particularly true in the absence of infection or other pelvic abnormalities.

Four syndromes have been described in regard to bladder abnormalities caused by disc derangement: total urinary retention, chronic long-standing partial retention, vesicular irritability, and loss of desire to void associated with an unawareness of the necessity to void. Jones and Moore[20] felt that the uninhibited type of neuropathic bladder dysfunction without loss of bladder sensation represents the incipient stage of an evolving bladder disorder due to increasing involvement of the sacral roots.

Sharr, Garfield and Jenkins[38] have recently emphasized the occurrence of bladder dysfunction with spinal stenosis, particularly of the degenerative variety. While the same neuropathic bladders were encountered as in the disc herniation group, the feature of intermittency of symptoms was emphasized, therefore adding another facet to the weakness, dysesthesia, and paresthesias already associated with intermittent neurogenic claudication.

If these symptoms, particularly in their more subtle forms, are not specifically sought out, they will often be overlooked.

Cystoscopy and a cystometrogram, in conjunction with the myelogram, are most helpful in obtaining a definite diagnosis. These clinical syndromes are unlikely to occur with monoradicular involvement.

References

1. Arnoldi, C. C., Brodsky, J., Cauchoix, H. V., et al: Lumbar spinal stenosis and nerve root entrapment syndromes. Clin. Orthop. *115*:4–5, 1976.
2. Abdullah, A. F., Ditto, E. W., Byrd, E. B., and Williams, R.: Extreme lateral lumbar disc herniations. J. Neurosurg. *41*:229–234, 1974.
3. Bernini, P. M., Rothman, R. H., and Simeone, F.: Sympathetic dystrophy complicating lumbar disc herniations. In press.
4. Bisla, R. S., Marchisello, P. J., Lockshin, M. D., et al.: Auto-immunological basis of disk degeneration. Clin. Orthop. *121*:205–211, 1976.
5. Bobechko, W. T., and Hirsh, C. Auto-immune response to nucleus pulposus in the rabbit. J. Bone Joint Surg. *47B*:574, 1965.
6. Bulos, S.: Herniated intervertebral lumbar disc in the teenager. J. Bone Joint Surg. *55B*:273–278, 1973.
7. Bradford, D. S., and Garcia, A.: Lumbar intervertebral disk herniations in children and adolescents. Orthop. Clin. North Am. *2*(2):583–592, 1971.
8. Brown, M. D., and Tsaltas, T. T.: Studies on the permeability of the intervertebral disc during skeletal maturation. Spine *1*(4):240–244, 1976.
9. Dyck, P., and Doyle, J. B.: "Bicycle test" of van Gelderen in diagnosis of intermittent cauda equina compression syndrome. J. Neurosurg. *46*:667–670, 1977.
10. Elliott, F. A., and Schutta, H. S.: The differential diagnosis of sciatica. Orthop. Clin. North Am. *2*(2):477–484, 1971.
11. Emmett, J., and Love, J.: Vesical dysfunction caused by protruded lumbar disc. J. Urol. *105*:80–91, 1971.
12. Epstein, B. S., Epstein, J. A., and Jones, M. D.: Lumbar spinal stenosis. Radiol. Clin. North Am. *15*(2):227–239, 1977.
13. Evans, J. G.: Neurogenic intermittent claudication. Br. Med. J. *5415*:985–987, 1964.
14. Farfan, H. S.: Mechanical Disorders of the Low Back. Philadelphia, Lea and Febiger, 1973.
15. Fidler, M. W., Jowett, R. L., and Troup, J. D. G.: Myosin ATPase activity in multifidus muscle from cases of lumbar spinal derangement. J. Bone Joint Surg. *57B*:220–227, 1975.
16. Friis, M. L., Gulliksen, G. C., Rasmussen, P., and Husby, J.: Pain and spinal root compression. Acta. Neurochir. *39*:241–249, 1977.
17. Gertzbein, S. D., Tait, J. H., and Devlin, S. R.: The stimulation of lymphocytes by nucleus pulposus in patients with degenerative disk disease of the lumbar spine. Clin. Orthop. *123*:149–154, 1977.
18. Hakelius, A., and Hindmarsh, J.: The significance of neurological signs and myelographic findings in the diagnosis of lumbar root compression. Acta Orthop. Scand. *43*:239–246, 1972.
19. Jayson, M. I., Herbert, C. M., and Barks, J. S.: Intervertebral discs: Nuclear morphology and bursting pressures. Ann. Rheum. Dis. *32*:308–315, 1973.
20. Jones, D. L., and Moore, T.: The types of neuropathic bladder dysfunction associated with prolapsed lumbar intervertebral discs. Br. J. Urol. *45*:39–43, 1973.
21. Keller, R. H.: Traumatic displacement of the cartilaginous vertebral rim: A sign of intervertebral disc prolapse. Radiology *110*:21–24, 1974.
22. Kellgren, J. H.: The anatomical source of back pain. Rheumatol. Rehabil. *16*:3–11, 1977.
23. Kulak, R. F., Schultz, A. B., and Belytschko, T. B.: Biomechanical characteristics of vertebral motion segments and intervertebral discs. Orthop. Clin. North Am. *6*(1):121–133, 1975.
24. Kulak, R. F., Belytschko, T. B., Schultz, A. B., and Galante, J.: Nonlinear behavior of the human intervertebral disc under axial load. Orthop. Clin. North Am. *9*:377–386, 1976.
25. Macnab, I.: Personal correspondence.
26. Markolf, K. L., and Morris, J. M.: The structural components of the intervertebral disc. J. Bone Joint Surg., *56-A*:675–687, 1974.
27. Maroudas, A., Nachemson, A., Stockwell, R., and Urban, J.: In vitro studies of the diffusion of glucose into the intervertebral disc. *In* Nachemson, A.: Towards a better understanding of low back pain: A review of the mechanics of the lumbar disc. Rheumatol. Rehabil. *14*:129–143, 1975.
28. Maury, M., Francois, N., and Skoda, A.: About the neurological sequelae of herniated intervertebral disc. Paraplegia, *11*:221–227, 1973.
29. Mooney, V., and Robertson, J.: The facet syndrome. Clin. Orthop. *115*:149–156, 1976.
30. Murphy, R. W.: Nerve roots and spinal nerves in degenerative disk disease. *129*:46–57, 1977.
31. Nachemson, A.: The load on lumbar disks in different positions of the body. Acta Orthop. Scand. *36*:426, 1965.
32. Nachemson, A.: Towards a better understanding of low-back pain: A review of the mechanics of the lumbar disc. Rheumatol. Rehabil. *14*:129–143, 1975.
33. Naylor, A.: Intervertebral disc prolapse and degeneration. The biochemical and biophysical approach. Spine *1*(2):108–114, 1976.
34. Peyser, E., and Harari, A.: Intradural rupture of lumbar intervertebral disk: Report of two cases with review of the literature. Surg. Neurol. *8*:95–98, 1977.
35. Raaf, J.: Some observations regarding 905 patients operated upon for protruded lumbar intervertebral disc. Am. J. Surg. *97*:388–399, 1959.
36. Resnick, D., and Niwayama, G.: Intervertebral disk herniations: Cartilaginous (Schmorl's) nodes. Radiology *126*:57–65, 1978.
37. Ross, J. C., and Jackson, R. M.: Vesical dysfunction due to prolapsed disc. Br. Med. J. *3*:752–754, 1971.
38. Sharr, M. M., Garfield, J. S., and Jenkins, J. D.: The association of bladder dysfunction with degenerative lumbar spondylosis. Br. J. Urol. *45*:616–620, 1973.
39. Spangfort, E. V.: The lumbar disc herniation. A computer-aided analysis of 2,504 operations. Acta Orthop. Scand. (Suppl.) *142*:61–77, 1972.
40. Smyth, M. J. and Wright, V. J.: Sciatica and the intervertebral disc. An experimental study. J. Bone Joint Surg. *40A*:1401, 1958.
41. Verbiest, H.: Radicular syndrome from developmental narrowing of lumbar vertebral canal. J. Bone Joint Surg. *36B*:230–237, 1954.
42. Verbiest, H.: Pathomorphologic aspects of developmental lumbar stenosis. Orthop. Clin. North Am. *6*(1):177–196, 1975.
43. Weber, H.: Lumbar disc herniations. A prospectus study of prognostic factors including a controlled trial. J. Oslo City Hosp. *28*:33–64, 89–120, 1978.

44. Wiley, A. M., and Trueta, J.: The vascular anatomy of the spine and its relationship to pyogenic vertebral osteomyelitis. J. Bone Joint Surg. *41B*(4):796–809, 1959.
45. Wilson, C. B., Ehni, G., and Grollimus, J.: Neurogenic intermittent claudication. Clin. Neurosurg. *18*:62–85, 1971.
46. Wiltse, L. L., Kirkaldy-Wills, W. H., and McIvor, G. W. D.: The treatment of spinal stenosis. Clin. Orthop. *115*:83–91, 1976.

Physical Examination

INSPECTION

Limitation of motion is usually noted during the symptomatic phase of lumbar disc disease. The range of motion should be noted not only in forward and lateral flexion and extension but also in rotation. The examiner must not equate flexion of the hips with flexion of the lumbar spine, and attention should be directed to whether reversal of the normal lumbar lordosis occurs. It has been previously noted that even in patients who have only sciatica, marked restriction of motion may be present in the lumbar spine.

When acute sciatica is present, the patient usually lists away from the side of the sciatica, producing a "sciatic scoliosis" (Fig. 9–18). When the disc herniation is lateral to the nerve root, the patient will incline away from the side of the irritated nerve in an attempt to draw the nerve root away from the

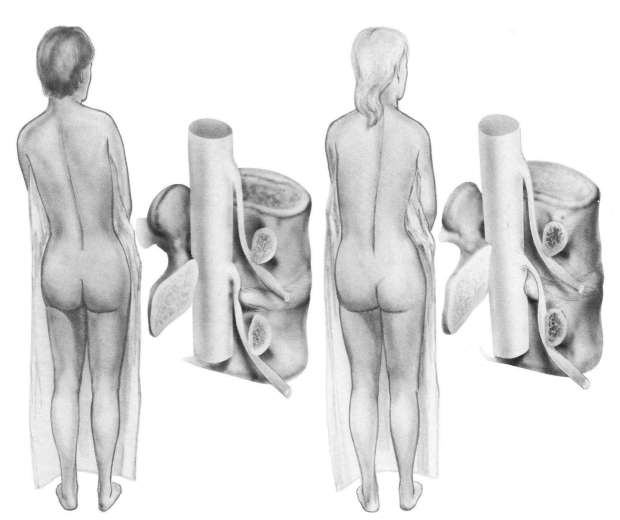

Figure 9–18. *A*, Herniation of the disc lateral to the nerve root. This will usually produce a sciatic list away from the side of the irritated nerve root. *B*, Herniation of the disc medial to the nerve root and in an axillary position. This will usually produce a sciatic list toward the side of the irritated nerve root.

disc fragment. This is dramatically demonstrated with extreme lateral disc herniations in that efforts at lateral bending to the side of the lesion will markedly exaggerate the patient's pain and paresthesias.[1, 13]

In a contrary fashion, when the herniation is in an axillary position medial to the nerve root, the patient will list toward the side of the lesion, also in an effort to decompress the nerve root.

The gait and stance of patients with acute disc syndrome are also characteristic. The patient usually holds the painful leg in a flexed position and is reluctant to place his foot directly on the floor. Presumably, flexion of the leg relaxes the sciatic nerve roots and is an involuntary effort at decompression of the root. When walking, the patient has an antalgic gait, putting as little weight as possible on the extremity and quickly transferring his weight to the unaffected side. Gait disturbances as well as significant loss of lumbar motility are very characteristic of disc herniation, particularly in adolescents.[2]

Loss of normal lumbar lordosis and paravertebral muscle spasm are also usually seen during the acute phase of the disease. These abnormalities are readily appreciated on inspection, particularly the contracted and spastic mass of the paravertebral muscles in extreme cases. Occasionally, in less acute situations, the muscle spasm can be elicited only when the patient is stressed by prolonged standing or forward flexion of the spine. Muscle spasm may on occasion be appreciated only unilaterally, and this is frequently strongly indicative of extreme lateral disc protrusion.[13]

PALPATION AND PERCUSSION

Palpation of the lumbar spine in the midline usually elicits pain at the level of the symptomatic degenerative disc. It is not unusual to find tenderness laterally along the iliac crest, the iliolumbar ligament, and over the sacroiliac joint. In many instances, this tenderness does not reflect disease in these lateral areas but rather hyperesthesia from nerve root irritation. Occasionally, no tenderness is elicited with palpation of the lumbar spine in the erect position, and it would be necessary to have the patient flex his spine to apply pressure in the midline and then to direct him to extend his spine. This may produce marked pain in certain instances.

When spasm is present, palpation will reveal significant hardness in the contracted muscle mass. This will frequently be exquisitely tender on firm palpation. In less marked cases of paravertebral muscle spasm, palpation should not be directed over the muscle belly but should start in the midline with pressure exerted laterally in order to appreciate more subtle differences in muscle tone.

Palpation over the facet joints 1 to 3 cm. from the midline will frequently elicit tenderness, particularly in patients with symptomatic degenerative joint disease with or without symptoms of spinal stenosis. This tenderness is exaggerated on palpation with extension of the spine, which increases the lumbar lordosis.

Percussion of the lumbar spine may either elicit local pain or, more significantly, may reproduce sciatica when nerve root compression is present. As with many of the previously noted findings, it is suggestive but not pathognomonic of herniated discs.

Palpation should also be performed in the sciatic notch, along the course of the sciatic nerve itself. Hyperesthesia along the nerve is often found, and, in addition, local tumors of the nerve may be discovered in this manner.

The presence of tender motor points (Fig. 9–19) in the lower extremity is probably of diagnostic and prognostic importance. These tender motor points represent the main neuromuscular junction in the involved muscle groups, and they are reliably constant in their anatomic position from one patient to another. Diagnostically, Gunn and others[6] have found that all patients with signs and symptoms of a radiculopathy had tender motor points in the myotome corresponding to the probable segmental level of nerve root involvement.

Prognostically, in the absence of radicular signs, back pain patients with tender motor points remain disabled nearly three times as long as those patients without tenderness. If a radiculopathy is present with the back pain, the disability is nearly four times as long. Frequently, this tenderness, particularly when it is in the calf, has been misinterpreted as a thrombophlebitis.[6]

NEUROLOGIC EXAMINATION

A meticulous neurologic examination will yield objective evidence of nerve root compression. It will suggest the level of disc herniation, but it is not conclusive in this regard. The two most common levels of disc herniation are L4-5 and L5-S1. The L3-4 disc

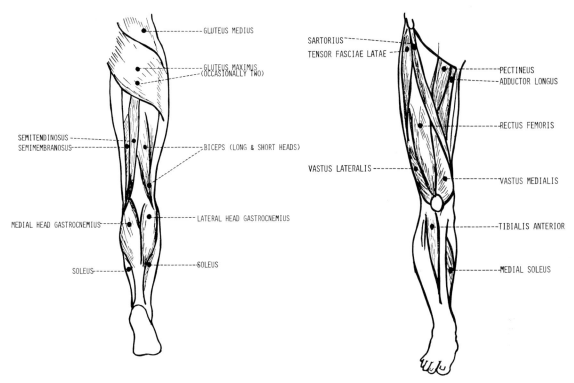

Figure 9–19. Motor points of the lower extremities. (From Gunn, C. C., Chir, B., and Milbrant, W. E.: Tenderness at motor points: A diagnostic and prognostic aid for low-back injury. J. Bone Joint Surg. (Am.) *58*:815, 1976.)

level is the next most common. Disc herniations at L5-S1 will usually compromise the first sacral nerve root. In a similar fashion, a disc herniation at L4-5 will most often compress the fifth lumbar root, while a herniation at L3-4 will more frequently involve the fourth lumbar root (Table 9–1). However, owing to variation in root configuration and the position of the herniation itself, disc herniation, particularly at L4-5, not only can affect the fifth lumbar nerve but also may involve the first sacral nerve. In extreme lateral herniations, the nerve exiting at the same level of the disc will be involved; that is, with an L4–5 disc herniation, the L4 nerve root would be compressed on its course out the neural foramen at that level. The pattern of neurologic involvement will be frequently more confusing when, in addition to a disc herniation, there is a superimposed facet arthritis with lateral encroachment of the foramina.

For this reason, it is the author's feeling that even though the neurologic picture is well defined, myelography should be performed to further localize the level of the lesion when surgery is indicated. If myelography cannot be performed, then exploration of at least L4-5

and L5-S1 is mandatory. This is particularly important in view of the fact that there may be a disc herniation at more than one level, although this would be most unusual.

TABLE 9–1. NERVE ROOT PATTERNS

L4 Nerve Root
 1. *Pain and numbness* — L4 dermatome, posterolateral aspect of thigh, across patella, anteromedial aspect of leg
 2. *Weakness and atrophy* — weak extension of knee and quadriceps muscle atrophy
 3. *Reflex* — depression of patellar reflex

L5 Nerve Root
 1. *Pain and numbness* — L5 dermatome, posterior aspect of thigh, anterolateral aspect of leg, medial aspect of foot and great toe
 2. *Weakness and atrophy* — weak dorsiflexion of foot and toes and atrophy of anterior compartment of leg
 3. *Reflex* — none, or absent posterior tibial tendon reflex

S1 Nerve Root
 1. *Pain and numbness* — S1 dermatome, posterior aspect of thigh, posterior aspect of leg, posterolateral aspect of foot, lateral toes
 2. *Weakness and atrophy* — weak plantar flexion of foot and toes and atrophy of posterior compartment of leg
 3. *Reflex* — depression of Achilles reflex

MOTOR FINDINGS

Compression of the motor fibers of the nerve root results in weakness or paralysis of the muscle group associated with loss of tone and loss of mass of the muscle belly. Usually, a group of muscles rather than a particular muscle is involved. The patient may not be aware of this weakness until the loss is rather profound. With compression of the first sacral nerve root, little motor involvement is noted other than an occasional weakness in flexion of the foot and great toe. With compromise of the fifth lumbar nerve root, weakness primarily of the great toe and other toe extensors and less often the evertors and dorsiflexors of the foot is noted with atrophy of the anterior and lateral compartment of the leg. With compression of the fourth lumbar nerve root, the quadriceps muscle is frequently affected, and the patient may note weakness of extension of the knee and more often instability of the knee. Atrophy is usually prominent.

One must keep in mind that motor weakness may be a manifestation of a metabolic peripheral neuropathy, such as diabetes. Clinically, the differentiation can be made since the paresis associated with compromise of the fifth lumbar nerve will frequently spare the tibialis anterior, whereas in the diabetic peroneal neuropathy, this muscle will usually be involved. Furthermore, the presence of a Trendelenburg sign due to gluteus medius denervation resulting from a fifth lumbar radiculopathy would not be present with a diabetic peroneal neuropathy.

SENSORY CHANGES

The pattern of sensory involvement when nerve root compression is present usually follows the dermatome of the affected nerve root. The sensory pattern of the thigh and buttocks is less specific than that in the leg and the foot. With compression of the fourth lumbar nerve root, sensory abnormalities may be noted in the anteromedial aspect of the leg. With compromise of the fifth lumbar nerve root, sensory abnormalities would be noted in the anterolateral portion of the leg and along the medial aspect of the foot to the great toe. S1 radiculopathy usually involves sensory abnormalities in the posterior aspect of the calf and lateral aspect of the foot.

REFLEX CHANGES

The deep tendon reflexes are frequently altered in nerve root compression syndromes. The Achilles reflex is diminished or absent with compression of the first sacral nerve root, although Hakelius[7] noted that the incidence of disc herniation among patients when the Achilles reflex was absent was higher than among those in whom this reflex was simply diminished. The compression of the fifth lumbar nerve root most commonly causes no reflex change, but on occasion a diminution in the posterior tibial reflex can be elicited. It is important to note, however, that the absence of this reflex must be asymmetrical to have any clinical significance. Involvement of the fourth lumbar nerve root classically results in a decrease or absence of a patellar tendon reflex; however, it is quite common to find an L4-5 disc herniation resulting in this patellar tendon abnormality.[7]

At the actual eliciting of the reflexes, it is suggested that several tendon taps should be performed in order to assess the true amplitude of a response. Frequently, one may actually be able to fatigue a reflex response when the involved reflex arc is compromised owing to disc herniation.

The reader should again be reminded that many etiologic factors other than disc herniation can produce abnormalities of the deep tendon reflexes. Indeed, on a statistical basis, absence of particularly the Achilles reflex is more often a concomitant of advanced age rather than of a radiculopathy.

STRAIGHT LEG RAISING TEST AND ITS VARIANTS

There are several maneuvers that tighten the sciatic nerve and in doing so further compress an inflamed nerve root against a herniated lumbar disc. An excellent comprehensive review of the so-called "tension signs" in lumbar disc prolapse has been presented by Scham and Taylor.[14] With the straight leg raising maneuver, the L5 and S1 nerve roots move 2 to 6 mm. at the level of the foramina. Whether this is a true sliding movement of the nerve or passive deformation of the nerve within the neural canal and foramina[3] is debatable. What is of importance, however, is that when the straight leg raising test is performed in a patient with a three-dimensionally compromised canal or foramen, the involved nerve is subject to a tensile or compressive force (or both) to which it cannot accommodate without producing radicular symptoms. The L4 nerve root moves a lesser distance, and the more proximal roots show little motion. Thus, the straight leg raising test is of most importance and value in lesions of the fifth lumbar and first sacral nerve roots.

Fahrni[5] has analyzed the dynamics of the straight leg raising test and has noted that tension is realized within the nerve roots contributing to the sciatic nerve at 35 to 70 degrees of elevation from the supine position. Since deformation after 70 degrees of elevation occurs in the sciatic nerve distal to the neural foramina, any radicular pain precipitated at this elevation should not be attributed to the sequela of degenerative disc disease (Fig. 9–20).

In a review of 2000 patients with operatively proved disc herniations, the straight leg raising sign was positive in 90 per cent. Younger patients were shown to have a marked propensity for straight leg raising test, although the test itself is not pathognomonic.[15] However, a negative test excludes with great probability the presence of a herniated disc. After the age of 30, the negative straight leg raising test no longer excludes this diagnosis (Fig. 9–21).

The straight leg raising test is performed with the patient supine with the head flat or on a low pillow. One of the examiner's hands is placed on the ilium to stabilize the pelvis, and the other hand slowly elevates the leg by the heel with the knee straight. The patient should be questioned as to whether this produces leg pain. Only when leg pain or radicular symptoms are produced is this test considered positive. Back pain alone is not a positive finding in this maneuver.

Many variations of this test have been described. The knee may first be flexed to 90 degrees and the hip then flexed to 90 degrees. Next, the knee is gradually extended. If this maneuver produces leg pain, the test is considered positive. Both this test and the straight leg raising test have been attributed to Lasègue. Fajersztajn[14] described a variation to the straight leg raising test in which the foot is dorsiflexed. This not only may produce an exacerbation of the pain in the straight leg raising test but also could reproduce radicular pain when the conventional straight leg raising test is negative.

Macnab[10] feels that the most reliable test of root tension is the bowstring sign, another manifestation of the straight leg raising test. The straight leg raising test is performed as usual until pain is elicited. At this point, however, the knee is flexed, and this will usually significantly reduce symptoms. Finger pressure is then applied to the popliteal space over the terminal aspect of the sciatic nerve, and this will reestablish the painful radicular symptoms.

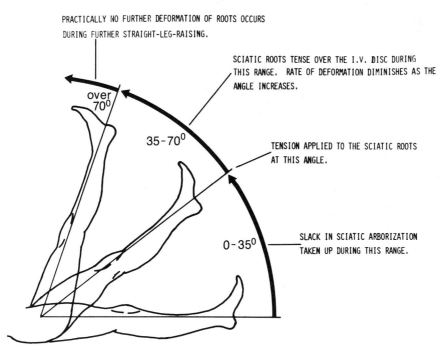

Figure 9–20 This figure illustrates the dynamics of the straight leg raising test. (Modified from Fahrni, W. H.: Observations on straight leg raising, with special reference to nerve root adhesions. Can. J. Surg. *9*:44, 1966.)

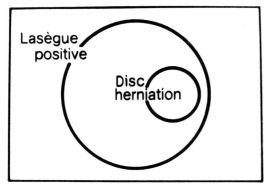

Age: under 30 years

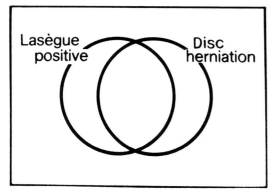

Age: over 30 years

Figure 9–21. These Venn diagrams illustrate the marked propensity for a positive Lasègue test with disc herniation in the young. Over the age of 30 the propensity decreases, although the specificity increases for this test in disc herniation. (From Spangfort, 1971.)

The sitting root test is yet another variation on this theme. With the patient sitting and the cervical spine flexed, the knee is extended while the hip remains flexed to 90 degrees. The patient may complain of leg pain or may attempt to extend his hip, again indicating nerve root tension.

Medial rotation of the hip joint can also apply tension to the sacral plexus in the supine posture. Troupe and Breig[16] reported that sciatic pain could be reproduced when medial hip rotation was performed at the pain-free limits of the straight leg raising test.

The contralateral straight leg raising test is performed in the same manner as the straight leg raising test, except that the non-painful leg is raised. If this produces the patient's sciatica in the opposite extremity, the test is considered positive. This is very suggestive of a herniated disc and also is an indication of the location of the extrusion.

Hudgins[8] reported that this sign was positive in 97 per cent of patients with surgically confirmed disc herniations. The prolapse will often be large but not in the usual lateral pattern. At surgery the disc will be noted usually medial to the nerve root in the axilla (Fig. 9–22).

It should be noted that when the roots of the femoral nerve are involved, they are tensed not by the straight leg raising test but by the reverse straight leg raising test, that is, by hip extension and knee flexion. This is usually performed while the patient is prone or laterally with the unaffected side down. As with the straight leg raising test, there is a contralateral femoral traction sign.[4]

PERIPHERAL VASCULAR EXAMINATION

No examination of a patient with back or leg pain can be considered complete without evaluation of the peripheral circulation. Examination of the posterior tibial and dorsalis pedis arteries should be performed, as well as an examination of the skin temperature and inspection for the presence of atrophic changes seen with ischemic disease.

In addition to the peripheral vascular examination, several other clinical findings as well as the history will usually help differentiate vascular claudication from intermittent neurogenic claudication. In the unusual case in which the patient's history and physical findings could be compatible with both types of claudication, quantitative studies of the arterial system and consultation with a vascular surgeon would then be indicated.

HIP JOINT EXAMINATION

One can usually differentiate intra-articular hip disease from symptomatic degenerative disc disease. Limitation of range of motion of the hip, particularly in rotation, along with groin discomfort, is most indicative of hip disease. Furthermore, with examination of the hip, coincident hip flexion and knee extension should not elicit any tension signs implicating nerve root tension.

It is of interest, however, that Magora[11] did find evidence of degenerative hip disease in 10 per cent of approximately 400 patients suffering from low back pain.

The piriformis muscle in external hip rotation has been implicated as a positive cause of sciatica-like symptoms.[9,12] This muscle runs in close proximity to the sciatic nerve, and any

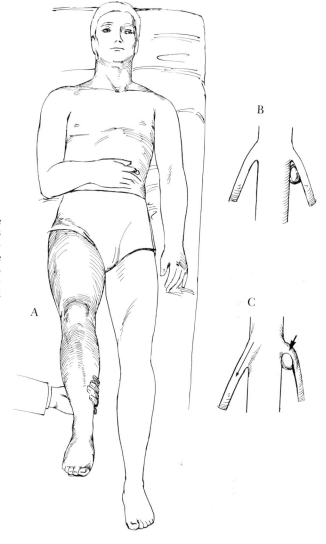

Figure 9–22. Movement of nerve roots when the leg on the opposite side is raised. *A*, When the leg is raised on the unaffected side the roots on the opposite side slide slightly downward and toward the midline. *B*, In the presence of a disc lesion, this movement increases the root tension. (From DePalma, A. F., and Rothman, R. H.: The Intervertebral Disc. Philadelphia, W. B. Saunders Co., 1970.)

injury to the muscle, particularly if it is anomalously bifurcated and surrounding the sciatic nerve, could precipitate local pain over the sciatic notch, as well as irritation along the course of the nerve. Tenderness over the piriformis muscle on rectal or vaginal examination, along with local and referred pain with weakness when the hip is abducted and externally rotated against resistance, is most suggestive of this syndrome. Bimanual injection of the muscle has yielded very satisfactory results.

ABDOMINAL AND RECTAL EXAMINATION

Many intra-abdominal and retroperitoneal abnormalities can result in back and leg pain. Careful palpation of the abdomen, together with rectal examination and pelvic examination, will disclose many of these lesions and will lead to a correct diagnosis.

References

1. Abudllah, A. F., Ditto, E. W., Byrd, E. B., and Williams, R.: Extreme lateral disc herniations. J. Neurosurg. *41*:229–234, 1974.
2. Boulos, S.: Herniated intervertebral lumbar disc in the teenager. J. Bone Joint Surg. *55B*(2):273–278, 1973.
3. Breig, A., and Marions, O.: Biomechanics of the lumbosacral nerve roots. Acta Radiol. *1*:1141, 1963.
4. Dyck, P.: The femoral nerve traction test with lumbar disc protrusions. Surg. Neurol. *6*:163, 1976.

5. Fahrni, W. H.: Observations on straight leg raising with special reference to nerve root adhesions. Can. J. Surg. 9:44–48, 1970.

6. Gunn, C. C., Chir, B., and Milbrand, W. E.: Tenderness at motor points: A diagnostic and prognostic aid to low back injury. J. Bone Joint Surg. 58A:815–825, 1976.

7. Hakelius, A., and Hindmarsh, J.: The significance of neurological signs and myelography findings in the diagnosis of lumbar root compression. Acta Orthop. Scand. 43:234–238, 1972.

8. Hudgins, W. R.: The crossed straight leg raising test. N. Engl. J. Med. 297:1127, 1977.

9. Kirkaldy-Willis, W. H., and Hill, R. J.: A more precise diagnosis for low back pain. Spine 4(2):102–109, 1979.

10. Macnab, I.: Backache. Baltimore, Williams and Wilkins Co., 1977.

11. Magora, A.: Investigation of the relation between low back pain and occupation. VII. Neurologic and orthopaedic condition. Scand. J. Rehabil. Med. 7:141–151, 1975.

12. Pace, J. B., and Neagle, D.: Piriformis syndrome. West J. Med. 124:435–439, 1976.

13. Patrick, B. S.: Extreme lateral ruptures of lumbar intervertebral discs. Surg. Neurol. 3:301–304, 1975.

14. Scham, S., and Taylor, T.: Tension signs in lumbar disc prolapse. Clin. Orthop. 44:163–170, 1966.

15. Spangfort, E.: Lasègue's sign in patients with lumbar disc herniation. Acta Orthop. 42:459, 1971.

16. Troupe, J. D. G., and Breig, A.: The effect of medial hip rotation on the sacral plexus and its significance in the straight leg raising test. Proceedings of the fifth annual meeting of the International Society for the Study of the Lumbar Spine. San Francisco, 1978.

Diagnostic Studies

ROUTINE RADIOGRAPHY

Radiographic examination of the lumbar spine is considered an integral part of the examination of the patient with low back pain. It should be emphasized, however, that the radiographic examination is only one facet of the total picture and that the treating physician should not allow his judgment to be superseded by the radiographic findings. Indeed, degenerative changes involving the facet joints or the vertebral body–intervertebral disc complex cannot definitively be approached as either causative of low back pain syndrome[74, 101] or predictive as to the development of low lumbar complaints.[64] In cases of degenerative spondylolisthesis, which is an advanced manifestation of both disc degeneration and degenerative subluxation of the zygoapophyseal joints, many patients are essentially symptom free.[31] Conversely, in young patients, a marked disc prolapse with incapacitating pain may be present with a completely normal radiograph.

The radiograph must be of excellent quality and must be taken with great attention to detail. It should routinely include anteroposterior, lateral, and oblique views. Special views will be necessary if visualization of the sacroiliac joints is indicated.

Thinning or loss of height of the disc space is frequently seen in disc degeneration. DePalma and Rothman found that in operatively proved disc degeneration at L5-S1 there was radiographic evidence of disc space narrowing in 41 per cent of cases. In disc degeneration at L4-5, radiographic evidence of disc space narrowing is found in 19 per cent of cases.[18] It should be emphasized that thinning of the disc space, while an indication of disc degeneration, may be noted at levels other than that producing the symptomatology and may not be present at all. It should also be recalled that narrowing of the disc space is not unique to disc degeneration but may also occur in metabolic and infectious diseases of the intervertebral disc. It is also frequently seen below a transitional lumbosacral vertebra.

With increasing age, one finds a greater incidence of degenerative changes in the lumbar motion segments,[64, 73, 101] exemplified by decreased vertebral height and increased vertebral width,[27, 28] sclerosis of the subchondral bone, and formation of peripheral osteophytes with disc degeneration[53] (Fig. 9–23). Again, bone spurs are not pathognomonic of disc degeneration but must be differentiated from other conditions, such as Reiter's syndrome, ankylosing spondylitis,[22] and ankylosing hyperostosis of the spine.[14] Osteophytes are usually more prominent anterolaterally than posterolaterally, and their phenomenon is most likely due to the nature of the anulus and ligamentous attachments to the body of the vertebrae above and below the degenerative disc space.[105] Macnab has described a unique osteophyte (Figs. 9–24 and 9–25) found 2 to 3 mm. from the disc space, which he terms the "traction spur." This is thought to arise from stress at the site of ligamentous insertion during the hypermobile phase of disc degeneration.[72]

The sclerosis seen adjacent to the end plate of the vertebrae may be thin, a diffuse zone, or it may be localized anteriorly or posteriorly. Occasionally, a considerable por-

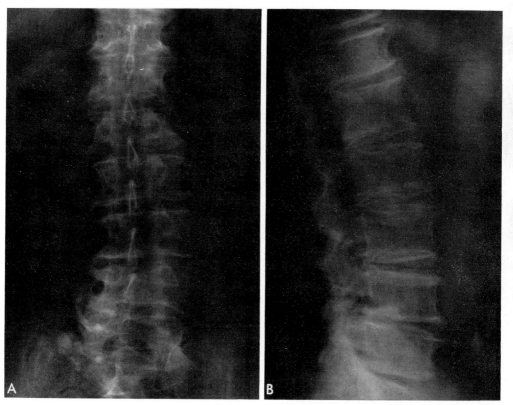

Figure 9–23. Radiographs of the lumbar spine illustrate advanced multilevel disc degeneration with loss of height of the disc space, marked osteophyte formation and sclerosis of the end plates. Foraminal encroachment is present.

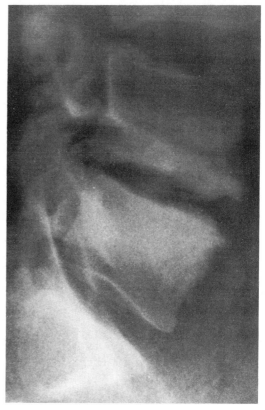

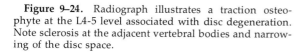

Figure 9–24. Radiograph illustrates a traction osteophyte at the L4-5 level associated with disc degeneration. Note sclerosis at the adjacent vertebral bodies and narrowing of the disc space.

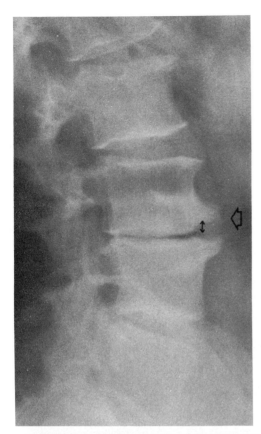

Figure 9–25. Radiograph illustrates traction osteophyte at the L3-4 level. Note that the osteophyte is horizontally oriented and 2 mm away from the disc space. Note the marked narrowing of the disc space and the vacuum phenomena at L3-4.

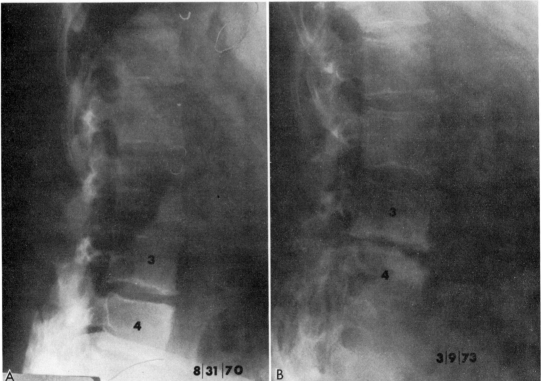

Figure 9–26. Radiographs illustrate the development of disc degeneration at the L3-L4 disc space over a period of three years. Note the loss of height of the disc space, osteophyte formation and sclerosis of the end plates. In this instance the radiographic appearance was suggestive of infection, and biopsy was performed but revealed only evidence of chronic disc degeneration. At times the sclerosis can be so marked as to simulate a neoplasm of the vertebral body.

tion of the vertebrae will be involved, and this can simulate a neoplastic or infectious process (Fig. 9–26).

Disc herniations may occur directly into the body of the vertebra (Schmorl's nodes) and are most commonly seen in the upper lumbar and lower thoracic areas, with frequency varying as a function of investigative techniques used.[83] They most often occur in the central and posterocentral portion of the body, surrounded by sclerotic bone. The herniation in all likelihood follows notochordal residual channels, vascular residual channels, or both types in the cartilaginous vertebral end plate. A limbus vertebra is also described[41, 90] as an anterosuperior herniation, which results in a triangular segment of vertebra separated from the parent bone by the displaced nucleus pulposus. A relative weakness at the interface of the vertebral body and cartilaginous end plate may predispose to this type of herniation. While there is no correlation between

this type of pathologic condition and posterior herniations causing spinal nerve encroachment, an association with disc disease has been suggested.[57]

One must also include in the differential diagnosis pathologic states such as trauma, infection, congenital defects, or metabolic disease that may weaken the cartilaginous end plate or the vertebral body itself and may precipitate an intervertebral herniation.[83]

During the course of disc degeneration, derangements may occur in the alignment of the vertebrae and their motion. A particular motion unit, that is, the disc and its two adjacent vertebrae, will often go through a hypermobile phase early in the course of disc degeneration and at a later state will achieve a hypomobile phase with focal suppression of motion. There is a wide variation of this tendency, but the end point roentgenographic appearance is referred to as a Type III or degenerative spondylolisthesis (Figs. 9–27 and

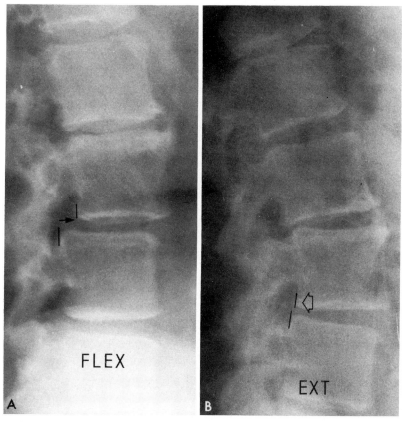

Figure 9–27. Radiographs illustrate segmental instability due to disc degeneration on flexion and extension views. *A*, Note that in flexion there is a 3.5 mm anterior migration of the cranial vertebra. *B*, In extension there is almost complete realignment of the vertebral body. This was productive of both back pain and sciatica.

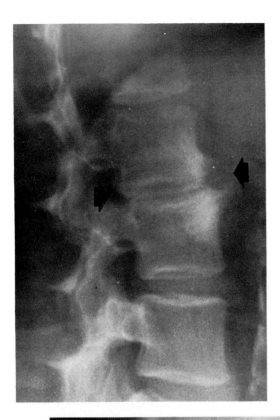

Figure 9–28. Radiograph illustrates marked disc degeneration at the L3-4 level. There is associated loss of height of the disc space, sclerosis of the adjacent vertebral body, osteophyte formation, and a 2 mm retrospondylolisthesis.

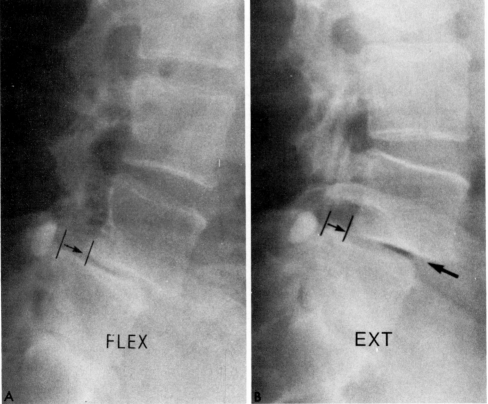

FLEX

EXT

A

B

Figure 9–29. Radiographs illustrate segmental instability at L4-5 secondary to disc degeneration. This is also termed degenerative spondylolisthesis. *A*, Note that in flexion there is a 5 mm anterior migration of L4 relative to L5. *B*, In extension there is only partial reduction of this subluxation together with production of a vacuum phenomenon at the affected level.

542

9–28). The tendency toward anterior migration (pseudospondylolisthesis) or posterior migration (pseudoretrospondylolisthesis) of one vertebral body over the subjacent vertebra is a function of the total force vector acting differently on separate motion units. The degree and direction of the olisthesis depends on the amount of degenerative disease present, inherent soft tissue stability present, and the segment of the lordotic lumbar curve involved.

Allbrook,[6] Farfan and colleagues,[30] and Fitzgerald and Newman[31] all emphasize the importance of the iliotransverse ligament in inhibiting olisthesis by acting as a guidewire in the lower vertebral segments. They furthermore have demonstrated that a deep-seated lumbar spine within the confines of the iliac wings will tend to put the L4-5 motion segment under increased stress and will contribute to the greater incidence of degenerative olisthesis generally found at that level (Fig. 9–29).

The hallmark of this phenomenon, however, is degeneration of the disc with slow insidious degeneration and subluxation of the facet joints, referred to as the "articular bolt" by Taillard.[99] These changes in alignment may produce significant symptoms of radiculopathy or intermittent neurogenic claudication, particularly in a congenitally narrow spinal canal. If this occurs at L3-4 or L4-5, one will not uncommonly see a complete myelographic block due to the phenomenon, even though the olisthesis will minimally range from a few millimeters to 1 to 1.5 cm. or up to 33 per cent with an average of a 17 per cent slip[31, 99] (Figs. 9–30 to 9–33).

Encroachment of the intervertebral foramina occurs, but it should be realized that the spatial relationships are such that more leeway is present for the nerve root or the spinal nerve in the lumbar foramina than in the cervical area. The dynamic compromise of the foramina with lordosis increased in extension, posterior osteophytes, hypertrophy of cap-

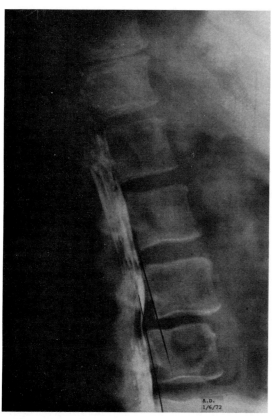

Figure 9–30 Flexion view of the lumbar spine reveals marked anterior migration of L3 on L4 secondary to disc degeneration. This is termed degenerative spondylolisthesis or pseudospondylolisthesis.

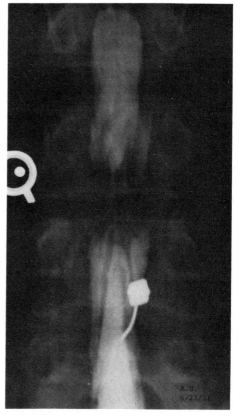

Figure 9–31. Myelogram reveals a complete block at the level of L3-L4 secondary to the pseudospondylolisthesis seen in Figure 9–30.

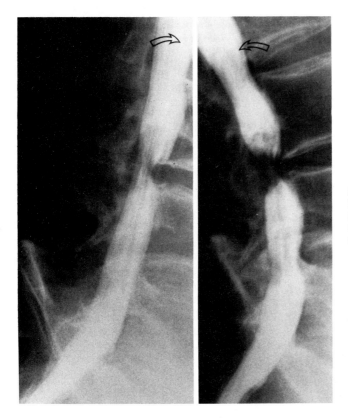

Figure 9–32. Metrizamide myelogram with flexion-extension lateral views reveals a partial block in flexion and a complete block in extension. Patient became markedly paretic in extension. This illustrates classic spinal stenosis secondary to disc degeneration.

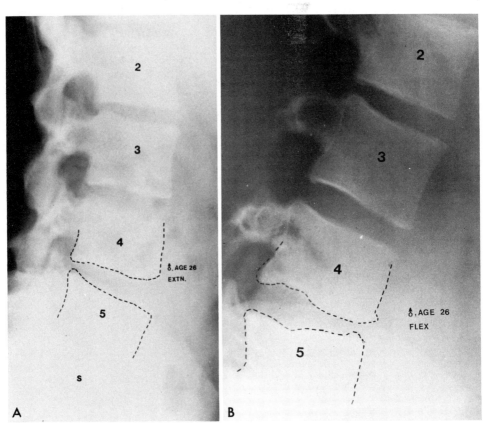

Figure 9–33. Radiographs illustrate segmental instability due to disc degeneration. *A*, Extension view and *B*, flexion view illustrate excessive angular motion indicative of the segmental instability.

sular ligaments, subluxation of the facets, and narrowing of the disc space with approximation of the pedicle will jointly compromise exiting spinal nerves and the theca. The spinal nerve rests in the uppermost portion of the foramina, usually well above the disc space, but the tip of the superior facet may impinge the spinal nerve as it subluxes in a cranial direction. In the presence of concomitant olisthesis, the foraminal compromise is increased.

Calcification of the nucleus does not occur often in lumbar disc degeneration, but it may be noted in the anulus fibrosus. In a postmortem study of human spines, Ratheke[82] found this type of calcification present in 71 per cent of spines examined. Magnussen[73] first called attention to the so-called "vacuum phenomenon" as a sign of disc degeneration. The vacuum phenomenon, accentuated in extension and diminished or eliminated in flexion of the spine, allows the free diffusion primarily of nitrogen from the extracellular fluid into nuclear recesses of the degenerative disc[32] (Fig. 9–34).

As previously noted, these stigmata of disc degeneration are seen in a very large percentage of the population, many of whom have no symptoms referable to the lumbar spine. For this reason, significance should be attached to their presence only when symptoms are present, and they should be carefully correlated with history and physical examination.

MYELOGRAPHY

GENERAL CONCEPTS. A carefully performed myelogram is an invaluable aid in the surgical treatment of lumbar disc disease, and the authors feel that this study should be performed in most instances before surgical intervention is undertaken. The rationale for performing myelography is that it will yield the following advantages:

1. Demonstration of tumors of the spinal cord that may clinically mimic symptomatic disc disease. Several striking examples have been seen in which the history and neurologic findings are characteristic of a herniated lumbar disc at the L4 or L5 level, and yet to the surprise of the treating surgeon, a myelogram revealed a tumor of the lower thoracic or upper lumbar spine. While the demonstration of a disc herniation occurring simultaneously with an intradural or intramedullary tumor is rare, this possibility remains. The authors also feel that in addition to myelography, CSF protein analysis should be performed at the time of lumbar puncture. Indeed, an abnormal myelogram that may be consistent with an intradural or epidural defect when combined with a markedly elevated CSF protein may help steer the wary surgeon away from inappropriate surgery and unsatisfactory results.[107]

2. A second advantage of routine myelography is the more exact localization of disc herniation and spinal nerve compromise. Edgar and Park[29] proposed a dual coordinate approach to symptomatic lumbar disc disease. Although they could accurately predict the horizontal location (either central, posterolateral or lateral) of a disc herniation, in 80 per cent of cases in this prospective study with straight leg raising, the vertical coordinate or level was identified without the use of myelography only 50 per cent of the time. Hakelius and Hindmarsh[50] found a comparable 46 per cent accuracy rate as to the involved level prediction on the basis of neurologic findings alone. Indeed, a variation in the nerve root configuration, that is, nerve root anomalies, and the location of the extrusions can lead to erroneous decisions if a neurologic deficit

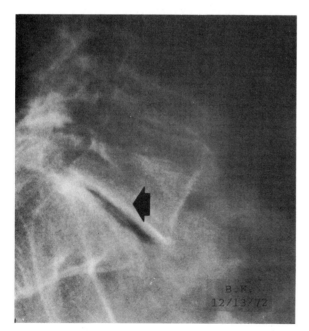

Figure 9–34. Radiograph illustrates the vacuum phenomenon at the L5-S1 disc space due to release of dissolved gas during extension stress on the spine.

alone is considered. An axillary or central protrusion at the L4-L5 level may well cause an S1 spinal nerve syndrome usually characteristic of an L5-S1 protrusion. Conversely, a very lateral L4 herniation or a central herniation with cranial migration of the fragment may well cause an L4 spinal nerve syndrome rather than the expected L5 syndrome. Double disc herniations (those at more than one level) can result in a confusing neurologic picture that may not be clarified and appropriately treated without myelographic definition.

A literature review[35] revealed an overall myelographic accuracy of 85 per cent. The shortcomings of this study were more often in sensitivity (false negative) than in specificity (false positive).[35, 71, 76] Improved accuracy of myelography is seen with the newer water-soluble dyes (see following section). Even the more viscous Pantopaque should obviate the need for multiple level explorations if used in the proper clinical setting.

It should be emphasized that neural and anatomic definition afforded by myelography can be completely realized only by proper technique and a complete series of exposures that include anteroposterior, oblique, and standing and prone lateral views. Flexion and extension films may also increase the yield, particularly when symptoms are dynamically exaggerated.

WATER-SOLUBLE VS. OIL LUMBAR MYELOGRAPHY

While oil myelography has traditionally been used in this country, recent FDA approval of the water-soluble agent metrizamide has made this contrast material the preferred agent for lumbar spine studies. Radiopaque water-soluble contrast media have been used extensively in arteriography and intravenous pyelography and in a variety of radiologic tests in order to visualize internal organs. These substances, when injected into the subarachnoid space, are absorbed in a few hours.[47] In light of the well-established relationship between symptomatic arachnoiditis and oil-base myelography, particularly when associated with surgical intervention,[98] efforts were made to develop a less toxic contrast medium. A variety of water-soluble media were used during the 1940s and 1950s, but all were too toxic for human investigation. Contact with the spinal cord or nerve roots in-

duced permanent damage, and extreme pain was also associated with their use.

In 1969 Ahlgren[2] reported the use of meglumine iothalamate (Conray) for lumbar radiculopathy. This agent was considered safe in contact with lumbar nerve roots, and in comparison with the other water-soluble contrast material was sufficiently nonirritating. In 1970, Ahlgren and Baumgartner reported on the use of meglumine iocarmate (Dimer X), the synthesized dimer of meglumine iothalamate — an agent developed to avoid the use of spinal anesthesia (previously required with water-soluble contrast agents) in lumbar radiculography.[3, 10] This substance was produced in order to achieve a less toxic agent by the conjugation of two molecules of meglumine iothalamate. In 1971, Skalpe[95] indicated that no serious complications were observed in a series of 100 lumbar radiculograms. He indicated that although 8 per cent of the patients in this series had chronic spasms of the lower extremities after radiculography, the spasms were less severe though not less frequent than those who had undergone meglumine iothalamate radiculography.

Metrizamide, a water-soluble tri-ionate contrast medium (Amopaque) was developed in Norway to overcome shortcomings of the previously used water-soluble dyes. Unlike other water-soluble dyes, metrizamide is nonionic and does not dissociate and therefore provides lower osmolality when in solution. While it is slightly hyperbaric, its isotonicity (when used with a suggested iodine concentration of 170 mg. per ml.) has been suggested as the reason for its fewer adverse affects and in particular for less arachnoiditis.[48, 85] To date, there have been no radiographically proved cases of arachnoiditis from the use of metrizamide.

Our experience as to patient tolerance of the dye has been excellent, although headaches and nausea and vomiting are frequent.[9, 13] Most recently, however, these adverse effects have been diminished when special attention is given to hydration of the patient per intravenous route prior to the study.

In addition to the acceptable level of short-term and long-term adverse signs and symptoms associated with metrizamide, this contrast material has provided a more facile technique of myelography and better resolution of the theca and the spinal nerves than are appreciated with oil contrast media.

Owing to the absorption of the metrizamide through the lumbar theca and primarily through the parasagittal arachnoid villi over the brain, the dye does not require removal. Therefore, the most time-consuming and uncomfortable part of the oil myelographic procedure is avoided.

The fully miscible metrizamide provides an excellent delineation of each spinal nerve subarachnoid extension out into the neural foramina as well as of the entire cauda equina stemming from the easily identifiable conus. Even subtle changes in the dimension or shape of a spinal nerve may be of significance if they fit the clinical presentation. Dynamic studies and supine filming are obviously easier since the spinal needle can be removed after dye injection because dye removal is obviated with this contrast medium.

Owing to its slow absorption rate (approximately 1 ml. per year), the authors still use oil-soluble contrast medium with steroid preparation for patients with definitely confirmed iodine allergies. Furthermore, in cases in which prolonged lower thoracic exposures are required or in cases in which an acute cauda equina syndrome develops, oil contrast myelography is still preferred.

ABNORMAL PATTERNS OF MYELOGRAPHY

Various patterns of myelographic abnormalities are noted, depending on the size and location of the protrusion as well as the contrast material used. Soft disc herniations will yield a pattern much different from the defects noted with chronic disc degeneration and osteophyte formation (spinal stenosis).

POSTEROLATERAL DISC HERNIATIONS. Defects most often noted with posterolateral disc herniations are incomplete filling or elevation of the spinal nerve sleeve, lateral indentation of the dural sac, and the double density of the sac noted in the lateral view. A large lateral herniation may also produce a complete myelographic block at the level of the disc space. Elevation of the nerve sleeve may be the only abnormality noted in the lateral disc protrusion, but it is the least reliable of the findings. This is particularly true in oil myelography, since the viscoid material may occasionally fail to completely fill the normal nerve sleeve. Owing to better radicular definition with metrizamide, subtle changes in the contour or location of the spinal nerve are more meaningful, particularly if there is asymmetrical proximal swelling of the nerve within the central dye column. Indentation of the dural sac seen in the AP or oblique views and the double density seen in the lateral view with either contrast medium are more convincing findings (Figs. 9–35 to 9–38).

CENTRAL HERNIATIONS. Large central disc herniations will often produce a characteristic complete myelographic block. The block will occur at the level of the disc space and in the anteroposterior view will show an irregular sawtooth or paintbrush appearance. The lateral view will show the anterior portion of the dural sac being compressed and elevated owing to ventral pressure from the disc herniation. Wasting defects are commonly noticed with small central discs as the origins of the nerve sleeves are forced laterally, preventing the dye from filling this area. More often than not, however, such "wasp waisting" defects are more compatible with roentgenographic spinal stenosis with or without contributing disc herniation (Figs. 9–39 and 9–40).

FREE FRAGMENTS. Free fragments of disc material may migrate in either a caudal or cranial direction and will be seen as well-circumscribed masses of varying diameters at a distance from the disc space (Figs. 9–41 and 9–42).

CHRONIC DISC DEGENERATION. Chronic disc degeneration will frequently be associated with spinal stenosis. Chronic disc degeneration will often produce myelographic defects due to diffuse posterior bulging of the anulus and osteophyte formation. In the anteroposterior views a symmetrical wasting of the dye column will be noted owing to obliteration of the lateral recess. In the lateral views the indentation of the dye column at the level of the disc space will be noted. If no osteophytes are present, this will usually be 2 to 3 mm. in height, or if osteophytes are present, they are easily seen and coincide with the defect in the dye column (Figs. 9–43 to 9–49).

ARTIFACTS

Many artifacts present in myelography can create defects not truly representative of disc degeneration. The defect created by the spinal needle can vary tremendously in size

Text continued on page 557

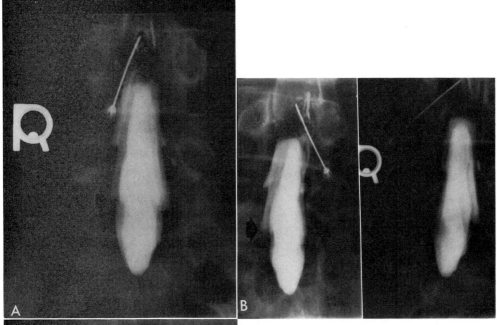

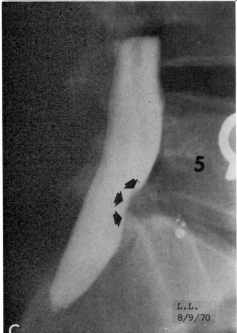

Figure 9–35. *A*, View of a lumbar oil myelogram reveals the typical defect from a lateral disc herniation. There is shortening and elevation of the S1 nerve root on the right. *B*, Oblique view again reveals shortening and elevation of the S1 root sleeve with displacement of dye along the swollen and edematous nerve root. There is also indentation of the dural sac. *C*, Lateral view reveals a ventral indentation of the dye column due to a disc herniation.

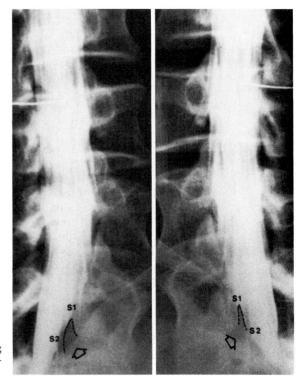

Figure 9–36. Metrizamide myelogram illustrating asymmetry of the S1 spinal nerve due to axillary herniation at L5-S1 on the left.

548

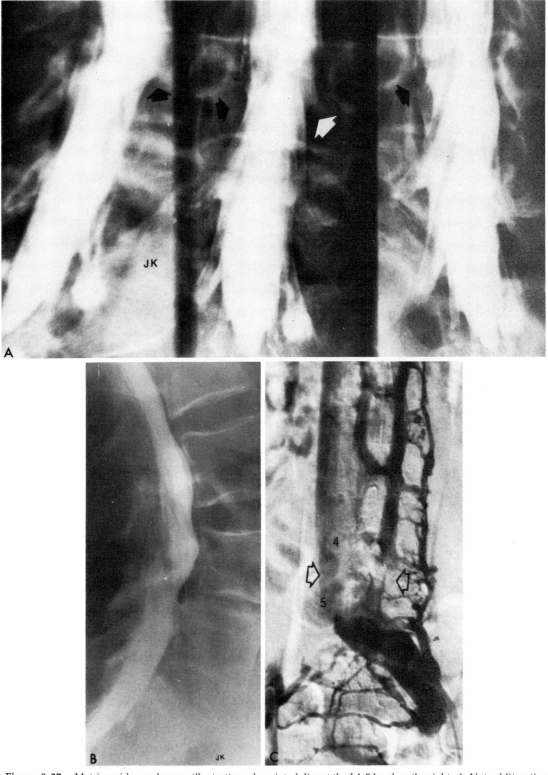

Figure 9–37. Metrizamide myelogram illustrating a herniated disc at the L4-5 level on the right. *A*, Note obliteration of the nerve root sleeve and indentation of the dural sac. *B*, Lateral view illustrates ventral indentation of the dural sac. *C*, Epidural venogram reveals occlusion of the anterior internal vertebral vein and radicular vein at the L4-5 level on the right.

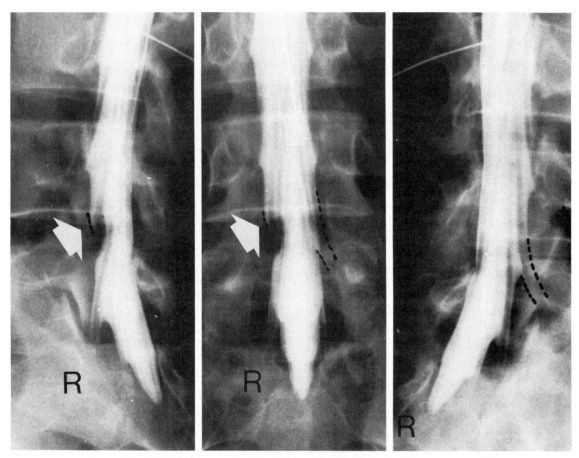

Figure 9–38.   Metrizamide myelogram illustrating a herniated disc at L4-5 on the right.
Note amputation of the nerve root sleeve and indentation of the dural sac.

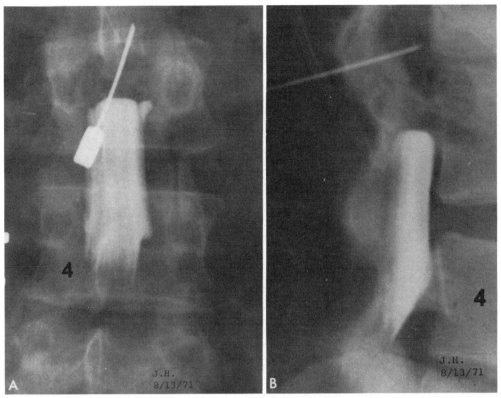

Figure 9–39. *A*, This oil myelogram illustrates a large central disc herniation. The anterior-posterior view reveals a complete block at the L4-L5 level, with an irregular sawtooth or paintbrush appearance characteristic of the block defect produced by disc herniation. *B*, Lateral view of the same patient reveals characteristic block pattern due to disc herniation with ventral pressure on the dye column producing a complete block at the level of the large central disc herniation.

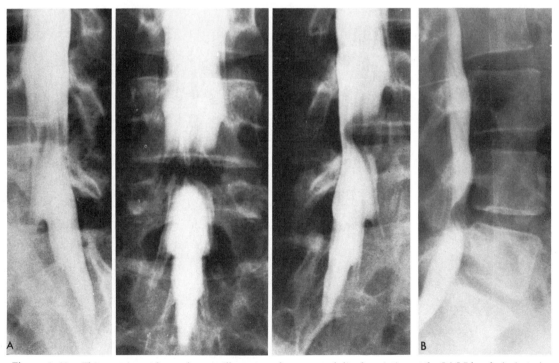

Figure 9–40. This metrizamide myelogram illustrates a large central disc herniation at the L4-L5 level. *A*, Anterior-posterior and oblique views reveal this prominent defect more marked on the right. *B*, This lateral view illustrates a "double density" prominent ventral indentation of the dye column.

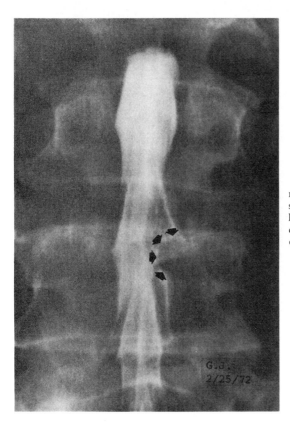

Figure 9–41. Free fragments of disc material produce a myelographic defect characterized by smooth, well circumscribed indentations in the dye column. They may be at the level of the disc space or migrate at a distance. They may be difficult to differentiate from neurofibromata. Oil was the contrast medium in this illustration.

Figure 9–42. Metrizamide myelogram illustrates a disc herniation with cephalic migration of a free fragment anterior to the mid-portion of the body of L3 on the left. Note swelling of the L3 root and absence of the L4 root. The patient had marked quadriceps atrophy and absence of patellar reflex.

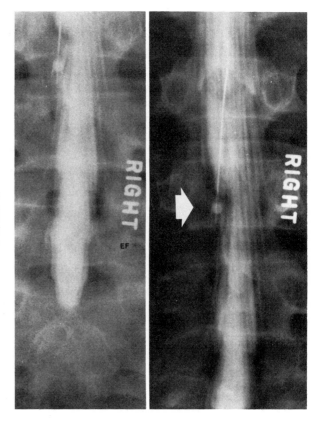

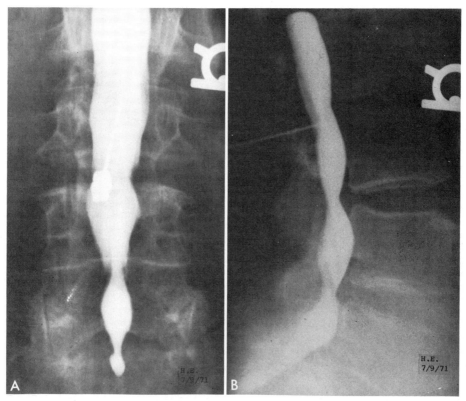

Figure 9–43. Oil myelograms show the characteristic appearance of chronic disc degeneration and spinal stenosis with diffuse posterior bulging of the anulus and osteophyte formation. There is symmetrical wasting of the dye column in the A-P view. The lateral view will show indentation of the dye column by the anulus anteriorly and the buckled ligamentum flavum and facet joints posteriorly.

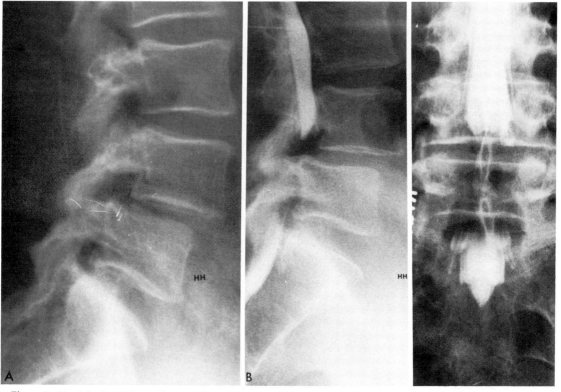

Figure 9–44, Metrizamide myelogram shows stenotic block at the L4-5 level due to degenerative spondylolisthesis and spinal stenosis at the L4-5 level. *A*, Note the 4 mm. anterior migration of L4 on L5 due to the degenerative spondylolisthesis. *B*, Note the extensive block on the metrizamide myelogram due to this spinal stenosis.

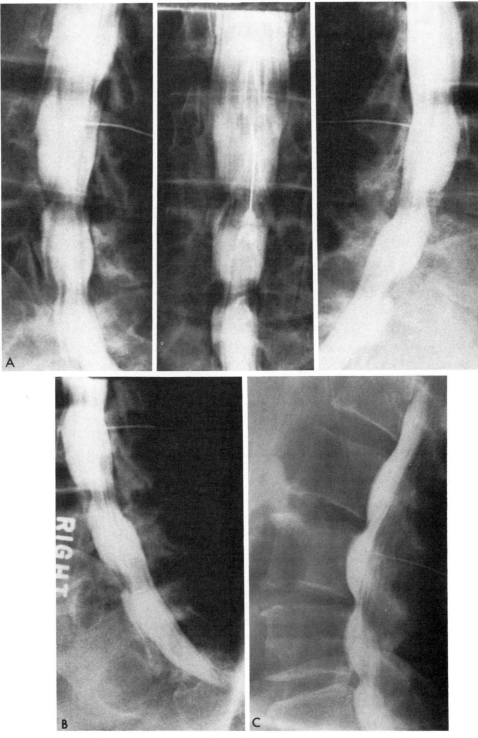

Figure 9–45. Metrizamide myelogram reveals this multiple-level spinal stenosis secondary to disc degeneration. *A* and *B*, The anterior-posterior and oblique views reveal the multiple wasting defects typical of spinal stenosis. *C*, Lateral view illustrates multiple ventral defects due to diffuse bulging at the anulus.

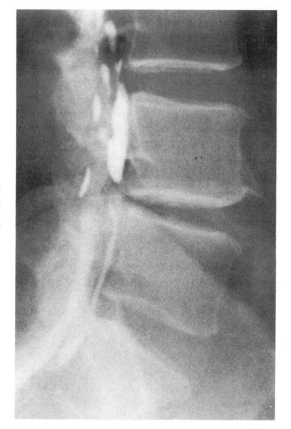

Figure 9–46. This oil myelogram reveals a complete block at the L4-5 level on the lateral view due to spinal stenosis. Note the traction osteophyte anteriorly associated with narrowing of the disc space and enlargement of the facet joints. The block is at the level of the disc space.

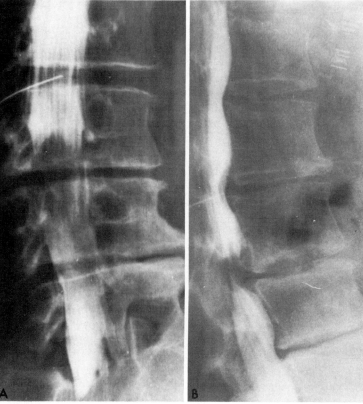

Figure 9–47. Metrizamide myelogram reveals a complete block at the L3-4 level due to spinal stenosis. *A*, In the anterior-posterior view note the block centered at the disc space with a paintbrush appearance. *B*, In the lateral view note that the compression is both anterior and posterior, is extradural in appearance, and is centered at the level of the disc space.

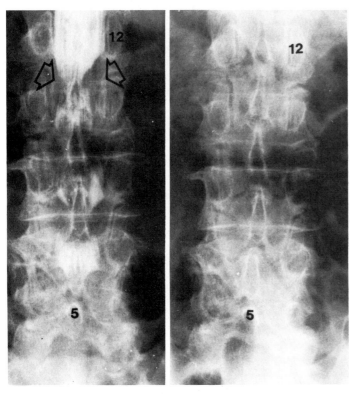

Figure 9–48. This metrizamide myelogram illustrates severe spinal stenosis from L1 to the sacrum. Note the enlarged facet joints, narrowing of the anterior laminar spaces, and tapering of the dye column at T12-L1.

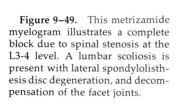

Figure 9–49. This metrizamide myelogram illustrates a complete block due to spinal stenosis at the L3-4 level. A lumbar scoliosis is present with lateral spondylolisthesis disc degeneration, and decompensation of the facet joints.

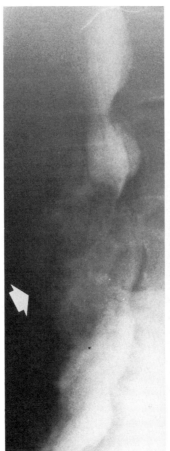

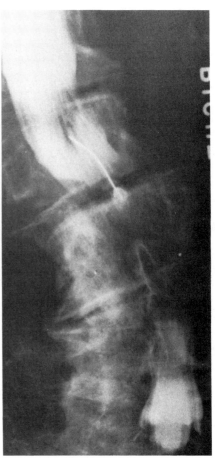

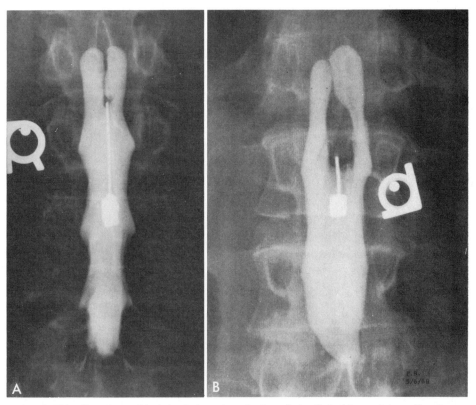

Figure 9–50. *A*, This oil myelographic defect is from the spinal needle itself. In this case it is small and symmetrical. *B*, A more dramatic needle defect which is larger and less symmetrical.

and occasionally is so dramatic as to mimic a space-occupying lesion (Fig. 9–50). An epidural hematoma resulting from a spinal needle advanced too far anteriorly can likewise produce a defect compatible with an epidural mass (Fig. 9–51). For this reason, the spinal puncture should be performed at a level well away from the expected site of disc herniation. The usual site of injection is the L2-3 level unless a high lumbar disc is suspected.

Artifacts are also commonly seen with previous oil contrast media myelography, particularly in the presence of previous surgery. Picard and others[79] reviewed 1950 studies and demonstrated an incidence of "scarring" in 14 per cent of patients not treated surgically and in 47 per cent of those subjected to operative intervention. The preference for the descriptive term "scarring" versus the anatomic terms of arachnoiditis and epiduritis avoids confusion and controversy (Fig. 9–52). Although epidural lesions without previous surgery are rarer, the myriad of possible artifacts in postsurgical patients from previous myelograms is extensive and can very easily obscure or mimic new pathologic conditions.

In conclusion, although it is appreciated that myelography is approximately 90 per cent

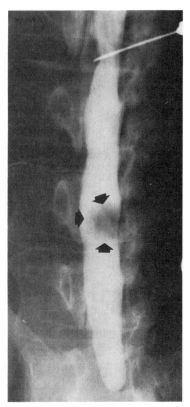

Figure 9–51. This myelographic defect represents a small extradural hematoma produced from a previous puncture.

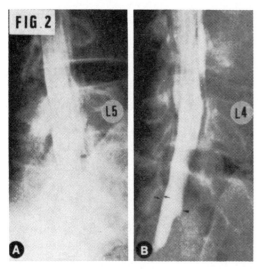

Figure 9–52. Various stages of arachnoid scarring. *A,* As arachnoiditis affects and eventually obliterates the root sleeves. *B,* Various stages of arachnoiditis as it affects the thecal sac. (From Picard, L., Roland, J., Blanchot, P., et al.: Scarring of the theca and the nerve roots as seen at radiculography. J. Neuroradiol. 41(1):29, 1977.)

accurate with both false positive and false negative results, it still remains extremely helpful and essential as a diagnostic tool in the preoperative evaluation of the patient with a suspected herniated disc. It should not be used in patients who are not surgical candidates in order to substantiate or disprove legal claims, nor should it be used as a primary deciding factor as to whether or not a particular patient should undergo surgical intervention. Other invasive studies mentioned in the following section can help verify the surgeon's suspicions. A patient with a classic history of a disc herniation with a clear-cut neurologic deficit and positive straight leg raising test who has not responded to conservative treatment should not be denied surgery simply on the basis of an equivocal or negative myelogram.

AIR LUMBAR MYELOGRAPHY

With the elucidation of the "ideal characteristics" of a contrast agent for lumbar myelography, one might indicate that air or some other safe gaseous medium would offer an obvious alternative. Although air is in fact safe and relatively quickly absorbed, the quality of radiographs of an air-filled lumbar theca

leaves much to be desired. In addition, a relatively large amount of spinal fluid must be exchanged so that the injected air will flow to the top of the spinal fluid column when the patient is in a marked head-down angulation. Some experienced clinicians still prefer the safety of this technique and indicate that its interpretation improves with experience. Recent work with double contrast using air and metrizamide in primates demonstrates better resolution of the cord and conus than with gas alone. There was, however, no advantage appreciated with definition of the spinal nerve.[54] Nevertheless, lumbar myelography with air is rarely done in the United States.

DISCOGRAPHY

Discography has not proved to be essential or reliable in our experience and that of others.[19, 60] Discography is performed by placing a fine-gauge spinal needle into a disc space under image intensification either posterolaterally or transdurally. Radiopaque dye is then injected into the interspace, and information is recorded about the amount of dye accepted, the pressure necessary to inject the material, the configuration of the opaque material, and the reproduction of the patient's pain. The diagnostic potential in the *lumbar* spine is therefore realized by the clinical response of the patient, resistance of the disc to infusion, and the roentgenographic appearance of the disc. A normal discogram may be helpful in ruling out disc degeneration, but abnormalities compatible with multiple degenerative discs are so common, particularly with increasing age,[78] that little significance can be placed on the presence of an abnormal discogram in terms of localizing the source of a patient's pain. Even though one might reliably reproduce the patient's spinal pain with a discogenic study, the results of spinal surgery for relief of back pain alone due to degenerative disc disease without herniations is disappointing.[97]

The study is essential in chymopapain therapy and may be helpful in documentation of significant lateral disc herniations not appreciated on myelography and in planning the extent of a fusion, particularly in spondylolisthesis.[94] It is our feeling, however, that in most cases the study is not essential, particularly in light of the diagnostic sensitivity afforded by water-soluble contrast myelography and epidural venography.

EPIDURAL VENOGRAPHY

It is possible, by the insertion of a large-gauge needle into the marrow of a lumbar spinous process and the subsequent injection of angiographic contrast material, to visualize the epidural venous plexus. In 1961, Schobinger, Krueger, and Sobel[91] were thereby able to demonstrate intervertebral disc herniations and certain intraspinal tumors. Patient discomfort and less than ideal perfusions are contraindications to this procedure. Catheterization of the iliac veins with sacrolumbar venous visualization was reported by Helender and Lendblem in 1955.[55] Bucheler and Janson in 1973,[15] Lepage in 1974,[65] and Gargano and others in 1974[35] improved on the technique and provided better visualization of the epidural veins through selected catheterization of the ascending lumbar veins.

The vertebral venous system can be divided into three major components. The first is the interosseous system, which is of no diagnostic value at this point in time. The second network is composed of the anterior internal vertebral vein, the ascending external vertebral vein, the emissary or radicular veins, and the posterior intervertebral veins. All but the latter are of diagnostic importance when mass lesions within the spinal canal are suspected. The third components are the external vertebral veins, particularly the ascending lumbar and lateral sacral veins, which allow access to the previously mentioned second venous network.

Concepts and facts that justify utilization of this well-tolerated but invasive technique follow.

1. There is a consistent and reliable epidural venous system in close proximity to the anterior limits of the spinal canal and neural foramina (Fig. 9–53). The variations in venous anatomy usually affect the number and caliber of the veins rather than their location within the confines of the spinal canal.

2. Since the easily compressible veins traverse the spinal canal in proximity to susceptible neural structures, abnormal venous filling can indirectly imply mass effect with encroachment.

3. Owing to the capacious anatomy of the spine at L4-5 and particularly at L5-S1 and owing to the limited subarachnoid extension along the spinal nerves, an ancillary study that can provide more sensitivity (fewer false negatives) than the myelogram should be available.

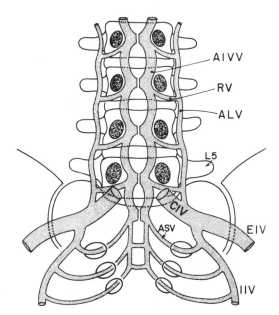

Figure 9–53. Schematic illustration of the vertebral venous system. AIVV — anterior internal vertebral veins; RV — radicular veins; ALV — ascending lumbar vein; ASV — ascending sacral vein; CIV — common iliac vein; EIV — external iliac vein; IIV — internal iliac vein. (From Macnab, I., St. Louis, E. L., Grabias, S. L., et al.: Selective ascending lumbo-sacral venography in the assessment of lumbar disc herniation. An anatomical study and clinical experience. J. Bone Joint Surg. (Am.) 58:1093, 1976.)

This is particularly true when the myelogram is equivocal in the presence of definitive neurologic findings and tension signs.

Several authors[35, 40, 71, 72] have demonstrated greater sensitivity with epidural venography than with myelography, particularly in the capacious L5-S1 segment. In the absence of previous surgery and in the presence of adequate filling, the following abnormalities (modified from Gargano[35] and Theron[100]) are felt to be compatible with disc herniations and other anatomic changes resulting in spinal canal compromise: (1) unilateral or bilateral complete or partial interruption of the anterior internal or anterior external vertebral veins; (2) increased contrast accumulation or enlargement of the anterior internal or anterior external vertebral vein above, below, or contiguous with the herniation secondary to venous stasis or bypass phenomenon; (3) deviation of the anterior vertebral veins without cessation of venous flow; and (4) deviation or occlusion of the emissary or radicular veins accompanying the spinal nerve indicative of lateral herniation or lateral encroachment (Figs. 9–54 to 9–60).

Text continued on page 564

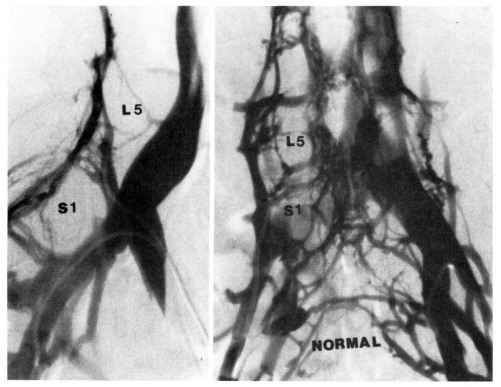

Figure 9–54. Normal epidural venogram.

Figure 9–55. Epidural venogram illustrates obliteration of the anterior internal vertebral vein at the L5-S1 level unilaterally. Lateral disc herniation was noted at this location.

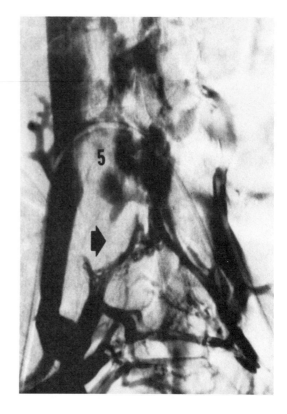

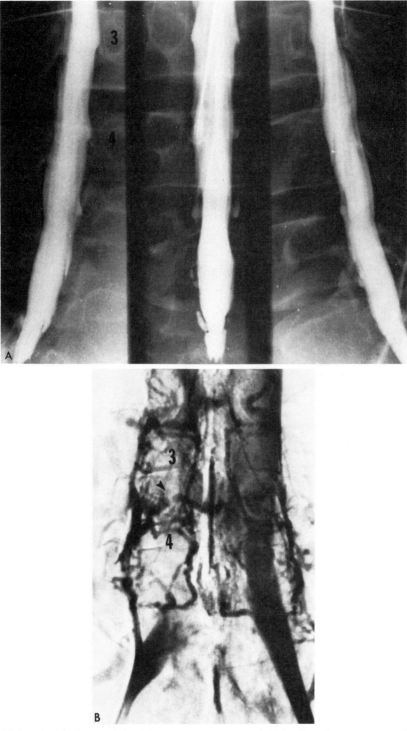

Figure 9–56. This patient had unremitting L4 nerve root symptoms. *A*, This oil myelogram was completely normal. *B*, The epidural venogram revealed a defect in the radicular vein at the L3-L4 level. A free disc fragment found in the foramen well laterally was the source of nerve root compression.

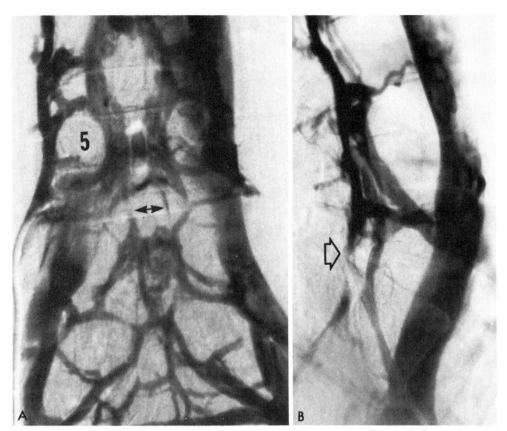

Figure 9–57. Epidural venogram reveals occlusion of the anterior internal vertebral veins bilaterally at L5-S1 due to a central disc herniation as seen in the anterior-posterior view (*A*) and in the lateral view *B*).

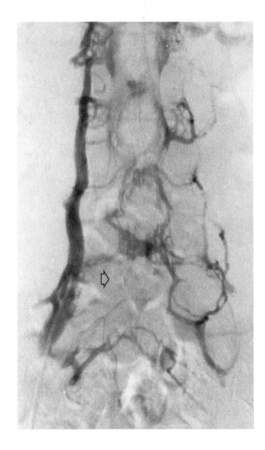

Figure 9–58. This epidural venogram illustrates interruption of the anterior intervertebral vein at L5-S1 on the right. This patient had unremitting right sciatica and a normal oil myelogram.

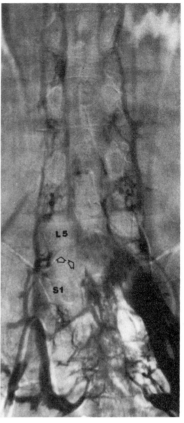

Figure 9–59. This epidural venogram reveals obliteration of the anterior intervertebral vein at L5-S1 associated with obliteration of the radicular vein at the same level. This patient had a large lateral disc herniation at L5-S1 compatible with this defect.

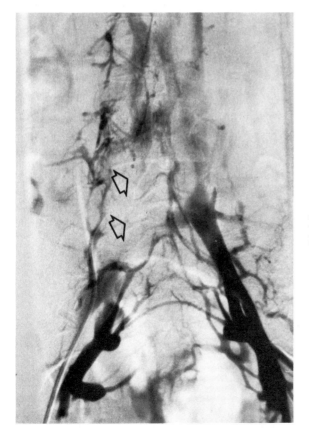

Figure 9–60. This epidural venogram reveals obliteration of the anterior internal vertebral vein and radicular vein at both L4-5 and L5-S1 secondary to narrowing of the lateral recess.

To avoid inadequate venous filling that would yield problems with reliable interpretation, patients are considered candidates for study if they have not had any previous spinal lumbar surgery. Furthermore, to avoid iatrogenic artifacts (particularly retrograde filling), bilateral transfemoral catheterization is performed using the ascending lumbar vein on the one side and the anterior lateral sacral vein on the contralateral side. We consider significant dye allergy and a previous history of thrombophlebitis as absolute contraindications to epidural venography. This study has been well tolerated by our patients; one case of nonlethal pulmonary embolism in over 100 cases has been the author's only significant complication.

The authors use this study primarily when myelography has been either equivocal or negative despite definitive neurologic findings or positive tension signs. It is important to realize that this study has not supplanted myelography but rather has increased the precision of our diagnostic capabilities when used in conjunction with it. The myelogram is still considered essential for localization and definition of subarachnoid space compromise and mass lesion.

AXIAL TOMOGRAPHY OF THE LUMBAR SPINE

FREDIE P. GARGANO, M.D.*

*Director of Radiology, Palmetto General Hospital, Hialeah, Florida; Clinical Professor of Radiology, Neurology and Neurosurgery, University of Miami School of Medicine.

INTRODUCTION. Transverse axial tomography is a well-established radiographic technique[7, 34, 36-39, 61, 80, 92] by which any segment of the spine can be viewed in cross-section. This method offers a nondistorted view of the spine that is ideally suited for evaluating constrictive pathologic conditions. Transverse axial tomography of the body[20, 21, 33, 56, 102] is not a new procdure, but its application in the evaluation of spinal constrictive disorders was initiated in 1972.[34, 38]

EQUIPMENT. The equipment originally used was the Toshiba transverse axial tomograph. The whole body CAT scanners are now being utilized to provide the same information.

The Toshiba unit consisted of (1) a sup-porting unit; (2) an x-ray unit; (3) a field defining device; (4) a cassette holder; (5) a wedge grid; and (6) a table. The magnification ratio was 1.33 with our Toshiba unit, and the image was recorded on x-ray film. Thickness of cut was 3 mm., and exposure dose was 1 to 1.4 R per radiograph.

In 1975 computed body scanners using x-ray sources, photomultiplier tubes for detectors, and computers to reconstruct images from density readings emerged on the medical scene. These units were readily utilized to evaluate pathologic conditions as defined by cross-sectional images of the spine.[16, 51, 62, 93, 106] At the present time this is the most common axial method to evaluate constrictive lesions of the spinal canal. The CAT equipment at our institution is an Ohio Nuclear Delta #50 Body Scanner. The specifications of this piece of equipment have been described in the literature.[5]

Originally we used 13 mm. collimation. These images proved to be too thick, and we had to use overlapping scans to better visualize the facets and foramina. Subsequently we changed to 8 mm. thick images, which provided better anatomic resolution owing to decreased volume averaging. New scanners allow 4 mm. thick sections, which further improves anatomic detail. The radiation dose with the Ohio Nuclear Scanner we have is 1.7 R per scan pair. The images are obtained in a sweep time of 2 minutes and 30 seconds. Newer units are available with scan times as short as one second, which further clarifies anatomic detail by eliminating patient motion.

In 1977 the Versagraph was developed by the Kermath Manufacturing Corporation. It is similar in design to the Toshiba x-ray unit but is much more flexible and versatile. It is a noncomputed machine using the traditional x-ray beam and film as a recording medium. The radiographs produced are superior to those of the Toshiba. The thickness of cut is 1 mm., which allows for excellent anatomic evaluation. The radiation dose is 1.3 R per exposure. The magnification ratio is 1.4 with the Versagraph.

POSITIONING. The patient is placed in the supine position for all examinations of the spine. Because the normal cervical spine has a lordotic curve, the patient is positioned to minimize or eliminate this curve. Ideally, the cervical spine should be parallel to the table. This can be partially accomplished by placing a piece of foam rubber underneath the occiput. The patient's chin is then flexed so the neck is in the military position.

To examine the thoracic area, the patient is supine in neutral position. If the patient has a severe kyphosis he may be examined in the prone position. In the lumbar area the hips should be in a flexed position to flatten the normal lordotic curve. The constant magnification ratio and reproducibility of the tomograms make possible accurate comparison of films at any given level with films from a previous examination in the same patient or with those taken at a similar level in a different patient.

To facilitate determination of the exact level of cut, markers are used. For the Toshiba unit the marker consists of multiple copper wires of varying length a fixed distance apart. In the cervical area, the marker has 10 wires; in the lumbar area, it has 20. The marker is placed over the area of interest, and a scout film is taken. The transverse axial tomograms are done, and then by counting the number of wires in cross-section, the exact level in the spine can be ascertained.

The Versagraph uses a grid-marked film to facilitate determination of the level of laminographic cut. With the CAT scanners most investigators use a series of parallel contrast-filled vascular catheters to form a localization grid.

NORMAL AXIAL ANATOMY. In the articulated spine (Fig. 9–61) it can be seen that the spine and spinal canal may be divided into an intraosseous or intrabody segment and the junctional or articular segment.[37, 49] Only the intraosseous segment is demonstrated in axial views of isolated vertebral bodies of which previous anatomic descriptions have been limited.[8, 12] Axial tomography allows both the intraosseous and the articular segment of the spinal canal to be studied in the living patient, giving a clearer appreciation of both the normal and pathologic anatomy of the spine (Fig. 9–62).

The intraosseous segment (Fig. 9–63) of the lumbar canal is formed by the continuous bony rim of the vertebral body, pedicles, pars interarticularis, laminae, and spinous process. Yet, in examining the articulated spine, it is obvious that only a small portion of the longitudinal extent of the spinal canal at each level is included in this segment. Actually, the intraosseous segments of two adjacent lumbar vertebral bodies delineate the superior and inferior limits of the larger articular segment of the canal.

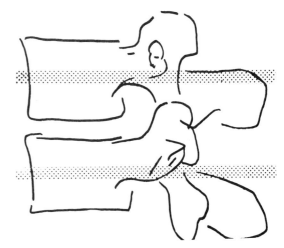

Figure 9–61. The dotted area represents the intraosseous segment of the vertebral body and canal. The segment betweeen the dotted areas is the junctional or articular segment of the vertebral canal.

The articular segment (Fig. 9–63) is formed by the vertebral body and intervertebral disc ventrally, the articular facets laterally and dorsolaterally, and the facets, laminae, and spinous process dorsally. The bony rim is incomplete. The articular segment contains the intervertebral disc, the intervertebral foramina, the articular processes, the articular facets, and the dorsal arch. These are the major anatomic components that are involved with most soft tissue and bony pathologic conditions affecting the lumbar spine.

The articular processes[8, 17, 26, 34, 44, 46, 49, 66] play a prominent role in both the normal and pathologic anatomy of the articular segment of the canal. In the normal canal, the inferior articular processes of the upper vertebra are always medial and dorsal to the subjacent superior articular processes. Both superior facets have a slightly concave medial surface facing the canal. The inferior articular processes are symmetrical, although divergent, as they join the laminae, completing the dorsal arch. This gives a biconvex configuration to the lateral and dorsal walls of the lumbar and lumbosacral articular segments of the spinal canal. The transition along the medial wall across the interfacet joint is always smooth. Thus, the articular segment of the canal is formed almost entirely by the articulating inferior and superior articular processes laterally, dorsolaterally, and dorsally. This entire facetal wall is vulnerable to either primary developmental change or secondary

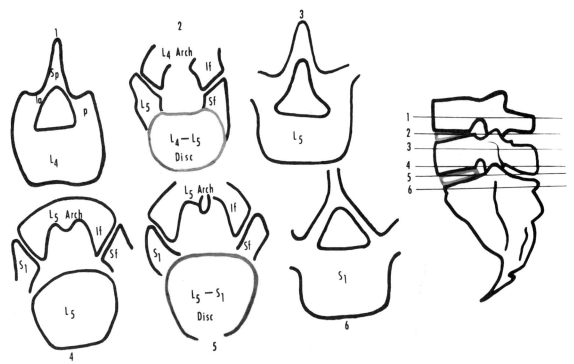

Figure 9–62. Line drawings of a series of normal lumbosacral axial tomograms. The lateral view shows the level of the tomographic cuts. It is noted that various components of adjacent vertebrae contribute to the axial tomogram at any level. The inferior articular processes of the superior vertebra are always dorsal and medial to the subjacent superior articular processes. Sp, la, p, If, and sf represent spinous process, lamina, pedicle, and inferior and superior articulating processes, respectively.

overgrowth associated with pathologic conditions of the intervertebral disc.[77, 88]

LUMBAR STENOSIS. The word "stenosis" implies narrowing of a hollow or tubular structure.

On this basis, lumbar spinal stenosis may be defined as any type of narrowing of the spinal canal, nerve root canals (or tunnels), or intervertebral foramina. It may be local, segmental, or generalized. It may be caused by bone or by soft tissue, and the narrowing may involve the bony canal alone, the dural sac, or both.

Herniations of the nucleus pulposus have in the past been considered as distinct and separate entities. They are included in this discussion since they occur not infrequently with stenosis. Space-occupying lesions due to the products of inflammation or neoplasm are in the strictest sense types of "stenosis" but are considered to be beyond the scope of this presentation.

DEVELOPMENTAL STENOSIS. In developmental stenosis (Fig. 9–64) there is a general narrowing of the canal[52, 63, 103, 104] This is always more marked within the articular segment of the canal regardless of the level of involvement. In many cases, the pedicles within the intraosseous segment are in normal position. It is the predominantly dorsal and dorsolateral overgrowth of the articular process and facets in the articular segment that leads to the anteroposterior foreshortening of the canal. This constriction and encroachment of the canal occurs at first within the dorsal half of the canal and is exaggerated with medial placement of the pedicles. Cross-sectional tomograms usually reveal the maximal stenosis to be within the L4-5 articular segment of the canal, in agreement with Verbiest's findings.[104] However, congenital stenosis is a diffuse problem in which evidence of narrowing can be demonstrated at multiple levels. Achondroplasia (Fig. 9–65) is the classic example of developmental stenosis. The dorsal arch is constricted medially and it is thickened. Normally, the ligamentum flavum is interposed between successive laminae in the interlaminar space, but with developmental stenosis, the entire dorsal wall of the canal

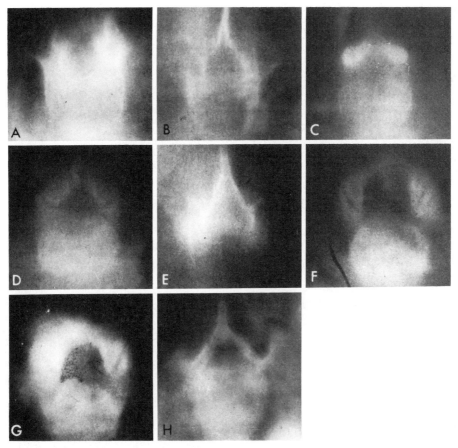

Figure 9–63. Serial tomograms from L4 to S1 in a normal lumbar spine. All sections of the canal demonstrate the symmetrical pattern of the normal canal. *A*, Upper body L4 with distinct pedicle marking the lateral border of the canal; *B*, L4 intraosseous section with a continuous rim of bone and a triangular shape; *C*, L4 laminar arch dorsally, with the L4-L5 disc faintly seen ventrally; *D*, Midsection of L4-L5 articular segment. The canal is still partly triangular in shape. The laminar arch and its extension into the inferior articular process form the lateral and dorsolateral walls. The superior articular process of L5 forms the most ventrolateral border of the canal. *E*, L5 intraosseous segment again demonstrating a solid bony rim and a triangular shape; *F* and *G*, Upper and lower sections through the L5-S1 articular segment of the canal. There is a marked change in shape, from triangular at L5 to parabolic at L5-S1, with definite enlargement of the entire lumbosacral canal. The laminar arch and inferior articular processes of L5 form the entire lateral and dorsolateral walls of the canal. The intervertebral foramina can be seen ventrolaterally. *H*, S1 intraosseous segment with an abrupt change to the triangular configuration and narrowing of the sacral canal.

is bony owing to overlapping and "shingling" of the thickened, distorted laminar arch. The articular processes, especially the inferior ones, which form the lateral and dorsolateral walls of the lower lumbar canal, are bulbous. The medial aspect of the inferior articular process bulges convexly into the dorsal half of the canal. The canal loses its normal outwardly convex shape, assuming a scalloped, biconvex configuration. A deep, constricted midline posterior recess develops between the articular facets.

ACQUIRED STENOSIS. Features of the spondylotic process that decrease the capacity of the spinal canal to accommodate the cauda equina are (1) posterior articulation (facet) arthrotic enlargments (facet hypertrophy); (2) thickening of laminae; (3) protrusions of discs; the compressive effects of these are augmented in lordosis or standing and are diminished in flexion or sitting; (4) forward movement of one vertebra on another (usually L4 on L5) owing to posterior articulation incompetence rather than pars interarticularis defects; (5) thickening and fibrosis ("hypertrophy") of the yellow ligaments.

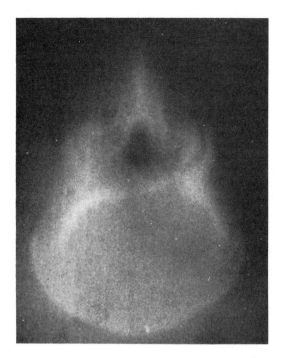

Figure 9–64. Small canal in a patient with developmental stenosis. All the diameters of the canal are constricted. Compare the size of the canal with the size of the vertebral body.

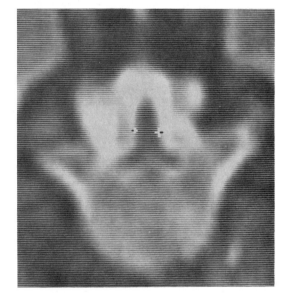

Figure 9–65. Small canal in a patient with achondroplasia. Note the short, thick pedicles and the keyhole shape of the spinal canal (arrows); also, note how deeply the vertebral body is recessed between the ilial wings.

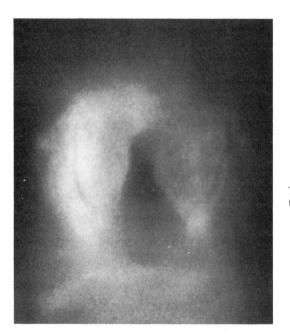

Figure 9–66. Transverse stenosis with posterior recess. The facets are bulbous and sclerotic. The facet joints are osteoarthritic.

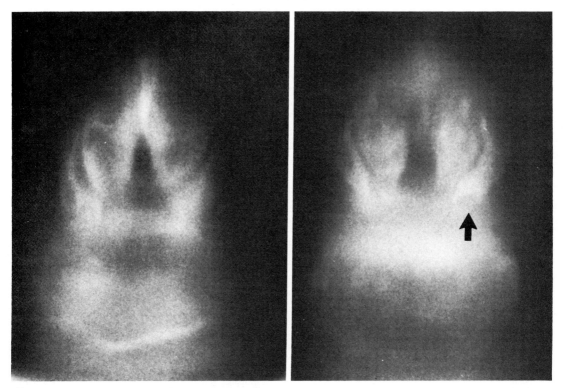

Figure 9–67. Lumbar stenosis in two adjacent radiographs through L4-L5. Note degenerative cystic changes in inferior facets bilaterally and in left superior facet (arrow).

The lumbosacral joint is thought to be the most stressed spinal joint, judging from the unfavorable inclined aspect of it in the standing position, but in spondylotic caudal radiculopathy, an ailment thought to be augmented by chronic spinal stress, this joint is less affected than L4-L5, which is the most vulnerable.

In acquired lumbar stenosis the most significant change is articular process hypertrophy primarily involving the inferior facets. The medial overgrowth of the articular processes leads to transverse narrowing, which is most prominent at the waist of the spinal canal (interfacet diameter). A posterior recess develops, giving the canal a trilobate appearance (Fig. 9–66). The inferior facet hypertrophy may be symmetrical (Figs. 9–67 and 9–68) or asymmetrical (Fig. 9–69), drastically changing the shape of the spinal canal. The shape of the canal may be concentrically narrowed (Figs. 9–70 and 9–71) or truncated (Figs. 9–72 and 9–73) due to unilateral medial constriction (hemiphypertrophy). Superior facet hypertrophy may also occur, causing more deformity of the canal. The molding of the facets and osteoarthritis differentiates acquired from developmental stenosis.

The "osteoarthritic" hypertrophied facet is bulbous and sclerotic. Besides contributing to lumbar stenosis, it may cause lateral recess encroachment. The lateral recess anatomical-

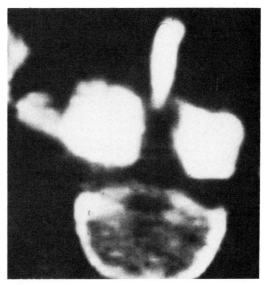

Figure 9–68. CAT scan through L4-L5 showing symmetrical stenosis.

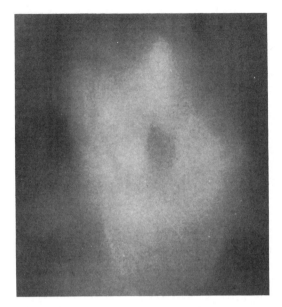

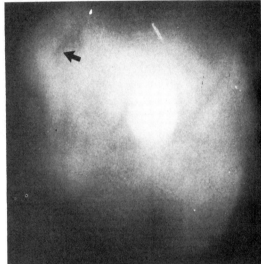

Figure 9–69. Transverse axial tomogram through L5-S1. The inferior and superior facets are sclerotic and hypertrophied. The entire facetal wall encroaches on the canal bilaterally but to a greater degree on the right.

Figure 9–70. Concentric lumbar stenosis with dural sac outlined by Pantopaque. The epidural space is markedly compressed by the bony overgrowth. Note the extreme molding due to superior facet overgrowth (arrow) to buttress the inferior facet hypertrophy.

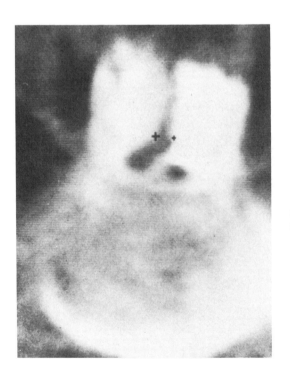

Figure 9–71. CAT scan through L4-L5 intra-articular segment showing spinal canal reduced to a small cleft between the hypertrophied facets (arrows).

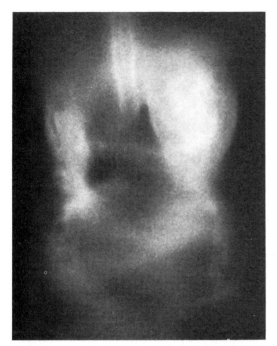

Figure 9–72. Hemihypertrophy of the left inferior facet of L4 transversely narrowing the spinal canal.

ly is medial to the pedicles and ventral to the superior facet. Any encroachment in the recess will compress the spinal nerve which traverses it. This lateral recess is anatomically different from that described with develop-

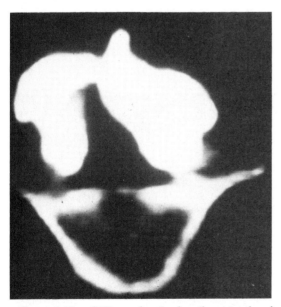

Figure 9–73. CAT scan showing hemihypertrophy of the left inferior facet at the level of L4-L5.

mental malrotation of the superior facet of S1.[8, 25, 88, 89] In this condition, the recess is due to medial overhang and frontal orientation of the superior articular process, the recess being ventral to this structure.

With osteoarthritic facets the recess is ventral to the inferior facet and medial to the superior facet. This acquired recess is more medial to the anatomic lateral recess and is termed the osteoarthritic gutter (Figs. 9–74 to 9–76).

Thus, primary degenerative spondylosis results in hypertrophied sclerotic articular processes that may constrict normal or developmentally small canals. The abnormalities may be focal, segmental, diffuse, symmetrical, or asymmetrical. The hypertrophy of the articular processes may be associated with sclerotic thickened laminae, prolapse of the intervertebral discs, hyperplasia of the ligamentum flavum, and osteophytes. In addition, the articular processes may be elongated, rotated, sclerotic, osteoarthritic, and too ventral in orientation. All these factors tend to decrease the size of the canal. The final degree of constriction of the canal and its segmental distribution determine the clinical symptoms and signs (level and degree of cauda equina compression).

VENTRAL OVERGROWTH OF SPINAL FUSIONS. Ventral overgrowth of posterior lumbar fusions into the lumbar canal leading to bony constriction and encasement of multiple lumbosacral roots is a recognized iatrogenic cause of lumbar stenosis.[11, 17, 86, 108] Macnab noted that more than 20 per cent of his patients subjected to posterior fusions required subsequent decompression for stenosis.

Patients subjected to a primary or secondary fusion may actually have unrecognized bony stenosis and facetal hypertrophy prior to the fusion. In these cases, axial tomograms reveal an abnormal canal typical of stenosis with an associated bony fusion mass presenting exterior to the laminar arch dorsally or dorsolaterally (Figs. 9–77 and 9–78).

Patients with a normal canal and dorsal fusion may develop progressive overgrowth of the fusion mass and the decorticated dorsal laminar arch into the canal (iatrogenic stenosis).[108] Cross-sectional studies in these cases are characterized by the loss of recognizable bony landmarks in the involved segment of the canal with bony distortion and constriction[38] (Figs. 9–79 and 9–80).

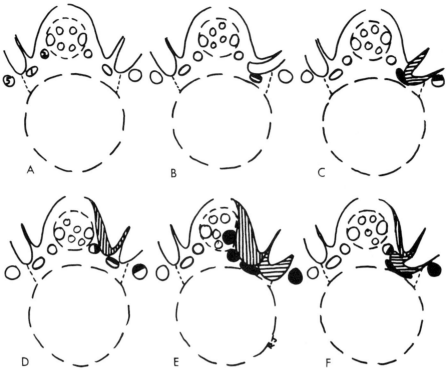

Figure 9–74. Diagrammatic cross-sections to demonstrate lateral recess abnormalities. Small circular broken line structure represents the dural sac with cauda equina. Large circular broken line structures represent compressed radicular nerves. Cross-hatched structures represent hypertrophy of facets. *A,* Normal; *B,* Medial rotation of superior facet; *C,* Isolated hypertrophy of superior facet; *D,* Isolated hypertrophy of inferior facet with formation of osteoarthritic gutter; *E,* Hemihypertrophy of inferior facet with large osteoarthritic gutter and concomitant hypertrophy of ipsilateral superior facet; *F,* Minimal hypertrophy of inferior facet with marked hypertrophy of the ipsilateral superior facet mimicking medial rotation of the superior facet (compare with *B*).

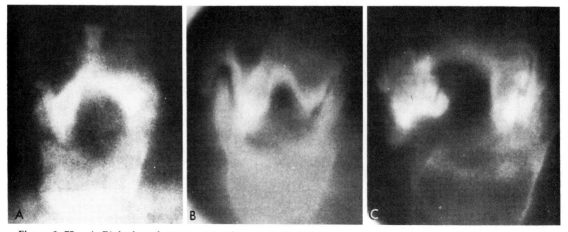

Figure 9–75. *A,* Right lateral recess encroachment. *B,* Right lateral recess encroachment with development of an osteoarthritic gutter. *C,* Left lateral recess encroachment with development of osteoarthritic gutter that extends to the vertebral body. In each case compare with opposite lateral recess.

Figure 9–76. CAT scan through intra-articular segment of L5-S1, showing right lateral recess encroachment.

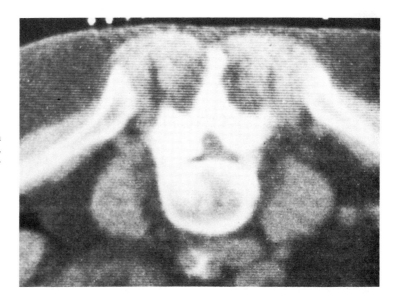

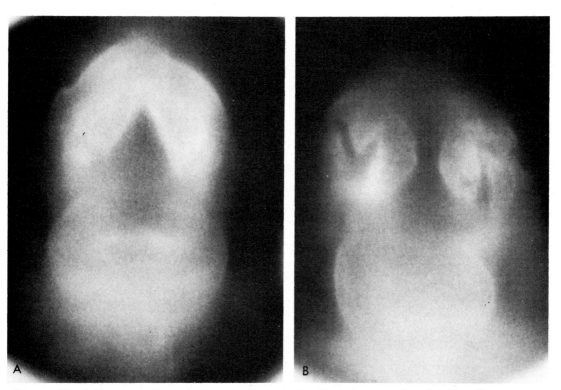

Figure 9–77. *A*, Dorsal operative bony fusion in a patient with a borderline normal canal. *B*, Dorsal lateral operative bony fusion with unrecognized stenosis. Note the narrow interfacet diameter.

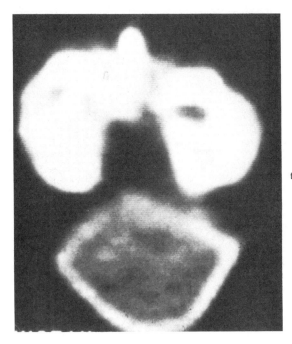

Figure 9–78. CAT scan showing dorsal fusion in a patient with unrecognized stenosis.

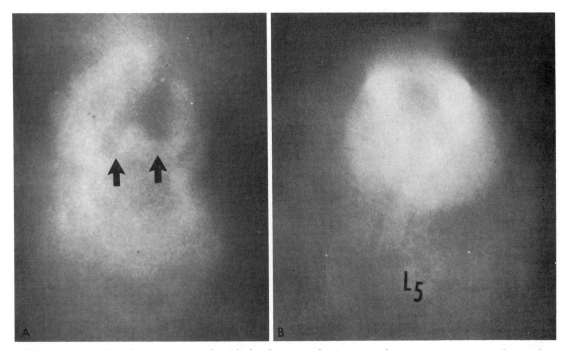

Figure 9–79. *A*, Bone fusion overgrowth with development of a transverse bar (arrows) separating the canal into dorsal and ventral compartments. *B*, Axial tomogram through L5. The dorsal symmetrical dense areas represent Herrington rods. The ventral dense areas are residual Pantopaque. The vertebral canal is completely obliterated secondary to bony fusion overgrowth.

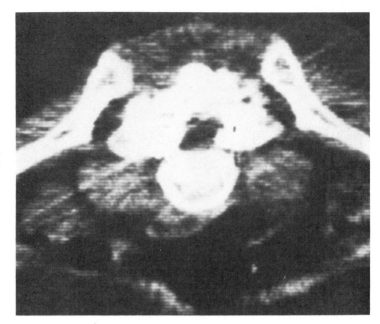

Figure 9–80. CAT scan through L5-S1, showing dorsal fusion with spinal canal encroachment.

The clinical diagnosis is often difficult in either group because of the diverse radicular symptoms and signs.[70, 109] Plain radiographs usually reveal dense sclerotic bone over the dorsal arches without an accurate way of ascertaining if the bone is encroaching on the canal. Axial tomography eliminates the overlap of the shadows and provides a cross-sectional view of the canal so that ventral overgrowth is easily detectable. The amount of overgrowth varies from moderate to complete obliteration of the canal by the fusion mass. At myelography the changes are usually erroneously attributed to arachnoiditis or dural adhesions.

SPONDYLOLISTHESIS. Spondylolisthesis has long been known to be a common cause of lumbar stenosis and intermittent claudication of the cauda equina[23, 25] Pathologically and radiologically, spondylolisthesis can be subdivided into spondylolytic spondylolisthesis[69] and pseudospondylolisthesis.[68] Pseudospondylolisthesis has a greater association with symptomatic lumbar stenosis.

Spondylolytic spondylolisthesis (Figs. 9–81 to 9–83) may occur at any level, although the great majority of cases are at L5.[42] In L5 spondylolytic spondylolisthesis, there is marked axial distortion of the canal in the anteroposterior plane. The articular facets have been abnormal in all cases studied. The superior articular processes of the caudal subluxed vertebra are densely sclerotic, hyper-

trophied, and irregular because these processes now assume the full brunt of weight bearing of the spine. There is obvious transverse narrowing of the canal by the abnormal articular processes.[42, 43]

The isthmic defect will be recognizable as

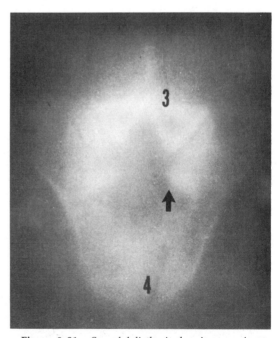

Figure 9–81. Spondylolisthesis showing superior articular process hypertrophy (arrow).

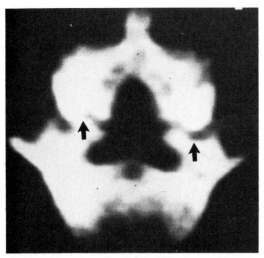

Figure 9–82. CAT scan through L5-S1 in a patient with both Paget's disease and spondylolisthesis. Note the defect in the pars articularis bilaterally (arrows).

a radiolucent defect on the CAT or TAT. There is also a transverse lucent band ventral to the spinal canal on the CAT scan, which is seen in spondylolisthesis[93] and in other disorders with malalignment of the vertebral bodies. When spondylolisthesis is seen at L5, the radiolucent transverse band is the posterior aspect of the L5-S1 disc uncovered by the slippage. It is bounded anteriorly by the posterior aspect of the L5 body and posteriorly by the superior margin of S1.

Pseudospondylolisthesis is due to degenerative molding of the articular processes and progressive slipping of the entire rostral vertebral body and its attached dorsal arch forward on the more caudal vertebra.[46, 53, 68] It is most commonly seen at L4-L5. Cross-sectional study of the canal at the involved level in several cases has demonstrated marked constriction of the canal. The dorsal arch and the attached inferior articular process slip forward until they are ventral to the adjacent superior facets (Fig. 9–84). There is associated sclerosis of the facets. The anterior displacement of the inferior processes relative to the subjacent superior facets has not been seen in other stenotic conditions or in the normal spine. It usually occurs in females in the fifth or sixth decade of life. It is more frequent in patients with an exaggerated lumbar lordosis and a sacralized L5 vertebral body. The slippage rarely exceeds 25 per cent of the superior surface of the subjacent vertebral body. These patients will also show the transverse radiolucent band in thin sections at the level of the pseudospondylolisthesis.

DISCUSSION. From the pathologic and surgical descriptions of developmental stenosis and primary degenerative spondylosis (acquired degenerative stenosis), it is apparent that the predominant source of encroachment is the hypertrophied articular process. Axial studies of the lumbar canal in both of these conditions demonstrate clearly that the major pathologic change is in the dorsal laminar arch and the articular processes, regardless of the presence or absence of abnormal pedicles, ventral body ridging, or soft disc disease. The most vulnerable borders of the vertebral canal are the articular processes and their extension into the dorsal laminal arch. Thus, the dorsal half of the canal, especially at L4-L5 and L5-S1, is particularly vulnerable to any change in the articular processes or dorsal arch. It is these structures that form and shape the lateral, dorsolateral, and dorsal walls of

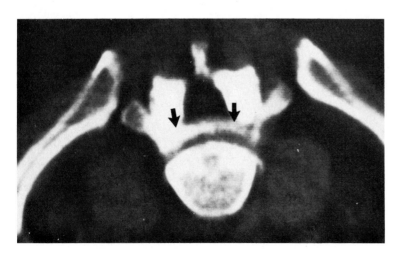

Figure 9–83. Spondylolisthesis at L5-S1. Note the posterior dense margin of S1 (arrows) with the more ventral radiolucency representing the L5-S1 intervertebral disc.

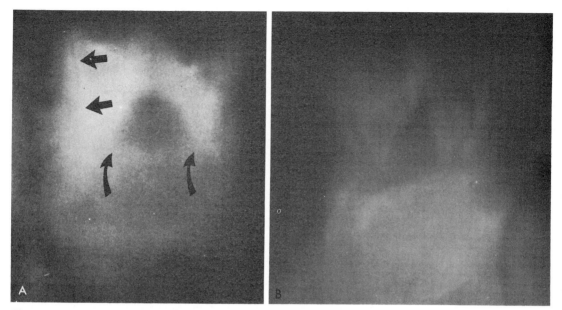

Figure 9–84. *A*, Pseudospondylolisthesis with ventral migration of the inferior facets encroaching on the lateral recesses bilaterally (lower arrows). The canal is concentrically narrowed owing to the anterior slippage of the superior adjacent vertebra. Note the vertical orientation of the facet joints (upper arrows). *B*, Pseudospondylolisthesis showing ventral migration of the inferior facets with secondary stenosis.

the lower lumbar canal and determine its configuration in both the normal and abnormal state. Since the epidural space is enlarging in the lumbosacral canal relative to the decrease in size of the tapering dural sac[17, 61] there may be significant narrowing of the canal and encroachment of the epidural space with infringements on its roots without the production of significant defects on myelographic examination.[11, 12]

By giving a cross-sectional tomographic view of the spinal canal, axial tomography reveals a bony pathologic condition, posterior and lateral recesses, and constriction of the canal that are not seen on plain radiographs or myelograms because of the overlapping of shadows. This allows the preoperative detection of the very common bony conditions which themselves mimic the lumbar disc syndrome[77, 81] or which are manifest occultly in association with herniated discs. Also, axial tomography offers a method of evaluating the patient with recurrent symptoms who has undergone previous laminectomy or fusion in whom the occult bony abnormality was not appreciated or has since been acquired.[53, 67, 70, 75]

MEASUREMENTS. In addition to evaluating the anatomic detail and configuration of the various vertebral components, measure-

ments are made routinely of the sagittal and transverse diameters.[38]

Transverse or interfacet measurement (Fig. 9–85) has been the most sensitive index of spinal canal narrowing.[24, 25, 58, 84, 87, 104]

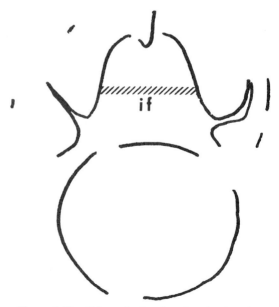

Figure 9–85. Schematic drawing showing interfacet diameter. The interfacet line (if) is the width of the canal measured at the midpoint of the sagittal diameter of the canal.

Since the primary pathologic condition in lumbar stenosis is articular process hypertrophy, the reliability of this measurement can be readily appreciated.[38] In some cases the interfacet distance was not the narrowest transverse diameter. These cases had more pronounced narrowing dorsal to the plane of the interfacet measurement.

The diagnosis of lumbar stenosis can most readily be made by studying the configuration of the canal on axial view and measuring the interfacet diameter. Interpediculate and sagittal diameters correlated poorly with lumbar stenosis, but their use should not be abandoned.[38] If the sagittal diameters or the interpediculate diameters on routine films are small, the patient probably has lumbar stenosis. However, if the sagittal or interpediculate measurements are normal, lumbar stenosis cannot be excluded.

Table 9–2 is a chart of normal measurements that we have developed to evaluate for lumbar stenosis.

CAT vs. TAT.   Patients of average habitus can be evaluated by both computed and noncomputed techniques equally well for suspected constrictive pathologic states.[80] Patients who are obese or osteoporotic are better examined with the CAT scanner. In addition, since CAT has the capacity to evaluate soft tissue densities inside and external to the canal, more information can be obtained by this technique. We routinely perform CAT examinations of the spinal canal rather than the radiographic noncomputed examination. Axial tomography is an excellent method to evaluate pathologic conditions of the spine, but it should be used in conjunction with plain films and myelography or extradural venography when clinically indicated.

HERNIATED LUMBAR DISCS.   In 1975, Alfidi and colleagues[5] raised the question of the usefulness of CAT scanning in the diagnosis of disc herniations. On plain CAT scanning, the diagnosis of a herniated disc is based on the presence of an asymmetric area of increased density in the ventral aspect of the spinal canal or by asymmetric loss of the normal epidural fat density. Accuracy is still limited but will improve as refinement of the CAT scanners occurs. Myelography and epidural venography still remain the definitive diagnostic studies for herniated lumbar discs.

SUMMARY.   Transverse axial tomography is a technique by which the spine is viewed radiographically in cross-section. By producing a cross-sectional tomographic view of the spinal canal, axial tomography reveals bony pathologic conditions, posterior and lateral recesses, and constriction of the canal that are not readily seen by plain radiography or myelography because of the overlapping of various shadows. Thus, axial tomography is able to detect the bony pathologic state of the lumbar canal in patients presenting initially with the "lumbar disc syndrome" or later as laminectomy failures.

Other abnormalities of the spine unrelated to constrictive pathologic conditions may also be demonstrated by axial tomography. These include congenital anomalies (Figs. 9–86 to 9–88), traumatic (Figs. 9–89 and 9–90) and surgical (Fig. 9–91) changes, neoplastic (Fig. 9–92) and inflammatory disease (Fig. 9–93), and occasionally disc abnormalities (Figs. 9–94 and 9–95).

TABLE 9–2. NORMAL AXIAL TOMOGRAPHIC MEASUREMENTS OF LUMBAR SPINE*

Level	Interpediculate	Sagittal	Interfacet
L4	23.6 (21–25)	16.5 (13.5–19)	
L4-L5	28 (25.5–32)	22 (19–30)	21 (16.5–23)
L5	25.5 (22.5–30)	18.5 (15–20)	
L5-S1 Upper portion	30 (24–41)	24 (19.5–28)	23 (20–27)
L5-S1 Lower portion	31 (26–40)	27 (22.5–31.5)	25.5 (22.5–28.5)
S1	29 (25–34.5)	20.5 (18–22.5)	

*Measurements in mm. corrected for magnification. Multiply by 1.33 for the Toshiba unit and 1.4 for the Kermath unit.

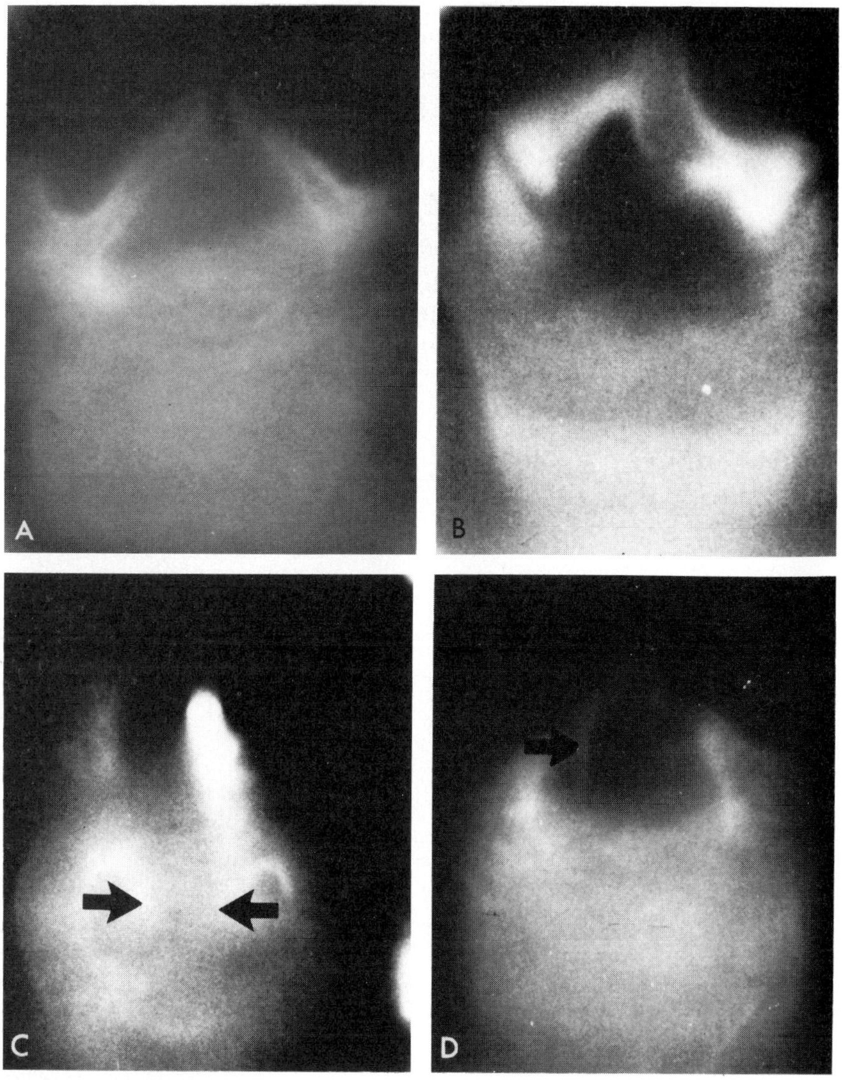

Figure 9–86. A, Spina bifida occulta; B, Deformed neural arch; C, Bifid vertebral body (arrows); D, Right dorsal spur (arrow) which impinged on underlying L5 nerve (demonstrated by myelography).

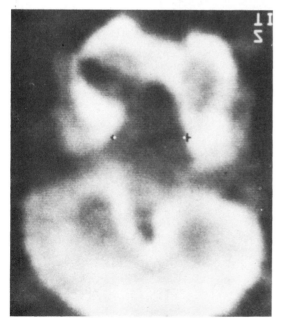

Figure 9–87. CAT scan corresponding to TAT on Figure 9–86C. The bifid vertebral body is better demonstrated by the CAT.

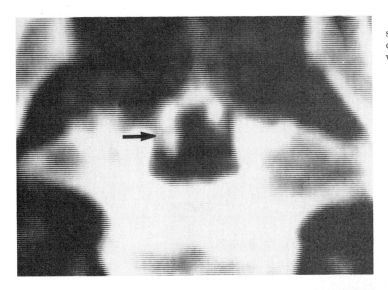

Figure 9–88. CAT scan, corresponding to TAT in Figure 9–86D, demonstrates the right dorsal spur (arrow) very well.

Figure 9–89. Unsuspected vertebral body fracture on TAT (arrows).

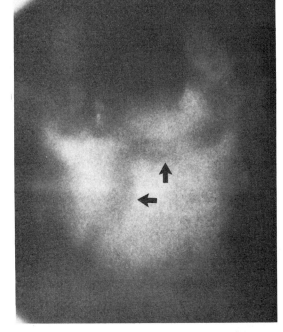

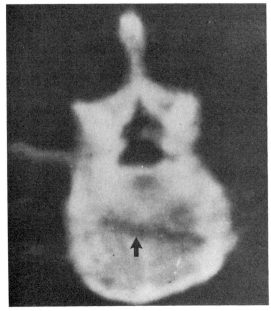

Figure 9–90. CAT scan showing transverse vertebral body fracture not demonstrable on routine radiographic studies (arrow).

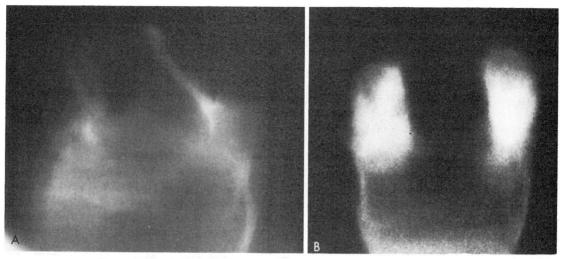

Figure 9–91. *A*, Right laminectomy defect; *B*, Bilateral laminectomy defects.

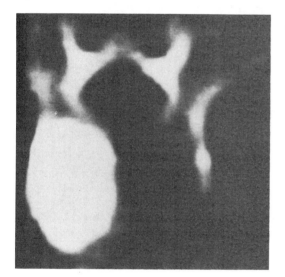

Figure 9–92. Osteoblastic metastatic lesion of vertebral body as demonstrated by CAT.

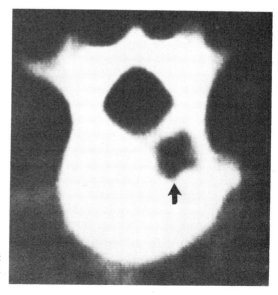

Figure 9–93. CAT scan through L1 showing radiolucent defect (arrow) due to tuberculous osteomyelitis. Changes on plain spine radiographs were minimal.

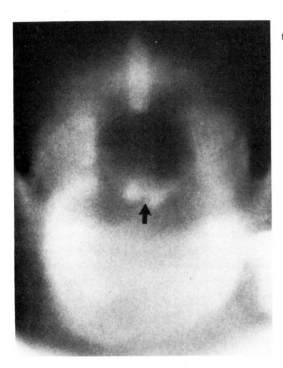

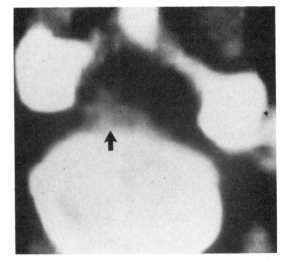

Figure 9–94. TAT showing a calcified herniated intervertebral disc (arrow).

Figure 9–95. CAT scan showing herniated disc (arrow).

ELECTROMYOGRAPHY

Electromyography documents the functional integrity of the motor unit, that is, the anterior horn cell, the axon, the neuromuscular junctions, and the muscle fibers innervated. When muscle groups of either anterior or posterior rami innervation demonstrate abnormal irritability (fibrillations), abnormally large motor unit action potentials, or an increased number of polyphasic motor unit action potentials on electromyography, abnormal acute or chronic neurofunction is implied.

Electromyography, however, does not define the altered anatomy causing neural dysfunction. The diagnostic specificity and sensitivity realized with the combination of a well-performed physical examination, epidural venography, and water-soluble myelography has obviated the authors' use of electromyography in the diagnosis of symptomatic lumbar disc disease.

However, when the suspicion of metabolic, ischemic, or heredofamilial peripheral neuropathies is being entertained, the electromyogram can be diagnostically helpful.

THE DIFFERENTIAL SPINAL BLOCK

Differential spinal anesthesia, as described by Ahlgren and colleagues,[1] involves the serial injection of increasing concentrations of an anesthetic into the subarachnoid space. This has proved to be a great aid in differentiating between organic and functional pain and is particularly useful in patients with strong emotional problems, in patients with a paucity of objective findings and the presence of severe pain, and in the patient who is suspected of malingering.[45]

A subarachnoid tap is done using a 20 gauge needle, with the patient in the lateral recumbent position and the painful side down.

Injections are made at 10 minute intervals of 5 ml. of isotonic saline (placebo), 10 ml. of 0.2 per cent procaine (sympathetic block), 10 ml. of 0.5 per cent procaine (sensory block), and 10 ml. of 1 per cent procaine (motor block). After each injection, the patient is asked to evaluate his pain at rest and then after a passive manipulation, such as the straight leg raising test. Evaluation of vasomotor sensory and motor function is also conducted to evaluate the efficacy of the anesthetic.

With the use of this test, the etiology of pain can usually be ascribed to either an organic lesion or a functional basis. It is further possible to determine if the organic pain is mediated principally by the sensory or sympathetic portion of the nervous system.

The results are most dramatic when the patient is either completely relieved of pain with only saline or when no relief is obtained with 1 per cent procaine when it produces motor paralysis or a sensory level several dermatomes above the pain site. In both of these circumstances, the etiology of the pain can be interpreted as nonorganic or functional in nature.

References

1. Ahlgren, E. W., et al.: Diagnosis of pain with a graduated spinal block technique. J.A.M.A. 195:125–128, 1966.
2. Ahlgren, P.: Lumbale Myelographie mit Conray meglumine 282. Fortschr. Rontgenstr. 111:270–276, 1969.
3. Ahlgren, P.: Lumbar myelography with dimer-X. IX Symposium Neuroradiologicum, Goteberg, August 1970. Book of abstracts. p. 135.
4. Ahlgren, P.: Postmyelografiske eller postoperative arachnoiditiske forandringer efter conturex-, Conray- og Dimer-X-myelografier (Danish).
5. Alfidi, R. J., Meany, T. F., et al.: Computed tomography of the thorax and abdomen: A preliminary report. Radiology 117:257–264, 1975.
6. Allbrook, D.: Movements of the lumbar spinal column. J. Bone Joint Surg. 39B:339–345, 1957.
7. Altman, R. D., Brown, M., and Gargano, F. P.: Etiology of back pain in Paget's disease of bone. In press.
8. Ayres, C.: Further use studies of lumbosacral pathology with consideration of involvement of intervertebal discs and articular facets, N. Engl. J. Med. 213:716, 1935.
9. Baker, R., Hillman, B. J., McLennan, J. E., et al.: Sequelae of metrizamide myelography in 200 examinations. Am. J. Roentgenol. 139:499–502, 1978.
10. Baumgartner, J., Bonte, G., Braun, J. P., et al.: La radiculographic lombosacrée a l'iothalamate de methyl glucamine (Contrix 28). Bilan de 847 examens. Rev. Rheumatol. 36:549–554, 1969.
11. Begg, C., Falconer, M., and McGeorge, M.: Myelography in lumbar intervertebral disc lesions. A correlation with operative findings, Br. J. Surg. 34:141, 1946.
12. Begg, C., and Falconer, M.: Plain radiography in intraspinal protrusion of lumbar intervertebral disc. A correlation with operative findings, Br. J. Surg. 36:225, 1949.
13. Bentson, J. R.: Comparison of metrizamide with other myelographic agents. Clin. Orthop. 127:111–119, 1977.
14. Bernini, P. M., Flandu, Y., Marvel, J., and Rothman, R.: Multiple thoracic spine fractures complicating anklyosing hyperostosis of the spine. J. Trauma, in press.
15. Bucheler, C., and Janson, R.: Combined catheter venography of the lumbar venous system and the inferior vena cava. Br. J. Radiol. 46:655–661, 1973.
16. Colley, D. P., and Kunsker, S. B.: Traumatic narrowing of the dorsolumbar spinal canal demonstrated by computer tomography. Radiology 129:95–98, 1978.
17. Danforth, M., and Wilson, P.: Anatomy of lumbosacral region in relation to sciatic pain. J. Bone Joint Surg. 7:109, 1925.
18. DePalma, A., and Rothman, R.: Surgery of the lumbar spine. Clin. Orthop. 63:162–170, 1969.
19. DePalma, A., and Rothman, R.: The Intervertebral Disc. Philadelphia. W. B. Saunders Co., 1970.
20. DiChiro, G.: Axial transverse encephalography. Am. J. Roentgenol. 92:441, 1964.
21. DiChiro, G.: Axial transverse encephalography with the radiotome. Medicamundi 10:92, 1965.
22. Edeiken, J., and Pitt, M. J.: The radiologic diagnosis of disc disease. Orthop. Clin. North Am. 2(2):405–417, 1971.
23. Ehni, G., Clark, K., Wilson, C., and Alexander, E.: Significance of the small lumbar spinal canal: Cauda equina compression syndrome due to spondylosis, J. Neurosurg. 31:490, 1969.
24. Epstein, J., Epstein, B., and Lavine, L.: Nerve root compression associated with narrowing of the lumbar spinal canal, J. Neurol. Neurosurg. Psychiatry 25:165, 1962.
25. Epstein, B., Epstein, J., and Lavine, L.: The effect of anatomic variations in lumbar vertebrae and spinal canal in cauda equina and nerve root syndromes. Am. J. Roentgenol. 91:1055, 1964.
26. Epstein, J. Epstein, B., Rosenthal, A., Carras, R., and Lavine, L.: Sciatica caused by nerve root entrapment in the lateral recess: The superior facet syndrome. J. Neurosurg. 36:583, 1972.
27. Ericksen, M. F.: Some aspects of aging in the lumbar spine. Am. J. Phys. Anthropol. 45:575–580, 1976.
28. Ericksen, M. F.: Aging in the lumbar spine (L1 and L2). Am. J. Phys. Anthropol. 48:241–246, 1978.
29. Edgar, M. A., and Park, W. M.: Induced pain patterns on passive straight leg raising in lower lumbar disc protrusion. J. Bone Joint Surg. 56B:658–667, 1974.
30. Farfan, H. F., Osteria, V., and Lamy C.: The mechanical etiology of spondylolysis and spondylolisthesis. Clin. Orthop. 117:40–55, 1976.
31. Fitzgerald, J. A. W., and Newman, P. H.: Degenerative spondylolisthesis. J. Bone Joint Surg. 58B:184–192, 1976.
32. Ford, L. T., Gilula, L. A., Murphy, W. A., and

Gado, M.: Analysis of gas in vacuum lumbar disc. Am. J. Roentgenol. *128*:1056–1057, 1977.

33. Frain, C., and Lacroix, F.: Effect stratigraphique et coupes horizontales. C. R. Acad. Sci. (Paris), *224*:973, 1947.

34. Gargano, F. P., Jacobson, R. E., and Rosomoff, H.: Transverse axial tomography of the spine. Neuroradiology, *6*:254, 1974.

35. Gargano, F. P., Meyer, J. D., and Sheldon, J. J.: Transfemoral ascending lumbar catheterization of the epidural veins in lumbar disk disease. Radiology *111*:329–335, 1974.

36. Gargano, F. P., Meyer, J., Houdek, P. V., and Charyulu, K. N.: Transverse axial tomography of the cervical spine. Radiology *113*(2):363, 1974.

37. Gargano, F. P.: Axial tomography of the lumbar spine. *In* Rothman, R. H., and Simeone, F. A. (eds.): The Spine, Vol. 2, Philadelphia, W. B. Saunders Co., 1975.

38. Gargano, F. P.: Transverse axial tomography of the spine. Crit. Rev. Clin. Radiol. Nucl. Med. *8*(3):279–328, 1976.

39. Gargano, F. P., Jacobson, R., Post, and Donovan, M. J., Transverse axial tomography of the spine. Orthop. Rev. *6*(2):77–80, 1977.

40. Gershater, R., and St. Louis, E. L.: Lumbar epidural venography. Radiology *131*:409–421, 1979.

41. Ghelman, B., and Freiberger, R. H.: The limbus vertebra: An anterior disc herniation demonstrated by discography. Am. J. Roentgenol. *127*:854–855, 1976.

42. Gill, G., Manning, J., and White, H.: Surgical treatment of spondylolisthesis without spinal fusion. J. Bone Joint Surg. *37A*:493, 1955.

43. Gill, G., and White, H.: Mechanism of nerve-root compression and irritation in backache. Clin. Orthop. *5*:66, 1955.

44. Ghormley, R.: Low back pain with special reference to the articular facets with presentation of an operative approach. J.A.M.A. *101*:1773, 1933.

45. Goldner, L. J.: Personal communication.

46. Goldthwait, J.: The lumbosacral articulation, an explanation of many cases of lumbago, sciatica, and paraplegia. Boston Med. Surg. J. *164*:365, 1911.

47. Gonsette, R.: An experimental and clinical assessment of water-soluble contrast medium in neuroradiology: A new medium-dimer-X. Clin. Radiol. *22*:44–56, 1971.

48. Grainger, R., G. Kendall, B. E., and Wylie, I. G.: Lumbar myelography with metrizamide — a new nonionic contrast medium. Br. J. Radiol. *49*:996–1003, 1976.

49. Hadley, L.: Anatomico-roentgenographic studies of posterior spinal articulation. Roentgenology *86*:270, 1961.

50. Hakelius, A., and Hindmarsh, J.: The comparative reliability of preoperative diagnostic methods in lumbar disc surgery. Acta Orthop. Scand. *43*:234–238, 1972.

51. Hammerschlag, S. B., Wolpert, S. M., and Corta, C. L.: Computed tomography of spinal canal. Radiology *121*:361–367, 1976.

52. Hancock, D.: Congenital narrowing of the spinal canal. Paraplegia *5*:89, 1967.

53. Harris, R., and Macnab, I.: Structural changes in the lumbar intervertebral discs. J. Bone Joint Surg. *35B*:304, 1954.

54. Haughton, V., and Correa-Paz, F.: Double contrast myelography. Invest. Radiol *12*:552–554, 1977.

55. Helender, C. G., and Lendblem, A.: Sacrolumbar venography. Acta Radiol. *44*:410–416, 1955.

56. Hertzog, E.: La tomomyelographie cervicale haute transversale. Acta Radiol. (Diagn.) *1*:721, 1963.

57. Hilton, R. C., Ball, J., and Benn, R. T.: Vertebral end-plate lesions (Schmorl's nodes) in the dorsolumbar spine. Ann. Rheumatol. *35*:127–132, 1976.

58. Hinck, V. C., Hopkins, C. E., and Clark, W. M.: Sagittal diameter of lumbar spinal canal in children and adults. Radiology *85*:929, 1965.

59. Hirsch, C. L.: On lumbar facetectomies, Acta Orthop. Scand. *17*:240, 1948.

60. Holt, E.: The question of lumbar discography. J. Bone Joint Surg. *50*:720–726, 1968.

61. Jacobson, R., Gargano, F., and Rosomoff, H. L.: Transverse axial tomography of the spine. J. Neurosurg. *42*:406, 1975.

62. James, H. E., and Cliff, M.: Computed tomography in spinal dysraphism. J. Comptr. Assisted Tomog. *1*:341–397, 1977.

63. Jones, R., and Thompson, J.: The narrow lumbar canal: A clinical and radiological review, J. Bone Joint Surg. *50B*:595, 1968.

64. LaRocca, H., and Macnab, I.: Value of pre-employment radiography assessment of the lumbar spine. R. Ind. Med. *39*(6):253–258, 1970.

65. LePage, J. R.: Transfemoral ascending lumbar catheterization of the epidural veins. Radiology *111*:337–339, 1974.

66. Lewin, T.: Osteoarthritis in lumbar synovial joints — a morphologic study, Acta Orthop. Scand. (Suppl.) *73*:5–108, 1964.

67. Loman, R., and Robinson, F.: Progressive vertebral interspace changes following lumbar disc surgery. Am. J. Roentgenol. Radium Ther. *97*:664, 1966.

68. Macnab, I.: Spondylolisthesis with an intact neural arch "pseudospondylolisthesis." J. Bone Joint Surg. *32B*:325, 1950.

69. Macnab, I.: The management of spondylolisthesis. Prog. Neurol. Surg. *4*:246, 1971.

70. Macnab, I., and Dall, D. E.: The blood supply of the lumbar spine and its application to the technique of intertransverse lumbar fusion. J. Bone Joint Surg. *50B*:628, 1971.

71. Macnab, I., St. Louis, E. L., Grabias, S. L., et al.: Selective ascending lumbosacral venography in the assessment of lumbar disc herniation. J. Bone Joint Surg. *58A*:1093–1098, 1976.

72. Macnab, I.: Backache. Baltimore, Williams and Wilkins Co., 1977.

73. Magnussen, W.: Über die Bedingungen des Herrortretons der Werkluken Gelenkspatte auf dem Rontgenbilde. Acta. Radiol. *18*:733–741, 1937.

74. Magora, A., and Schwartz, A.: Relation between the low back pain syndrome and x-ray findings. Scand. J. Rehabil. Med. *8*:115–125, 1976.

75. Nashold, B., and Hrubec, A.: Lumbar Disc Disease. A Twenty-Year Clinical Follow-up Study. St. Louis, The C. V. Mosby Co., 1971.

76. O'Dell, C. W., Coel, M. N., and Ignelzi, R. J.: Ascending lumbar venography in lumbar disc disease. J. Bone Joint Surg. *59A*:159–163, 1977.

77. Paine, K., and Haung, P.: Lumbar disc syndrome, J. Neurosurg. *37*:75, 1972.

78. Patrick, B. S.: Lumbar discography: A five year study. Surg. Neurol. *1*:267–273, 1973.

79. Picard, L., et al.: Scarring of the theca. Neuroradiol. *4*(1):29–48, 1977.

80. Post, M. J., Gargano, F. P., Vining, D. Q., and

Rosomoff, H. L.: A comparison of radiographic methods of diagnosing constrictive lesions of the spinal canal. J. Neurosurg. *48*:360–368, 1978.

81. Putti, V.: New conceptions in the pathogenesis of sciatic pain. Lancet *2*:53, 1927.

82. Ratheke, L.: Über Kalkablagerungen in den Zwischenwirbelscheiben. Fortschr. Roint. Gentstr. *45*, 1932.

83. Resnick, D., and Niwayama, G.: Intervertebral disk herniations: Cartilaginious (Schmorl's) nodes. Radiology *126*:57–65, 1978.

84. Roberson, G. H., Llewellyn, H. J., and Taveras, J. M.: The narrow lumbar spinal canal syndrome. Radiology *107*:89, 1973.

85. Roland, J., Treil, J., Larde, D., et al.: Lumbar phlebography in the diagnosis of disc herniations. J. Neurosurg. *49*:544–550, 1978.

86. Schatzker, J., and Pennal, G.: Spinal stenosis, a cause of cauda equina compression. J. Bone Joint Surg. *50B*:606, 1968.

87. Schlesinger, E. B., and Taveras, J. M.: Factors in the production of "cauda equina" syndromes in lumbar discs. Trans. Am. Neurol. Assoc. *78*:263, 1953.

88. Schlesinger, P.: Incarceration of the first sacral nerve in a lateral bony recess of the spinal canal as a cause of sciatica. J. Bone Joint Surg. *37A*:115, 1955.

89. Schlesinger, P.: Low lumbar nerve-root compression and adequate operative exposure, J. Bone Joint Surg. *39A*:541, 1957.

90. Schmorl, G., and Jungham, H.: The Human Spine in Health and Diseases. New York, Grune and Stratton, 1971.

91. Schobinger, R. A.., Krueger, E., and Sobel, G.: Comparison of intraosseous vertebral venography and Pantopaque myelography in the diagnosis of surgical conditions of the lumbar spine and nerve roots. Radiology *77*:397, 1961.

92. Sheldon, J. J., Russin, L. A., and Gargano, F. P.: Lumbar spinal stenosis. Clin. Orthop. *115*:53–67, 1976.

93. Sheldon, J. J., Sersland, T., and Leborgne, J.: Computed tomography of the lower lumbar vertebral column. Radiology *124*:113–118, 1977.

94. Simmons, E. H., and Segil, C. M.: An evaluation of discography in the localization of symptomatic levels in discogenic disease of the spine. Clin. Orthop. *108*:57–69, 1975.

95. Skalpe, I. O.: Lumbar myelography with Conray melgumine 282. Report of 100 examinations with special reference to the adverse effects. Acta Neurol. (Scand.) *47*:569–578, 1971.

96. Skalpe, I. O.: Adhesive arachnoiditis following lumbar radiculography with water soluble contrast agents. Radiology *121*;647–651, 1976.

97. Spangfort, E. V.: The lumbar disc herniation. A computer-aided analysis of 2504 operations. Acta Orthop. Scand. (Suppl.) *142*:61–77, 1972.

98. Symposium: Lumbar arachnoiditis: Nomenclature, etiology and pathology. Spine *3*(1):21–92, 1978.

99. Taillard, W.: Etiology of spondylolisthesis. Clin. Orthop.. *117*:30–39, 1976.

100. Theron, J., Houtteville, J. P., Ammerich, H., et al.: Lumbar phlebography by catheterization of the lateral sacral and ascending lumbar veins with abdominal compression. Neuroradiology *11*:175–182, 1976.

101. Torgerson, W. R., and Dotter, W. E.: Comparative roentgenographic study of the asymptomatic and symptomatic lumbar spine. J. Bone Joint Surg. *58A*:850–853, 1976.

102. Vallebona, A.: Nouvelle methode roentgenstratigraphique. Radiol. Clin. (Basel) *16*:279, 1947.

103. Verbiest, H.: A radicular syndrome from developmental narrowing of the lumbar vertebral cord. J. Bone Joint Surg. *36B*:230, 1954.

104. Verbiest, H.: Further experiences on the pathological influence of a developmental narrowness of the bony lumbar vertebral canal. J. Bone Joint Surg. *37B*:576, 1955.

105. Vernon-Roberts, B., and Pirie, C. J.: Degenerative changes in the intervertebral discs of the lumbar spine and their sequelae. Rheumatol. Rehabil. *16*:13–21, 1977.

106. Weinstein, M. A., Ruthner, A. D., Duchesneau, P., and Dohn, D. F.: Computed tomography in diastematomyelia. Radiology *11*:609–611, 1975.

107. Wiesel, S., Ignatius, P., Marvel, J. P., et al.: Intradural neurofibroma stimulating lumbar disc disease. J. Bone Joint Surg. *58A*:1040–1042, 1976.

108. Williams, P., and Yglesias, L.: Lumbosacral facetectomy for post-fusion persistent sciatica. J. Bone Joint Surg. *15*:579, 1933.

109. Woolsey, R.: The mechanism of neurological symptoms in spondylolisthesis. J. Neurosurg., *11*:67, 1954.

CONGENITAL ABNORMALITIES OF THE LUMBAR SPINE AND THEIR RELATIONSHIP TO DISC DISEASE

The relationship between congenital structural abnormalities of the spine to disc degeneration is poorly understood. Too often, fallacious reasoning has created misunderstandings in this field. A patient with back pain shows a structural abnormality on his radiograph, and, therefore, it is assumed that the abnormality is the cause of the pain. Recent epidemiologic studies have dispensed with many of these misunderstandings.[2, 3] Only through large-scale radiographic investigation of both symptomatic and asymptomatic individuals can knowledge useful in terms of the etiology of the back symptoms be generated. Relating one group of abnormalities, such as the congenital structural changes, to a second group of abnormalities, such as disc degeneration, either or both of which may be asymptomatic, becomes rather difficult.

Increased Lumbar Lordosis

Theoretically, one might expect an increased lumbar lordosis to subject a lower

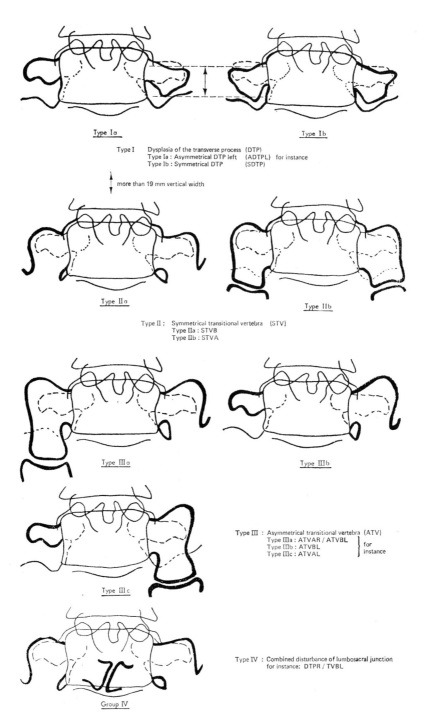

Figure 9–96. Classification of lumbosacral transitional vertebra. (From Timmi, P. G., Wieser, C., and Zinn, W.: The transitional vertebra of the lumbosacral spine: Its radiological classification, incidence, prevalence and clinical significance. Rheumatol. Rehabil. *16*:180, 1977.)

lumbar disc to excessive shearing and stresses and thereby to lead to the early onset of lumbar disc degeneration. Several population studies have given no support to this hypothesis. Magora and Schwartz[5] did appreciate a higher roentgenographic incidence of degenerative disc disease in patients with increased lumbar lordosis, but importantly, this was not associated with increased symptomatology.

Somewhat surprisingly, increased inclination of the lumbosacral joints seem to protect it against anular damage.[2, 3, 9] As previously stated, rotatory stress seems to have greater significance than flexion and extension stress, and thus the part played by lordosis may be minor.

Sacralization and Lumbarization

The transitional vertebrae may be either lumbarized sacral vertebrae or sacralized lumbar vertebrae. There is a great variation in both symmetry and degree. The normal lumbar transverse process may be slightly increased in size, or it may be solidly fused to the sacrum. This may occur either unilaterally or bilaterally. Timmi and colleagues[11] presented a detailed classification of the anomalies of segmentation found at the lumbosacral joint (Fig. 9–96). While their findings suggested a genetic factor working in the production of the anomaly, they did not find any relationship between the presence of an anomaly and low back pain. The more completely sacralized the lumbar vertebrae is, the more stable it will be. The discs between the transitional vertebrae and the sacrum will usually be vestigial. Ruptures and degeneration of this disc are extremely uncommon. When disc degeneration or rupture occurs in relationship to a transitional vertebra, it is almost always above the level of the transitional vertebra.

Spina Bifida

There is no evidence to indicate that spina bifida statistically predisposes an individual to back pain or disc degeneration. It is being found more frequently in patients with spondylolisthesis,[8] but whether this is coinicidental or causal is uncertain.

A few isolated cases have been reported in which a spina bifida occulta associated with a prominent spinous process of L5 produced compression of the cauda equina in extension.[10]

Tropism of the Facets

Asymmetrical orientation of the lumbosacral facets is termed "tropism." The studies of Farfan and Sullivan[1] indicate that the incidence of anular tears is related to the orientation of the facets. They found that asymmetrical articular processes led to asymmetrical degeneration. This protrusion tended to be on the side of the more oblique joint surface. Theoretically, this occurs because of an abnormal rotatory stress acting on the anulus, producing degenerative changes. Approximately half of the torque resistance of the intervertebral joint is supplied by the posterior elements, and of this, the greatest percentage is by the facet joints themselves. When both facets are oriented in the sagittal direction, rotational forces are inhibited and there is decreased torque. Theoretically, this is the best configuration. Conversely, when one facet is oriented in the sagittal direction and the other in the coronal direction, one not only loses rotational stability, but a cam action is present as well. These suppositions are supported by studies relating facet orientation to disc herniation,[1] but the presence of facet tropism in and of itself is probably not related to the presence of back pain.[6]

The specific facet anomaly that has been frequently confused with facet fracture has been called the ossicle of Oppenheimer. This free ossicle, best appreciated on oblique radiographs of the lumbosacral spine, involves the inferior articular facets, usually around the L3 level.[7] This anomaly has no clinical significance and bears no known relationship to degenerative disc disease.[4]

Lumbosacral Tilt and Leg Length Discrepancy

Tilting of the pelvis may occur with abnormal development of the lumbosacral facets, with abnormal development of the sacrum and pelvis, and with inequality of leg lengths. There is no evidence to indicate that these entities contribute to back pain or disc degeneration.[2, 3]

References

1. Farfan, H. F., and Sullivan, J. D.: The relationship of facet orientation to intervertebral disc failure. Can. J. Surg. *10*:179–185, 1967.
2. Horal, J.: The clinical appearance of low back dis-

orders. Acta Orthop. Scand. (Suppl.) *118*:7–109, 1969.

3. Hult, L.: The Munkfors investigation. Acta Orthop. Scan. (Suppl.) *16*:5–102, 1954.
4. LaRocca, H., and Macnab, I.: Value of pre-employment radiographic assessment of the lumbar spine. Industr. Med. *39*:31–36, 1970.
5. Magora, A., and Schwartz, A.: Relation between the low back pain syndrome and x-ray findings. Scan. J. Rehabil. Med. *8*:115–125, 1976.
6. Nachemson, A.: The lumbar spine — an orthopaedic challenge. Spine *1*:59, 1976.
7. Oppenheimer, A.: The apophyseal intervertebral articulations, roentgenologically considered. Radiology *30*:724, 1938.
8. Roche, M. D., and Rowe, G. G.: The incidence of separate neural arch in coincident bone variations. J. Bone Joint Surg. *34A*:491, 1952.
9. Splitoff, C.: Roentgenographic comparison of patients with or without backache. J.A.M.A. *152*:1610, 1953.
10. Stark, W. A.: Spina bifida occulta and engagement of the fifth lumbar spinous process. Clin. Orthop. *81*:71–72, 1971.
11. Timmi, P. G., Wieser, C., and Zinn, W. M.: The transitional vertebra of the lumbosacral spine: Its radiological classification, incidence, prevalence and clinical significance. Rheumatol. Rehabil. *16*:180–185, 1977.

ALGORITHM FOR TREATMENT OF LUMBAR DISC DEGENERATION

The task of the spinal surgeon, as he approaches the patient with low back pain, is to return that patient as promptly as possible to a normal functional existence. The ability to achieve that idealized goal is dependent not so much on technical excellence in the operating room as it is on the precision and accuracy of decision-making. In an effort to help physicians improve their decision-making capacities, the authors have developed a treatment algorithm at Pennsylvania Hospital to analyze these very difficult and complex situations.

The plan outlined is derived not only from evaluating their therapeutic successes but also, and probably of greater significance, from evaluating the clinical course of the patients who have failed to respond to operative measures of treatment — the so-called "salvage back." By relying heavily on this clinical data, a format and an approach have been developed that will optimize therapeutic efforts by basing decision-making on well-delineated rules rather than on emotion and intuition. Webster defines an algorithm (Fig. 9–97) as "a set of rules for solving a particular problem in a finite number of steps."

The algorithm can then be followed in sequence. Assume that a treating physician has examined these individuals and has come to the conclusion after this initial interview and examination that the symptoms are secondary to lumbar disc degeneration. Assuming that these patients have not been previously treated, the overwhelming majority should be instructed to begin a course of conservative therapy. Only the patient with a frank cauda equina syndrome or unequivocal progressive motor weakness should proceed along the more aggressive line of myelography and possible surgery. The early stage of treatment of lumbar disc disease is a waiting game. The passage of time, the use of salicylates, and bedrest are the modalities that have proved themselves safest and most effective. We advise an initial period of conservative treatment along these lines for up to six weeks. In our experience, only one or two patients per year justify following the pathway towards initial surgical intervention.

However, in the face of a frank cauda equina syndrome or truly progressive motor weakness, equivocation and procrastination are not warranted, and a vigorous recommendation for myelography is indicated. In these instances, the myelogram will almost always be clearly positive and should be promptly followed by lumbar laminectomy. One can almost always expect dramatic resolution of pain, if not motor deficit, with prompt return to normal life patterns. Even in these patients, one might argue that the data substantiating this aggressive surgical posture are not adequate; however, at the present time, our recommendation remains as stated.

Those individuals who respond to conservative treatment after their initial encounter should be mobilized with the use of a lightweight flexible corset when they have achieved approximately 80 per cent relief of their symptoms. Once they have been able to return to increased function and are more comfortable, we would begin a program of isometric lumbar flexion exercises with subsequent return to a normal life pattern. The pathways along this portion of the algorithm are two-way streets, and should regression occur with exacerbation of symptoms, one can simply resort to more stringent conservative measures, returning to the use of a corset and, if necessary, further bedrest. The vast majority of patients with acute low back pain will proceed along this pathway, returning to a normal life pattern within two months from the onset of their symptoms.

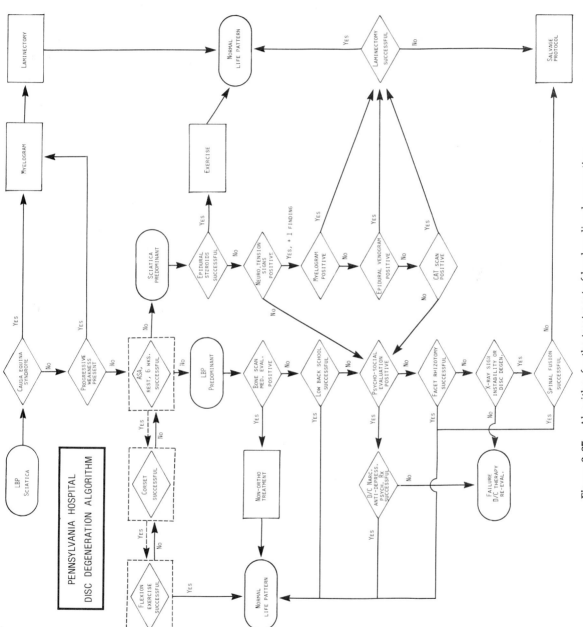

Figure 9–97. Algorithm for the treatment of lumbar disc degeneration.

If this initial battery of conservative measures has failed and six weeks have passed, then we would advise sorting these patients into two groups; the first in which sciatica is predominant and the second in which low back pain predominates. In those patients in whom *low back pain* is the predominant and persisting symptom despite six weeks of conservative measures, we would advise a technetium bone scan and complete medical evaluation by an internist. In those patients in whom *sciatica* is the predominant and persisting symptom, we would escalate our conservative therapy to include the use of epidural steroids on either an inpatient or outpatient basis. There are a multitude of alternate types of conservative treatment available, such as traction and manipulation, but unfortunately they have *not* stood the test of scientific scrutiny and thus should not become a routine part of the treatment program. Occasionally, there may be a patient in whom traction will be utilized and even in whom it is helpful, but as a group, patients treated with traction improve at no more rapid a rate than those treated simply by bedrest alone. In patients who undergo epidural steroid therapy, this treatment may be repeated on one or two occasions. We will usually allow an additional six weeks to pass before considering epidural steroid therapy a failure.

If the epidural steroids are effective in alleviating sciatica, then the patient should be started on a program of isometric lumbar flexion exercises and should be promptly encouraged to return to a normal life pattern. Again, this pathway will usually be complete in less than three months. If the epidural steroids have not shown themselves to be effective and if three months have passed with persistent and intolerable sciatica, then surgery should be considered. At this point, one must carefully reevaluate the patient in terms of the presence of a neurologic deficit and a tension sign, such as the straight leg raising test or sitting root test.

It has been repeatedly documented that for surgery to be effective in the treatment of sciatica, the surgeon must find unequivocal evidence of nerve root compression at surgery. In order to predict this mechanical root compression, he must have firm substantiation, not only in the neurologic examination but also in terms of radiographic data, before proceeding with laminectomy. If the patient has neither a neurologic deficit nor a positive tension sign, then we feel that regardless of the radiographic findings, there is inadequate evidence of root compression to proceed with surgery. Those individuals who have unremitting complaints but a paucity of findings will then be directed toward a psychosocial evaluation in an effort to explain this discrepancy. Those individuals who have either a neurologic deficit or a positive tension sign are subjected to a myelogram. If the myelogram is clearly positive, then surgery should be promptly undertaken. If the myelogram is negative, it is possible that a lateral disc herniation that lies beyond the dural pouch and root sleeve is present. An epidural venogram should be performed for these individuals, and it may reveal lateral herniation. If this is positive, surgery would then be indicated. If the epidural venogram is unrevealing, we would then proceed to computer assisted tomography to substantiate that bony foraminal encroachment may be present but not seen either on the myelogram or venogram. If the scan is positive, surgery in the form of foraminotomy would be recommended. If all these radiographic modalities are unrevealing, then the patient would be denied surgery and would proceed to a psychological evaluation. Exceptions to these operative criteria should be few and far between. In the authors' experience, when sympathy for the patient's complaints has outweighed the objective evaluation, surgical endeavors have been fraught with great difficulty. The explorations have been almost always unrevealing and thus unrewarding. In individuals who have met these firm criteria for lumbar laminectomy, the results are overwhelmingly satisfactory, and one could expect 95 per cent of these patients to have a good or excellent result.

Let us now return to those patients who were originally classified as predominantly having back pain and who failed to respond to the initial program of conservative treatment. They will undergo a bone scan and medical evaluation by an internist. The bone scan has been found to be an excellent survey tool, often identifying early spinal tumors and infections not seen on routine radiographic examination. In actuality, if the authors had one diagnostic study available in patient management, they would prefer the bone scan to routine radiographic examination. The internist's thorough search will also frequently reveal problems, such as the posterior penetrating ulcer, pancreatitis, and abdominal aneurysms, that we as orthopaedists may not have the expertise or facility to diagnose. If these diagnostic studies are positive, the patient would be transferred into nonorthopaedic treatment and no longer would be in our therapeutic algorithm. If these patients are not found to have an abnormality on their bone scan and are not shown to have other medical disease as a cause for their back pain, they then would be referred for a second level of therapy, which is the low back school. This concept has as its basis the belief that patients with low back pain, given proper education and understanding as to their disease and the proper forms of self-administered conservative therapy, can often return to a productive and functional life. Ergonomics, the proper and efficient use of the body in work and recreation, is stressed. This type of educational process is both inexpensive and effective, a most desired set of qualities.

If the low back school is effective during its four week curriculum, then the patient may return to a normal life pattern and is discharged. It is critical that before a patient is referred to this type of facility, he must be thoroughly screened, as has been outlined, so that one is not in the position of treating tumors and infections in classrooms.

If, however, the low back school has failed, then these patients should undergo a thorough psychosocial evaluation in an attempt to explain the failure of the usually effective therapeutic measures for low back pain. The use of a psychosocial evaluation is predicated on the knowledge and belief that a patient's disability is related not only to the pathologic anatomy but also to his perception of pain and his stability in relationship to his sociologic environment. Only the most myopic physician would deny that the patient's psychologic profile and ability to function in a specific environment have a part to play in the treatment of low back pain. All spinal surgeons see the patient with a frank herniated disc who is able to continue working and who regards this as only a trivial and annoying problem. At the other end of the spectrum, one sees the hysterical patient who takes to bed immediately upon the slightest twinge of lumbago. The type of psychosocial evaluation utilized would depend on the needs of the patient and the facilities available to the treating physician. The type of symptoms would also dictate in part the studies required. The Minnesota Multiphasic Personality Inventory

and consultation by a psychiatrist expert in the treatment of chronic low back disorders are routinely utilized. In addition, the differential spinal block is utilized for those persons with a significant component of leg pain, and the thiopental (Pentothal) interview is used for those whose symptoms are primarily axial in nature. At this point it is not uncommon to uncover drug habituation, depression, and other psychiatric and psychologic causes for magnification and propagation of the pain complaint. If the evaluation is revealing of this type of pathologic emotional state, then proper measures are instituted to overcome the disability. It is shocking to note the numbers of ambulatory patients who present with addiction to oxycodone hydrochloride (Percodan) and diazepam (Valium), alone or in combination. The authors strongly feel that the use of these drugs should be kept at an absolute minimum. Percodan is truly addicting, and Valium is both habituating and depressing. The complaint of low back pain is a common expression of depression, and to treat these individuals with Valium is not only foolish but also detrimental to their welfare. In a patient whose symptoms seem primarily an expression of depression, great usefulness has been found in the antidepressant drugs such as amitriptyline (Elavil). Because of the moderate side effects with the use of Elavil, this drug has been utilized with the tranquilizer–antidepressant combination of perphazine and amitriptyline (Triavil). It has been the most effective antidepressant with the least number of unpleasant side effects. The type of psychiatric and psychologic treatment indicated will depend on the background of the patient, his intelligence and insight, and the means available to afford this type of treatment. Unfortunately, psychiatric therapy is expensive and demanding of a high level of insight and motivation. Psychologists and psychiatric clinics with ancillary personnel such as psychiatric social workers are often a reasonable answer. Programs of behavior modification such as operant conditioning have shown themselves to be useful in certain situations in returning patients to a more productive way of life, but conclusive data supporting their use are not available at the present time. If the patient is unwilling or unable to follow the program outlined, continues the use of narcotics, and rejects or fails the recommended psychiatric treatment, then the patient must be considered a failure. Discontinuation of medical therapy would be advocated at that time. To continue random measures of treatment for these individuals without correcting their underlying psychosocial disorder is a waste of time, money, and medical facilities. They should be discharged from therapy with the offer to reevaluate them in one year should they wish to reenter the treatment protocol. If patients are able to rid themselves of the use of narcotics and respond to the psychiatric counseling offered, they will usually be able to return to a normal life pattern without further orthopaedic treatment.

Returning to those patients who have persistent back and leg pain and in whom no psychosocial abnormality was detected, facet rhizotomy might be utilized. The candidate for this procedure should be a patient with persistent back pain, with or without referred leg pain, and without documentation of nerve root compression. This therapeutic measure has not faced the scrutiny of a double-blind prospective study, but our early investigations do show some usefulness and little potential for harm. It must be stated that the ultimate role of this modality is not yet defined and is still under study. If this treatment measure is successful, then the patient can return promptly to a normal life pattern. If, on the other hand, the facet rhizotomy fails to alleviate back pain, the lumbar spine radiographs should be carefully studied for unequivocal evidence of instability or localized disc degeneration. For these purposes, instability would be defined as to and fro motion with flexion and extension, reversal of the normal lordotic position of the motion segment, or traction osteophytes at one level. In patients with unremitting mechanical back pain who have not responded to prolonged conservative treatment and in whom no psychosocial disorder is found, spinal fusion may be of help.

If these radiographic stigmata of instability or localized disc degeneration are not present, then the patient must be considered a failure of treatment, and therapy should be discontinued. There are no further measures that will benefit these individuals, and they should be offered reevaluation in one year to be certain their clinical picture has not changed and to determine if any occult disease process can be uncovered. If the decision to proceed with spinal fusion is undertaken, the surgeon and the patient must both be ready to accept a level of effectiveness of approximately 75 per cent. The failure rate after spinal fusion in these patients is considerably higher than the failure rate after laminectomy for the criteria outlined earlier. If success is gained with the use of spinal fusion, the patient should be encouraged to promptly return to a normal life pattern. If the spinal fusion has failed, then the patient will proceed to the salvage protocol discussed earlier. It should be emphasized that few patients will be candidates for spinal fusion at this point in the algorithm, and in the authors' practice, only three or four patients per year will require arthrodesis for disc degeneration. By far the greater number of patients with low back pain will have improved with conservative measures or will have been found to have non-orthopaedic causes for the low back pain or psychosocial disturbances.

The authors have found that with the use of this decision-making algorithm, their patients receive the therapeutic measures most helpful at the optimal time and are neither denied helpful surgery nor submitted to operations that are useless surgical exercises.

CONSERVATIVE TREATMENT OF LUMBAR DISC DISEASE

The goals to be established in the nonoperative treatment of lumbar disc disease should be threefold: (1) relief of pain, (2) increase of functional capacity, and (3) slowing of disease progression.

At our present state of knowledge the first two goals are frequently within the reach of the treating physician. The last and most important is not. Reports on the efficacy of various types of conservative therapy vary tremendously. One of the most optimistic of these reports claims that in a group of 400 patients with acute disc lesions, only two required operative intervention after conservative therapy.[15] Our own experience has led us to become more cautious in responding to inquiries about the possible failure of conservative therapy and the necessity for operative intervention. Approximately 20 per cent of patients with a firm diagnosis of an acute disc hernia will ultimately require surgery when followed over a period of years. This is in agreement with several reports in the literature.[4, 12, 13]

The results of conservative treatment of patients with disc disease will depend in part on the criteria for including a patient in this study group. Colonna and Friedenberg,[4] utilizing the strict criteria of myelographic demonstration of disc protrusion, found a relatively low recovery rate of about 30 per cent. In a similar vein, Weber's prospective study utilizing strict clinical and roentgenographic prerequisites also found that results at one year following conservative management were not as good as those results following surgery.[21] After four years of follow-up study, however, there was no statistically significant difference between surgery and conservative management. It is of interest that the neurologic deficits remaining (excluding cauda equina syndrome and rapidly progressive deficits) at four years of follow-up study were independent of the treatment modality utilized.

The question of efficacy of nonoperative treatment depends not only on the diagnostic and intellectual capabilities of the physician but also on his ability to educate the patient and provide proper emotional support during his problem. Success will depend on the willingness of the patient to accept not only various levels of chronic and acute pain but also altered functional capacity. It must be kept in mind and emphasized to the patient that disc degeneration is not a lethal disease. If the patient is willing to live with the pain, it is his prerogative to persist with the course of conservative therapy despite the treating physician's feeling that it has failed and operative intervention is required. A decision for surgical intervention should not be made ex cathedra but by the patient and the physician on the basis of mutual understanding, confidence, and trust. The patient with a bona fide disc lesion who does not respond to conservative therapy in a reasonable length of time should be granted the benefit of surgical intervention to allow him a more comfortable and active life.

The course of conservative therapy will be presented here as it evolved over a period of years and was found to be effective in a large patient population. The reasons for its efficacy are often hypothetical, but it has been shown on an empiric basis to be the most efficient approach to problems of acute and chronic disc lesions.

Bedrest

The most important element of therapy in acute lumbar disc lesions is an adequate period of bedrest. This conclusion has been derived empirically over the years and has received support through biomechanical and clinical studies.

Nachemson has established in vivo data verifying that in the vertebral disc, pressure can be significantly reduced with the supine posture.[18] Related work by Anderson and Ortengren[1] has demonstrated a reduction of dorsal and abdominal muscle activity as one assumes a more horizontal position. Assuming the validity of the clinical correlation of increasing pressure and increasing symptoms in the lumbar spine, bedrest would seem to be the rational first line in conservative management. Indeed, disc pressures and facet joint reactive forces in the lumbar spine are due to the summation of the force of gravity as well as associated muscle force vectors called upon to provide stability in the upright stance.

Clinically, Wiesel and Rothman[23] conducted a randomized study on the efficacy of bedrest in acute low back pain in 80 basic combat trainees. All patients had back pain, but none had tension signs or neural deficits indicative of radiculopathy. While one group of 40 patients were kept at complete bedrest, the second group of 40 patients were kept ambulatory but excused from any physical activity. Both groups received acetaminophen. The bedrest group returned to full duty 50 per cent faster and experienced 60 per cent less pain than the ambulatory group.

Prescribed bedrest can be accomplished most effectively at home, where the patient is in comfortable and familiar surroundings and is cared for by his family. Should he lack adequate facilities of good home care, he should be admitted to the hospital for this treatment. It is expected that the patient will remain in bed with the exception of bathroom privileges for bowel movements once or twice a day either with the use of a bedside commode or a nearby toilet facility. A short period of ambulation necessary to reach the bathroom is frequently less stressful than the acrobatics required to utilize a bedpan. If a firm mattress is available, we feel that bedboards are not necessary and in many instances will actually increase the level of discomfort noted by the patient.

While in bed, the patient should be placed in a position so that the hips and knees are flexed to a moderate but comfortable degree. This has been found to be particularly necessary in disc herniations at the L4-5 level. The patient is cautioned against sleeping in a prone position, which will result in hyperextension of the lumbar spine. A natural or synthetic "sheepskin" will provide additional comfort if prolonged periods of bedrest are required.

The duration of this period of bedrest is of prime importance. Too frequently patients are mobilized and allowed to return to work before the inflammatory reaction of disc herniation or musculotendinous strain has subsided. When the disability is due to an acute disc herniation, a minimum of two weeks is required at complete bedrest whether at home or in the hospital. Subsequent to this, a week to 10 days of gradual mobilization is instituted if the patient has had substantial relief of pain and is free of list and paravertebral muscle spasm. It should be mentioned parenthetically that the patient with profound motor loss or with a progressive neurologic deficit should undergo operative intervention. These patients are not candidates for conservative therapy. It is unrealistic to expect a patient with frank disc herniation to return to full activities in less than one month. Compromise on this point is frequently sought by the patient but in the long run will not be to his benefit. It should be pointed out to the patient that operative intervention in itself requires a prolonged period of rehabilitation and that strict adherence to a conservative program may preclude the necessity of operative intervention.

Based on our present knowledge of the pathophysiology of disc degeneration, it is the authors' feeling that bedrest is important so that the secondary inflammatory reaction to disc degeneration may subside. Bedrest is not instituted with the expectation that an extruded fragment will return to its original place within the anulus. Once extruded into the anulus beneath the posterior longitudal ligament, a fragment of nuclear material does not return to its original location. In many instances, however, if the edema and hyperemia of the soft tissues and nerve roots surrounding the extruded fragment are allowed to subside, the patient will become free of acute back pain and sciatica. This relief may or may not be permanent. As noted earlier, the work of Nachemson has shown that only in the horizontal position is the disc free of significant stress. The sitting position places substantial burden upon the lumbar disc; therefore, patients should be clearly informed that sitting at a desk or in an armchair does not provide adequate relief from stress on the lumbar spine.

Traction

Traction is a popular nonstandardized conservative treatment modality for low back pain and sciatica that has been used over the centuries. The principle behind its utilization is that of unloading the spine by stretching muscles and ligaments and eventually significantly decreasing the intradiscal pressures. The realization of this goal, however, is not easily achieved. Nachemson and Elfstrom[19] concluded that a distraction force equivalent to 60 per cent of body weight is necessary to reduce intradiscal pressure at L3 only 25 per cent when the patient is standing. Moreover, even in the supine posture a reduction of only 20 to 30 per cent of intradiscal pressure when as much as 30 kilos of traction are applied for three seconds can be accomplished.[19] Since the discs are prestressed owing to the advantageous position of the posterior ligaments of the spine,[20] zero intradiscal pressures have not been realized with actual traction.

These methodologic limitations and the clinical and empirical acceptance of this treatment modality has led to double-blind studies on the effects of actual traction on patients suffering from sciatica.[21, 22] No significant statistical differences were appreciated between the groups receiving real and only apparent traction in terms of relieving symptoms. Furthermore, Weber[21] found that traction had no effect on spinal mobility, tension signs, deep tendon reflexes, paresis, sensory deficit, or the consumption of analgesics. In some cases one might not only accomplish little amelioration of symptoms but also actually may aggravate symptoms,[7] although the treatment is usually well tolerated.

The use of traction, however, should not be totally discredited. Weber[21] appreciated a positive psychologic effect as to the patient's expectations for recovery while in traction. The authors, however, have found that traction is occasionally helpful in enforcing a prescription of bedrest, which is the most important facet of conservative management utilized.

Manipulation

Empicirism has also fostered popularity of the use of spinal manipulation as a conservative modality in treating the low back pain syndrome. The principle behind its use is based on the assumption that subluxation of the vertebrae precipitates low back complaints and that these complaints can be reduced with correction of the "misalignment." There is, however, "no scientific proof for or against either the efficacy of this spinal manipulation therapy or the pathophysiological foundation from which it is derived."[2]

Separate randomized studies in England designed to evaluate the efficacy of spinal manipulation therapy when compared to other conservative therapy failed to demonstrate any significant difference at one and three weeks after treatment.[6, 9] It was of interest, however, that a more rapid relief of pain was realized with manipulative therapy. Kirkaldy-Willis and Hull[14] have also found manipulation effective in well-defined posterior facet and sacroiliac joint syndromes.

Manipulative reduction of small disc protrusions has been reported,[5, 17] and reductions in the severity of the straight leg raising tension have also been demonstrated, but much skepticism remains.[3]

Grieve[10] has hypothesized the following mechanism that may contribute to the short-term effects of manipulation: (1) relief of pain by an inhibitory effect on afferent painful stimuli; (2) relief of muscle spasm; (3) effect on tissue fluid exchange in collagenous tissue; (4) restoration of movement; and (5) placebo effect.

At this point in time, however, there are no scientific data to support its use on a regular basis with low back pain or sciatica secondary to degenerative disc disease. It has not been shown to shorten the course of symptomatic disc disease or lessen the morbidity. In cases of pathologic bone disease involving the lumbosacral spine, manipulation may be harmful.

References

1. Andersson, B. J. G., and Ortengren, R.: Myoelectric back muscle activity during sitting. Scand. J. Rehabil. Med. (Suppl.) 3:73–90, 1974.
2. Anonymous: The scientific status of the fundamentals of chiropractic analysis and recommendations. National Institute of Neurological and Communicative Disorders and Stroke. April 8, 1975.
3. Chrisman, O. D., Mittrracht, A., and Snook, G. A.: A study of the results following rotatory manipulation in the lumbar intervertebral disc syndrome. J. Bone Joint Surg., 46A:517, 1964.
4. Colonna, P. C., and Friedenberg, Z.: The disc syndrome. J. Bone Joint Surg. 31A:614–618, 1949.
5. Cyriax, J.: Dural pain. Lancet 1:919–921, 1978.
6. Doran, D. M., and Newell, D. J.: Manipulation in treatment of low back pain. A multi-center study. Br. Med. J. 1:161–164, 1975.
7. Eie, N., and Kristiansen, K.: Komplikasjouer os farer sed tzakljoulehandling av lumbale skiveprolape. T. Morske Loejeforen 81:1517–1520, 1961.
8. Fink, J. W.: The straight leg raising test. Its relevance to possible disc pathology. N. Z. Med. J. 81:557–560, 1975.
9. Glover, J. R., Morris, J. G., and Khosla, T.: Back pain: A randomized clinical trial of rotational manipulation of the trunk. Br. J. Ind. Med. 31:59–64, 1974.
10. Grieve, G. P.: Manipulation. Physiotherapy 61:11–18, 1975.
11. Hakelius, A.: Prognosis in sciatica. Acta Orthop. Scand. 129:6–76, 1970.
12. Henderson, R. S.: The treatment of lumbar intervertebral disc protrusion. Br. Med. J. 2:597–598,1952.
13. Key, J. A.: The conservative and operative treatment of lesions of the intervertebral discs in the low back. Surgery 17:291–303, 1945.
14. Kirkaldy-Willis, W. M., and Hull, R. J.: A more precise diagnosis for low back pain. Spine 4(1):102–109, 1979.
15. Marshall, L. L.: Conservative management of low back pain: A review of 700 cases. Med. J. Aust. 1:266–267, 1967.
16. Mathews, J. A., and Hickling, J.: Lumbar traction: A double blind controlled study for sciatica. Rheumatol. Rehabil. 14:222–225, 1975.
17. Mathews, J. A., and Yater, D. A. H.: Reduction of lumbar disc prolapse by manipulation. Br. Med. J. 3:696–697, 1969.
18. Nachemson, A.: The load on lumbar disks in different positions of the body. Acta Orthop. Scand. 36:426, 1965.
19. Nachemson, A., and Elfstrom, G.: Intravital dynamic pressure measurements in lumbar disc. Scand. J. Rehabil. Med. (Suppl.) 1:5–40, 1970.
20. Nachemson, A.:Rheumatology and Rheumatism.
21. Weber, H.: Lumbar disc herniation. A prospective study of prognostic factors including a controlled trial. J. Oslo City Hosp. 28:36–61, 89–103, 1978.
22. Weber, H.: Traction therapy in sciatica due to disc prolapse. J. Oslo City Hosp. 23:167–179, 1973.
23. Wiesel, S. W., and Rothman, R. H.: Acute low back pain. An objective analysis of conservative therapy. Clin. Orthop. 143:290, 1979.

Flexion Exercises

Lumbar flexion exercise becomes important in the subacute or chronic phases of lumbar disc degeneration (Fig. 9–98). The use of lumbar flexion exercise is based on the theory expounded by Williams.[6] The overall aim is to reduce the lumbar lordosis. The reversal of the lumbar curve and full flexion of the lumbosacral joint will accomplish this goal. Subluxed overriding facet joints are

Lumbar spine exercises.

Two exercise sessions every day: (Morning and night *OR* afternoon and night).

Start with two (2) of each and gradually increase to ten (10) of each (twice a day), over a period of 10 days to two weeks.

1. Stand with back against wall and heels flat on the floor. Flatten "small" of back against wall by rotating pelvis up and forward.

   NOTE: No space between small of back and wall.

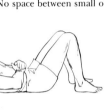

2. Lie on back with knees bent and feet flat on floor. Place hands on abdomen. Raise head and upper part of spinal column while contracting abdominal muscles.

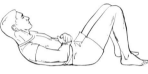

3. Lie on back. Separate legs. Bend knees and hips, and draw knees up toward axillae by clasping them with hands. *NOT TO BE DONE BY POSTOPERATIVE SPINE FUSION PATIENTS.*

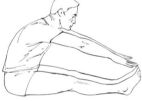

4. Sit on floor with legs outstretched. Touch toes without bending knees. When able to touch toes, stretch beyond toes. "Spring."

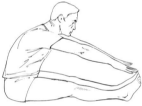

5. Lie flat on back. Without bending knees, lift one leg straight up, bending at hip; then the other; then both together.

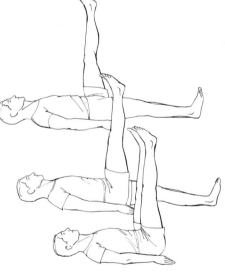

Figure 9–98. Lumbar spine exercises.

placed in the position where they no longer overlap. Second, the spine is placed in a position of greater stability where the shearing stresses are minimized at the lower lumbar levels. Third, the intervertebral foramina are widened, allowing maximal room for exit of the nerve roots. A fourth goal of lumbar flexion exercises is to strengthen the abdominal musculature and the flexors to the spine. Both of these muscle groups have been shown to be important in supporting the spine and alleviating stress on the intervertebral disc. All the goals and the reasons for the effectiveness of a lumbar flexion exercise program are open to question. Their efficacy, however, on an empiric and clinical basis has been clearly shown.

Lumbar flexion exercise should not be instituted in acute disc herniation until the patient's symptoms have subsided to the point at which list and paravertebral muscle spasm are no longer noted and the major part of the acute symptomatology has subsided. This will usually be two to three weeks after the initiation of conservative therapy. Exercises are then started in a very gentle manner and are immediately discontinued if a flareup of the patient's symptomatology appears. They may be reinstituted at a later date when the patient's tolerance for them has increased. It is not necessary, however, to wait until the patient is asymptomatic before instituting this program of exercise.

General Measures of Back Hygiene

Along with a program of lumbar flexion exercises, the patient with lumbar disc degeneration should be educated in certain measures of back hygiene that are in accord with flexion management of these disorders. He should be instructed to sleep on his side or back with his legs and hips in a position of flexion. He should be cautioned against the prone position, which hyperextends the lumbar spine. If this patient is in a hospital bed, Fowler's position should be utilized. When sitting in a chair, he should sit with the buttocks well forward and the spine in a flexed position. This position is sometimes referred to as "slumping" and is regarded with a sense of horror by many physical therapists. It is our feeling, however, that people will habitually assume this situation because of the comfort it provides. Crossing the legs while seated will add further flexion to this position and is also desirable. Lifting heavy loads above the waist should be prohibited, particularly those in which the patient is forced to rock back in a position of hyperextension. When picking up a load from the floor, the patient must be cautioned to utilize the musculature of the legs and bend from the knee and hip rather than from the thoracic and lumbar spine. It is most important, however, that the length of the lever arm (the distance between the lumbar spine and the object being lifted) utilized during lifting be kept at a minimum.[1] While most patients can be instructed on these prophylactic aspects of back hygiene at an office visit, a structured, multifaceted approach has been designed particularly for the chronic and subacute low back pain patient. The concept of the back school was conceived in 1970 by Zachrisson-Forcel, a physiotherapist at the Danderyd Hospital in Sweden.[3, 8] The audiovisual program that evolved found its data base in the currently appreciated anatomic, epidemiologic, and biomechanical factors that give rise to low back pain.

Initially, the patient is introduced to the goals of the back school and the anatomy and physiology contributing to the various back disorders. The various treatment modalities described all emphasize natural healing processes which, if allowed, would lead to amelioration of symptoms.

The patient is then instructed in the applied biomechanics of the spine and how posture analysis can allow one to reduce the forces that come to bear on the lumbar spine and precipitate symptoms. Muscle function, particularly of the abdomen, is emphasized as the intrinsic dynamic support that one can actively utilize to improve low back function.

The final goal of the program is to emphasize that back hygiene can most effectively be realized if the patient remains physically and socially active despite the apparent physical handicap. Thus far, this multifaceted approach has yielded more encouraging results than routine physiotherapeutic modalities.[7]

Physical Therapy

The use of local heat and light massage are well tolerated and pleasant for most patients with low back pain syndrome, but aside from their relaxing capabilities, they add little to the efficacy of bedrest alone.

BRACES AND CORSETS

Routine immobilization of the lumbar spine will rapidly lead to soft tissue contracture and muscle atrophy. For this reason, the use of rigid lumbar braces is seldom recommended. The young patient with degenerative disease is more advantageously treated with a program designed to increase range of motion, strength, and musculature rather than one based upon immobilization.

There are, however, certain instances in which the external support plays a useful role. The obese patient with poor abdominal musculature is frequently fitted with a firm corset with flexible metal stays (Fig. 9–99). This corset serves the function of reinforcing the abdominal musculature and thereby increases the patient's efficiency in utilizing the thoracic and abdominal cavities to support and extend the spine.[4] Nachemson and Morris[5] demonstrated that the support realized with the lumbosacral corset is reflected in diminution of intradiscal pressure of approximately 30 per cent.

The mechanism by which the thoracic and abdominal cavities act as an extension of the spine is discussed in Chapter 2, Anatomy of the Spine. It would, of course, be preferable to train these patients to develop their abdominal musculature and shed unneeded adipose tissue.

The second category of individuals for whom braces are utilized are elderly individuals with advanced multilevel degenerative changes. These patients will not tolerate an exercise program, and, indeed, their symptoms are frequently intensified by a program of mobilization. Depending upon the extent of their disease, a Knight-Taylor brace with shoulder straps or possibly a short lumbosacral brace with rigid metal stays is utilized to partially immobilize the spine and place these arthritic joints at rest (Fig. 9–100). With bracing, marked relief of pain is rapidly achieved in these individuals. It is frequently possible to wean these people from this support, and this should be attempted if possible after their acute symptoms subside. This is to prevent further loss of muscle tone and stiffness in an already weakened spine.

Bracing is no longer utilized in the postoperative management of patients who have undergone spinal fusion. If more than a two level spinal fusion is undertaken (that is, L3 to the sacrum or longer), the brace may be utilized.

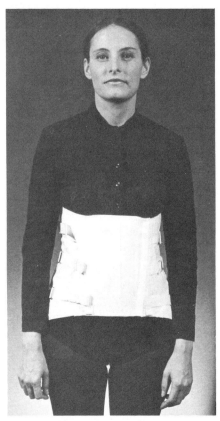

Figure 9–99. The lumbosacral corset with flexible metal stays utilized for abdominal and spinal support.

Pregnancy and Lumbar Disc Problems

One of the most challenging problems confronting the orthopaedic surgeon is the pregnant patient presenting with symptoms of disc degeneration. It is our feeling that the intervertebral disc is placed under excessive stress during pregnancy for two reasons. The first of these is the obvious extra burden of carrying the fetus, and the second is the unusual ligamentous laxity found during pregnancy. The laxity is caused by maternal production of relaxin and relaxin-like hormones. Relaxin is a hormone found in many mammals that produces the ligamentous laxity about the pelvis necessary for the birth of offspring that may be larger than the bony pelvic outlet. It is possible that a similar hormone produced near term in humans may contribute to the development of congenital hip dislocation and can certainly be of importance in producing relaxation of the ligamentous supporting structures of the spine.

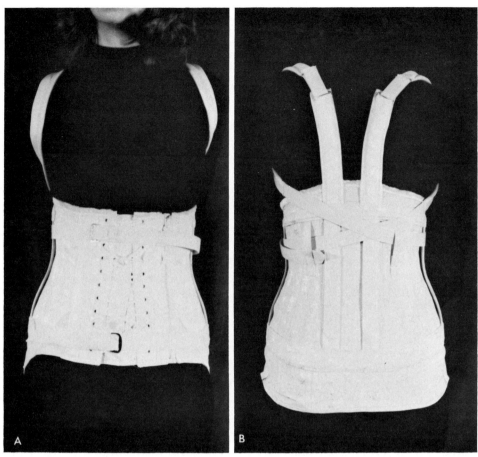

Figure 9–100. Knight-Taylor brace; *A*, front, *B*, back.

Therapeutic modalities available during pregnancy are somewhat limited. For the most part, one must depend upon bedrest and the use of a supporting corset, although the latter method is frequently very uncomfortable. A very well tolerated alternative is a century-old supporting corset that has been used by the Japanese during the latter months of pregnancy. This "Iwata-Obi" is a Japanese maternity support that is made up of approximately five yards of eight inch cotton cloth with the lateral third being made of soft elastic material. The terminal four inches of cotton are tapered to allow for easy tucking or pinning after it has been wrapped around the lower abdomen to provide for greater support. Empirically, this device seems to increase abdominal support that has been lost by the attenuated muscle fibers, particularly in the latter months of pregnancy.[2]

The physician hesitates to prescribe potent and potentially teratogenic drugs during pregnancy. Diagnosis is also somewhat hampered by the limited use of radiography during the first trimester of pregnancy. Surgery, of course, is the last resort during pregnancy and is indicated only in the presence of serious neurologic findings. It is often necessary to prescribe long periods of bedrest for a pregnant patient in order for her to obtain a measure of relief. The use of a firm, flexible corset or the Japanese modification is of great help in relieving the spine of excessive stress.

References

1. Andersson, B. J. G., Ortengren, R., and Nachemson, A.: Quantitative study of back loads in lifting. Spine *1*(3):178–185, 1976.
2. Hecter, A. W., Budd, F. W., and Curlin, J. P.: "Iwata Obi" (Japanese maternity lumbosacral support). Military Medicine 359–360, 1972.
3. Lidstrom, A., and Zachrissen, M.: Physical therapy on

low back pain and sciatica. An attempt at evaluation. Scand. J. Rehabil. Med. 2:37–42, 1970.

4. Morris, J. M.: Low back bracing. Clin. Orthop. 102:120–132, 1974.

5. Nachemson, A., and Morris, J. M.: In vivo measurements of intradiscal pressure: Discometry, a method for determination of pressure in the lower lumbar disc. J. Bone Joint Surg. 46A:1077, 1964.

6. Williams, R. C.: Examination and conservative treatment for disc lesions of the lower spine. Clin. Orthop. 5:28–35, 1955.

7. Williams, S. J.: Back school. Physiotherapy 63:590, 1977.

8. Zachrissen, M.: The low back pain school. Danderyd's Hospital, Danderyd, Sweden, 1972.

Drug Therapy

The intelligent use of drug therapy is an important modality in the treatment of lumbar disc disease. Three categories of pharmacologic agents are utilized: (1) anti-inflammatory drugs, (2) analgesics, and (3) muscle relaxants.

Both mechanical compression of neural structures and inflammatory reaction contribute to the symptoms of low back pain and sciatica. The inflammatory reaction is most likely due to the local irritant sequela of nerve compression as well as the poorly understood autoimmune phenomenon.

Gertzbein and others[2] have summarized the following clinical observations that support the contention that an inflammatory reaction contributes to the pathogenesis of the various degenerative disc syndromes:

1. In entrapment syndromes, the predominant feature is numbness and paresthesiae as opposed to pain, which is predominantly a feature of inflammation.

2. The findings at surgery are compatible with perineural inflammation and in a later stage with perineural fibrosis.

3. The microscopic picture of vascular ingrowth, granulation, and fibrosis in degenerative discs is compatible with an inflammatory reaction.

4. Patients treated with local or systemic anti-inflammatory drugs report dramatic relief.

Several double-blind studies have compared various anti-inflammatory drugs in treatment of low back pain with or without sciatica, and generally no difference in their efficacy was demonstrated.[1, 4, 5, 8, 9] Most of these studies, however, do not quantify the contributing beneficial effects of bedrest prescribed along with the various medications.

Wiesel and Rothman[9] concluded that aspirin or phenylbutazone (Butazolidin) in conjunction with bedrest were no more effective in relieving symptoms of acute lumbago than bedrest with the non-anti-inflammatory acetaminophen. Green,[3] however, found that initially high but tapering doses of the steroid dexamethasone was beneficial in the treatment of sciatica from myelographically proved disc hernia that had failed to respond to bedrest alone.

In principle, the authors feel that anti-inflammatory medication, particularly aspirin, 10 to 15 grains every four hours, should be utilized in conjunction with bedrest for treatment of low back pain due to disc disease with sciatica. In those individuals with gastrointestinal intolerance, buffered or enteric coated aspirin or the liquid methyl salicylate can be safely used.

It has been the authors' experience, as well as others',[3, 7] that certain patients who fail to show a response to aspirin may get dramatic relief from the use of short-course systemic steroids. They can be administered either in the hospital or at home with the patient aware that he must adhere to the prescription instructions explicitly. The dosages of dexamethasone prescribed are 6 mgs. four times on day 1, 4 mgs. four times on day 2, 2 mgs. four times on day 3, 1 mg. three times on day 4, 0.75 mg. twice on day 5, 0.5 mg. twice on day 6, and 0.5 mg. once on day 7. This regimen has been well tolerated even in patients with a history of peptic ulcer disease and diabetes when used with appropriate precautions.

As patients resolve their acute disc symptoms, they may have residual chronic symptomatology of low back pain that will require anti-inflammatory medications, usually in doses lower than those used for the acute episodes.

The judicious use of analgesics is of extreme importance during the acute phase of disc disease. It is our feeling that if pain is of such severe nature that parenteral narcotics are required, then morphine sulfate is the drug of choice. The dosage should be adequate to insure substantial relief of the patient's symptoms. Patients must be reassured that pain medication is available for their use and that a stoic attitude is therefore not essential. Many times during the acute early phases of treatment, the narcotics will be ordered on a regular basis rather than as the patient requests them. This will relieve the patient of the burden of summoning and waiting for nurses to obtain pain medication. Constipation is an untoward side effect of many of the opiates, and a stool softener should be added to the regimen if prolonged use of narcotics is required. As pain subsides, oral codeine or non-narcotic analgesics may be substituted for more potent drugs.

The authors infrequently use muscle relaxants, which may be effective at times in acute disc lesions in which muscle spasm is a prominent finding. Methocarbamol and carisoprodol are the drugs most commonly used for this purpose. Either of them may cause drowsiness. Carisoprodol is used in a dosage of 350 mg. two times daily, and methocarbamol is used in a dosage of 1.5 gm. four times daily. Occasionally, in an extreme acute problem of marked paravertebral muscle spasm, therapy will be initiated with the use of 10 ml. of intravenous methocarbamol, which is then continued with the oral form of the drug. This will frequently produce striking relief of both pain and limitation of motion. Muscle relaxants are rarely used in the chronic or subacute phase of disc degeneration.

It has been found useful to add a sedative or a mild tranquilizer to the patient's regimen to alleviate any anxiety and make a prolonged period of bedrest more tolerable. Phenobarbital in 15 to 30 mgm. doses four times daily will accomplish this goal. The use of diazepam in chronic and acute low back pain as either a muscle relaxant or tranquilizer should be discouraged[6] since it is actually a depressant and will accentuate the depression that is often an integral feature of an individual's symptom complex. In contrast, the cautious use of antidepressants, such as amitriptyline or thioridazine, is often of great help in the depressed patient who expresses inner conflict as low back pain.

References

1. Barretter, R. R.: A double blind comparative study of carisoprodol, propoxyphene and placebo in the management of low back syndromes. Curr. Ther. Res. *20*:233–240, 1976.
2. Gertzbein, S. D., Tile, M., Gross, A., and Falk, R.: Autoimmunity and degenerative disc disease of the lumbar spine. Orthop. Clin. North Am. *6*:67, 1975.
3. Green, L. N.: Dexamethasone in the management of symptoms due to herniated lumbar disc. J. Neurol. Neurosurg. Psychiatry *38*:1211–1217, 1975.
4. Hingorani, K., and Templeton, J. S.: A comparative trial of azapropazone and ketoprofen in the treatment of acute backache. Curr. Med. Res. Opin. *3*:407–412, 1975.
5. Jaffe, G.: A double blind multi-center comparison of naproxen and indomethacin in acute musculoskeletal disorders. Current Med. Res. Opin. *4*:373–380, 1976.
6. Mooney, V., and Cairns, D.: Management of patient with chronic low back pain. Orthop. Clin. North Am. *9*:543–557, 1978.
7. Naylor, A., and Turner, R.: ACTH in treatment of lumbar disc prolapse. Proc. R. Soc. Med. *54*:15–16, 1961.
8. Vignon, G.: Comparative study of intravenous ketoprofen versus aspirin. Rheumatol. Rehabil. *15*:83–84, 1976.
9. Wiesel, S. W., and Rothman, R. H.: Acute low back pain. An objective analysis of conservative therapy. Clin. Orthop. *143*:290, 1979.

THE OPERATIVE TREATMENT OF LUMBAR DISC DISEASE

Indications for Surgery

If the various nonsurgical treatment modalities discussed in the section on conservative management are not successful, then surgery becomes the "conservative management" of choice.

PROFOUND OR PROGRESSIVE NEUROLOGIC DEFICIT

The most dramatic presentation of an acute disc herniation is the cauda equina syndrome, and this is the most certain indication for immediate surgical intervention. If bowel, bladder, and sexual function are to be preserved, immediate decompression of the cauda equina is imperative. The complex interplay of compression, edema, and vascular insult to the cauda equina secondary to disc herniation alone or in combination with surgical intervention makes a prediction as to outcome difficult. The temporal framework within which the syndrome develops and within which surgical treatment is realized are likewise factors that affect the prognosis.

In any event, the rarity of spontaneous recovery of sexual and sphincter function[5] makes myelographic definition and rapid surgical decompression of paramount importance.

Motor weakness requires more judgment in terms of urgency as a criterion for surgical intervention. Owing to their functional importance, acute complete paralysis of the quadriceps muscle or acute complete paralysis of the dorsiflexors of the foot are indications for surgical decompression of the involved spinal nerves. The more prolonged the pressure on the spinal nerve and the more intense the compression, the less likely is the return of function. It should be stated, however, that this guideline is not absolute, and in the authors' experience, several cases have been seen in which the recommended decompression under these circumstances was not undertaken and the patient had complete restoration of function with time.

In Weber's[8] excellent prospective study, the degree of residual paresis was similar in the surgically and conservatively treated groups after three years. It is possible that the surgical results were compromised by an initial period of nonoperative management. The authors agree with Weber — with acute profound motor weakness, decompression should be performed as soon as possible. When lesser degrees of motor weakness are present, judgment must be exercised as to when surgery should be recommended. If the weakness is mild to moderate and compatible with adequate function of the extremity, a period of observation and conservative treatment is indicated. This is particularly true in subacute and chronic situations. However, if the motor weakness is progressive in nature and becomes significant in terms of function, then surgical intervention is mandatory.

Sensory and reflex changes are helpful in terms of diagnosis but are not in themselves indications for surgical intervention and are of no prognostic value in predicting the ultimate outcome of the disease. Weber found sensory dysfunction in nearly 46 per cent of his total series of patients after four years. The abnormalities encountered existed either prior to treatment or developed subsequent to either surgical or conservative management. It is interesting to note that no patient was disabled because of sensory deficits. Similarly, a diminution or loss of reflex in the face of lessening pain would certainly not be an indication for surgery.

UNRELENTING SCIATICA

Occasionally, an acute attack of sciatica will fail to respond to all forms of conservative treatment. The exact time after which surgery should be recommended will vary from patient to patient according to their pain tolerance,

emotional stability, and the demands of their socioeconomic environment. In general, the authors do not recommend surgical consideration in acute sciatica before a period of four to six weeks has elapsed.

Since 80 per cent of Weber's nonsurgically managed group showed "good" or "fair" results within three months, observation is justified for this period of time. After this period of conservative treatment with little or no improvement, surgical intervention should be undertaken. Further procrastination will adversely affect the results of surgery.

RECURRENT EPISODES OF SCIATICA

In certain individuals, after an initial successful course of conservative treatment, they will have recurrent sciatica that becomes incapacitating. There may be a complete absence of symptoms between the acute episodes, or low-grade sciatica may continue to a greater or lesser extent. If the recurrent episodes are not disabling and if the intensity of the symptoms is within the patient's emotional tolerance, then persistent conservative therapy is indicated. However, if the frequency and intensity of the attacks are severe enough to interfere with the individual's ability to follow gainful employment and enjoy normal activities of daily living, then surgery should be undertaken. In general, the authors would consider surgery only after three recurrent episodes, but there is variation in this regard.

PERSONALITY FACTORS

Care must be taken to evaluate both the emotional stability of these patients and their reaction to pain. A person who continues to have minor symptoms with conservative therapy but who has an overwhelming emotional reaction to this pain, particularly if an element of hostility is present, will usually do poorly even after surgery.

The authors, however, emphasize that this admonition is not proposed in order to differentiate the "functional" from the "organic" back pain patient. Indeed, it would be naive to overlook the reciprocal interaction between the patient's somatic and emotional state. Rather, effective management of this disabling episode of pain may rest on coincident psychotherapeutic support, carefully monitored antidepressant medication, or both.[4]

An efficient and rapid psychiatric assessment[10] can be elicited using the following points of subjectivity:

1. Has the patient's pain precipitated adverse mood changes? (That is, are the patient's "spirits down?")

2. Has there been an onset of vegetative behavioral changes (appetite alterations, sleep disturbances, and diminution in libido)?

3. Has the pain created problems at home or work?

4. Has the patient demonstrated an appropriate response to management thus far?

The use of the MMPI Conversion 5 profile as demonstrated by Hanvick,[2] its modified form,[9] or the pain drawing screening test introduced by Ransford and others[7] may shed some light on the psychiatric factors involved. In and of themselves, however, these ancillary studies are more a temporal indication of the patient's intensity of the fear of pain rather than a statement about the etiology of that pain.[1, 6]

If any uncertainty as to the emotional stability of the patient is present, psychiatric consultation is mandatory. This is not to say that all patients with emotional problems, particularly those with long-standing pain, should be denied surgical relief. It has been well demonstrated that long-standing pain will lead to depression even in basically stable individuals and that depression will sometimes lift after the pain is alleviated. In general, it is a good rule of thumb to treat the emotional factors prior to rendering a surgical decision. More often than not, intolerable pain becomes quite tolerable once depression has lifted.

In most instances, surgery will be undertaken for the relief of sciatic pain, and its effectiveness will depend on the discovery and relief of pressure upon the neural elements. Ideally, every operative procedure undertaken to relieve sciatica would reveal mechanical compromise of the nerve roots. This is often not the case, and in these instances, surgery will often fail. One might assume that failure to discover mechanical compression is due to one of two factors, either an inadequate exploration or a nonmechanical cause of the sciatica. The former factor may be remedied by more thorough exploration and more complete understanding of the pathologic condition. The nonmechanical sciatica can best be appreciated by an analysis of those factors present in the preoperative evaluation that best correlate with the presence or absence of demonstrable nerve root compression. The most thorough study in this regard is that of Hirsch[3] in a review of some 3000 low back operations. He found that the most significant preoperative factors in the determination of mechanical paraspinal nerve compression were (1) a well-defined neurologic deficit, (2) a positive myelogram, and (3) a positive straight leg raising test. When all these factors are present, surgery will usually uncover mechanical compression and will be followed by a good result. If one or more of these factors is absent, much deliberation should take place before surgery is undertaken. This is not to say that one should not recommend surgery in the absence of a positive myelogram or in the absence of a neurologic deficit but that careful evaluation of these cases should be undertaken. If, for instance, the patient has a well-defined neurologic deficit (such as an absent Achilles reflex), a positive straight leg raising test, and a positive contralateral straight leg raising test, one might expect to find a herniated L5 disc compromising the S1 spinal nerve despite the presence of a normal myelogram. However, if two of three critical factors are missing, such as a positive myelogram and neurologic deficit, one might well expect a negative exploration and failure to relieve sciatica postoperatively.

The authors have recently modified these guidelines as follows. In order to predict mechanical root compression, the patient must have (1) *either* a positive tension sign or a neurologic deficit *and* (2) a correlative finding on contrast studies (metrizamide myelography or epidural venography). With the use of both water-soluble myelography and epidural venography, both of which are highly sensitive, it would be most unusual for us to undertake exploration without radiographic confirmation of root compression. False negative studies are becoming increasingly rare.

References

1. Caldwell, A. B., and Chase, C.: Diagnosis and treatment of personality factors in chronic low back pain. Clin. Orthop. *129*:141–149, 1977.
2. Hanvick, L. J.: MMPI profiles in patients with low back pain. J. Consult. Psychol. *15*:350–353, 1951.
3. Hirsch, C.: Efficiency of surgery in low back disorders. J. Bone Joint Surg. *47A*:991, 1965.
4. Maruta, T., Swanson, D. W., and Swenson, W. M.: Low back pain patients in a psychiatric population. Mayo Clin. Proc. *51*:57–61, 1976.
5. Maury, M., Francois, N., and Skoda, A.: About the

neurological sequelae of herniated interverebral disc. Paraplegia *11*:221–227, 1973.

6. Mooney, V., Cairns, D., and Robertson, J.: A system for evaluating and treating chronic back disability. West. J. Med. *124*(5):370–376, 1976.

7. Ransford, A. O., Cairns, D., and Mooney, V.: The pain drawing as an aid to the psychologic evaluation of patients with low-back pain. Spine *1*(2):127–134, 1976.

8. Weber, H.: Lumbar disc herniation: A prospective study of prognostic factors including a controlled trial. J. Oslo City Hosp. *28*:33–64, 89–120, 1978.

9. Wiltse, L. L., and Rocchio, P. D.: Pre-operative psychological tests as predictors of success of chemonucleolysis treatment of the low back syndrome. J. Bone Joint Surg. *57A*:478–483, 1975.

10. Wolkind, S. N.: Psychiatric aspects of low back pain. Psychotherapy *60*(3):75–77, 1974.

Selection of the Operation

ACUTE DISC HERNIATION

In most individuals with acute disc herniations, the primary compelling symptom that leads to surgery is sciatica. Although the patient may have had many years of preceding troublesome but tolerable back pain, the leg symptoms ultimately will force him toward surgery. In individuals such as this, limited laminectomy with excision of the herniated material as well as excision of the nucleus of the abnormal disc is the procedure of choice. The approach may be limited, and in cases with a wide interlaminar space, little or no bone need be removed. It is essential that the nerve root be completely explored well out through the foramen and be free of all external pressure and tension at the termination of the procedure.

CHRONIC DISC DEGENERATION AND SPINAL STENOSIS

BACK PAIN ONLY. Most individuals with chronic disc degeneration and back pain can be managed effectively with nonoperative treatment. The authors advocate a very conservative posture in regard to surgical treatment of patients with disc degeneration and back pain only. The rationale for this is that disc degeneration often becomes a diffuse process throughout the entire lumbar spine with the passage of time and, furthermore, it is extremely difficult to ascertain which of the several levels may be the source of the patient's pain. Occasionally an individual will develop severe incapacitating back pain that is intractable to medical therapy and is clearly limited to one or two disc spaces. These individuals will obtain relief through arthrodesis of the spine. The procedure of choice is a bilateral spine fusion from the affected level to the sacrum. When surgery is undertaken for this type of diagnostic category, a fusion of L4 to the sacrum is usually undertaken. A bone graft should not be placed in the midline over the lamina, as this will lead to thickening of the lamina with the possible late formation of spinal stenosis (Fig. 9–107). This diagnostic entity of spinal stenosis after midline spinal fusions is seen with greater frequency as experience with spinal fusion increases.

BACK AND LEG PAIN. Patients with chronic disc degeneration will present with a wide variety of ratios of back to leg pain. One extreme is the individual with florid sciatica and negligible back pain. This individual requires decompression only if it can be accomplished without creation of instability during the operation. If a strong component of back pain is present, stabilization at the same time should be undertaken, with a bilateral lateral spinal fusion incorporating the degenerated levels down through the sacrum. This combined procedure of decompression and fusion is also indicated if iatrogenic instability is created (bilateral foraminotomy at one level) or if demonstrable radiographic instability is evident.

The type of pathologic condition present will dictate the extent and type of decompression required. If midline ridging is the only abnormality present and if the nerve roots are free in the foramen, then complete laminectomy of the affected levels with preservation of the facet joints will suffice. If an extrusion of disc material is present, this obviously should be removed, but this is not usually the case in end stage disc degeneration. The disc space need not be entered in the majority of these individuals, since little nuclear material will be present.

Although the symptoms may be unilateral, the authors would advise a complete bilateral laminectomy to prevent contralateral symptomatology in the future. If foraminal encroachment is present, complete foraminotomy is indicated. If a narrow lateral recess is present, this must be unroofed completely out to the pedicle. When possible, the lateral portion of the facet joint is maintained intact. Often this is not possible, particularly on the symptomatic side, and then complete removal of the facets and complete foraminotomy should be undertaken.

In certain individuals, even after foraminotomy and unroofing of the lateral recesses, the nerve root will still be tightly tethered around a pedicle that has undergone a relative descent during disc degeneration. In these individuals, excision of the pedicle must be undertaken. Occasionally, a lateral herniation or the presence of an aberrant ligament, such as the corporotransverse ligament, will cause a nerve root compression distal to the foramen. These sources of nerve root compression, of course, must be corrected.

In the majority of these patients with chronic disc degeneration, a minimum of two levels of decompression are undertaken, i.e., at L5 and L4, but in developmental spinal stenosis a minimum of three levels are decompressed, extending up to L3. The decision as to how far craniad to proceed with decompression will also depend upon the operative findings, and we would not hesitate to advocate complete lumbar decompression from L1 to L5 if the pathologic condition warrants it.

It should be reiterated that laminectomy per se does not create sufficient instability to warrant the combined procedure of decompression and spinal fusion. Only demonstrable segmental instability or iatrogenic instability due to bilateral foraminotomy at the same level are indications for spinal fusion in addition to the decompression.

INDICATIONS FOR FUSION

The questions as to what is the ideal surgical procedure and what is the role of spinal fusion in a degenerated intervertebral disc are as yet unanswered. When reviewing the literature in this field, one is reminded of Josh Billings' cryptic statement, "It ain't what a man don't know that makes him a fool, but what he does know that ain't so." Semmes reviewed 1500 patients in whom only disc excision had been performed and found that 98 per cent considered themselves to have been benefited from their operation.[13] At the other end of the spectrum, Young and Love reviewed a series of 450 patients with a combined procedure and 558 patients with disc excision alone and found that the combined operation relieved both symptoms in 20 per cent more patients than did the operation for removal of the disc alone and that there were three times as many failures to obtain relief of either back or leg pain when the fusion was not performed.[16] There are innumerable other follow-up studies in the literature that fail to resolve these questions. The answers will not be forthcoming until long-term prospective studies are undertaken in which patients in a definite diagnostic category are treated in a random and variable pattern. Until this is done, the proposed benefits of a considered spinal fusion will rest on less than solid ground.

At our present state of knowledge, spinal fusion should be undertaken for the following indications:

1. Acute disc herniations with a protracted significant component of back pain.

2. Chronic disc degeneration with significant back pain and degeneration limited to one or two disc levels.

3. Surgical instability created during decompression with bilateral removal of the facet joints.

4. The presence of neural arch defects coincident with disc disease.

5. The presence of symptomatic and radiographically demonstrable segmental instability.

Surgical Technique

SIMPLE DISC EXCISION

It must be emphasized that the procedure described below is used in young people with evidence of acute, single level soft disc herniation in whom radicular symptoms predominate. This method is designed to minimize the postoperative recovery time yet effectively treat the source of nerve root compression, which is anticipated to be frankly herniated or extruded disc material.

ANESTHESIA. This operation may be performed under spinal, epidural, local, or general endotracheal anesthesia. The authors' preference is for the use of spinal anesthesia. The patient may be awake or asleep as he prefers, but in any event, the patient is able to breathe and cough for himself with minimal disturbance to his physiology. This policy has proved itself to be quite safe and satisfactory during the past 10 years.

POSITION AT OPERATION. The patient is placed in a kneeling position as described on page 171. The abdomen lies free, and the intra-abdominal pressure is reduced, thereby minimizing epidural venous bleeding. This position has proved to be of benefit, and since its adoption epidural bleeding has virtually been eliminated as a cause of concern during surgery. When operative procedures were done in a prone position with pressure on the abdomen, it was not infrequent for the surgeon to visualize distended epidural veins in the operative field. With the use of the abdomen-free kneeling position, however, the epidural veins are collapsed and offer little problem when encountered. Elastic stockings are used routinely.

PREPARATION AND ANTIBIOTICS. Prophylactic antibiotics are utilized in the form of intravenous cefazolin sodium (Ancef). A test dose is administered the night prior to surgery to be certain that no allergy is present. The morning of surgery, the patient is given 0.5 gram of Ancef intravenously and the second 0.5 gram immediately before the incision is made. Intravenous Ancef is continued for 72 hours postoperatively at a dosage of 0.5 gram IV every six hours. The back is widely shaved and scrubbed with an antiseptic soap solution such as Betadine the night prior to surgery and again on the morning of surgery. Betadine solution is used as skin preparation in the operating room.

INCISION. Because this technique emphasizes a minimum of soft tissue dissection, to enhance early ambulation and recovery, accurate placement of the incision is required. Three criteria are utilized to place the incision, which is ordinarily 4 cm. long, directly over the affected disc:

1. Notation of the level of the iliac crest on the plain lumbar spine films.

2. Observation of the skin mark by the myelographic spinal puncture needle and correlation of this scar with the level of needle insertion on the myelographic studies.

3. Palpation of the last spinous process, which is usually S1. By a combination of these landmarks, the operator can ordinarily satisfactorily locate the precise spinous process of concern. The incision runs from the centers of the spinous processes of the vertebrae between which the affected disc lies. Through this small incision the paraspinous muscles are dissected free from the lamina on the appropriate side and held in place with a Taylor retractor. This retractor fits nicely through the incision, and its point comes to rest on the lateral-most extension of the lamina, just beneath the facet joints. The Taylor retractor may either be fixed to the drape or held by a roller gauze looped under the surgeon's foot. Palpation of the lamina at this point will ascer-

tain the appropriate level, since L5 is the lowest vertebra to have a definitive lamina or ligamentum flavum, or both. In addition, the operator may grasp the spinous process with a large towel clip. The sacral spinous process does not move, whereas the other lumbar lamina will be somewhat mobile on normal articulations. This maneuver, incidentally, can demonstrate a particularly "loose" lamina suggestive of spinal instability or spondylolisthesis (Fig. 9–101).

The ligamentum flavum beneath the superior lamina is separated, and a thumbnail-sized opening is rongeured on the inferior margin of the superior lamina (Fig. 9–102). At this point, magnifying loupes of two and one-half power are applied, which greatly enhance the surgeon's ability to delineate fine structures. The ligamentum flavum is opened with a #15 scalpel blade, and a long cottonoid pattie is inserted between the ligamentum flavum and the epidural tissue (Fig. 9–103). A long, thin cottonoid pattie is easily accepted in this space, thereby separating the dura from the subsequent dissection of the ligamentum flavum. The remaining ligament can be excised by sharp dissection or removed piecemeal with the Kerrison punch rongeur. Epidural fat, if present, is removed gently with forceps. At this point, the dura is clearly evident through the laminectomy incision. A separate thin band of ligamentum flavum, which runs along the lateral-most portion of the spinal canal, may have to be removed separately.

The operator is now prepared to inspect the nerve root (Fig. 9–104). This is the most significant portion of the procedure because only by palpation can one assume that the appropriate nerve root is under pressure and thereby responsible for the radicular symptoms. Under loupe magnification, the nerve root is retracted medially with a Freer nasal septum elevator. A thinner instrument with similar contour, the Penfield dissector, can separate the inferior surface of the nerve root dura from the floor of the spinal canal. When there is a significant disc herniation, these two structures are frequently adherent. If difficulty is encountered in retraction of the nerve root, the operator can assume that there is pressure caused by bulging or extruding disc material. If frank extrusion is encountered at this point, an effort should be made to remove it fairly early in the dissection in order to avoid retraction injury to the nerve root. The extruded fragment should be removed intact, if pos-

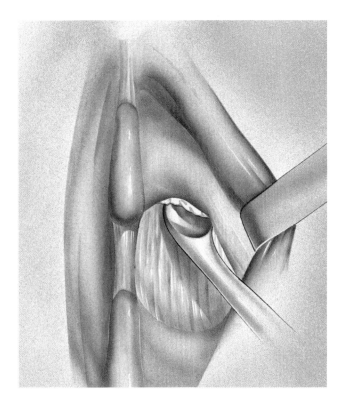

Figure 9–101. The posterior elements of the spine are cleaned of all soft tissue using sharp curets.

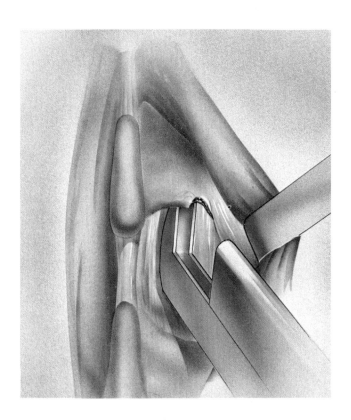

Figure 9–102. The limits of the ligamentum flavum are well defined as are the bony landmarks.

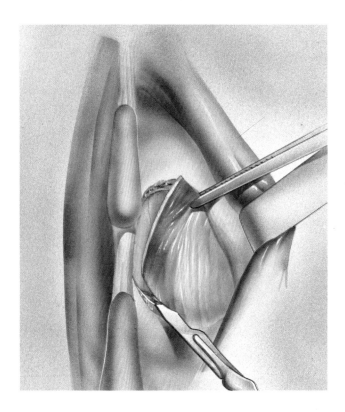

Figure 9–103. The ligamentum flavum is turned down with a fine forceps and excised using a small scalpel. The point of the knife is under direct vision.

Figure 9–104. The extent of bone removal and ligamentum flavum removal prior to nerve root retraction. The lateral border of the nerve root is well seen before the nerve is retracted. Note the extruded nucleus beneath the nerve root.

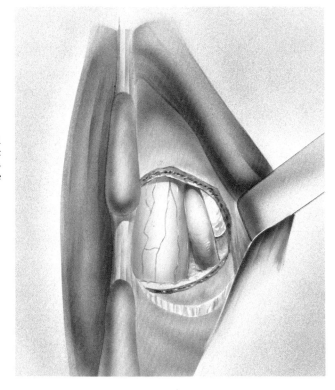

sible, since portions of a fragmented extrusion may be difficult to find subsequently. If a bulging disc is encountered, as is most frequently the case, 1 × 1 cm. cottonoid patties with radiopaque strings can be put in the epidural space after the nerve root is gently retracted over the dome of the disc. Such patties, above and below the disc herniation, can gently retract the nerve root and thereby avoid the hazards of a metal root retractor in the hands of an assistant. Ultimately, with nerve root retractor in place, an area of herniated disc at least 1 cm.^{2} should be visible. It may be necessary to extend the laminectomy lateralward to get sufficient room. Removal of significant portions of the intervertebral facet joint is not necessary in order to expose the usual disc herniation.

The largest possible incision into the anulus fibrosus and disc material is made with a number 15 knife blade on a long thin handle. This is often accompanied by a spontaneous extrusion of the nucleus pulposus. Straight and angled intervertebral disc rongeurs are inserted into the disc material (Fig. 9–105). The surgeon should at all times be aware of the depth to which the rongeur is being inserted. Although the jaws of the rongeur are

operated by the right hand (for a right-handed surgeon) the left hand holds the shaft of the disc rongeur and prevents it from plunging when vigorous "bites" of disc material are extracted. A sense of bottoming is felt when the jaws of the rongeur are closed. The jaws are then opened and advanced a few millimeters into the disc material prior to its excision. The jaws of the disc material should be in contact with the cartilaginous plates of the superior or inferior vertebra during the piecemeal removal of disc material. This technique, along with the surgeon's undivided concentration, will prevent plunging of the disc rongeur into the retroperitoneal space. When the central and lateral-most portions of the nucleus pulposus have been removed, the interspace is entered with a right angled dural separator, and the residual, more fibrotic disc material is separated from the anulus. It is forced into the center of the interspace and retrieved separately with disc rongeurs. Angled curets are then inserted into the interspace, and the disc material is scraped from the cartilaginous plates and again retrieved. Care is taken to effect as complete an excision of the disc material as is possible. The right angled dural elevator is then placed between the nerve root

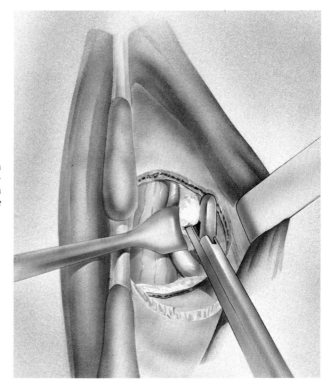

Figure 9–105. Removal of the disc extrusion while the nerve is retracted. The authors recommend retraction of the nerve root with cotton pledgets whenever possible to avoid trauma to the nerve root.

and the site of the former disc herniation in the epidural space. Any residual bulging is flattened by forceful collapse of the elevated area into the interspace.

At this point a careful inspection of the epidural space around the nerve root is made with an appropriate instrument. The nerve root should now be movable with a minimum of force. If there is a resistance to movement or tension the procedure is not complete: A search must be made for extruded disc fragments, perhaps more remote from the laminectomy (Fig. 9–106). If the nerve root continues to be tense, a "foraminotomy" may be performed. With a Kerrison punch rongeur, bone is excised along the course of the exiting nerve root. This could require removal of the medial portion of the interarticular facet joint. This sacrifice must be made, however, if the nerve root cannot be freed in any other way. Our experience indicates that significant portions of this joint can be excised at one level, unilaterally, without subsequent problems. If persistent tension on this nerve root is due to an underlying spondylotic spur, foraminotomy may be the only technique by which the nerve root can be decompressed. Ultimately, the foraminotomy may extend well out beyond

the confines of the spinal canal to the point at which the nerve root curves around the pedicle. If there is evidence of nerve root tension at this point, pedicle removal may be required. At this point, the nerve root is usually quite free. It is not unusual, however, to expose 2 to 3 cm. of nerve root prior to effecting the desired "loose" feeling.

WOUND CLOSURE. After the disc material has been radically removed and the nerve root is free, the entire exposed dura is covered with an autogenous fat graft. This graft is removed with scalpel by dissection from the subcutaneous area, utilizing great care not to interfere with the blood supply to the skin. If no fat is available, then Gelfoam is utilized. The paraspinous muscles are approximated with 00 chromic suture, and the subcutaneous closure is obtained with 00 chromic suture and wire staples for the skin. The postoperative management is the same as described for the other laminectomy techniques discussed in the next section.

LUMBAR DECOMPRESSIVE LAMINECTOMY AND FORAMINOTOMY

This procedure is applied for most cases of symptomatic spinal stenosis, for large acute

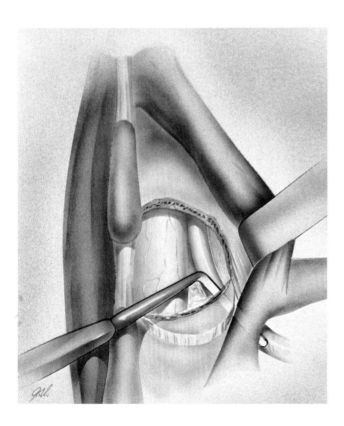

Figure 9–106. Exploration of the intervertebral foramen with a Fraser or malleable uterine probe. The nerve root should be free of both compression and tension.

disc herniations with high degree myelographic block, for multiple myelographic disc defects, particularly when the symptomatic disc is uncertain, and for situations of multiple nerve root involvement. The operation is designed to decompress the lumbar theca and appropriate nerve roots, especially when it may be impossible to actually remove the anteriorly placed source of compression.

ANESTHESIA. As with simple disc excisions, spinal anesthesia is the authors' method of choice.

POSITION AT OPERATION. Again the kneeling position, with abdomen free, is preferred (as previously described).

INCISION. The incision is made at midline and ordinarily covers several of the lower lumbar vertebrae. When the edges of the incision are open and retracted with hemostats, the fascia of the paraspinous muscles is incised at its point of contact to the spinous processes. With a broad, sharp periosteal elevator, the paraspinous muscles are stripped subperiosteally from the spine. Frequent packing with dry sponges maintains hemostasis as the dissection continues. Large, self-retaining retractors are then applied, and the appropriate spinous processes and laminae are identified (Figs. 9–107 to 9–113).

Using the sharp-angled bone cutter, the spinous processes of the appropriate laminae are removed. Using large curets, soft tissue between the laminae is scraped free, and the laminae themselves are gently rongeured. When there is evidence of great pressure, this procedure must be done very carefully with pointed rongeurs. When the myelogram indicates foraminal involvement, particularly with a relatively compression-free central lumbar theca, the laminae and ligamentum flavum can be removed with a large, right-angled Kerrison punch rongeur. Ultimately, the appropriate laminae are removed to the level of the medial surface of the pedicles. If a central decompression is desired and if there has been no significant evidence of radiculopathy, the nerve roots may be inspected for looseness, and the procedure can then be terminated. If there have been radicular symptoms, as is usually the case with the ordinary indications for surgery, the appropriate nerve roots should be inspected. Almost without exception we will inspect the L4, L5, and S1 nerve roots on the involved side. If difficulty in retracting the nerve root is encountered, one ordinarily palpates an an-

teriorly placed, bulging, chronically degenerated disc. Although it may be possible to remove portions of this disc material or even an extruded fragment, it is frequently feasible to decompress the root only by the performance of an extended foraminotomy (as described earlier). The history, neurologic examination, and myelogram will indicate which nerve roots must be explored and which foramina must be opened. If multiple, extensive, bilateral foraminotomies must be done, the procedure is ordinarily followed by a lateral spinal fusion. When the nerve roots are free, the entire exposed dura is covered with an autogenous fat graft.

WOUND CLOSURES. After a sponge count, the paraspinous muscles are approximated with 0 chromic gut, and the skin is closed in two layers. If meticulous hemostasis is obtained, closed drainage is not necessary. Postoperative management is similar to that indicated for the fusion procedure.

INTERPOSITION MEMBRANE

Scar formation about the dural sac and nerve roots after surgical intervention constitutes one of the most frequent causes of postoperative pain. In our experience, this scar formation is almost always present to some extent. It acts as a constrictive force about the neural elements and also tethers the nerve roots to the spine. For reasons that are not well explained, this scar formation causes symptomatology in certain patients and not in others. It may be present for several months or a year before the symptoms become apparent. Surgical removal of this scar tissue in the past has usually led to its recurrence in a short time. Thus, it was with great interest that surgeons concerned with the spine greeted the recent research of Macnab[12] on the etiology and prevention of postoperative scar formation in the neural canal. In the experimental animal, he clearly showed the relationship of postoperative dural scar to surgically exposed muscle. This tendency toward scar formation could be markedly inhibited by the interposition of a resorbable Gelfoam membrane. Attention to atraumatic technique and complete hemostasis were also of obvious importance.

No clinical reports are as yet available on the use of Gelfoam membranes. The authors have used this type of Gelfoam membrane interposed about all areas of the dura and nerve roots for a period of four years in over

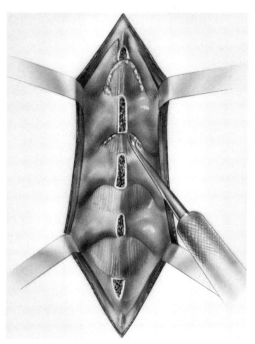

Figure 9–107. Preliminary step for performance of a lumbar decompressive laminectomy. Using sharp curets, all soft tissues are removed from the lamina and interlaminar spaces down to the superficial layers of the ligamentum flavum. The curets used must be sharp and ventral pressure must be avoided. Curettage should be performed against the bony surfaces.

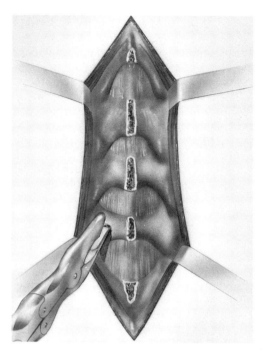

Figure 9–108. Removal of the lamina using a Lexcel rongeur. The rongeur jaws should be closed, then lifted in a ventral direction. Downward pressure must never be exerted against a compromised neural canal.

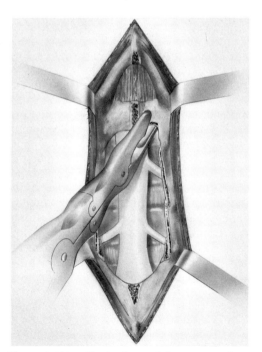

Figure 9–109. The lamina and ligamentum flavum are completely removed. The lateral portion of the facet joints are preserved if possible to retain the structural integrity and stability of the spine. With removal of the fifth, fourth, and a portion of the third lamina, the surgeon should be able to inspect the L4, L5, and S1 nerve roots bilaterally without difficulty.

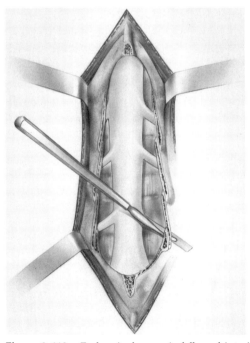

Figure 9–110. Each spinal nerve is followed into its foramen with a uterine probe or Fraser right-angled elevator to be certain that the root is under neither compression nor tension in the area of the lateral recess or foramen.

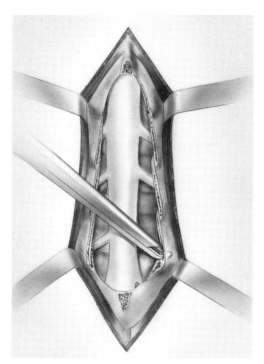

Figure 9–111. Performance of a foraminotomy by removal of the dorsal portion of the facet joints with an angled Schlessinger punch. The instruments follow the path of the spinal nerve with great caution never to exert ventral compression on the neural elements. If the Schlessinger punch will not fit in the foramen, a Sella punch or air drill can be utilized.

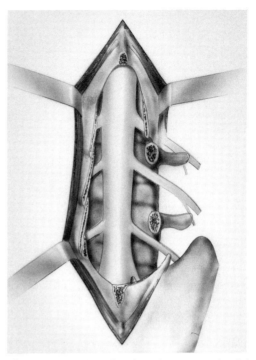

Figure 9–112. Complete foraminotomy on the right, unroofing the L4 and L5 spinal nerves. The lateral portion of the facet joints are preserved on the left to avoid spinal instability.

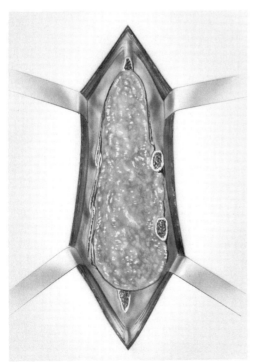

Figure 9–113. At the conclusion of the decompression, an autogenous fat graft is placed about the exposed surface of the dura and spinal nerve to prevent scar tissue formation.

300 cases of nerve root decompression. No ill effects have become evident, although the period of follow-up evaluation is still too short to make a general conclusion.

More recently, during the past two years, the authors have utilized an autogenous fat graft, where available, rather than Gelfoam membranes. This is based on the laboratory studies of Langenskold, Gill, and Jacobs that have indicated that autogenous fat is a more effective deterrent to scar tissue formation than is Gelfoam.[5, 9, 11] Where fat is not available, Gelfoam continues to be utilized.

LATERAL SPINE FUSION

When arthrodesis of the spine is necessary, the authors currently recommend the use of bilateral lateral fusion. Many variations of this technique have been reported in the past.[3, 14, 15] There are several advantages in the use of a lateral fusion. Foremost among these are the certainty of obtaining a solid fusion, the ability to perform the fusion in the absence of the posterior elements, and the prevention of iatrogenic spinal stenosis (Figs. 9–114 and 9–115).

613

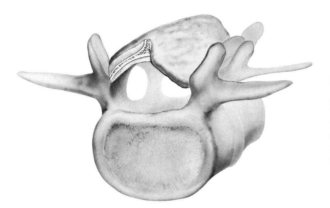

Figure 9–114. This drawing illustrates iatrogenic spinal stenosis due to a midline spinal fusion. The decortication of lamina and application of bone graft in the midline created spinal stenosis through two mechanisms. The first of these is thickening of the lamina and the second is overgrowth of the fusion mass at the cranial end of the fusion dipping into the interspace and compressing the neural elements.

ANESTHESIA. This operation is performed under spinal anesthesia. Cardiac monitors are used on elderly individuals and in the presence of a history of cardiovascular disease.

POSITION AT OPERATION. This procedure is performed in the prone position. If decompressive laminectomy or disc excision

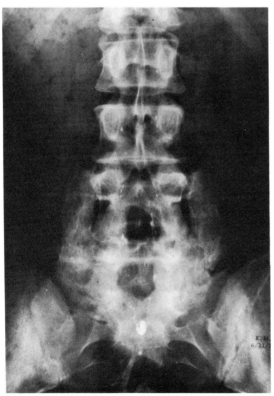

Figure 9–115. Well formed bilateral lateral spinal fusion from L4 to the sacrum. Note the massive appearance of the bone graft from the transverse process of L4 to the ala of the sacrum. No graft material is placed in the midline.

is to be performed at the same time, the kneeling position is utilized to ensure collapse of the epidural veins and to minimize abdominal compression (Fig. 9–116). If only a spinal fusion is to be performed, the patient is placed on a flat operating table with lateral rolls beneath the chest and abdomen to allow breathing space. The anterior iliac crest is centered over the kidney rest, permitting flexion of the table if desired to reduce the lumbar lordosis. Elastic stockings are placed on the patient to prevent thrombophlebitis.

ANTIBIOTICS. The use of antibiotics is advised prophylactically as outlined before.

INCISION. A hockey stick incision is utilized, with the lower pole deviating to the side where the iliac crest graft will be obtained. If an L4 to the sacrum fusion is to be performed, the incision starts above the third lumbar spinous process, continues in a caudal direction to the sacral spinous process, and then deviates gradually 2 inches in a lateral direction (Fig. 9–117). The horizontal component of the lower end of the incision allows easy access to the ilium to obtain graft material. The vertical limb of the incision is carried directly down to the fascia in the midline, without the creation of layers. Absolute hemostasis is obtained at this step. Then, utilizing the electric cutting knife, the fascia is incised from above the third spinous process to the lower portion of the sacrum. Subsequently, utilizing a broad sharp periosteal elevator, the paraspinal muscles are stripped subperiosteally from the spine. This dissection is carried to the facet joints. As this dissection progresses, the wound is packed tightly with sponges to control bleeding. When this is completed, the sponges are removed, and large self-retaining retractors are placed to expose the posterior elements of the spine. At this point, the

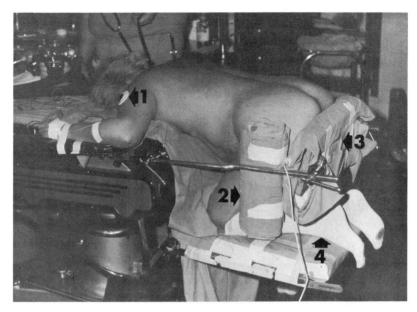

Figure 9–116. Kneeling position utilized for laminectomy and spinal fusion. Note how, even in this obese patient, the abdomen is completely free preventing any pressure on the vena cava.

1. EKG monitoring is used because of the difficulty of listening to the heart sounds in this position.

2. Lateral padding is used to stabilize the patient and prevent pressure on the side bars.

3. The patient is stabilized caudally by the use of a seat to prevent extreme flexion at the knees and hips.

4. Elastic stockings or elastic bandages are used to prevent pooling of blood in the calf area.

surgeon should orient himself carefully through the sacrum and the lower lumbar vertebrae to be certain he is working at the correct levels.

Utilizing a large, sharp-angled bone biter, the spinous processes of the sacrum, the fourth and fifth lumbar vertebrae, and a por-

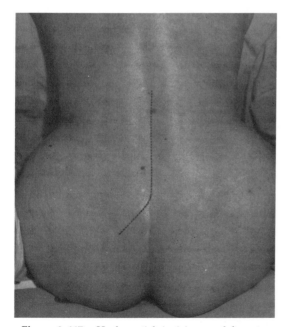

Figure 9–117. Hockey stick incision used for a two level spinal fusion from L4 to the sacrum. Incision extends from the third lumbar spinous process to the sacrum and then deviates laterally to allow exposure of the iliac crest.

tion of the third spinous process are removed. The soft tissues are then meticulously dissected and removed from the posterior elements of the spine down to the ligamentum flavum. This is accomplished with large sharp curets. This dissection is most easily accomplished when started laterally at the facet joints and when the tissues are swept toward the midline, where they are removed with the scalpel. The correct use of the curet is mandatory. Pressure should never be exerted in a downward direction. Rather, the curet should be directed cranially or caudally, allowing it to cut the soft tissues cleanly from bone. It should be stressed that a large curet is infinitely safer than a small one in this area.

If nerve root exploration and decompression are to be undertaken, they may start at this juncture. If not, attention is then turned to exposure of the transverse processes. Using either the electric knife or a sharp periosteal elevator, the fascia is incised directly laterally to the facet joints of L3-L4. As this fascia is incised, the periosteal elevator can sweep laterally along the superior articular facet of L4 and down onto the fourth transverse process. Paraspinal muscles can then be swept laterally, exposing the entire length of the transverse process. When the process is cleaned of soft tissue and completely exposed on its dorsal aspect, this area should be packed with a sponge to control bleeding. The incision in the fascia should then be continued in a caudal direction, and, utilizing the L4-L5 facet joint as a landmark, the fifth transverse process should be exposed in a similar manner. All ligaments and muscles should be dissected well laterally, forming an uninterrupted gutter between the transverse processes and the ala of the sacrum. After the fifth transverse process is exposed, cleaned, and packed, the fascia incision is continued down to a point distal and lateral to the superior articular facet of the sacrum. Dissection lateral to this element will expose the ala of the sacrum. Many dense ligaments are adherent in this area and must be dissected from the sacrum in order to clearly expose the ala. It is essential to clearly visualize both the transverse processes and the ala in order to obtain an optimal preparation of the fusion bed. The sponges previously used to obtain hemostasis about the transverse processes and the ala of the sacrum are then removed, and a careful decortication of the transverse processes, the lateral portion of the pedicle, and the lateral portion of the articular facets is performed. This is best accomplished with large, sharp curets. Some care is required in order not to fracture the transverse process.

The ala of the sacrum is best decorticated with a narrow, round gouge. The lateral portion of the superior articular facet of the sacrum should also be decorticated. A hole is created in the cranial portion of the ala of the sacrum using a large curet, which will ultimately receive a portion of the graft material. This process of exposure and decortication is repeated on both sides of the spine. The wound is again carefully packed, and the midline fascia is closed with a towel clip.

BONE GRAFT. The posterior iliac crest is exposed by dissecting away the layer of adipose tissue with a large sponge. The fascia is incised in line with the posterior iliac crest, and the crest is then dissected subperiosteally. The gluteal muscles are carefully dissected from the lateral wing of the ilium. Care must be taken to remain beneath the periosteum, or dramatic bleeding that is difficult to control can occur. A broad reverse retractor is then inserted to clearly expose the lateral portion of the ilium. Utilizing sharp, curved gouges, long strips of cortical and cancellous bone are removed from the ilium until the inner wall of the ilium is exposed. Large amounts of bone are readily obtained from this area. This graft material should be cut into strips approximately 1 to 2 mm. in width and saved in blood-soaked sponges (Fig. 9–118).

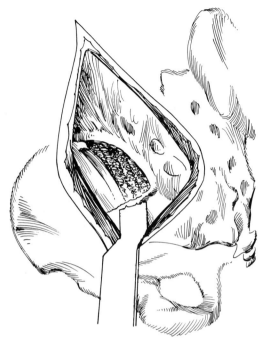

Figure 9–118. Technique of obtaining autogenous graft material from the posterior iliac crest. A large spiked retractor is utilized to expose the posterior surface of the ilium. Long strips of cortical and cancellous bone are then obtained, utilizing curved gouges. The graft material is saved in blood-soaked sponges and transferred to the previously prepared bed within five minutes.

PLACEMENT OF THE GRAFT MATERIAL AND CLOSURE OF THE WOUND. The midline wound is then reexposed, and the self-retaining retractors are reinserted. All the sponges are removed from the wound, and the wound is checked with careful finger palpation to be certain that none of the recesses harbor a hidden sponge. At this point, the preliminary sponge count should be obtained. The graft material is then placed in the trough that has been created from the fourth transverse process to the ala of the sacrum bilaterally (Fig. 9–119).

The wounds should be frequently irrigated with antibiotic solution, and at this point all devitalized tissue should be debrided. The double limb suction drain is inserted with one limb deep in the midline wound and the other at the iliac crest donor site. The fascia is then closed using #1 chromic suture. Subcutaneous closure is obtained with 00 chromic suture, and the skin edges are approximated with metallic staples.

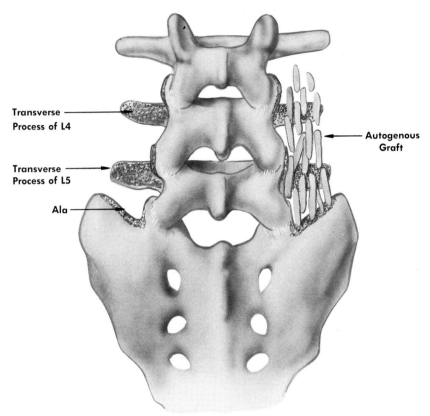

Transverse Process of L4

Autogenous Graft

Transverse Process of L5

Ala

Figure 9–119. Area of the bed of raw cancellous bone for a lateral spine fusion from L4 to the sacrum. The bed is shown on the left and the graft material is in place on the right. In actuality a much larger volume of graft material is utilized. The bed includes the transverse processes, the ala of the sacrum, the lateral portion of the pedicle and the lateral portion of the superior articular facets.

POSTOPERATIVE MANAGEMENT. The patient is allowed out of bed and walking the day after surgery. If there is difficulty in voiding, the patient may be allowed to stand at his bedside on the night of surgery. This may circumvent the need for catheterization with its attendant risk of infection. An exercise program is started on the second or third postoperative day, with deep knee bends and tuck exercises with the knees being drawn to the chest. No external support is utilized in the way of braces or corsets. This program of early mobilization has not been shown to lower the rate of successful fusion and has many dramatic advantages. Psychologically, the patient becomes attuned to an optimistic course and early return to productive life. The paraspinal muscles rapidly resume their normal tone, and the resolution of edema and hematoma occurs quickly.

The suction drains are withdrawn and the dressings removed at 48 hours. The wound remains exposed to the air after this point. It is sprayed with Betadine (povidone-iodine) twice daily. Narcotics or mild analgesics are utilized for the first few postoperative days as needed. Antibiotics, as previously noted, are administered for 72 hours postoperatively. The staples are removed and the patient is discharged in 10 days.

Subsequent to discharge, the patient is encouraged to gradually increase his level of activity. He is advised that the pain in his spine should be his guideline to his level of activity and that this should not be exceeded. Automobile riding is prohibited for the first several weeks. Heavy lifting is also discouraged. After four to six weeks, the patient may return to light work, at least on a part-time basis. After three months, most patients are able to return full time to sedentary and moderately active employment. Heavy physical labor is prohibited for six months. The same is true of vigorous athletics.

The patient is reevaluated at six-week intervals for the first three months and then at three-month intervals for the first year. As recovery progresses, the patient is placed on a more vigorous program of flexion exercises and is again instructed as to the essential aspects of back hygiene. He is encouraged to return to a normal way of life as rapidly as possible.

ANTERIOR INTERBODY FUSION

This type of fusion should be reserved for certain patients who have had multiple surgical procedures through the posterior approach to the spine that have failed. Dense posterior scarring, wide resection of the posterior elements of the spine, and a failed lateral spinal fusion are indications for consideration of this technique. The major disadvantage inherent in this surgical approach is the inability to carefully explore and decompress nerve roots when this is required.

This operation should be performed by a spinal surgeon and an abdominal surgeon together, unless the spinal surgeon has had extensive experience with the anterior approach.

ANESTHESIA. A nasogastric tube is utilized to prevent abdominal distention. Endotracheal anesthesia is preferred with the patient in the Trendelenburg position.

APPROACH. The retroperitoneal approach described by Harmon is utilized. A left paramedian incision is made, the anterior rectus sheath is opened, and the muscle is retracted laterally. The retroperitoneal space is entered, and the peritoneum is dissected bluntly from the undersurface of the posterior rectus sheath.[7] The peritoneum is mobilized, and as the lower lumbar spine is exposed, the ureter is left in its peritoneal bed and reflected to the right. The sacral promontory is identified by palpation. It is essential not to damage the sympathetic nerves coursing over the sacrum. The major sympathetic chains on either side of the lumbar vertebrae are carefully dissected and retracted in a lateral direction. The L5 interspace is exposed by retracting the left iliac artery and vein to the left and the right iliac artery and vein to the right. To expose the fourth lumbar vertebra, the left artery and vein are displaced to the right side of the spine. Spiked retractors are driven into the body of the vertebra to maintain exposure.

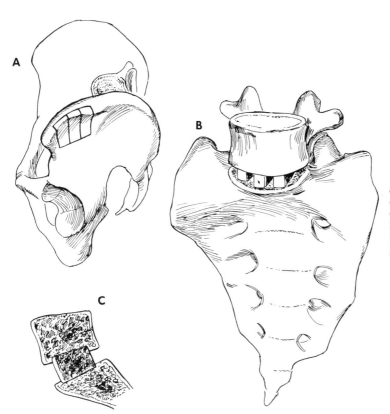

Figure 9–120. Technique of anterior lumbar fusion. After excision of the intervertebral disc, cortical cancellous grafts from the iliac crest are inserted into countersunk panels created in the adjacent vertebral end plates.

ANTERIOR DISC EXCISION AND FUSION. The anterior longitudinal ligament is elevated as a flap, with the base attached on the left. Exposure can be improved at this time by hyerextension of the operating table and spine. Then, utilizing the sharp osteotome, curets, and rongeurs, the entire disc is excised, and a trough is created in the opposing surfaces of the vertebral body above and below. The dimensions of this space are then measured, and three corticocancellous grafts are obtained from the left iliac crest. The grafts should be slightly larger than the notch so that firm impaction can be obtained. After insertion of the three grafts the spine can be brought to a neutral position, locking the grafts in place (Fig. 9–120). The previously created flap of anterior longitudinal ligament can be reattached or, if this is not possible, excised. The wound is closed in a routine manner after hemostasis is obtained. An excellent comprehensive discussion of the role, techniques, and results of anterior disc excision and fusion was presented by Goldner.

POSTOPERATIVE MANAGEMENT. The nasogastric tube is removed after peristalsis returns. Elastic stockings, early ambulation, and prophylactic anticoagulants are utilized to prevent thrombophlebitis. The management in other respects is similar to that after lateral spinal fusion.

Results of Operative Treatment of Lumbar Disc Disease

Over three decades have passed since the advent of surgical treatment of lumbar disc disease. Improvement in the efficiency of surgical treatment must be predicated on accurate knowledge of the quality of result that can be expected with each technique and diagnosis. Long-term follow-up is essential in this area, and studies of this type are now available in the literature.[2, 16] The pressing need at the present time is for an accurately constructed prospective study using various surgical techniques for each of the specific diagnostic entities under consideration. Retrospective studies grouping all disc diseases into one diagnostic category are of limited value.

DePalma and Rothman have reported their experience over a period of 20 years with over 1500 patients who had undergone surgery for lumbar disc degenerations.[2] These patients were called back for personal interview,

TABLE 9–3. POPULATION

Mean age surgery	40 years
Mean age follow up	48 years
Mean follow up	8 years
Range follow up	1–20 years
Ten year or greater follow up	195 patients

physical examination, and repeat radiographic examination, including stress films. In order to minimize bias, the evaluations were performed by physicians other than the operating surgeon.

Examination of the population distribution curve revealed that the average age at surgery was 40, with a normal frequency distribution above and below this level. This age distribution is in keeping with the more recent pathologic concepts of disc degeneration. The average age of follow-up evaluation was 48, the average follow-up period was 8 years. One hundred and ninety-five patients were followed for a period of 10 years or longer (Table 9–3).

Relief of symptoms was the most important criterion for success in terms of low back surgery. Patients were questioned about the degree and temporal nature of their relief of back and leg pain. Their evaluation as to the subjective worth of their surgery was also elicited.

In individuals with L5 disc degeneration, 15 per cent had persistent back pain, 7 per cent had persistent sciatica, and 14 per cent had both back pain and sciatica. The results are approximately the same with L4 disc degeneration and two-level disc degeneration (Table 9–4). When questioned as to overall relief of their pain, approximately 60 per cent of individuals in each category stated that they had obtained complete relief of back and leg

TABLE 9–4. PERCENTAGES OF DISC DEGENERATION PATIENTS SHOWING SYMPTOMS AT FOLLOW UP

	L5–S1	L4–L5	Both
Preoperative			
Back pain	10	7	7
Leg pain	5	0	4
Both	85	93	89
Postoperative			
Back pain	15	17	11
Leg pain	7	7	4
Both	14	17	20

TABLE 9–5.   PATIENTS WITH DISC DEGENERATION SHOWING SUBJECTIVE RELIEF AT FOLLOW UP

	L5–S1	L4–L5	Both
Total	62	67	59
Partial	30	24	28
Temporary	4	7	11
None	3	3	2
Surgery worthwhile	88	88	75

pain, approximately 30 per cent considered themselves partially relieved, and 2 to 3 per cent were a total failure with no relief whatsoever. Of the patients with disc degeneration at L4 or L5, 88 per cent felt their surgery worthwhile; the percentage was less when both disc spaces were affected (Table 9–5).

Physical findings were evaluated at follow-up and compared to preoperative findings. The nonspecific findings such as muscle spasm, tenderness, and limitation of motion, and straight leg raising disappeared in 90 per cent of those individuals who showed these findings preoperatively. Neurologic deficits returned to normal less often postoperatively. Motor and sensory deficits that had been present preoperatively disappeared in 50 per cent of the patients. Only 25 per cent of the patients lost their preoperative reflex changes. This is somewhat better than the results reported by Knutsson, in which only 33 per cent of patients lost their sensory deficit, 24 per cent lost their motor deficit and 2½ per cent lost their reflex abnormalities[10] (Table 9–6).

Certain general observations were noted that are also of interest. An attempt was made to select those factors that would be of poor prognostic significance for the patient undergoing back surgery.

In regard to diagnosis, high discs (i.e., above the L4-L5 level) did more poorly in regard to relief of symptomatology. One oper-

ative category appeared to fare more poorly: lumbosacral fusion combined with disc excision alone at the L4-L5 level. At one time this operation was felt to be appropriate when a degenerated L4-L5 disc was found together with evidence of an unstable lumbosacral mechanism. The correlation of physical findings with quality of result revealed that a negative straight leg raising test in the preoperative examination tended to correlate with a poor result. This observation was also noted by Hirsch.[8] He noted that laminectomy and exploration were negative more often when the straight leg raising test, neurologic examination, and myelogram were negative. He further observed that with negative exploration the quality of result was poor regardless of the operative procedure performed.

PSEUDARTHROSIS

The overall rate of solid fusion in the previous series was 92 per cent, with an incidence of pseudarthrosis of 8 per cent. Following the advent of the lateral fusion technique, the incidence of pseudarthrosis in two level fusions is 6 per cent.[1] The incidence of pseudarthrosis in one-level fusions utilizing the lateral technique is less than 1 per cent. In our study group, 39 patients were discovered whom we could classify radiographically as having definite pseudarthrosis. In the hope of learning in detail what the diagnosis of pseudarthrosis portends for a patient, we studied these individuals in detail. They were compared with a matched group of 39 patients, each having an identical diagnosis and operation in whom the fusion was solid. By comparing these two matched groups, we can state with some degree of precision the implication of pseudarthrosis for the patient who has undergone a spinal fusion.

In an overall subjective evaluation of the worth of their surgery, 82 per cent of the patients who had developed pseudarthrosis felt that their surgery was worthwhile, whereas 92 per cent of the group who had solid fusions felt that their surgery was worthwhile (Table 9–7). Little difference was found

TABLE 9–6.   PERCENTAGE CHANGES IN PHYSICAL FINDINGS AFTER SURGERY

Loss of all reflex change	25
Loss of all motor deficit	50
Loss of all sensory deficit	50
Loss of abnormal curve	
Muscle spasm	
Tenderness	⎡90 or
Limited motion	⎣more
Straight leg raising	

TABLE 9–7.   PERCENTAGE OF PATIENTS WHO CONSIDERED SURGERY WORTHWHILE

Pseudarthrosis	Solid Fusion
82	92

TABLE 9–8. PERCENTAGE OF PATIENTS RECEIVING RELIEF FROM SYMPTOMS

	Pseudarthrosis	Solid Fusion
Total	56	61
Partial	34	26
Temporary	10	5
None	0	8

TABLE 9–10. PERCENTAGE OF PATIENTS WITH SCIATICA AT FOLLOW UP

	Pseudarthrosis	Solid Fusion
Preoperative	79	85
Postoperative	25	20

between the pseudarthrosis group and the solid fusion group when they were asked specifically about their overall relief from symptomatology. Fifty-six per cent of patients in the former group and 61 per cent in the latter group obtained total relief. It is interesting to note that, although there was a slight decrease in the number who obtained total relief in the pseudarthrosis group, three patients who achieved solid fusions obtained no relief, and all patients who developed pseudarthrosis obtained at least partial or temporary relief (Table 9–8).

When back pain alone was considered, of the 92 per cent of patients in the pseudarthrosis group who originally had back pain, 44 per cent still had the symptoms at follow-up evaluation. In the solid fusion group, of the 97 per cent of patients who originally had back pain, 38 per cent had significant back pain at follow-up evaluation (Table 9–9).

Sciatica was eliminated more consistently than back pain at follow-up evaluation. Of the 79 per cent of patients in the pseudarthrosis group who had sciatica, only 25 per cent had their symptoms at follow-up evaluation. In the solid fusion group, of the 85 per cent of patients who originally had sciatica, only 20 per cent had their symptoms at follow-up evaluation (Table 9–10). The subjective factors noted above were submitted to chi-square analysis and in no case was a significant difference noted between the pseudarthrosis and the solid fusion group. It seems justifiable to draw certain conclusions from the preceding information. One of two situations must exist: either the pseudarthrosis

represents a fibrous stabilization, which is essentially as effective as bony fusion, or the fusion component of these procedures was not essential. The former is not unreasonable, as the amount of motion demonstrated on flexion-extension films of pseudarthrosis is usually minimal and is often less than 2 ml. The latter conclusion, however, remains in question.

It would furthermore seem prudent to carefully observe patients with pseudarthrosis for a rather prolonged period of time before reoperating in an attempt to achieve union. There seems little rationale for submitting patients to multiple attempts at repair of pseudarthrosis if, as a group, there is little difference in their subjective result when solid fusion is obtained.

The overall picture obtained is that a certain number of patients who have undergone spinal fusion continue to have back pain and less frequently sciatica, whether or not their fusion has become solid. The success rate, as judged by objective evaluation, is slightly greater in that group that has achieved solid fusion. Pseudarthrosis, of itself, does not appear to be the dreaded complication that is often portrayed. A more precise definition of the role of spinal fusion and evaluation of the essentiality of achieving this fusion will depend on the availability of long-term prospective studies of spinal surgery.

As one reviews the overwhelming amount of written material pertaining to spinal surgery, certain precepts become clear, and certain requirements evident, if good results are to be obtained.

REQUIREMENTS FOR SUCCESSFUL SPINAL SURGERY

1. Accurate knowledge of the variable pathology of disc degeneration.
2. Accurate diagnosis of nerve root compression.
3. Adherence to the proper criteria for surgical intervention.

TABLE 9–9. PERCENTAGES OF PATIENTS WITH BACK PAIN AT FOLLOW UP

	Pseudarthrosis	Solid Fusion
Preoperative	92	97
Postoperative	44	38

4. Selection of the proper operative procedure.

5. Skillful execution of the surgical procedure by an experienced spinal surgeon.

6. The prompt recognition and treatment of complications.

7. Careful postoperative care and rehabilitation.

If every patient undergoing spine surgery had the benefit of these principles, the quality of surgical result would improve dramatically, and the grey veil of apprehension, fear, and anxiety that has surrounded spinal surgery for years would be lifted.

References

1. DePalma, A., and Rothman, R.: The nature of pseudarthrosis. Clin. Orthop. 59:113–118, 1968.
2. DePalma, A., and Rothman, R.: Surgery of the lumbar spine. Clin. Orthop. 63:162–170, 1969.
3. DePalma, A., and Rothman, R.: The Intervertebral Disc. Philadelphia, W. B. Saunders Co., 1970.
4. DiStefano, V. J., et al.: Intra-operative analysis of the effects of position body habitus on surgery of the low back. Clin. Orthop. 99:51–56, 1974.
5. Gill, G. C., et al.: Pedicle fat graft for the prevention of scar formation after laminectomy. Proceedings of the fifth annual meeting of the International Society for Study of the Lumbar Spine. San Francisco, 1978.
6. Goldner, J. L., et al.: Anterior disc excision and interbody spine fusion for chronic low back pain. Orthop. Clin. North Am. 2:543–568, 1971.
7. Harmon, P. H., and Abel, M.: Correlation of multiple objective diagnostic methods in lower lumbar disc disease. Clin. Orthop. 28:132–151, 1963.
8. Hirsch, C.: Efficiency of surgery in low back disorders. J. Bone Joint Surg. 47A:991, 1965.
9. Jacobs, R., McClain, O., and Neff, J.: Control of post-laminectomy scar formation: An experimental and clinical evaluation. Spine 5:223–229, 1980.
10. Knutsson, B.: Aspects of the neurogenic electromyographic records of voluntary contraction in cases of nerve root compression. Electromyography 2:238–242, 1962.
11. Langenskold, A., et al.: Prevention of epidural scar formation after operation on the lumbar spine by means of a free fat transplant. Clin. Orthop. 115:92–95, 1976.
12. Macnab, I.: The laminectomy membrane. J. Bone Joint Surg. 56B:545–550, 1974.
13. Semmes, E.: Ruptures of the Lumbar Intervertebral Disc. Springfield, C C Thomas Co., 1964.
14. Truchly, G., et al.: Posterolateral fusion of the lumbosacral spine. J. Bone Joint Surg. (A) 44A:505–512, 1962.
15. Watkins, M. B.: Lumbosacral fusion results with early ambulation. Surg. Gynecol. Obstet. 102:604–606, 1956.
16. Young, H., and Love, J.: End results of removal of protruded lumbar intervertebral discs with and without fusion. AAOS Instructional Course Lecture 16:213–216, 1959.

Complications of Lumbar Disc Surgery

The basic precept of all surgeons is, "above all, do no harm." The prevention of complications in spine surgery demands an awareness of all the potential hazards, a thorough knowledge of standard and variational anatomy, and meticulous surgical technique. Despite elaborate precautions and great care, however, these complications may occur but should be recognized early and treated appropriately.

COMPLICATIONS DURING OPERATION

VASCULAR AND VISCERAL INJURIES. Injuries to the great vessels, including the aorta, inferior vena cava, and iliac vessels, as well as other visceral structures, occur from penetration of the inferior portion of the anulus with surgical instruments. These injuries can carry serious implications with mortality rates of up to 78 per cent if the injury is arterial and up to 89 per cent if the injury is venous.[8]

The majority of these injuries occur while trying to clean the anterior portion of the disc space with a curet or pituitary rongeur. An erroneous estimation of the depth of the interspace will lead to the instrument's penetrating the anulus and traumatizing one of the large vessels. It is important to remember that the anterior anulus does not have to be necessarily violated by surgical instruments since the degenerative disc process affects not only the posterior aspect of the anulus but also the anterior aspect.[18]

The aorta and vena cava lie in approximation to the L4-L5 disc space, while the iliac vessels lie in approximation to the L5-S1 disc space (Fig. 9–121).[20]

Immediate laceration violating the lumen of these vessels may occur with massive hemorrhage; partial injuries to the wall of a vessel with delayed hemorrhage may occur, or laceration of both artery and vein may occur with a resultant arteriovenous fistula.

There tends to be a delay in the diagnosis of arteriovenous fistula following discectomy, primarily since in the majority of cases reported, no bleeding was appreciated from the disc space at the time of surgery.[14] This unique complication more often occurs at the L4-5 interspace because of the close proximity of the iliac artery and vein. The right common iliac artery has been most susceptible to injury, with venous injuries equally distributed

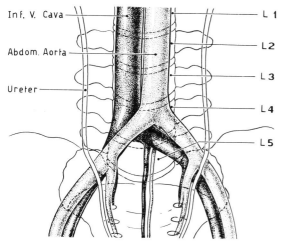

Figure 9–121. Relationship between the great vessels and the lumbar disc spaces. (From Montorsi, W., and Ghiringhelli, C.: Genesis, diagnosis, and treatment of vascular complications after intervertebral disc surgery. Int. Surg. *58*:233, 1973.)

among the left and right iliac veins and the inferior vena cava. Approximately half of the cases reported were diagnosed within one month of surgery, and 70 per cent were diagnosed within six months. A majority of patients presented with signs and symptoms of high output cardiac decompensation, specifically tachycardia with or without cardiomegaly, orthopnea due to congestive heart failure, and a to and fro, machinery-type lower abdominal bruit.[14] Injury to the ureter[21] and the appendix[4] have also been reported and have been associated with arteriovenous fistulas. Fortunately, despite the delay in diagnosis and treatment, a comparatively low mortality rate of only approximately 8 per cent has been reported.

Prevention of these injuries will be enhanced if adequate exposure is undertaken during surgery. If adequate exposure and hemostasis are not obtained prior to entering the disc space, continuous epidural bleeding will obscure the field of vision and will make it difficult to estimate the depth of the disc space. The depth with which an instrument penetrates the disc space should never exceed 1⅛ inches. The surgeon who occasionally performs spine surgery should have his instruments marked in this regard. Even skilled surgeons, however, must constantly keep this dimension in mind while working in the depths of the disc space. A third and most important precaution is that every instrument tip should

be against bone while cleaning a disc space. Pituitary rongeurs should not be closed unless the rasp of metal upon bone is felt, nor should the stroke of a curet be continued unless this reassuring sensation is felt.

Further avoidance of these dreaded complications is provided by the kneeling or tucked position utilized by the authors, since it decreases epidural pressure and subsequently affords better exposure of the disc space, but also importantly, the abdominal contents, including the major vessels, will tend to drift ventrally away from the spine during the course of surgery.

Awareness of the possibility of this complication is important, and prompt surgical intervention is the only effective treatment. Profuse bleeding from the disc space or hypovolemic shock disproportionate to the observable blood loss should alert the surgeon to this possibility. The management of this complication is immediate laparotomy and repair of the vascular injury. The spinal wound should be closed immediately with towel clips and a sterile plastic drape. Blood and fluid replacement should begin immediately, and the patient should be turned to the supine position while a vascular surgeon is summoned.

AIR EMBOLISM. While very rare, the kneeling position advocated for lumbar surgery can give rise to air embolism, since negative pressures can be realized in the vena cava with this position. Consequently, some surgeons advocate the use of intraoperative right arterial catheters with Doppler ultrasonic transducers to monitor the possible occurrence of air embolism.[1]

INJURIES TO THE NEURAL ELEMENTS. Tears of the dura may occur during laminectomy and decompression while gaining access to the spinal canal. Packing cottonoids between the dura and bony elements of the canal will prevent this mishap. Much more difficulty will be found in cases in which previous surgery has been performed with the formation of extensive scar tissue around the dura. Even with utmost care, tears of the dura occasionally will occur. Should this injury occur, it is important to promptly repair the defect with continuous fine silk sutures, preferably with a non-cutting needle. Failure to perform an adequate repair may result in the formation of a fistula or spinal extradural cyst.

Nerve root injuries may occur from excessive retraction, laceration, or thermal burns. Excessive retraction with metallic instruments can be avoided by gently packing the nerve roots with cotton pledgets. If this is properly performed, the nerve root can be adequately displaced medially without the necessity of repeated instrumentation as described in the section on the technique of disc excision. This should prevent the "battered" root syndrome that has been reported.[3]

Lacerations of the nerve root usually occur through inadequate visualization and failure to recognize a flattened nerve root over an extruded disc. These injuries can be prevented through adequate visualization and careful control of bleeding. There is no particular advantage in attempting to identify a nerve root and disc herniations through a minute opening in the spinal canal. When any difficulty whatsoever is encountered in recognizing pertinent anatomic features, such as the shoulder of the nerve root and disc herniations, the laminectomy should be widened so that the nerve root can be identified with confidence proximal to the disc herniation. An excision into the anulus should never be made until the nerve root at that level is positively identified and retracted. A wide exposure, particularly laterally, will facilitate this procedure.

Thermal burns can be prevented by employing fine tip, bipolar electrocautery. This, however, should be used only when the nerve root has been identified and protected. Extreme care should also be used when setting the current level, and this should be checked on muscle tissue before coagulation within the spinal canal.

COMPLICATIONS DURING THE IMMEDIATE POSTOPERATIVE PERIOD

These complications are not unique to spine surgery and follow the basic precepts of good surgical physiology. Pulmonary atelectasis with failure to adequately expand the lungs postoperatively is frequently seen in patients with endotracheal anesthesia. This is seen in the first three postoperative days, and it is a common cause for temperature elevations. Physical findings may be minimal, and even chest radiographs may not be revealing with minimal episodes of atelectasis. The best prevention and treatment is early mobilization of the patient, encouragement to cough frequently, and deep breathing. The anxious patient or one who cannot be rapidly mobilized should be routinely placed on intermittent positive pressure breathing. Blow bottles are some help. The authors' use of spinal anesthesia for most cases involving lumbar surgery has obviated the problem of pulmonary atelectasis to a great degree, although patient cooperation to improve ventilation is still encouraged.

Intestinal ileus is occasionally a complication of low back surgery. It will produce abdominal distention, nausea and vomiting, and respiratory distress, and auscultation will reveal the absence of bowel sounds. When the syndrome is appreciated, treatment should include nasogastric suction with administration of intravenous fluids and electrolytes until restoration of bowel function is indicated by peristalsis and the passage of flatus. It is our custom not to feed postlaminectomy patients for 24 hours postoperatively and to resume meals once we are confident of restitution of normal bowel function.

URINARY RETENTION. This complication is seen in the immediate postoperative course and is due to a combination of anxiety, pain in the supine position, and nerve root irritation prior to and during surgery. The use of narcotics is also somewhat contributory to this retention. The great danger is the excessive use of urethral catheters with some danger of infection. Great efforts are made to manage this problem without the use of catheterization. Male patients are allowed to stand at the bedside as early as the night of surgery, and female patients are allowed to use a bedside commode. If this is unsuccessful, parenteral bethanechol chloride (Urecholine) should be utilized. Only when these two measures fail is catheterization undertaken, and when it is undertaken, the intermittent variety rather than an indwelling approach has proved successful.

WOUND INFECTION. Wound infection is a complication dreaded by all surgeons. It should be suspected when pain or temperature elevation occurs during the latter part of the first postoperative week. If there is any significant suspicion of infection, the wound should be cultured either through needle aspiration or swab, and immediate Gram stain with culture and minimal inhibitory sensitivities should be obtained. If an organism is identified, treatment should be instituted immediately. In the presence of a significant infection, the patient should be returned to the operating room, and the wound should be reopened, thoroughly debrided, and irrigated. The authors prefer leaving the wound wide open and attending to daily wound care in isolation in the patient's room. If the dura is exposed, a closed irrigation system is utilized. In addition to this local care, parenteral antibiotics appropriate for the specific organism cultured should, of course, be administered. Minor infection should be drained promptly and treated with specific antibiotics. It should be emphasized that the primary treatment of surgical infection is surgery. Antibiotics are not adequate by themselves for collection of purulent material.

Spangfort[23] in his computerized review of over 10,000 procedures reported a postlaminectomy infection rate of approximately 2.9 per cent. Of the more recent cases reported in his monograph, however, the infection rate had been reduced to less than 2 per cent. Occasionally lumbar epidural abscesses will develop and characteristically will present with a progression from spinal pain to root pain to frank paresis and paralysis.[2, 15] Under this circumstance, immediate myelography, culture, sensitivity, and decompressive laminectomy would then be indicated.

CAUDA EQUINA SYNDROME. This is the most dreaded complication short of death that can occur in lumbar disc surgery. The exact mechanism is uncertain, although mechanical trauma, hematoma, or vascular injury has been implicated. The artery of Adamkowitz (arteria radicularis anteria magna) is the largest feeder of the lumbar spinal cord and has been reported entering the spinal canal between T7 and as low as the L4 level.[9] While its predilection is for the left side between T9 and T11, injury to this vessel while retracting or cauterizing about lumbar nerves may explain this rare and unexpected complication.

Spangfort[23] reported on five patients developing a complication of cauda equina syndrome, which represented 0.2 per cent of his computerized series undergoing lumbar discectomy. The severity of the syndrome is further reinforced in that only 40 per cent of these patients recovered completely.

THROMBOPHLEBITIS. Thrombophlebitis is seen with decreasing frequency since the routine use of early mobilization. Its onset is heralded by a feeling of pain, tightness, and swelling in the affected extremity. Physical examination will reveal tenderness along the course of the vein and swelling of one or both extremities. A temperature elevation will frequently be seen, and a positive Homans' sign may or may not be present. Treatment is immediately instituted with intravenous heparin, warm compresses to the leg, and elevation of the extremity. The incidence of this complication is so low after spinal surgery that routine postoperative anticoagulation therapy is not indicated unless the patient has had a prior episode of thrombophlebitis or is extremely obese. Spangfort[23] reported an incidence of thrombophlebitis of only 1 per cent following laminectomy, and less than half of these patients showed any evidence of an embolic phenomenon.

TECHNICAL COMPLICATIONS RESULTING IN PERSISTENT SYMPTOMS

INADEQUATE NERVE ROOT DECOMPRESSION. Not infrequently a patient continues with unrelenting sciatica postoperatively, and upon reexploration it becomes evident that the true pathologic condition was not uncovered at the time of surgery. This complication can be prevented only if the variety of pathologic entities causing nerve root compression are understood and appreciated by the surgeon. To simply look for an acute disc herniation through a small fenestration and consider this adequate treatment in all cases is to invite persistent pain. The most common conditions in which nerve root compression is not relieved are unrecognized disc lesions at another level, unrecognized lateral recess syndrome, an unappreciated migrated free fragment of disc material, foraminal encroachment, tethering of the nerve root about a pedicle, or anomalous root anatomy. These oversights can be avoided with a generous laminectomy and wide exposure whenever doubt exists as to the true nature of the pathologic state. Careful exploration of the nerve root should be undertaken from its origin at the dural sac, well out into the foramen. A large, malleable cervical dilator is found useful in exploring foramina. Right angle nerve root elevators can be used with advantage to explore beneath the nerve root and dural sac and will rule out central protrusions and migrated fragments. When doubt exists as to the level of protrusion, exploration of two or three disc levels should be undertaken. An additional half hour spent in careful exploration could save the patient years of misery and disability. The importance of an adequate meticulous exploration cannot be overemphasized. It should be emphasized parenthetically that no additional morbidity has been experienced with wide laminectomy.[13]

FIBROSIS AROUND THE NERVE ROOTS AND DURA. Scar formation will occur with great regularity about the dura and nerve roots after surgical exploration. The reason why this may cause symptoms in one patient and not in another is not understood at the present time. The scar tissue connection is a tethering force as well as a constricting force about the nerve roots.

Early enthusiasm for the use of a Gelfoam membrane, advocated by LaRocca and Macnab,[17] has given way to the introduction of the concept of the free fat graft by Langenskiöld and Kiviluoto.[16] The principle of maintaining a fat–dural interface is that it would not only inhibit perineural fibrosis and symptoms of nerve encroachment but also would allow for safer dissection if reoperation in the future became necessary. No statistical data are available yet as to the efficacy of this method; however, in the three cases personally explored by the authors where fat grafts were utilized, all were viable and little scarring was noted. More recently, Gill and others[12] suggested that a pedicle fat graft may actually be superior to the free fat graft. Careful hemostasis, as well as gentle handling of the neural tissue, will also decrease the amount of scar tissue formation.

PSEUDARTHROSIS. Pseudarthrosis is an undesirable complication of spinal fusion. The incidence of this complication has been decreased markedly with the advent of the lateral spine fusion. In a study by DePalma and Rothman,[7] a group of 39 patients with radiographically demonstrable pseudarthrosis were studied. Of this group, only 17 per cent were symptomatic. Thus, it is the authors' recommendation that a significant trial of conservative therapy be instituted before surgical correction is undertaken. The prevention of pseudarthrosis is based on adequate surgical technique and attention to the general physiology of the patient and particularly to the treatment of anemia.[22]

DISC SPACE INFECTION. Disc space infection should be considered when there is a rapid dramatic occurrence of severe back pain one to six weeks after excision of an intervertebral disc. This may be accompanied by recurrence of sciatica or femoral neuritis, as well as severe muscle cramping.[10] Straight leg raising or reverse straight leg raising will frequently become more limited than prior to the operation. The patient may or may not have a temperature elevation, and frequently the only laboratory abnormality would be an elevated sedimentation rate.

Serial radiographic examination will reveal loss of height of the disc space, irregular destruction of the end plate, and, ultimately, sclerotic reaction[25] (Fig. 9–122).

Diagnosis can usually be made by radiographic and clinical findings without biopsy or needle aspiration of the disc space. Treatment consists of complete immobilization, preferably in a plastic spica from the lower rib cage to above the knees. Large doses of parenteral antibiotics effective against staphylococcus organisms are utilized for a period of two to three months. Those patients, however, who do not respond to conservative therapy within a short period of time after the institution of antibiotics should undergo debridement of the disc space either through a retroperitoneal approach or a direct posterior approach, particularly if a neurologic deficit is appreciated. Spangfort[24] estimated an incidence of approximately 2 per cent in his computerized study.

SUBARACHNOID CYST. If dural tears are unrecognized or are not repaired, then arachnoid cysts may be formed and can, on occasion, assume dramatic size. Frequently, the symptoms of an extradural pseudocyst are the same as those experienced in acute disc herniations. Occasionally, however, meningeal signs may be present, as well as headache and neck pain. Myelography will usually disclose the true nature of the patient's symptoms.[26]

Treatment of these lesions usually necessitates operation and complete excision of the cyst with closure at the dural margins either primarily or with the aid of fascial grafting. Mayfield[19] reported on 11 patients who developed this complication in a series of over 1000 operations. Most of these resulted from rents near the dural sleeve, and it was found that free fat plugs would successfully seal such rents.

INSTABILITY OF A MOTOR UNIT. Instability of a motor unit may be present preoperatively or after the excision of an intervertebral disc and associated facet joints. There is some evidence to suggest that this instability is associated with failure of relief of symptoms after disc excision.[11]

In the face of persistent back pain and sciatica after disc excision and radiographically proved instability, lateral spine fusion should be undertaken to stabilize the spine. The instability may be manifest in either a forward or reversed translation in the sagittal plane of one vertebral body or another or may be represented by wedging of the disc space with flexion and extension films. This potential for instability is not in itself an adequate

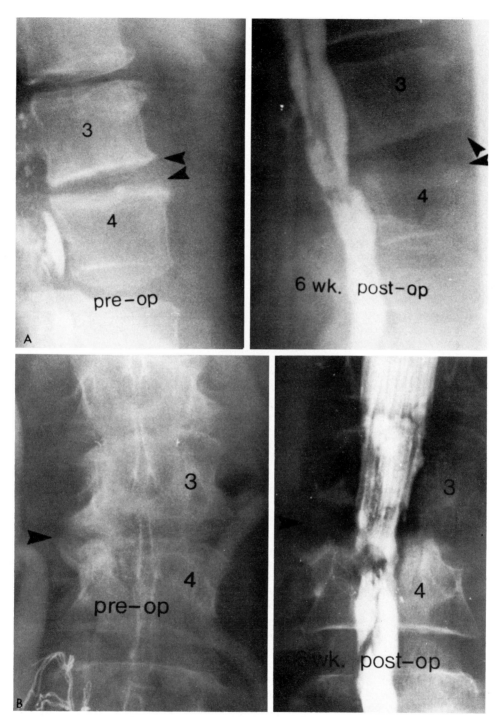

Figure 9–122. Radiographs illustrate a postoperative disc space infection at the L3-4 level. *A*, On the left preoperative lateral and on the right six weeks postoperative lateral. Note the loss of definition of the endplate and irregular destruction of the endplate and osteophytes. *B*, On the left the preoperative AP and on the right the six weeks postoperative AP revealing loss of the endplate, osteoporosis, and erosion of the osteophyte.

justification for fusion of all spines after disc excision. The criteria for a combined procedure and spinal fusion are outlined in the discussion on indications for spinal surgery and the selection of the appropriate operative procedure.

IMPINGEMENT SYNDROME. After midline spinal fusion, certain patients develop symptoms at the site of contact of the fusion mass against the spinous processes of the vertebra directly cranial to the fusion. This clinical picture is one of pain on extension of the spine with point tenderness at the area of impingement. This usually also can be demonstrated radiographically. Treatment of this entity requires section of the lower portion of the involved spinous process if local injection is not therapeutic.

RETAINED FOREIGN BODIES. With the use of accurate sponge counts and radiographic tagging of sponges and cotton pledgets, this complication should be rather rare. Occasionally a cotton pledget will get detached from its identifying string and if unrecognized may be retained in the wound. These foreign bodies may cause a local inflammatory reaction, and for this reason reexploration and removal of the foreign body should be undertaken. Bone wax, as well as starch granules from the glove packaging, may sometimes cause a granulomatous reaction and persistent drainage from the wound. Bone wax should, therefore, be used sparingly, if at all, and the starch on the gloves should be wiped off with a moist towel prior to surgery.

IATROGENIC SPINAL STENOSIS. As our temporal perspective increases, many instances are being noted of cauda equina compression secondary to overgrowth of lamina and fusion masses when midline fusion techniques have been utilized.[5] Not only will the bone graft material hypertrophy, but also the lamina will appear to increase in thickness under the stimulus of decortication and grafting (Fig. 9–107). The neural canal and foramina may be encroached, presenting a classic spinal stenotic syndrome. The clinical syndrome is usually quite apparent, but computerized axial tomography may provide a diagnostic clue as to this entity. Treatment in either case would require satisfactory decompression of the neural elements.

PELVIC INSTABILITY. The creation of pelvic instability after removing iliac bone for grafting and fatigue fractures at the site of the bone removed are rare complications of spinal fusion but should be considered in patients with persistent back pain after fusion.[6] Fatigue fractures will heal spontaneously. Symptomatic pelvic instability may require a sacroiliac fusion.

References

1. Albin, M. S.: Venous air embolism and lumbar disk surgery. Letter to the Editor, J.A.M.A. *240*:1713, 1978.
2. Baker, A. S., Ojemann, R. G., Schwartz, M. N., and Richardson, E. P.: Spinal epidural abscess. N. Engl. J. Med. *293*:(10):463–469, 1975.
3. Bertrand, G.: The "battered" root problem. Orthop. Clin. North Am. *6*:305–309, 1975.
4. Birkeland, I. W., and Taylor, T. K. F.: Major vascular injuries in lumbar disc surgery. J. Bone Joint Surg. *51B*(1):4–19, 1969.
5. Brodsky, A. E.: Post-laminectomy and post-fusion stenosis of the lumbar spine. Clin. Orthop. *115*:130–139, 1976.
6. Coventry, M. B., and Tapper, E.: Pelvic instability. J. Bone Joint Surg. *54A*:83–101, 1972.
7. DePalma, A., and Rothman, R.: The nature of pseudoarthrosis. Clin. Orthop. *59*:113–118, 1968.
8. Desausseure, R. L.: Vascular injuries coincident to disc surgery. J. Neurosurg. *16*:222–229, 1959.
9. Dommisse, G. F.: The blood supply of the spinal cord. J. Bone Joint Surg. *56B*:225–235, 1974.
10. El-Gindi, S., Aref, S., Salama, M., and Andrew, J.: Infection of intervertebral discs after operation. J. Bone Joint Surg. *58*:114–116, 1976.
11. Froning, E. C., and Frohman, B.: Motion of the lumbosacral spine after laminectomy and spine fusion. J. Bone Joint Surg. *50A*:897–918, 1968.
12. Gill, G. C., Sakovich, L., and Thompson, E.: Pedicle fat graft for the prevention of scar formation after laminectomy: An experimental study in dogs. Proceedings of the 5th annual meeting of the International Society for the Study of the Lumbar Spine. San Francisco, 1978.
13. Jackson, R. K.: The long term effects of wide laminectomy for lumbar disc excision. J. Bone Joint Surg. *53B*:609–616, 1971.
14. Jarstfer, B. S., and Rich, N. M.: The challenge of arteriovenous fistula formation following disk surgery: A collective review. J. Trauma *16*:(9):726–733, 1976.
15. Keon-Cohen, B. T.: Epidural abscess simulating disc herniation. J. Bone Joint Surg. *50B*:128–130, 1968.
16. Langenskiöld, A., and Kiviluoto, O.: Prevention of epidural scar formation after operations on the lumbar spine by means of free fat transplants. Clin. Orthop. *115*:92–95, 1976.
17. LaRocca, H., and MacNab, I.: The laminectomy membrane, J. Bone Joint Surg. *56B*:545–550, 1974.
18. Lindblom, K.: Intervertebral disc degeneration as a pressure atrophy. J. Bone Joint Surg. *39A*:933, 1957.
19. Mayfield, F. H.: Complications of laminectomy. Clin. Neurosurg. *23*:435–439, 1976.
20. Montorsi, W., and Ghiringhelli, C.: Genesis, diagnosis and treatment of vascular complications after intervertebral disc surgery. Int. Surg. *58*(4):233–235, 1973.

21. Moore, C. A., and Cohen, A.: Combined arterial venous and urethral injuries complicating disc surgery. Am. J. Surg. *115*:574, 1968.
22. Rothman, R., et al.: The effect of iron deficiency anemia on fracture healing. Clin. Orthop. *77*:276–283, 1971.
23. Spangfort, E. V.: The lumbar disc herniation — a computerized analysis of 2,504 operations. Acta Orthop. Scand. (Suppl.) *142*:52–78, 1972.
24. Spangfort, E. V.: Postoperative discitis. Nord. Med. *71*:162, 1964.
25. Thibodeau, A. A.: Closed space infection following removal of lumbar intervertebral disc. J. Bone Joint Surg. *50A*:400–410, 1968.
26. Borgesen, S. E., and Vang, P. J.: Extradural pseudocysts: A cause of pain after lumbar disc operation. Acta Orthop. Scand. *44*:12–20, 1973.

INDUSTRIAL COMPENSATION AND LEGAL BACK INJURIES

The economics of industrial lumbar disability has prompted efforts towards a comprehensive study of the prevention and treatment of these injuries. Epidemiologically, it is estimated that annually 1.25 million Americans sustain actual skeletal injuries.[4] In the United Kingdom greater than one third of the working days lost to sickness were attributed to back injuries.[11] Furthermore, Chafin and Parke[5] concluded that the proportion of valid medical claims precipitated by low back disability ranged from 10 per cent in the American industry to as high as 36 per cent in certain industries in Sweden.

Efforts at prevention of lumbar disability have taken two major pathways in industry. The first involves preemployment data collection, including appropriate history and roentgenograms to identify the susceptible worker. The second avenue utilized has been ergonomics, defined as the precise application of human anatomic, physiologic, psychologic, and mechanical principles to "insure the maximum efficiency of operation, to minimize the possibility of human error, reduce fatigue and eliminate as far as possible the risk to the operator."[10]

Lumbar spine roentgenography has been used as a preemployment baseline for evaluating subsequent injury as well as to identify anatomic features that may accurately predict potential lumbar disability. LaRocca and MacNab[18] found no developmental or degenerative criteria that can reliably predict the potential for lumbar disability. While their data did indicate that degenerative changes are associated with symptom production, they emphasize, however, that those changes could not accurately predict the risk of developing an industrial disability. Magora and Schwartz[30] add further credence to this conclusion by noting that roentgenographic hallmarks of degenerative arthritis of the spine will be found in symptomatic as well as asymptomatic subjects in a variety of occupations demanding the full spectrum of physical activity. Montgomery[31] concluded after extensive review of the literature that he could not substantiate the hypothesis that the incidence of low back injury would be increased in the presence of developmental abnormalities. Nachemson[33] qualified roentgenographic findings in regard to their significance in the causation of lumbosacral pain, but while those proposed guidelines may be used prognostically, they should not be utilized as the sole screening method but rather in conjunction with a comprehensive physical examination and careful medical history.[13]

The precise utilization of ergonomics should allow for the avoidance of precipitating factors that would initiate pain and lumbar disability. Indeed, the ideal working environment for each individual at each specific job should allow for a safe arc of motion of the spine under tolerable compressive, tensile, and sheer forces in an atmosphere psychologically conducive to productive work. Furthermore, these forces should ideally be computed for each of the components of the motion segments of the spine, that is the intervertebral disc, the facet joints, the vertebrae themselves, the ligaments, and the muscle tendon units.

While such data are not currently available, the *in vivo* dorsal and abdominal myoelectric activity range reported by Andersson and others[1, 2, 3] under various postural loads and the intervertebral pressures demonstrated by Nachemson[32] (see Clinical Syndromes) have provided guidelines that enable environmental manipulation aimed at avoiding extreme joint reactive forces on the lumbar spine. Fiorini and McCammond's[9] analysis of the forces on the zygoapophyseal joint utilizing the principles of engineering statistics as well as Farfan's[7] definition of the structural integrity role of the posterior longitudinal system underscores the importance of the facets and ligaments in our understanding of the biomechanics and pathophysiology of the lumbar spine. Indeed, these investigators have in separate fashion supported Schultz and others'[34] conclusions that motion coupling in the vertebral segments is a function of the inherent kinematics of the segment and the position of that segment in the body under load.

Ergonomics has also benefited from empirical studies dealing with lumbosacral disabilities found in various occupations specifically chosen to demonstrate the full spectrum of physical and psychological demands on the individual in industry.

Magora[23-29] studied the relationship between low back pain and occupation in eight preselected occupations chosen to represent the spectrum of physical, psychological, and socioeconomic demands encountered in the industrial population. Occupations that demand marked physical activity through a full spinal arc of motion have a higher incidence of back pain. Lifting, bending, and reaching per se were not culpable; rather, improper lifting, unexpected maximal physical effort, or lifting with a long lever arm[2] are all provocative factors. Furthermore, occupations that require prolonged sitting or standing and did not allow for variations in posture are likewise more susceptible to complaints of back pain.

Kelsey[15-17] in her epidemiologic study of the relationship between occupation and acute herniation of lumbar intervertebral discs, mirrored Magora's findings of prolonged sitting as a risk factor with the higher incidence found in sedentary workers, particularly drivers of motor vehicles. It is important to note that Kelsey's failure to implicate heavy manual labor as did Magora as a risk to the lumbar spine was based on the absence of signs and symptoms of disc herniation. Magora's study, on the other hand, was derived primarily from back pain as a symptom and not disc herniations per se. Magora found that gender per se was not significant except when inadequate physical ability or improper physical training was apparent. Most likely, Kelsey's findings of susceptibility of disc disease in women who had full-term pregnancies perhaps reflects inadequate physical strength secondary to abdominal muscle insufficiency as well as postpartum ligamentous laxity. Magora furthermore found that low back pain increased in linear proportion to age, and both his study and Kelsey's demonstrate an early manifestation of lumbar disability when found in combination with the previously noted physical demands.

Magora suggested that one's subjective assessment of an occupation's physical demands and greater overall mental and physical responsibilities can also affect the incidence of low back pain. Those with low back pain felt their jobs were physically demanding, while an inverse ratio was found in their matched controls. Furthermore, the greater the occupational seniority, the higher the incidence of low back pain occurs, particularly when age and the previously listed physical attributes of the job were considered. Not only was the perception of physical demands greater in the symptomatic group, but when subjects were not satisfied with their occupation and social status, they also felt that the mental demands of the job, exemplified by concentration and responsibility requirements, were also greater than in those appreciated by the controls.

These conclusions were supported in Dehlin and Berg's[6] study of nursing aides in which actual skeletal complaints were greater in those who had a lower level of overall satisfaction with the job and perceived greater physical and mental demands in their job description. The fact that Magora found a higher incidence of low back pain with a higher level of education and a lower degree of religious conviction adds further credence to self-assessment of one's occupational role in contributing to back pain, although the exact psychodynamic mechanism manifested can only be speculated on at this time.

It is quite obvious that a complex interaction of dynamic physical and psychosocial factors contributes to the production and interpretation of painful lumbar stimuli in the industrial environment.

Hadler,[12] in critically reviewing industrial medical literature, concludes that the morbidity of various regional musculoskeletal diseases and their pattern of usage are clinical correlates that are anecdotal and do not define the pathophysiologic role of the physical activity involved. While cross-sectional studies like Magora's and Kelsey's provide trends, they do not provide a cause-and-effect relationship, and Hadler therefore recommends prospective studies in which there are few and definable variables that will allow for reliable interpretation of causality.

Once lumbar disability has occurred in industry, the process of recovery is more costly and of longer duration than the disability occurring in the general population.[10, 14, 19-22]

Leavitt and associates[19-22] made an in-depth study of the process of recovery in industrial back injuries and presented several sobering conclusions.

1. Concerning costs, a large proportion of the effort and expense emanating from industrial injuries is focused on a minority of cases with compensation expense consuming approximately ¾ of the total cost. The latter is understandable in that consultation and diagnostic efforts are frequently deemed necessary prior to the assessment of compensatory benefits. Furthermore, an average of 50 days of sick leave were required prior to the first attempts at return to work, while 16 per cent of the cases had not returned to work three years after the injury.

2. Variables that are available within two weeks of documentation of the injury that are predictable or indicative of the total costs of a particular case were females with a history of previous lumbar disability and currently carrying a specific diagnosis, such as disc herniation or fracture. Other factors not available two weeks from the date of injury but also predictive include a prolonged delay between injury and the second physician referral as well as prolonged delay between injury and the last day worked. The need to hospitalize the patient and discussion of surgery as well as litigation were all predictive.

In summary, it was concluded by Leavitt that since the actual determinants of morbidity were made manifest during the assessment of compensation benefits, the major deficit in the process of recovery was in the hands of the health care delivery process itself.

Even the novice physician quickly becomes aware that the patient who has sustained low back injury at work in a compensation setting or in a circumstance with legal involvement may be much less responsive to operative or nonoperative treatment than the patient who sustained the injury in a less complex and encumbered situation. There have been a multitude of studies dealing with this problem that have reinforced this observation. One of the more recent comprehensive and concise reviews of this topic is that of Beals and Hickman.[4] The more jaded observer will feel that these patients are only frank malingerers, whereas the more psychiatrically oriented physician will feel that these patients are attempting to answer their emotional problems through their somatic complaints. There

is little doubt that in addition to the patient's physical injury, a number of other aspects of this problem, including the psychiatric, sociologic, economic, and vocational variables, will determine the patient's recovery and return to work.

Several key factors must be understood and appreciated in the approach to the patient with significant industrial back pain.

1. As time progresses from the time of the injury, patients often increasingly elaborate and exaggerate their symptoms with less evidence of depression. The neurotic triad of hypochondriasis, depression, and hysteria displays an evolutionary pattern, which early is shown as severe depressive reactions with mild hypochondriasis and hysteria and later is shown with less depression and greater hypochondriasis and hysteria. Paradoxically, a study of Westrin dealing with the reliability of autoanamnesis and its occurrence with industrial back problems found that with recovery from a low back syndrome episode, nearly 25 per cent of the employees who missed at least eight days of work in the previous three to four years denied (autoanamnesis) being on the sick list because of low back trouble.[37]

2. The chronically neurotic individual's condition is often aggravated by surgical intervention.

3. Emotional and sociologic inadequacy of patients with back symptoms may predispose them to conversion symptoms. Through this mechanism, they resolve their psychological conflicts and convert them to somatic presentation.

4. Patients who are psychologically disabled will not return to work despite recovery from physical disability.

5. Operative intervention may be helpful in these patients when medically indicated by the strict criteria outlined earlier in this chapter and when not contraindicated by gross psychopathology. The role of surgery must be highly selective and requires great judgment. The modulating effect of secondary gain should be recognized as a negative prognostic feature as to recovery time consumed and ultimate functional outcome.[8, 36] When less than the most rigid criteria of surgical intervention are utilized, failure is preordained.

Thus, it would seem quite clear that industrial back injuries are complex problems involving not only anatomic but also psychiatric considerations, sociologic fragility, and the economic and legal milieu of the patient. Effective recovery of these individuals is predicated upon appreciation of the situation by the treating physician and a multidisciplinary approach to these problem cases.

References

1. Andersson, J. G., Ortengren, R., and Nachemson, A.: Intradiskal pressure, intra-abdominal pressure and myoelectric back muscle activity related to posture and loading. Clin. Orthop. *129*:156–164, 1977.
2. Andersson, B. J. G., Ortengren, R., and Nachemson, A.: Quantitative studies of back loads in lifting. Spine *1*(3):178–185, 1976.
3. Andersson, B. J. G., and Ortengren, R.: Myoelectric back muscle activity during sitting. Scand. J. Rehab. Med. (Suppl.) *3*:73–90, 1974.
4. Beals, R. K., and Hickman, N. W.: Industrial injuries of the back and extremities. J. Bone Joint Surg. *54A*:1593–1611, 1972.
5. Chafin, D. D., and Park, K. S.: A longitudinal study of low back pain as associated with occupational weight lifting factors. Am. Ind. Hyg. Assoc. J. *34*:513–525, 1973.
6. Dehlin, O., and Berg, S.: Back symptoms and psychological perception of work. Scand. J. Rehab. Med. *9*:61–65, 1977.
7. Farfan, H. F., Osteria, V., and Lamy, C.: The mechanical etiology of spondylolysis and spondylolisthesis. Clin. Orthop. *117*:40–55, 1976.
8. Finneson, B. E.: Modulating effect of secondary gain on the low back pain syndrome. *In* Advances in Pain Research and Therapy; Vol. 1. New York, Raven Press, 1976, pp. 949–952.
9. Fiorini, G. T., and McCammond, D.: Forces on Lumbo Vertebral Facets. New York, Academic Press, Inc., 1976, pp. 354–363.
10. Garrett, J. T., and Ahmad, I.: The industrial back problem: Role of the industrial hygienist and ergonomics. Am. Ind. Hyg. Assoc. J. *38*:560–562, 1977.
11. Glover, J. R.: Occupational health research and the problem of back pain. Trans. Soc. Occup. Med. *21*:2–12, 1970.
12. Hadler, N. M.: Industrial rheumatology. Arthritis Rheum. *20*(4):1019–1025, 1977.
13. Harley, W. J.: Lost time back injuries, their relationship to heavy work and preplacement back x-rays. J.O.M. *14*(38):611–614, 1972.
14. Jewell, W. S., and Leavitt, S. S.: Scientific disability management systems. C. Teknekron, Inc., April 15, 1970 (unpublished).
15. Kelsey, J. L.: An epidemiological study of the relationship between occupations and acute herniated lumbar intervertebral discs. Int. J. Epidemiol. *4*(3):197–205, 1975.
16. Kelsey, J. L.: An epidemiological study of acute herniated lumbar intervertebral discs. Rheum. Rehabil. *14*:144, 1975.
17. Kelsey, J. L., and Hardy, R. J.: Driving of motor vehicles as a risk factor for acute herniated lumbar intervertebral disc. Am. J. Epidemiol. *102*(1):63–72, 1975.
18. LaRocca, H., and MacNab, I.: Value of pre-employment radiographic assessment of the lumbar spine. Ind. Med. *39*(6):253–258, 1970.
19. Leavitt, S. S., Johnston, T. L., and Beyer, R. D.: The process of recovery: Patterns in industrial back injury, part 1. Ind. Med. *40*(8):7–14, 1971.
20. Leavitt, S. S., Johnston, T. L., and Beyer, R. D.: The process of recovery: Patterns in industrial back injury, part 2. Ind. Med. *40*(9):7–15, 1971.
21. Leavitt, S. S., Johnston, T. L., and Beyer, R. D.: The process of recovery: Patterns in industrial back injury, part 3. Ind. Med. *41*(1):7–11, 1972.
22. Leavitt, S. S., Johnston, T. L., and Beyer, R. D.: The process of recovery: Patterns in industrial back injury, part 4. Ind. Med. *41*(2):5–9, 1972.
23. Magora, A.: Investigation of the relation between low back pain and occupation, part I. Ind. Med. *39*(11):31–37, 1970.
24. Magora, A.: Investigation of the relation between low back pain and occupation, part II. Ind. Med. *39*(12):28–34, 1970.
25. Magora, A.: Investigation of the relation between low back pain and occupation, part III. Ind. Med. *41*(12):5–9, 1972.
26. Magora, A.: Investigation of the relation between low back pain and occupation, part IV. Scand. J. Rehabil. Med. *5*:186–190, 1973.
27. Magora, A.: Investigation of the relation between low back pain and occupation, part V. Scand. J. Rehabil. Med. *5*:191–196, 1973.
28. Magora, A.: Investigation of the relation between low back pain and occupation, part VI. Scand. J. Rehabil. Med. *6*:81–88, 1974.
29. Magora, A.: Investigation of the relation between low back pain and occupation, part VII. Scand. J. Rehabil. Med. *7*:146–151, 1975.
30. Magora, A., and Schwartz, A.: Relationship between the low back pain syndrome and x-ray findings. Scand. J. Rehabil. Med. *8*:115–125, 1976.
31. Montgomery, C. H.: Pre-employment back x-rays. J. Occup. Med. *18*(7):495–498, 1976.
32. Nachemson, A.: The load on lumbar disks in different positions of the body. Acta Orthop. Scand. *36*:426, 1965.
33. Nachemson, A.: The lumbar spine — an orthopedic challenge. Spine *1*:59, 1976.
34. Schultz, A. B., Belytschko, T. B., and Andriacchi, T. P.: Analog studies of forces in the human spine: Mechanical properties and motion segment behavior. J. Biomech. *6*:373–383, 1973.
35. Singleton, W. T.: Introduction to Ergonomics. Geneva, W.H.O., 1972.
36. Waring, E. M., Weisz, G. M., and Bailey, S. I.: Predictive factors in the treatment of low back pain by surgical intervention. *In* Advances in Pain Research and Therapy; Vol. 1. New York, Raven Press, 1976, pp. 939–942.
37. Westrin, C.: The reliability of auto-anamnesis. Scand. J. Soc. Med. *2*:23–35, 1974.

CHEMONUCLEOLYSIS

Chemonucleolysis is the term used to describe injection of the enzyme chymopapain into the intervertebral disc as a method of treatment of back pain and sciatica. The use of

TABLE 9–11. TREATMENT OF BACK PAIN AND SCIATICA BY
CHEMONUCLEOLYSIS—TABULATION BY YEAR

Year	1963	1964	1965	1966	1967	1968	1969	1970	1971	1972	1973	1974	1975	Total	%
Safety Data*															
Cases/Year	41	19	25	66	288	376	502	1221	1775	2863	3462	4499	1848	16,985	
Cumulative Total	41	60	85	151	439	815	1317	2538	4313	7176	10,638	15,137	16,985	16,985	
Adverse Reactions/ Year															
Sensitivity	2	1	0	0	3	6	10	23	14	42	50	80	34	265	1.5
Previously Described	0	0	0	1	1	1	1	5	5	5	14	10	6	49	0.3
Unanticipated	3	0	0	2	10	5	5	15	13	11	13	25	11	113	0.7
Procedure Related	7	0	0	0	3	1	9	14	7	12	19	32	14	118	0.7
														545	3.2
Efficacy Data**															
Cases/Year	18	5	0	31	179	154	316	877	1433	2498	3043	3860	1571	13,985	
Cumulative Total	18	23	23	54	233	387	703	1580	3013	5511	8554	12,414	13,985	13,985	
Response to Treatment															
Marked	12	3	0	13	105	89	191	576	936	1692	2092	2660	1097	9466	
%	67	60	0	42	59	58	60	66	65	68	69	69	70	68	
Slight	3	1	0	10	24	30	44	100	213	345	420	613	263	2066	
%	17	20	0	32	13	19	14	11	15	14	14	16	17	15	
None	3	1	0	8	50	35	81	201	284	461	531	587	211	2453	
%	17	20	0	26	28	23	26	23	20	18	17	15	13	17	

*Safety data include all patients injected by all investigators (16,985 patients).
**Efficacy data include all patients, 16,985, minus those injected by the three terminated investigators, 2,491, minus those patients whose response to treatment is not known, 509 (13,985 patients).
(Modified from Travenol Laboratories).

this technique in humans was first described by Lyman Smith.[19, 20, 21] This chemical decompression for symptomatic lumbar disc disease has been proposed as an acceptable alternative to surgical decompression when nonoperative treatment fails to relieve radicular symptoms.

Despite the report of "marked" relief in nearly 70 per cent of 16,985 patients treated with the enzyme in the decade following Smith's initial report (Table 9–11), the FDA has withdrawn its initial acceptance of the drug for clinical use in the United States.[3]

This reversal stemmed in part from a rising skepticism as to the actual therapeutic efficacy of chymopapain, which was never subjected to an objective double-blind protocol.[16] Schwetschenau and others[8, 17] subjected patients with myelographically confirmed symptomatic lumbar disc herniations to the scientific scrutiny of a double-blind study. The chymopapain used was the commercially available preparation (Discase), while the placebo utilized was the stabilizing vehicle in that same preparation (sodium etitate, cystine hydrochloride, and iothalamate). Early clinical results after at least two months of follow-up study reveal no statistical difference between the treatment and control groups. A reactive criticism of this study by proponents of chemonucleolytic therapy was precipitated with questions raised as to the pharmacologic activity of the placebo used[9] and the adequacy of the dose of the active enzyme employed.[2] The pharmacologic controversy was then complicated by medical, legal, political, and economic factors fostered by both the medical community and lay press.

A second factor leading to the FDA reversal was the number and variety of complications reported, ranging from minor allergic reactions to irreversible paraplegia and anaphylactic death.[24]

A new multicenter double-blind study has been established[23] to study the effectiveness of chymopapain when compared with the preparation's commercial vehicle and saline. It is hoped that this will definitively resolve the emotional controversy over the enzyme's efficacy.

Indications for Chemonucleolysis

Chemonucleolysis may serve as an intermediate treatment level between conservative therapy and operative intervention. It may be thought of as the last step of conservative treatment. The same criteria utilized for surgical intervention in acute soft disc herniations are utilized for chemonucleolysis (Fig. 9–97). In general, those patients who were expected to fare best with laminectomy have also shown the best results with chemonucleolysis. Patients with multiple previous operative interventions and those with advanced bony structural degenerative changes and those with predominant back pain have responded less well than have patients with acute disc herniations. The patient should be prepared to undergo surgical laminectomy if the sciatica is not relieved by chemonucleolysis.

Mode of Action

Chymopapain, the major proteolytic component of papaya latex, rapidly dissolves portions of the water-insoluble, noncollagenous components of nucleus pulposus from normal or prolapsed discs *in vitro*.[22] Injection of this enzyme into the disc is thought to hasten the degradation of chondromucoprotein[22] to relieve excessive and uneven intradiscal pressure and therefore realize a chemical decompression of the neural canal contents.

Macnab, however, after myelographic and surgical study of patients who have undergone chemonucleolysis, states that this structural concept, while useful, may not be significant in realizing the relief of sciatica.[7] Indeed, activity at a more cellular level in the form of alteration of surface charges,[7] a "chemical rhizotomy" secondary to chymopapain's effects on neural tissue,[15] and enzymatic disruption of the neurovascular supply, subsequently altering the associated inflammatory response found with degenerative disc disease,[27] have all been hypothesized.

Safety

As with any new therapeutic procedure, the desire of the treating physician to do no harm is paramount. It appears that the technique is proving itself extremely safe. The major problems encountered to date are related either to allergy to the chymopapain that may exist and inadvertent neural injury due to the enzyme or the spinal needles used.

The incidence of allergic reaction is approximately 2 to 4 per cent,[24] but fortunately, the immediate anaphylactic response is much less.

Veterinary studies have demonstrated good subject tolerance of the enzyme when injected epidurally, intradiscally, or intravenously in doses far in excess of what is clinically used to dissolve nuclear and anular disc material.[6] Intrathecal injections, however, have caused subarachnoid hemorrhage[6, 18] as well as intraneural edema and subsequent degeneration and fibrosis that have increased the threshold voltage needed to elicit action potentials.[15] Neurotoxic effects have been reported by others[11] but have not been universally documented.[5, 6]

Various other complications not unique to chemonucleolysis have been reported, and subsequently it has been suggested that this form of therapy should not be approached as a conservative modality but rather as an alternative to surgery.[24]

Technique

The basic technique of chemonucleolysis has been outlined by Lyman Smith[19] and has been changed little to the present time. General anesthesia is usually employed, although McCulloch[10] performs the procedure under local anesthesia with an intravenous line so that when symptoms of anaphylaxis appear, they are not masked by the general anesthesia and can be appropriately treated. The patient is placed right side up on the radiograph table, and a bolster or plastic kidney rest is placed under the left flank. Although this procedure can be performed with routine x-ray equipment, an image intensifier is desirable. The skin is prepared and draped as for a surgical procedure. Eighteen gauge, 6 inch needles are introduced into the lower three lumbar discs. The lateral approach is recommended rather than the transdural approach to decrease the chance of neurologic injury, although a midline approach may on occasion be necessary because of the structural configuration of the lower disc spaces. The needles are directed from a point 8 cm. lateral to the posterior spine of L4, 45 degrees caudal for the L5-S1 disc. At the higher disc levels, the 45 degree anterior inclination of the needle is utilized at the appropriate level. The needles are placed, and using the image intensifier, check roentgenograms are taken confirming their exact position in both planes. One-half to 1 ml. of Renografin is then injected into the disc to be investigated. A period of observation is useful to allow detection of any allergic reaction to the contrast material. Depending on the result of this discogram and the previous myelogram, the appropriate discs are then injected with chymopapain in a dose of 2 to 4 mg. Smaller doses are utilized for degenerated discs and larger doses for a protruded disc. A further period of observation after the injection of chymopapain is also important to rule out allergic reactions to chymopapain. The patient is then taken to the recovery room for observation and is subsequently returned to bed. Postoperative management is similar to that after laminectomy.

Recommended Precautions

Certain precautions are advised to prevent problems that have been described with chemonucleolysis. Careful history of allergies is important, particularly to radiographic dyes, iodine, and meat tenderizer.

If the procedure is performed under local anesthesia, then signs or symptoms that may herald anaphylaxis would merit prompt treatment. Indeed, if nausea, pruritus, paresthesias, incipient syncope, or respiratory distress develops, then 0.5 cc. of epinephrine, 1:1000 concentration, should be given through the intravenous line for a short period of time and supplemented with steroids and fluids. Sterile procedure is mandatory during this procedure to decrease the risk of discitis.

Results

UNCONTROLLED STUDIES

The results to be expected after chemonucleolysis have been described by several clinical investigators.[1, 4, 5, 12, 20, 21] A classification of end results has been proposed by Macnab with four end result categories: excellent — no pain, no restriction of activities; good — occasional back or leg pain of severity insufficient to interfere with the patient's ability to do his normal work or the capacity to enjoy himself in his leisure hours; fair — improved functional capacity, but handicapped by intermittent pain of severity sufficient to curtail or modify work or leisure activities; poor — no improvement or improvement insufficient to enable increase in activities, further operative intervention required.

Table 9–12 allows for comparison of the various series reported by investigators in this

TABLE 9–12. EFFECTIVENESS OF CHEMONUCLEOLYSIS

	Author			
	Nordby	*Smith*	*Ford*	*Day*
Result (per cent)				
Excellent	13	>88	>59	33
Good	61			44
Fair	16	4	22	8
Poor	10	8	19	1
No. of patients	100	112	126	86

area. Satisfactory results are reported in approximately 70 per cent of the patients studied. Less satisfactory results, however, have been reported in patients with previous back surgery,[6, 26] or when symptoms were due to spinal stenosis or were aggravated by psychogenic factors.[26]

CHYMOPAPAIN AND SURGERY

Uncontrolled studies comparing the efficacy of chymopapain compared with surgery realized similar satisfactory results with both treatment modalities.[19, 25] In "classical" disc herniations, however, Watts and others found that 80 per cent of patients had good results following surgery versus a 60 per cent good result with the enzyme.

DOUBLE-BLIND STUDIES

While double-blind studies[4, 5] thus far found no statistically significant difference between chymopapain and placebo treated patients, controversy over protocol design prevents definitive conclusions. The results of a new multicenter double-blind study[23] should help clarify questions as to the efficacy of chymopapain.

Summary

The clinical results available to date do not yet demonstrate with certainty the worth of this modality of treatment. With time and further carefully controlled clinical research, perhaps the enthusiasm of the earlier works in this field will be validated. If it is found to be a useful tool in the treatment of lumbar disc degeneration, it should probably then be utilized on an intermediate level between traditional conservative care and surgical excision of the offending disc.

The advantages that may evolve from chemonucleolysis are (1) decreased perineural scar formation; (2) avoidance of surgical complications, such as wound infection, nerve root injury, and blood transfusion; (3) decreased morbidity and faster recovery; and (4) few patients are made worse by this procedure.

The disadvantages are (1) possibility of not discovering an intraspinal neoplasm that would be apparent on laminectomy; (2) inability to deal effectively with osseous pathologic conditions and extruded migrated disc material; and (3) the possibility of allergic reaction.

References

1. Brown, J. E.: Clinical studies on chemonucleolysis. Clin. Orthop. *67*:94–99, 1969.
2. Brown, M. D., and Daroff, R. B.: The double blind study comparing Discase to placebo. Spine *2*(3):233–236, 1977.
3. Clark, M. A.: Statement from the Office of Scientific Evaluation, U.S. Food and Drug Administration (position statement on chymopapain). J. Neurosurg. *42*:373, 1975.
4. Day, P. L.: Lateral approach for lumbar diskogram and chemonucleolysis. Clin. Orthop. *67*:90, 1969.
5. Ford, L.: Clinical use of chymopapain in lumbar and dorsal disc lesions. Clin. Orthop. *67*:81–87, 1969.
6. Garvin, P. J., Jennings, R. B., Smith, L. Z., and Gesler, R. N.: Chymopapain: A pharmacologic and toxicologic evaluation in experimental animals. Clin. Orthop. *41*:204–223, 1965.
7. Macnab, I., et al.: Chemonucleolysis. Can. J. Surg. *14*:280–289, 1971.
8. Martins, A. N., Ramirez, A., Johnson, J., and Schwetschenau, P. R.: Double blind evaluation of chemonucleolysis for herniated lumbar discs. J. Neurosurg. *49*:816–827, 1978.
9. Massaro, T. A., and Jovid, M.: Chemonucleolysis. J. Neurosurg. *46*:696–697, 1977.
10. McCulloch, J. A.: Chemonucleolysis. J. Bone Joint Surg. *59B*:45–52, 1977.
11. Nachemson, A.: *Cited in* Present status of chymopapain and chemonucleolysis. Clin. Orthop. *129*:79–83, 1977.
12. Nordby, E. J., and Lucas, G. L.: A comparative analysis of lumbar disc disease treated by laminectomy or chemonucleolysis. Clin. Orthop. *90*:119–129, 1973.

13. Nordby, E. J., and Brown, M. D.: Present status of chymopapain and chemonucleolysis. Clin. Orthop. *129*:79–83, 1977.
14. Onofrio, B.: Injecting chymopapain into intervertebral disks. J. Neurosurg. *42*:384, 1975.
15. Rydevik, B., Branemark, P., Nordborg, C., et al.: Effects of chymopapain on nerve tissue. Spine *1*(3):137–148, 1976.
16. Schneider, R. C.: Statement from the American Association of Neurological Surgeons. (Position statement on chymopapain). J. Neurosurg. *42*:373, 1975.
17. Schwetschenau, P. R., Ramirez, A., Johnson, J., et al.: Double blind evaluation of intradiscal chymopapain for herniated lumbar discs. J. Neurosurg. *45*:622–627, 1976.
18. Shealy, C. N.: Reaction to chymopapain in cats. J. Neurosurg. *26*:327–330, 1967.
19. Smith, L.: Chemonucleolysis. Clin. Orthop. *67*:72–80, 1969.
20. Smith, L.: Enzyme dissolution of the nucleus pulposus in humans. J.A.M.A. *187*:137, 1964.
21. Smith, L., Garvin, P. J., Gesler, R. M., and Jennings, R. B.: Enzyme dissolution of the nucleus pulposus. Nature *198*:1311, 1963.
22. Stein, I. J.: Biochemistry of chymopapain. Clin. Orthop. *67*:42–46, 1969.
23. Travenol Laboratories (Flint Laboratories of Canada): Chemonucleolysis Seminar. Montreal, Quebec, November 19, 1977.
24. Watts, C., Knighton, R., and Roulhac, G.: Chymopapain treatment of intervertebral disc disease. J. Neurosurg. *42*:374–383, 1975.
25. Watts, C., Hutchison, G., Stern, J., and Clark, K.: Comparison of intervertebral disc disease treatment by chymopapain injection and open surgery. J. Neurosurg. *42*:397–400, 1975.
26. Wiltse, L. L., Widell, E. H., and Yuan, H. A.: Chymopapain chemonucleolysis in lumbar disk disease. J.A.M.A. *231*(5):474–479, 1975.
27. Zaleske, D. J., Ehrlich, M. G., and Huddleston, J. I.: Combined biochemical and clinical investigation of chemonucleolysis failures. Clin. Orthop. *126*:121–126, 1977.

MANAGEMENT OF FAILURES OF LUMBAR DISC SURGERY

One of the most difficult tasks in medicine is the management of the patient who has failed to gain lasting relief from spinal surgery. These patients often present with a perplexing history and physical examination, show evidence of both depression and anxiety, and, understandably, are reluctant to put faith in their treating physician. Having once gone through a major surgical procedure with unsatisfactory results, they are torn between continuing with a life of pain and disability or seeking salvation through operative treatment that has on at least one occasion fallen short of its goals. They not infrequently fall into the hands of unscrupulous practitioners and charlatans, only to meet further disappointment. If a physician is to accept responsibility for these individuals, he must be willing to invest many hours in their evaluation, develop a methodical approach to their diagnosis and treatment, and, finally, be willing to accept less than perfect results. These problems are indeed a trial for both the patient and the treating physician.

Algorithm for the Management of Failures of Lumbar Disc Surgery

The inherent complexity of the case of the patient who presents after one or more failed spinal operations demands a method of problem solving that is precise and unambiguous. An algorithm for the diagnosis and treatment of this group of patients will not only allow us careful measurement of our present methods of treatment but also will allow us to develop and evaluate new approaches to treatment. An algorithm is defined as a method of solving a particular problem in a finite number of steps (Fig. 9–123).

The goals utilized in creating this algorithm are as follows:

1. It should allow the treating physician to diagnose and treat psychosocial problems without extensive orthopaedic evaluation.

2. It should allow the diagnosis and treatment of medical disorders that present as back pain without prolonged and extensive involvement in orthopaedic or neurosurgical testing.

3. It should allow for selection of those patients requiring inpatient evaluation.

4. Surgery should be reserved for those very few patients who will show benefit. In the authors' experience this is only 1 in 20 new patients.

5. Inpatient evaluation design should be efficient and cost effective.

6. The algorithm should guide us in such a way that prompt surgery will be performed on those who are appropriate candidates without inordinate procrastination.

7. It should allow discontinuation of therapy on those patients for whom medicine has no answer, such as patients with arachnoiditis, patients who are addicted and are unwilling or unable to shed their drug addiction, and patients who have pain without a definable cause.

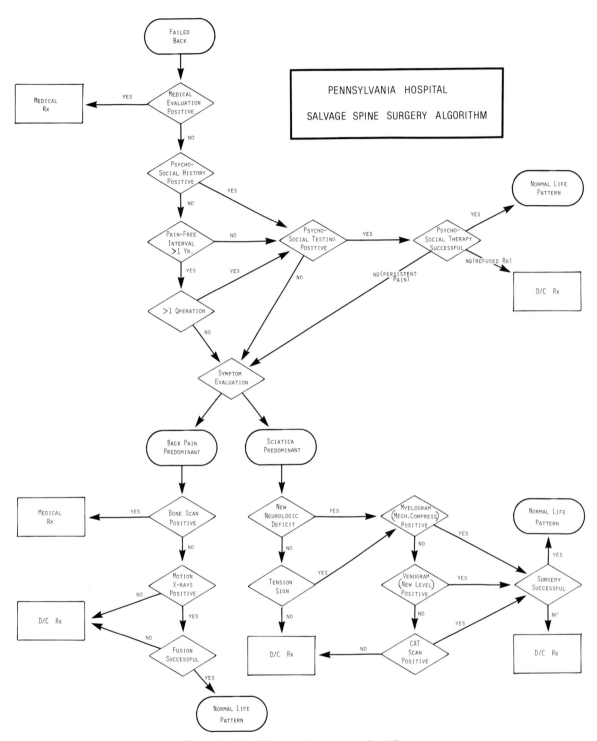

Figure 9–123. Salvage spine surgery algorithm.

The algorithm has been evolved through careful evaluation of the authors' personal experience with salvage surgery, their failures as well as their successes.

MEDICAL EVALUATION

The algorithm begins with a broad universe of patients presenting with failed spinal surgery. The first effort should be a thorough medical evaluation, which defines those patients whose back and leg pain emanates from a nonskeletal cause, such as pancreatitis, diabetes, or an abdominal aneurysm. Clearly those individuals deserve primary treatment in nonorthopaedic areas.

OTHER NONSURGICAL CONDITIONS

Certain other categories of patients are shunted away from the mainstream of possible reoperation early in their evaluation. The patient with psychosocial instability, as evidenced by alcoholism, drug dependence, depression, and litigious involvement clearly deserve a thorough psychosocial evaluation before considering further surgery. It has been clearly demonstrated that persons with profound emotional disturbance or those in the midst of active litigation do not derive observable benefit from surgery aimed at the relief of pain.

Patients who have not gained at least a one year interval of freedom from pain tend to do poorly with reoperation. Their diagnosis is often arachnoiditis and scarring, and on a statistical basis, they have been most resistant to benefits from reoperation. Those patients are also referred for thorough psychosocial testing before further diagnostic studies and consideration for surgery is undertaken.

Finally, patients with more than one prior operation present a barrier that is also almost insurmountable.

These three factors, that is, psychosocial instability, lack of a pain-free interval, and multiple previous surgery, are among the most ominous factors found in the authors' evaluation. If thorough psychosocial testing reveals these patients to have no underlying disorder that would preclude successful surgery, then they may reenter the diagnostic algorithm. If, however, their psychosocial evaluation gives evidence of an underlying personality problem, then treatment of this disorder should be undertaken. If these recommendations are refused, then treatment should be discontinued.

If the appropriate therapy is followed, frequently the somatic complaints and disability will disappear.

MECHANICAL VS. NONMECHANICAL SCIATICA

If none of the previous confounding factors are evident, then symptom evaluation should proceed, and the patient's problem should be categorized either as primarily sciatica or primarily low back pain. In first considering patients with sciatica, the physician must demonstrate definitive abnormalities on the neurologic examination before contrast studies are undertaken. Pain, in and of itself, is inadequate justification for myelography. The authors insist upon the presence of a new deficit since stable or residual neurologic deficits may simply be the result of prior surgical intrusions. In the absence of an evolutionary or new neurologic deficit, a positive tension sign, such as the straight leg raising test or sitting root test, would have to be present before proceeding with myelography. If neither a new neurologic deficit nor a tension sign is present, then discontinuation of therapy is advocated. In these situations, invariably no mechanical compression is present, and the cause of pain will be arachnoiditis or perineural fibrosis, neither of which are amenable to treatment at the present time.

CONTRAST STUDIES AND CT SCAN

If definitive findings are present on the physical examination, then myelography is undertaken, and if this reveals unequivocal mechanical compression of the neural elements, then decompressive surgery is recommended. If the myelogram is negative, then epidural venography may be of help, particularly with lateral disc hernias. Since previously operated disc levels will almost always show abnormalities on the venogram, only deficits at unoperated levels caudal to prior surgery have significance. A normal venogram, however, is most helpful. If the venogram is unrevealing, a CAT scan would be recommended in order to rule out bony encroachment in the lateral recesses and foramina. Positive findings on the myelogram, venogram, or CAT scan in the presence of correlative neurologic deficits would lead to a recommendation for reoperation. If neither the contrast studies nor CAT scan were positive, then discontinuation of treatment would be advocated for the sciatic complaints since medical therapy of the nonmechanical causes of sciatica have no proven merit.

BONE SCAN

In those patients in whom back pain predominates, we would advocate a technetium bone scan in the hope of defining treatable disorders such as neoplasm, infection, or inflammatory disease of the spine. These patients would, of course, receive the appropriate therapy after diagnosis is achieved.

SEGMENTAL INSTABILITY

If the bone scan is not revealing, then analysis of flexion-extension stress films would be undertaken in the hope of diagnosing segmental instability.

In the presence of unequivocal segmental instability, spinal arthrodesis could be considered. If this is successful in terms of achieving arthrodesis and relief of pain, then the patient would return to a normal life pattern. If the low back pain continues despite an anatomically successful fusion, then treatment would be discontinued.

Careful adherence to this plan will prevent the treating physician from advising those unfortunate patients who have already suffered one unsuccessful operation from undergoing yet another futile exercise and yet will allow the pleasure of promptly helping those who would benefit from their operative skill.

Diagnosis

As in all other areas of medicine, the first step in effective treatment is rendering an accurate diagnosis. A thorough differential diagnosis of the causes of persistent back pain after surgery must be pursued, with each cause being considered or eliminated on a rational basis.

ERRORS IN ORIGINAL DIAGNOSIS

Lumbar laminectomy and disc excision will obviously fail to alleviate a patient's symptomatology if a herniated disc and root compression were not the true causes for the symptoms. This statement, although obvious, needs great emphasis. Disc degeneration, with or without herniation, is such a ubiquitous process that its very presence does not imply that it is the cause for a patient's disability. We have seen many instances in which a myelogram revealed a herniated disc in the lower lumbar spine when in actuality the cause of the patient's symptoms was either tumor or infection in the upper lumbar or lower thoracic area. One cannot end the diagnostic search with the appearance of an abnormal myelogram. If there is any inconsistency between the myelographic appearance and the patient's symptomatology, further diagnostic investigation must be considered. After a failed back operation, this problem becomes compounded. The authors have made it a policy to personally telephone the surgeon who performed the original operation in order to obtain an accurate description of the pathology found. All too often operative reports fail to yield a true description of the operative findings. Usually greater candor will be obtained in personal discussions. If this type of information is not obtained, one can fall into the trap of "operating on operations." By this we mean the patient who is reexplored after failed disc surgery and in whom at the time of reexploration only perineural scarring is found and removed. A spine fusion is performed at this operation only to have the patient continue with symptoms. At some future date, a nonunion of the fusion occurs, and further surgical intervention is undertaken to repair the nonunion. As might be expected, this also fails to alleviate the patient's symptoms, with the further specters of cordotomy, thalamic surgery, and insertion of dorsal column stimulators appearing on the horizon. This entire cycle, of course, might have been prevented if it had been ascertained that no nerve root compression was demonstrated at the original laminectomy. The point of this is that great effort must be made to ascertain whether at any time definite evidence of disc herniation with nerve root compression was demonstrated. If not, further search must be made for nonmechanical causes of the patient's back pain and sciatica. Tumor, infection, and arthritic disorders of the spine must be considered as well as the other nondiscogenic problems.

Technical Causes for Failure of Lumbar Disc Surgery

The technical complications that may lead to persistent symptomatology after surgery have been described in detail earlier but will be outlined here.

1. Inadequate nerve root decompression.
2. Fibrosis about the nerve roots and dura.
3. Pseudarthrosis.
4. Disc space infection.
5. Arachnoid cyst.
6. Instability of a motor unit.
7. Impingement syndrome.
8. Retained foreign bodies.
9. Iatrogenic spinal stenosis.
10. Pelvic instability.

Other Causes for Recurrent Symptoms

NEW HERNIATION AT ANOTHER LEVEL. One will on occasion see patients who have had a disc herniation treated successfully, with complete relief of symptoms, and who after a pain-free interval, develop signs and symptoms of a further disc herniation at a different level. These patients should not be considered in the category of failed spinal surgery. Their diagnosis is usually clear-cut and should respond well to the appropriate treatment, whether nonoperative or surgical.

RECURRENT HERNIATION AT THE SAME LEVEL. If the nuclear material is incompletely evacuated at the first operation, patients may develop recurrent herniations at the original site. These patients, after a period of pain relief, develop recurrent sciatica in the original nerve root distribution. It is difficult, if not impossible, to differentiate these symptoms from those of perineural scar formation. On occasion, myelography may be helpful, but often it is not, owing to scar formation that has formed and tethers the nerve root.

CONTRALATERAL NERVE ROOT IRRITATION DUE TO BUCKLING OF THE ANULUS AT THE LEVEL OF DISC EXCISION. Certain patients during their first two to three months of convalescence after discectomy will note symptoms of nerve root irritation in the contralateral leg. This is often due to settling of the disc space after excision of nuclear material, with buckling of the anulus and irritation of the contralateral nerve root. In our experience, these symptoms usually subside with rest and anti-inflammatory drugs and do not require further surgical intervention.

PSYCHONEUROSES. Anxiety and depression frequently cause failures of spinal surgery. On the other hand, failed spine surgery, not too surprisingly, often leads to profound depression. Understanding and analysis of the problem is essential in the successful management of these patients and cannot be ignored. A complete discussion of this problem will be found in Chapter 18.

Diagnostic Evaluation

A logical and systematic approach to failed spinal surgery, as indicated in the previous section, is undertaken frequently on an inpatient basis with a multidisciplinary approach. Despite the wide spectrum of physicians involved and the multitude of special tests undertaken, one individual must assume overall responsibility for the patient's care and must develop a meaningful relationship with the patient.

As a routine, we advise inpatient evaluation by our medical, neurosurgical, orthopedic, and psychiatric services. Each adds a valuable facet to our understanding of the patient, and all have been helpful in our experience.

Radiographic examination of the lumbar spine is routinely performed with anterior, posterior, oblique, and lateral views. Flexion-extension films are helpful in demonstrating instability or nonunions of fusions. Tomography will further define the possibility of a nonunion of a fusion. Despite the known shortcomings of postoperative myelograms, we almost routinely repeat this procedure to rule out spinal neoplasms, spinal stenosis, or recurrent disc herniation.

Electromyography is not performed routinely but may be useful in certain instances to document neurologic deficit. This study may also help to differentiate functional from organic motor weakness.

Subsequent to psychiatric consultation, psychological testing may be performed at the psychiatrist's discretion. The differential spinal block and Pentothal interview are particularly helpful in differentiating organic from nonorganic causes for the patient's symptoms.

CAT scanning will help to define more precisely the presence of spinal stenosis, foraminal encroachment, or lateral recess narrowing.

Therapy

The recurrence of symptoms, in and of itself, is not justification for repeated surgical intervention. Conservative therapy should be instituted as outlined earlier (see page 592). If conservative treatment is successful in achieving an acceptable level of pain relief to the patient, no further consideration of surgical intervention need be undertaken.

If pain persists despite conservative treatment, the patient must then decide if the level of pain is enough to warrant further surgical intervention. This presumes that the diagnostic entity under consideration is amenable to surgical treatment. At this point, the limitations of surgical intervention must be clearly spelled out to the patient. We caution that one of three patients undergoing salvage surgery of this type will receive little or no benefit from their procedure. Although this may be somewhat pessimistic, we are anxious that patients realize that surgical intervention at this point cannot guarantee success. It should be pointed out to patients that with permanent limitation of their activities, they may be able to bring their symptoms within tolerable bounds.

There will be a group of patients whose pain is intolerable and has not responded to conservative treatment, who would in all likelihood not respond to further surgical intervention in the lumbar spine. They should be considered for procedures designed primarily for pain relief as discussed in Chapter 17.

OPERATIVE PROCEDURE FOR FAILED DISC SURGERY

When called upon to reexplore a nerve root and disc space that has had previous surgery, it is not uncommon for us to find a mixed type of pathologic conditions. Usually, extensive fibrosis is present about the dura and nerve root, extending well into the foramen. Protrusions at the disc space itself may consist of both a bulging anulus and nuclear material. Varying amounts of bone will have been resected at the time of the primary or secondary laminectomy. We feel compelled to excise scar tissue and perform a radical exploration of the nerve root well beyond the foramen. This will often call for a foraminotomy and wide laminectomy. All nerve roots that are involved clinically and myelographically are explored. At this juncture, the amount of instability created is difficult to evaluate. In an attempt to render a definitive operation to the patient, we will usually perform a lateral spinal fusion at the completion of the decompressive portion of the operation.

In those patients whose primary symptom is back pain, nerve root exploration may not be mandatory. The indications for spinal fusion in the absence of sciatica should be reviewed. The first of these is severe, incapacitating back pain after disc excision. Assuming no other pathologic process is present other than disc degeneration and the patient is free of psychosocial disorder, one has a reasonable chance of success with arthrodesis of the lumbar spine. Because of the difficulty in proving that a degenerated disc is the cause of a particular patient's back pain, we rarely reoperate on this particular basis. Perhaps once yearly in our practice we will permit reoperation under these circumstances.

Iatrogenic instability produced through the intervention of the surgeon at the time of the primary procedure is a second indication for spinal fusion. With the more complete knowledge of the pathology of the spine and more radical exploration of nerve roots, the spinal surgeon will often find it necessary to resect facet joints, complete laminae, and pedicles. While resection of these elements is not often necessary to achieve nerve root decompression, the resultant spine may be quite unstable. Certain individuals will also develop instability after a simple disc excision. Careful statistical analysis of this problem would indicate that extensive motion after discectomy will tend toward persistent back pain, while restriction of interspace motion will tend toward a more satisfactory result. If one is to utilize this criteria of instability for reoperation, there must be absolute certainty that radiographically demonstrable instability is present on motion films.

The third indication for spinal fusion is the presence of a neural arch defect that was not stabilized at the time of the primary operation.

The Surgical Treatment of Spondylolisthesis in Adults

The clinical picture of spondylolisthesis evolves gradually as one studies the transition from late adolescence to early adulthood. For a complete discussion of etiologic classification and treatment of this disorder in childhood and adolescence, the reader is referred

TABLE 9–13. TYPES OF
SPONDYLOLISTHESIS

I—Dysplastic—in this type of congenital abnormality, the upper sacrum or arch of L5 permits the olisthesis to occur.

II—Isthmic—the lesion is in the pars interarticularis. Three types can be recognized.
    a. Lytic—fatigue fracture of the pars
    b. Elongated but intact pars
    c. Acute fracture

III—Degenerative—due to long-standing intersegmental instability.

IV—Traumatic—due to fractures in other areas of the bony hook and the pars.

V—Pathologic—there is a generalized or localized bone disease.

to Chapter 5, Congenital Anomalies of the Spine.

Spondylolisthesis merits discussion in a chapter dealing with lumbar disc disease since Type III[24] (degenerative spondylolisthesis) (Table 9–13) is secondary to degenerative changes in the intervertebral disc and the facet joint with subsequent motion segment instability.[3, 7, 10, 14] Furthermore, any of the classified forms of spondylolisthesis not only can give rise to low back pain syndromes but also can contribute to a radicular syndrome and the intermittent neurogenic claudication syndrome discussed previously in this chapter.[10]

TYPE I AND TYPE II

It is important to differentiate the clinical syndrome and pathologic condition in the skeletally immature spine from that found in the adult. In the former, the growth potential merits different management.[6, 25]

Upon reaching maturity, the fear of further anterior migration of Type I and Type II spondylolisthesis is no longer present and is only a minor consideration in terms of surgical treatment.

There is, however, significant evidence that individuals with a pars defect will have a 25 per cent greater likelihood of back disability than an individual without the defect.[8, 20, 26] Macnab,[10] after studying 1000 patients with back pain, concluded that spondylolisthesis is most likely the cause of pain in patients under 26 years of age but is rarely the sole cause of complaints after 40. The various pain syndromes that can occur are most likely due to disc degeneration, presumably due to abnormal movement between the involved motion segments.[15]

The mechanical stress, particularly torsional stresses, which are most detrimental to the disc, are exerted upon the anuli with resultant early breakdown. Interestingly enough, extrusion of nuclear material at this level is very uncommon. In the author's experience with the operative treatment of spondylolisthesis, extrusions have been noted above the level of the spondylolisthesis but only rarely at the same level. Scoville and others,[19] however, described 11 of 15 patients with a herniation occurring at the same level as the spondylolisthesis.

After emphasizing the usual forms of nonoperative therapy, such as limitation of stressful activities, lumbosacral corseting, and spinal and abdominal exercises, certain individuals will remain incapacitated by low back pain and leg pain secondary to spondylolisthesis. It is these individuals who should be considered candidates for surgery.[12] Progressive deformity and neurologic deficit are subsidiary considerations in terms of management decisions.

It is unrealistic to recommend any one surgical procedure for the entire spectrum of clinical disorders associated with spondylolisthesis. Great confusion has existed in the literature. Advocates are found for simple nerve root decompression by resection of the loose neural arch for Type I (many can have associated pars defects) and Type II slips with or without fusion. When selecting the optimal type of surgical treatment, one must consider the age of the patient, his functional demands, the clinical pain pattern, evidence of dynamic instability, and the anatomic configuration of the spine (type of olisthesis) in regard to degree of slip and size of the transverse processes. The decision to fuse may also depend on the degree of iatrogenic instability created intraoperatively in order to achieve satisfactory neural decompression.

Despite the frequency of this disorder and the large amounts of surgery performed on an annual basis for this problem, there exist in the literature no randomized prospective studies of the surgical treatment of spondylolisthesis. In the absence of this essential information, one must be guided by one's personal experience and skill as well as by the limited amount of information available from the retrospective studies conducted in the literature.

A plan of approach to this problem in

adults is outlined below; the authors have found it to be generally satisfactory, and it has been supported by the work of others interested in this problem.

BACK PAIN ONLY

The existence of spondylolisthesis and of spondylolysis has been correlated with lumbosacral complaints.[13, 22] The source of back pain is not certain, but a recent anatomic investigation of 485 skeletons by Eisenstein[2] found without exception abnormally enlarged superior facets of the affected spondylotic vertebra in 3.5 per cent of involved specimens, implicating facet overload as a pain pathway in Type II olisthesis. Most patients with spondylolisthesis have back pain and lumbar insufficiency as primary symptoms. Approximately one third will, in addition, have sciatica, a ratio constant in both children and adults.[9] A successful spinal fusion will usually alleviate symptoms in those individuals who have only back pain.[5, 18, 21] The relief of pain with solid fusion is most effectively achieved by the technique of posterolateral fusion, since it provides for a large graft bed with inclusion of the facet joints and incidental obliteration of the medial branch of the posterior rami as it courses over the intersection of the transverse process and the superior facet of the involved vertebra.[17] The extent of the fusion will depend on both the degree of slip and the size of the fifth transverse process. When the degree of slip is minor and the fifth transverse process is large, the fusion need extend only from L5 to the sacrum.[27] If the degree of slip is large and the transverse process is small, the fusion should be carried from the sacrum to the fourth transverse process. When any doubt exists as to the adequacy of the transverse process, the surgeon should not hesitate to extend the fusion to L4 in order to obtain a more adequate bed.

BACK PAIN AND LEG PAIN

Those skeletally mature individuals with both back and leg pain require both central and foraminal decompression by excision of the loose neural arch and the fibrocartilaginous mass at the defect site and stabilization of the spine by fusion for optimal relief of symptoms. This appears to combine the excellent relief of sciatica produced by the decompression, as advocated by Gill and colleagues, with the stability and relief of back pain offered by the spinal fusion.[4]

Osterman and others[16] provided long-term follow-up study of patients who underwent the Gill procedure without stabilization and found an unsatisfactory result in 19 of 75 patients between the ages of 30 and 59. They attributed the rise from 17 per cent unsatisfactory results after one year to 25 per cent after five years to disc degeneration that they appreciated roentgenographically at the level of the decompression.

This combined procedure, therefore, is the most common operation utilized by the authors for symptomatic spondylolisthesis in the physiologically young or functionally active adult. It has yielded excellent results in our hands as well as others: Rombold[18] reported 93 per cent satisfactory long-term results with this approach. As previously stated, the extent of the fusion should be determined by the size and accessibility of the fifth transverse process.

PATIENTS OVER AGE 60 WITH PREDOMINANT LEG PAIN

In older patients in whom leg pain is a predominant symptom, simple resection of the loose posterior elements and nerve root decompression as advocated by Gill appears to be a satisfactory approach. At times, resection of the caudal portion of the ventral part of the pedicle may also be necessary to adequately decompress the spinal nerve.[23] The enthusiastic reports by Gill for the treatment of spondylolisthesis have not been uniformly supported. Amuso and coauthors[1] noted only 65 per cent satisfactory results utilizing the same criteria for grading as Gill; however, the older individuals with limited demands on the spine and greater intrinsic stability at the level of the spondylolisthesis will usually obtain satisfactory relief of pain. Further progression of the slip after resection of the posterior elements, a valid fear in children, does not appear to be a problem in adults.[1, 4] Indeed, while Osterman and colleagues[16] and Vestad and Naes[23] reported progression of olisthesis in many skeletally mature patients (the increased slip actually decreasing in absolute terms with increasing age) subjected to decompression only, neither reported any correlation between the final results and the degree of postoperative slip.

NONUNION OF SPINAL FUSION

Those individuals who have a pseudarthrosis after a midline spinal fusion and whose symptoms justify the need for further surgery are recommended to have a lateral spinal fusion. In those who have had a lateral spinal fusion that has failed, the anterior approach to the spine is then utilized as described in Chapter 4. If the primary approach to the spondylolisthesis has been the anterior approach and nonunion has resulted, a posterolateral spinal fusion is then utilized.

TYPE III DEGENERATIVE SPONDYLOLISTHESIS

Degenerative spondylolisthesis (and retro-olisthesis) represents a true migration of one vertebral body on another in the sagittal plane but does not represent the true defect in the posterior neural arch. Rather, malalignment of the vertebrae is associated with and due to disc degeneration and instability of both the disc itself and the facet joints subjected to static and dynamic forces acting in the lumbar spine. The surgical treatment of the disorder is considered together with disc degeneration and spinal stenosis.

Types IV and V spondylolisthesis are unusual types of olisthesis that merit individualized discussion beyond the scope of this chapter. The principles that guide treatment, however, which are similar to those applicable to the other forms of spondylolisthesis, rest on diagnosis, relief of pain (both osseous and neural in origin), and stabilization.

References

1. Amuso, S., et al.: The surgical treatment of spondylolisthesis by posterior element resection. J. Bone Joint Surg. *52A*:529–536, 1970.
2. Eisenstein, S.: The morphology and pathological anatomy of the lumbar spine in South African Negros and Caucasoids with specific reference to spinal stenosis. J. Bone Joint Surg. *60B*, 1976.
3. Fitzgerald, J. A. W., and Newman, P. H.: Degenerative spondylolisthesis. J. Bone Joint Surg. *58B*:184–192, 1976.
4. Gill, G., Manning, J. G., and White, H. L.: Surgical treatment of spondylolisthesis without spine fusion. J. Bone Joint Surg. *37A*:493–520, 1955.
5. Henderson, E. D.: Results of the surgical treatment of spondylolisthesis. J. Bone Joint Surg. *48A*:619, 1966.
6. Hensinger, R. N., Lange, J. R., and MacEwen, G. D.: Surgical management of spondylolisthesis in children and adolescents. Spine *1*:207–216, 1976.
7. Junghanns, H.: Spondylolisthesen ohne Spalt im Zwischengelenstuck. Archiv fur Orthopadische und Unfall-Chirurgie. *29*:118–127, 1930–31.
8. Kettelkamp, D., and Wright, D.: Spondylolisthesis in the Alaskan Eskimo. Paper presented at the meeting of the Western Orthopedic Association, Portland, Oregon, October 6, 1970.
9. Laurent, L., and Einola, S.: Spondylolisthesis in children and adolescents. Acta Orthop. Scand. *31*:45–64, 1961.
10. Macnab, I.: Spondylolisthesis with an intact neural arch—the so-called pseudospondylolisthesis. J. Bone Joint Surg. *32B*:325–333, 1950.
11. Macnab, I.: Backache. Baltimore, Williams and Wilkins Co., 1977.
12. Magora, A.: Conservative treatment in spondylolisthesis. Clin. Orthop. *117*:74–79, 1976.
13. Nachemson, A.: The lumbar spine: An orthopaedic challenge. Spine *1*:59, 1976.
14. Newman, P. H., and Stone, K. H.: The etiology of spondylolisthesis. J. Bone Joint Surg. *45B*:39–59, 1963.
15. Olsson, T. H., Selvik, G., and Willner, S.: Vertebral motion in spondylolisthesis. Acta Radiol. (Diagn.) *17*:6, November, 1976.
16. Osterman, K., Lindholm, M. D., and Laurent, L. E.: Late results of removal of the loose posterior element (Gill's operation) in the treatment of lytic lumbar spondylolisthesis. Clin. Orthop. *117*:121–128, 1976.
17. Penderson, H. E., Blunk, L. F. J., and Garnder, E.: Anatomy of lumbosacral posterior rami and meningeal branches of spinal nerves. J. Bone Joint Surg. *38A*:377, 1956.
18. Rombold, C.: Treatment of spondylolisthesis by posterolateral fusion. J. Bone Joint Surg. *48A*:1282, 1966.
19. Scoville, W. B., and Corkill, G.: Lumbar spondylolisthesis with ruptured disc. J. Neurosurg. *40*:529–554, 1974.
20. Splitoff, C.: Roentgenographic comparison of patients with and without backache. J.A.M.A. *152*:1610, 1953.
21. Stauffer, R., and Coventry, M.: Posterolateral lumbar spine fusion. J. Bone Joint Surg. *54A*:1195–1204, 1972.
22. Jorgensen, W. R., and Dotter, W. E.: Comparative roentgenographic study of the asymptomatic and symptomatic lumbar spine. J. Bone Joint Surg. *58A*:850–853, 1976.
23. Vestad, E., and Naes, B.: Spondylolisthesis. Acta Orthop. Scand. *48*:472–478, 1977.
24. Wiltse, L. L., Newman, P. H., and Macnab, I.: Classification of spondylolysis and spondylolisthesis. Clin. Orthop. *117*:23–29, 1976.
25. Wiltse, L. L., and Jackson, D. W.: Treatment of spondylolisthesis and spondylolysis in children. Clin. Orthop. *117*:92–100, 1976.
26. Wiltse, L. L.: The effect of common anomalies of the lumbar spine upon disc degeneration and low back pain. Orthop. Clin. North Am. *2*:569, 1971.
27. Wiltse, L. L., and Hutchison, R.: Surgical treatment of spondylolisthesis. Clin. Orthop. *35*:116–135, 1964.

INDEX

Page numbers in *italics* refer to illustrations; page numbers followed by (t) refer to tables.